System of Orthopaedics and Fractures

System of Orthopaedics and Fractures

Fifth edition

A. Graham Apley

M.B., B.S., F.R.C.S.
*Honorary Director, Department of
Orthopaedics, St. Thomas' Hospital, London;
Consultant Orthopaedic Surgeon,
The Rowley Bristow Orthopaedic Hospital, Pyrford,
and St. Peter's Hospital,
Chertsey, Surrey*

Butterworths

London and Boston

THE BUTTERWORTH GROUP

ENGLAND

Butterworth & Co (Publishers) Ltd
London: 88 Kingsway, WC2B 6AB

AUSTRALIA

Butterworths Pty Ltd
Sydney: 586 Pacific Highway, NSW 2067
Also at Melbourne, Brisbane, Adelaide
 and Perth

SOUTH AFRICA

Butterworth & Co (South Africa) (Pty) Ltd
Durban: 152–154 Gale Street

NEW ZEALAND

Butterworths of New Zealand Ltd
Wellington: T & W Young Building.
 77–85 Customhouse Quay, CPO Box 472

CANADA

Butterworth & Co (Canada) Ltd
Toronto: 2265 Midland Avenue,
 Scarborough, Ontario, M1P 4S1

USA

Butterworth (Publishers) Inc
Boston: 19 Cummings Park, Woburn,
 Mass. 01801

First published	*1959*
Second Edition	*1963*
Third Edition	*1968*
Reprinted	*1970*
Reprinted	*1972*
Fourth Edition	*1973*
Reprinted	*1975*
Reprinted	*1977*
Fifth Edition	*1977*
Reprinted	*1978*

ISBN 0 407 40653 0

©
Butterworth & Co (Publishers) Ltd
1977

British Library Cataloguing in Publication Data

Apley, Alan Graham

 System of orthopaedics and fractures. — 5th ed.
  1. Orthopedia
  I. Title
  617'.3   RD731   77–30243

 ISBN 0 407 40653 0

Made and printed in Great Britain by
The Whitefriars Press Ltd, London and Tonbridge

CONTENTS

PREFACE

I first wrote the outline of this book in 1954. The F.R.C.S. course at Pyrford was then six years old; but as it became more comprehensive the students could either pay attention or scribble notes — they couldn't do both. The only answer was to give them summaries of all the lectures. These were revised and retyped annually, but as the course grew longer typed notes became unmanageable (and secretaries rebellious) so in 1959 the publishers had to take over.

For the printed version I tried to convert the notes into more readable English, but decided to stick to the original systematic approach. Students seemed to like the idea of a standard pattern of headings for orthopaedics and fractures alike, and welcomed the logic of a constant sequence for describing physical signs; learning to *look*, *feel* and *move* before turning to x-rays is a habit they can profitably carry over from the lecture room (via the examination hall) to the consulting room.

Illustrations were a big problem — I wanted so many that the book threatened to become unwieldy. I therefore set about pruning the many x-rays and pictures (so that, by excision of all unwanted material, even small illustrations could display what was needed), and arranging groups of them into what were called ' composites ', each of which would tell its own story. This idea fitted in well with something every teacher knows: that, no matter how good a single illustration may be, it is more effective when combined with others in meaningful groups. Composites are the natural way of showing stages in a process, of contrasting varying methods of treatment, of highlighting important clinical signs, and of summing up differential diagnosis. There is a total of 1932 illustrations arranged into 372 composites. The illustrations can be used by themselves for quick revision; together with the text I hope they provide a substantial yet concise presentation of orthopaedics and fractures in a single volume.

For this fifth edition the entire text and illustrations have again been revised. There are, naturally, many areas with no change other than minor alterations and updating, but some growing points of orthopaedic interest have been included for the first time, while others have been rewritten. These include: chondromalacia patellae, metabolic bone disease, haemophilia, venous thrombosis and some aspects of osteoarthritis; new work on the treatment of Perthes' disease, scoliosis, spina bifida, tuberculosis, and malignant bone tumours has been incorporated; technical advances in knee-joint replacement and micro-surgery are described; and, in the sections on trauma, stress fractures, knee ligament injuries, cast bracing, external fixation and spinal injuries, all receive fresh or more detailed attention, as do a number of individual fractures, particularly in the lower limb.

London   A. Graham Apley
June 1977

ACKNOWLEDGMENTS

I owe and gratefully acknowledge an immeasurable debt to my teacher George Perkins, whose influence has, I hope, pervaded both my work and my teaching. He has also generously allowed me to use a number of the illustrations from his classic book on orthopaedics; Athlone Press, his publishers, have kindly added their permission.

My colleagues and friends at Pyrford (G. Hadfield, W. Murphy and R. P. Hollingsworth) and those at St. Thomas' Hospital (D. R. Urquhart, D. A. Reynolds and F. W. Heatley) have allowed me to use illustrations of their patients, and given valuable help. In particular Liam Murphy has been a tower of strength with the whole process of revision and new writing, and Gordon Hadfield a splendid shoulder on which to lean at all times. It is also a pleasure to thank those who helped with individual sections, notably Philip Cheong-Leen (Paralytic Disorders), Robin Hollingsworth (Major Accidents and Bone Infections), Fred Heatley (Osteoarthritis), John Mathews (Rheumatoid Arthritis), Min Mehta (Scoliosis), Ronald Urquhart (Haemophilia) and Peter Johnson (Spine Fractures). I am also grateful for valuable help from Jim Pemberton and Nigel Grieve (radiologists) and from a number of registrars and senior registrars (some now consultants) including George Adams, Rolfe Birch, Jim Buchanan, Tony Cross, Rob Grey, John Shepperd, Mike Smith and Ken Walker.

The exacting requirements of photography have been carried out with superb skill by Ken Fensom at Pyrford (who did the bulk of the work), Mrs Barry at St. Peter's Hospital and George Brandon at St. Thomas' Hospital. David Seaton drew all the new diagrams and prepared the new composites; his artistry and patience, combined with a total lack of ' artistic temperament ' made it a pleasure to work with him. The arduous secretarial work has been performed punctiliously and uncomplainingly by Beryl Wheldon; her contributions, including keeping the notes (and their author) in order, have been greatly appreciated. For proof reading I am indebted to Mrs Mary Love, George Raine and Rolfe Birch. The publishers have been unfailingly co-operative; they have had a lot to put up with, but I am happy to say we are still friends.

I am grateful also to colleagues elsewhere who so willingly loaned x-rays or photographs to fill some inevitable gaps. They include the following, but I apologize in advance if, inadvertently, the name of some generous contributor has been omitted.

Chace Farm Hospital, Enfield and Highlands Hospital, Winchmore Hill. Orthopaedic department **Mr B. Helal;** X-ray departments **Dr K. Lavers, Dr L. Pell.**—Figs. 3.1(a), 3.7(a), 6.8(c,d), 6.10(a), 6.11(g), 7.1(a), 7.4(d), 11.4, 15.3(e) 18.5(b), 20.16(d) 21.13(f), 21.18(a), 24.8(a,b), 25.25(c).

Einstein Medical College, New York. **Prof. A. J. Helfet.**—Fig. 25.19(a,b).

King's College, Hospital, London. **Mr H. L.-C. Woods, Mr R. C. F. Catterall, Mr R. Q. Crellin.**—Figs. 6.6(a,b), 23.21(g).

Letterman Army Medical Center, San Francisco. **Col. H. A. Feagin.**—Fig. 25.12.

Norfolk and Norwich Hospital. **Mr R. C. Howard.**—Fig. 11.2(d).

Princess Alexandra Hospital, Harlow. **Mr G. R. Fisk.**—Fig. 25.35(a,b).

Princess Margaret Rose Hospital, Edinburgh. **Mr G. E. Fulford.**—Fig. 6.4(a).
Queen Mary's Hospital for Children, Carshalton. The late **Mr T. L. Bowen.**— Fig. 1.9.
Redhill Group of Hospitals. **Mr P. A. Ring.**—Fig. 18.32(b).
Royal Adelaide Hospital, S. Australia. **Mr G. A. Jose.**—Fig. 6.10(b,c).
Royal Portsmouth Hospital **Mr R. A. Denham.**—Figs. 1.7(d), 6.7, 6.16(b,c), 7.4(a,b,c), 8.8(a), 11.7, 21.14.
Royal Hospital for Sick Children, Aberdeen. **Dr A. M. Stewart.**—Fig. 8.8(c).
Royal National Orthopaedic Hospital, Stanmore. **Dr R. O. Murray.**—Fig. 6.8(b).
Royal Victoria Infirmary, Newcastle-upon-Tyne. **Mr J. K. Stanger.**—Fig. 8.3(a).
St. Peter's Hospital, Chertsey. **Dr N. W. T. Grieve.**—Fig. 21.20.
United Bristol Hospitals. **Dr R. S. Gordon.**—Figs. 2.1(a,b,c), 2.2, 6.4(c), 7.1(c), 7.3(c), 21.25(f,g,h).
Westminster Hospital, London. **Mr D. L. Evans.**—Fig. 25.2(c).
Winchester Group of Hospitals. **Prof. J. S. Ellis.**—Fig. 23.27(e).
Wrightington Centre for Hip Surgery, Wigan. **Prof. Sir J. Charnley.**—Figs. 11.2(c), 18.31(d).

The following have been reproduced or redrawn from the original articles or books in which they appeared, and I gratefully acknowledge the courtesy of the respective authors, editors and publishers for permission to do this.

Fig. 1.6: Miss R. Wynne-Davies, *Journal of Bone & Joint Surgery*, **52B**, 704.
Fig. 15.8: D. A. Bailey, *The Infected Hand*. London: H. K. Lewis.
Fig. 15.9: R. J. Furlong, *Injuries of the Hand*. London: Churchill.
Fig. 19.19: J. W. Goodfellow, *Journal of Bone & Joint Surgery*, **58B**, 291.
Figs. 24.1—24.12 have also appeared in the *Annals of the Royal College of Surgeons*, **46**, 210.

CHAPTER 1

DIAGNOSIS IN ORTHOPAEDICS

An orthopaedic disorder does not exist in isolation. It is part of a patient who has a personality, a mind and a body; a job and hobbies; a family and a home. Any of these factors may have an important bearing upon the disorder and its treatment. They will not be considered at length, but are stressed here as they should be at the beginning of any clinical examination. It would also be out of place to discuss in detail the symptoms and signs of general illness in patients with orthopaedic disorders. Their importance is obvious, and in subsequent chapters they take pride of place before the symptoms and signs of local disorder.

Orthopaedics is concerned with disorders of bones, joints, muscles, tendons and nerves. The field is wide, yet limited. When a diagnosis appears elusive it is sometimes helpful to review the pathological entities likely to be encountered. They fall into easily remembered pairs: injury and inflammation; tumour and degeneration; muscle weakness and mechanical derangement; congenital deformity and acquired dystrophy.

LOCAL SYMPTOMS

A thorough history demands patience. Unless the doctor allows the patient to tell his story more or less in his own way, important facts may be missed and the patient may feel justifiably aggrieved.

The common symptoms in orthopaedics fall into three groups. The patient may complain that something *looks* wrong (deformity, shortening, swelling or a lump); that something *feels* wrong (pain, tingling or numbness); or that *movement* is wrong (limp, weakness, flailness, stiffness or mechanical derangement). Pain, local or referred, is the most common and important symptom.

Although the patient must be allowed to tell his own story, he needs guidance. Of any particular symptom it may be necessary to enquire if the onset was sudden or gradual, or preceded by injury or illness; if it is constant or intermittent, static or increasing, and whether anything makes it better or worse; finally, the occupation and any previous illness or injury may be important.

LOCAL SIGNS

For examination, a patient must be suitably undressed; no mere rolling up of a trouser leg is sufficient. Where one limb is to be examined, the opposite one must be adequately exposed, so that the two may be compared.

EXAMINATION OF A JOINT

LOOK

The student, or inexperienced doctor, is inclined to rush in with his hands—a temptation which must be resisted. His motto should be 'look before you feel'. And in looking he must follow a purposeful orderly system; otherwise he will miss vital clues.

GENERAL FEATURES		A brisk general appraisal of the patient is imperative
LOCAL SYMPTOMS		Let the patient tell his story (with guidance), and point to the site of pain
LOCAL SIGNS		A system is the key to accurate diagnosis
Look	Skin Shape Position	At this stage *shortening* is assessed
Feel	Skin Soft tissues Bones	Localized tenderness may be diagnostic. Be gentle — watch the patient's face
Move	Active Passive Power	Examine the good limb first or both simultaneously At this stage *function* is assessed
X-ray		Plus other investigations

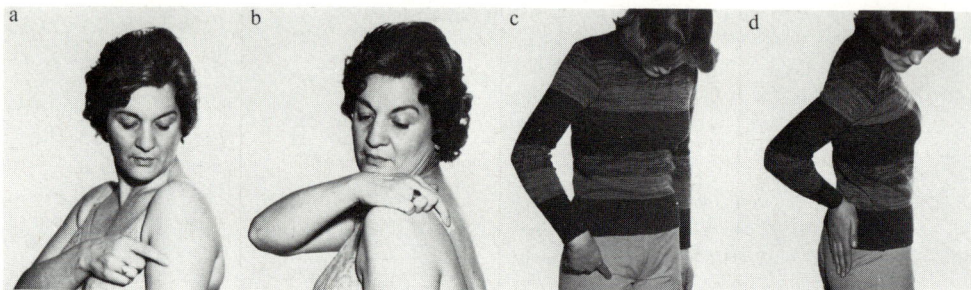

1.1 'POINT TO WHERE IT HURTS'
In (a) and (b) the complaint would be of 'shoulder' pain, in (c) and (d) of 'hip' pain. The likely diagnoses are (a) supraspinatus tendinitis, (b) cervical spondylosis, (c) a disorder of the hip joint itself, (d) a prolapsed lumbar disc.

Skin — This naturally comes first. Colour changes, abnormal creases, and scars (operative or accidental) often point the way to diagnosis.
Shape — 'Shape' means what it says. A mis-shapen limb may be too fat (think of fluid or a lump), or too thin (think of wasting).
Position — While the position in which a joint is held may vary, if the joint is normal, it 'looks natural'; any deviation from this natural appearance demands investigation. In many joint disorders and in most nerve lesions the limb adopts a characteristic attitude.

FEEL

We must feel (as we should have looked) systematically: the good limb then the bad; and the skin before the deep tissues.
Skin — Is the skin warm or cold, moist or dry, rough or smooth? and—equally important —can the patient feel you touching him, or is sensation abnormal?
Soft tissues — Deep to the skin we may encounter tenderness, which is important—in two ways. First, we must avoid hurting the patient; and so we watch his face and not our hands while examining him. Secondly, tenderness is often sharply localized; if so we know immediately the precise anatomical site of the lesion.

With superficial joints we can also feel if the synovial membrane is thickened (by rolling its edge under the fingers) and we can detect excess fluid. The methods of demonstrating fluid are shown in Fig. 1.2.

A soft tissue lump always demands careful examination to determine its size, shape, surface, consistency, edge and attachments.

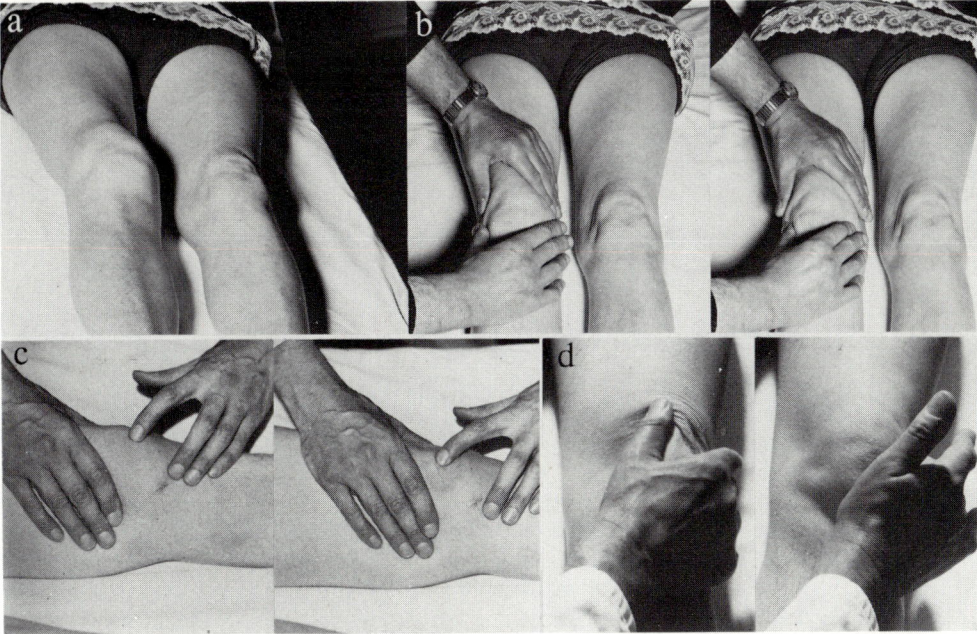

1.2 FLUID IN THE KNEE
(a) The suprapatellar pouch is bulging and the thigh wasted; (b) cross fluctuation;
(c) the patellar tap; (d) the bulge test — fluid is expelled from one side, pressed back
from the other, and watched returning.

Bony lumps are discussed on page 8; but the entire bone should always be palpated for tenderness, abnormal thickening or any irregularity of surface.

MOVE
Active — The advantage of testing active movements first is that the patient is not likely to hurt himself; he stops when the point of pain is reached.
Passive — We need to know if a particular movement is limited (and by how much), or painful (and at what angle); we must also be on the lookout for increased movement and for abnormal movements.
Power — Muscle testing is not as easy as it sounds; few patients have mastered *Gray's Anatomy*, and we must make ourselves understood. The easiest way is shown in Fig. 1.3. The sequence is important: you lift — he holds — you push — he resists while you feel. The normal limb is examined first, then the affected limb and the two are compared.

Examination of the muscle tells us something about the function of the limb. We can learn even more by watching the patient perform certain specific activities. In the upper limb he can try reaching for a high object or we can test him picking up weights and handling fine objects. In the lower limb we can watch him stand, walk, run or hop.

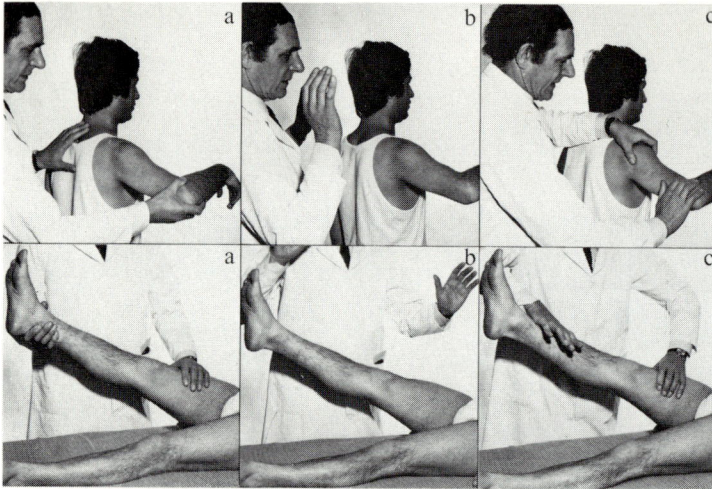

1.3   TESTING MUSCLE POWER
The sequence is always the same, no matter whether the deltoid, quadriceps, or any other muscle is being examined: (a) 'Let me lift it'. (b) 'Hold it there'. (c) 'Keep it there'.

JOINT DEFORMITY

A postural deformity is one which the patient himself can, if properly instructed, correct by his own muscular effort.

A fixed or structural deformity is one in which a joint cannot be restored to its anatomical position without anaesthetic or operation.

An idiopathic deformity has no known cause; examples are scoliosis, knock knee, flat feet.

Hysterical deformity is usually gross and should not be diagnosed unless other causes of deformity have been excluded and other stigmata of hysteria are present.

CAUSES

Deformities affecting many joints may be due to congenital disorders (e.g., Morquio–Brailsford disease), or to acquired disease (especially rheumatoid arthritis).

In deformity of a single joint or localized group of joints, it is often possible to identify the responsible factor, which may be one of the following.

Skin — Contracture (for example, after a burn, operation or injury) may limit movement and produce deformity.

Fascia — This is rarely a cause of joint deformity, but in Dupuytren's contracture fibrosis of the palmar fascia pulls the fingers into fixed flexion (page 177).

Muscle — Paralysis, spasm or fibrosis may lead to joint deformity.

Unbalanced paralysis may, if a strong muscle is unopposed, pull a joint into a deformed position. Peripheral nerve lesions give characteristic deformities but usually the deformity is not fixed and is essentially an abnormal attitude. After poliomyelitis, deformity due to unopposed muscle action often becomes fixed.

Prolonged muscle spasm occurs with chronic joint inflammation and flexion deformities result. In spastic paralysis also muscle imbalance leads to joint deformities.

Shrinkage of fibrosed muscle is the cause of contracture following Volkmann's ischaemia. For example, if the forearm muscles have contracted the fingers are held flexed, and can only be straightened by flexing the wrist, thus allowing the muscle to 'pay out'.

Tendon — Division, especially in the hand, may lead to deformity (page 176) and deformity may also result from adhesions within a tendon sheath (page 177).

Ligaments — These may be overstretched permitting such deformities as knock knee or flat foot. In Charcot's disease deformity is associated with gross ligament laxity.

Capsule — Fibrosis occurs in osteoarthritis, producing fixed deformity.

Bone — A bent bone may produce deformity at or near a joint; and faulty position of the bones (that is, dislocation or subluxation) is an obvious cause of deformity.

SHORTENING

Shortness of stature (dwarfism) may be due to short limbs (as in achondroplasia), a short trunk (as in severe scoliosis or kyphosis), or to short limbs and a short trunk (as in diaphyseal aclasis or in brittle bones).

1.4   REAL AND APPARENT SHORTENING (*see also* Fig. 18.2, page 230).

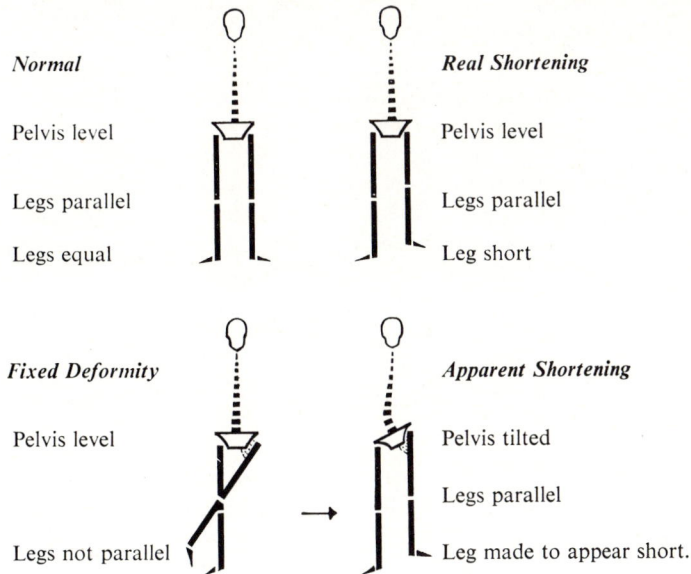

Normal

Pelvis level

Legs parallel

Legs equal

Real Shortening

Pelvis level

Legs parallel

Leg short

Fixed Deformity

Pelvis level

Legs not parallel

Apparent Shortening

Pelvis tilted

Legs parallel

Leg made to appear short.

Shortening of the arm is rarely a problem in orthopaedics, but shortening of the leg often is.   Bilateral shortening of the lower limbs, because it is symmetrical, is rarely a symptom.   It occurs with bilateral hip dislocation or infantile coxa vara.

Shortening of the whole of one lower limb — The whole of one limb, that is, both femur and tibia, may be short. As a rule the leg is also thin and the foot small.   Causes include: congenital abnormalities, sometimes associated with spina bifida; and paralysis, either a spastic hemiplegia, or poliomyelitis occurring in childhood.

Shortening of part of one lower limb — Part of one limb may be short.   The shortening is analysed and measured in three stages.

(1) Is it real, or apparent, or both?
(2) Is it above or below the knee?
(3) Is it above or below the greater trochanter?

Above the greater trochanter— Here shortening may be due to:
   Hip joint dislocation, or fixed deformity (giving apparent shortening).
   A femoral head which has been flattened (by Perthes' disease), or destroyed (by tuberculosis).
   In the upper epiphysis, coxa vara (infantile or adolescent).
   In the femoral neck, coxa vara (due to a mal-united trochanteric fracture), non-union of a transcervical fracture, or bending of soft bone (rickets or Paget's disease).
Below the greater trochanter — Here shortening may be due to one of the following disorders:

In the femoral shaft, congenital abnormalities, bending of soft bone (rickets, Paget's disease or fibrous dysplasia), mal-union of a fracture, or epiphyseal arrest.

In the tibia the causes are the same as in the shaft of the femur.

Below the medial malleolus tarsal injuries, especially calcaneal fractures, may cause slight shortening.

JOINT STIFFNESS

The term 'stiffness' is used to cover a wide variety of limitations of movement. It is convenient to consider three grades.

All movements absent — Complete absence of movement may result from a suppurative arthritis in which articular cartilage has been destroyed and bony trabeculae cross the joint (bony ankylosis); or from operation (arthrodesis).

All movements limited — With active inflammation of synovium, extremes of all movements are limited and the joint is said to be 'irritable'. With active arthritis there is joint rigidity, spasm preventing all but a few degrees of movement.

Tuberculous arthritis heals by fibrosis, leading to an unsound joint, that is, one in which forced movement causes spasm or pain, and deformity may increase with time. The term 'fibrous ankylosis' is used when fibrous tissue across the joint is so short that only a few degrees of movement exist. With longer fibrous tissue and more movement, the term 'ankylosis' is best avoided and 'long fibrous joint' is better.

In osteoarthritis the capsule fibroses and as the fibrous tissue matures it shrinks, limiting movement. In rheumatoid arthritis movement at several joints may be limited by pain; subsequent fibrosis may perpetuate the limitation.

After severe injury, especially compound fractures near a joint, movement in all directions may be limited as a result of infection, adhesions, or loss of muscle extensibility.

Some movements limited — When movement in at least one direction is full and painless the cause is usually mechanical. Thus a torn and displaced meniscus may prevent extension of the knee but not flexion.

Again, if one group of muscles acting on a joint is paralysed, the opposing group eventually loses the ability to stretch fully and fixed deformity with stiffness in one direction results.

Bone deformity may alter the arc of movement, so that it is limited in one direction (loss of abduction in coxa vara is an example) but movement in the opposite direction is full or even increased.

MYOSITIS OSSIFICANS

This term covers a group of disorders with limited movement at one or many joints.

Myositis ossificans traumatica affects a single joint (page 340). It may follow one definite injury such as an elbow fracture or a kick on the thigh; or repeated minor strains, for example, to the adductor region in jockeys; similar changes may follow operations on the hip (page 135).

Myositis ossificans circumscripta affects several joints, especially the hips, knees and shoulders. The condition particularly affects patients with traumatic paraplegia or brain damage. Massive heterotopic ossification may abolish movement at the affected joints.

Myositis ossificans progressiva, a rare disorder, is not the sequel to injury; indeed the cause is unknown. In the first few years of life episodes of fever occur and tender swellings appear, chiefly in the head, neck or trunk. Subsequently, plates of bone develop in muscles, mainly of the trunk. An associated anomaly is undue shortness of the halluces and sometimes also of the thumbs. The muscle ossification gradually extends, limiting movement more and more and, until recently, the outcome was inevitably fatal. Treatment with diphosphonates, however, seems to halt the ossification and it may be hoped that the outlook will now be better.

ARTHROGRYPOSIS MULTIPLEX CONGENITA

This is characterized by stiffness of many joints dating from birth. Almost certainly the term represents a group of arrested intra-uterine myopathies and neuropathies. The deformities (which reflect the foetal posture) do not progress after birth. The lack of skin creases, the pipe-stem appearance of some affected limbs, and the multiple deformities are characteristic. Some stiff joints are extended, others flexed and bridged by webs of skin. Hip dislocation, scoliosis and severe talipes may further complicate the picture.

Treatment is arduous and prolonged, but may be surprisingly rewarding, no doubt because the children are often highly intelligent. A programme of stretching and strapping

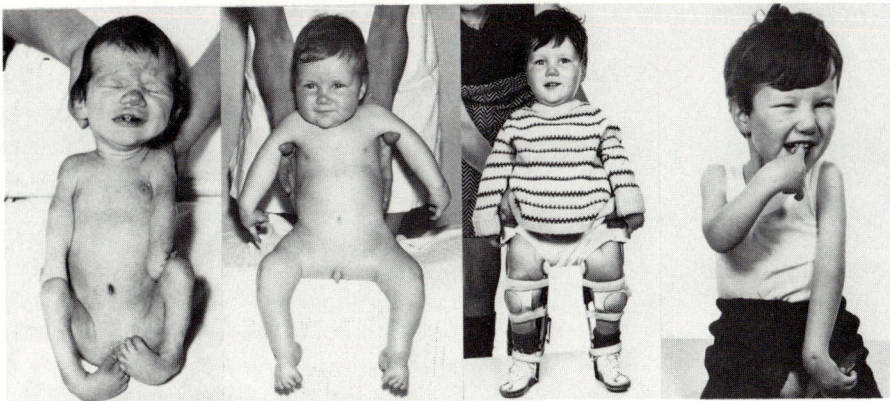

1.5 ARTHROGRYPOSIS MULTIPLEX CONGENITA
Severe deformities are present at birth but surgery is possible and, as this bright lad shows, worthwhile.

begins soon after birth; but after the first year severe deformities usually demand drastic surgery. Lloyd-Roberts (1971) advises correcting the lower limbs first; the aim is straight legs with plantigrade feet. Upper limb surgery is best postponed until the child's considerable powers of adaptation can be assessed; then the minimum aim is getting a hand to the mouth (Fig. 1.5).

JOINT LAXITY

Increased movement at a single joint may result from muscle paralysis (especially when a joint is flail), from ligamentous injury, or from ligamentous stretching after chronic or repeated joint swelling.

Increased movement at one or only a few joints also may follow paralysis, or it may be the sequel to polyarthritis. But the possibility of Charcot's disease must be borne in mind (page 52).

Generalized joint hypermobility is the term applied to a disorder, usually familial, in which undue ligament laxity is combined with relative frequency of herniae and ganglia. Because of the laxity the knees and elbows can be hyperextended, and the hands and feet can attain unusual positions. Orthopaedic interest centres on the well-recognized association with congenital hip dislocation and with recurrent dislocation of the patella and the shoulder. Another penalty of hypermobility is early joint degeneration.

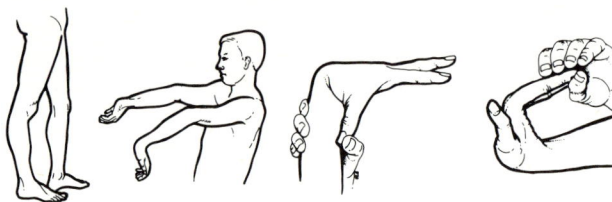

1.6 GENERALIZED JOINT HYPERMOBILITY
Being 'double-jointed' is not an unmixed blessing: recurrent dislocation and late degeneration are likely sequels. (Re-drawn from *Journal of Bone and Joint Surgery*, Vol. 52B, No. 4, page 704, by courtesy of Miss R. Wynne-Davies, and the Editor.)

Generalized joint hypermobility may occur as an isolated phenomenon or be associated with disorders such as Marfan's disease and brittle bones. In *Ehlers–Danlos syndrome* ligament laxity is combined with other connective tissue disorders: the skin is hyperextensile and splits easily to leave tissue-paper scars; and because blood-vessel walls are weak the patient bruises readily and may develop aneurysms. In *Larsen's disease* these connective tissue disorders are not present, but there is congenital dislocation of several joints.

BONY LUMPS

Multiple bony lumps are uncommon. They occur in diaphyseal aclasis as squat knobs of bone around one or several joints. In syphilis and yaws there may be two or more diffuse swellings on the shaft of a bone.

A single bony lump may be due to faulty development, injury, inflammation or a tumour. Although x-ray examination is essential, a diagnosis can usually be made clinically by considering the following factors.

Size — A large lump attached to bone, or a lump which is getting bigger is nearly always a tumour.

Site — A lump near a joint may be a cancellous osteoma (if small), an osteochondroma (if large), a benign giant-cell tumour (if ill-defined and at the very end of the bone), or a sarcoma (if ill-defined, tender and near the metaphysis). A lump in the shaft itself may be callus (which extends all round the bone), inflammatory (if tender and ill-defined), or a tumour.

Shape — A benign tumour sticks out from one aspect of the bone, malignant tumours or callus extend all round it.

Tenderness — Lumps due to active inflammation, recent callus or a rapidly growing sarcoma are tender.

Edge — A benign tumour has a well-defined margin; malignant tumours, inflammatory lumps and callus have a vague edge.

Consistency — A benign tumour feels bony hard; malignant tumours often give the impression that they can be indented. Occasionally a small ganglion or a cyst (especially of the lateral meniscus) feels almost bony hard.

EXAMINATION OF A BONE

Bones, like joints, should be examined systematically, and the pattern of headings is similar.

LOOK

Skin — First look for scars or colour changes.

Shape — The bone may be bent (page 9); or unduly wide as in Paget's disease or Caffey's disease.

Position — Distortion at either end of the bone should be noted.

FEEL
Skin — This may feel unduly warm or cool; sensory changes may be present.
Soft tissues — Lumps or swellings may be palpable.
The bone itself — The bone may feel too wide, surface irregularities or lumps may be palpable, and there may be localized tenderness.

MOVE

The appropriate headings are: joint above, joint below and the bone itself.

Not only should the joints be examined, but it is wise also to examine the bone itself for movement; otherwise non-union in the forearm or leg (often painless) may go undetected.

BENT BONES

The long bones are straight or have slight natural curves. If a bone is abnormally bent it must have broken, or been soft at some time, or have grown faultily.

If several bones are bent, the likely causes are multiple injury (for example, to brittle bones) or a general bone-softening disease (such as rickets or Paget's disease).

Bending of a single bone may follow injury, localized Paget's disease, fibrous dysplasia or faulty growth. It should be noted that fracture-separation of an epiphysis hardly ever affects growth, whereas an apparently minor fracture through the substance of the epiphysis frequently does.

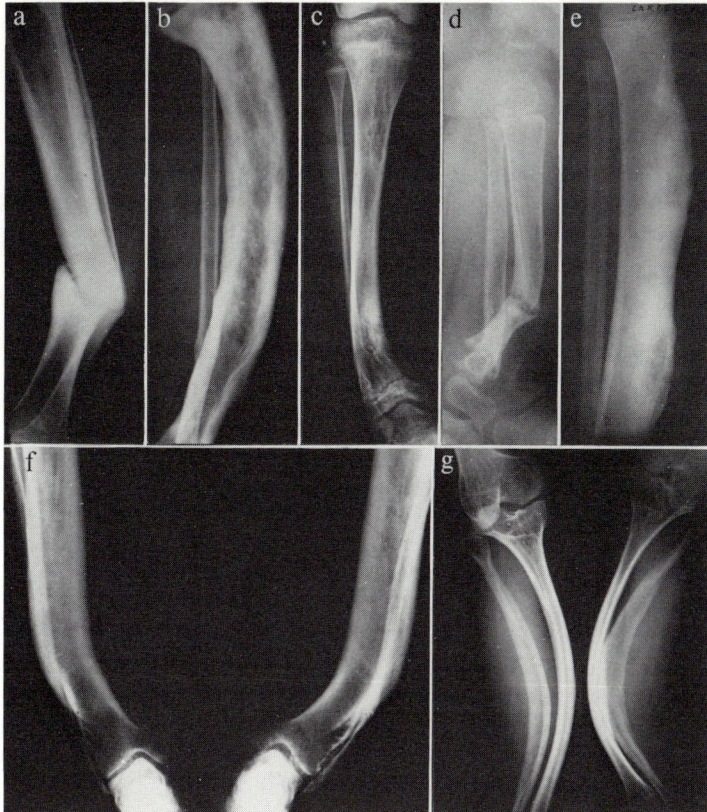

1.7 BENT TIBIAE
(a) Malunited fracture, (b) Paget's disease, (c) fibrous dysplasia, (d) congenital pseudarthrosis, (e) syphilitic sabre tibia.

(f) Old rickets, (g) brittle bones.

THE BENT TIBIA

The causes include:

Injury — With mal-union of a fracture the bone is angulated rather than curved.

Paget's disease — The curve is uniform over the whole bone, and the bone is thickened. Often only one tibia is affected.

Dysplasias — Fibrous dysplasia, especially of the lower third of the tibia often results in bending, and a similar deformity can occur with neurofibromatosis. *Congenital pseudarthrosis* is probably a special variety of dysplasia: a baby may be born with a tibia fractured at the junction of the middle and lower thirds, or with a tibia bent at that level and which subsequently breaks.

Syphilitic osteitis — The bone is not really curved, but new periosteal bone laid down on its anterior border makes it look bent (sabre tibia). The posterior border remains straight.

Rickets — Near the lower end the tibia bends backwards and inwards. Both tibiae are symmetrically affected.

Brittle bones — The bending is usually bilateral and often gross. It may result from a combination of mal-united fractures and osteoporosis.

X-RAY EXAMINATION

The minimum requirement is two views of the affected area: antero-posterior and lateral. Occasionally oblique views are valuable. Often it is necessary to compare films of two limbs and, where bone density is important, these should if possible be taken on one x-ray plate. Occasionally, as with dystrophies and tumours, other parts of the body need to be x-rayed. Special techniques, such as tomograms, stereoscopic views, radio-opaque injections and radio-isotope scanning are sometimes helpful.

The examination of x-ray films needs to be just as methodical as that of a patient, and the following headings are useful.

X-RAY OF A BONE

General features	The bone as a whole	Components of the bone
Patient	Shape	Periosteum
Site	Density	Cortex
Soft tissues	Architecture	Medulla

GENERAL FEATURES

Patient — Try to 'look through' the film and to visualize a living patient, particularly the build and age: thus, solitary bone cysts are seen only before skeletal maturity, giant-cell tumours only after it.

Site — Which part of the body is seen and which part of the bone is involved? Thus acute osteomyelitis usually begins in the metaphysis, whereas Perthes' disease affects the epiphysis.

Soft tissues — These merit a separate heading, because they are otherwise liable to be forgotten. Metallic foreign bodies are always strikingly self evident, but even wood or glass may show in suitable films. Loose bodies in a joint are sometimes less obvious, but it is always worth trying to identify their source. Extra-osseous calcification may occur in a haematoma (myositis ossificans), in a cold abscess, in a tendon (especially supraspinatus), in a tendon sheath (peritendinitis calcarea), and in veins (phleboliths). Occasionally a damaged ligament calcifies and huge masses of calcium may be seen round joints in the rare condition called tumoral calcinosis. If the soft tissues are unduly translucent, think of a lipoma.

THE BONE AS A WHOLE

Shape — This is clearly important. The bone may be too wide, as in Paget's disease; too narrow, as in osteogenesis imperfecta; or it may be bent (page 9).

Density — Bone density must be assessed with caution, for illusions can be created by variations in radiography. Generalized increase of density is seen in marble bones (page 66); generalized decrease in osteoporosis (page 82) and osteomalacia (page 78). More localized changes follow alterations in the amount of blood reaching the bone: thus avascular necrosis following injury or bone infection causes increased density ('dead bone is dense bone'); and rarefaction follows the increased vascularity of a joint chronically inflamed in tuberculosis or rheumatoid arthritis. 'Osteolysis' is the term used when bone disappears for no obvious reason.

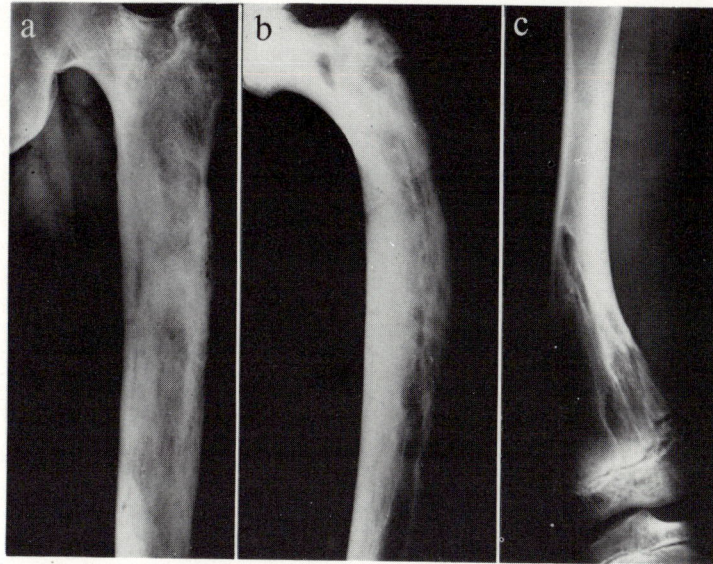

1.8 BONE ARCHITECTURE (a) In chronic osteomyelitis the normal architecture is lost and the bone is thickened but straight. (b) Paget's disease looks somewhat similar except that the bone is bent. (c) In fibrous dysplasia the bone contains 'bubbles and stripes': it is bent but not thick.

Architecture — This term is difficult to define, but refers to the general structural appearance of the bone. The three examples in Fig. 1.8 are relatively common and important, although unimportant rarities such as osteopoikilosis and osteopathia striata (page 67) may be more striking.

COMPONENTS OF THE BONE

Periosteum — Except in young infants periosteum is not visible on x-ray; but once it is lifted away from the cortex of the bone calcification occurs (Fig. 1.9). Widespread periosteal changes are seen in syphilis and in Caffey's disease (page 16).

Cortex — The cortex of pipe bone should be uniform in thickness throughout the diaphysis but tapering at both ends. Any alteration is noteworthy. The cortex may look thinner because it has been partly eroded (e.g. by a cyst, tumour or aneurysm); or it may be thickened in conditions such as Paget's disease. Actual perforation of the cortex is more sinister, suggesting malignancy, although in syphilis the appearances can be strikingly similar ('syphilis can mimic anything').

Medulla — The medulla needs to be inspected purposefully for areas of increased or diminished density, which may be single or multiple.

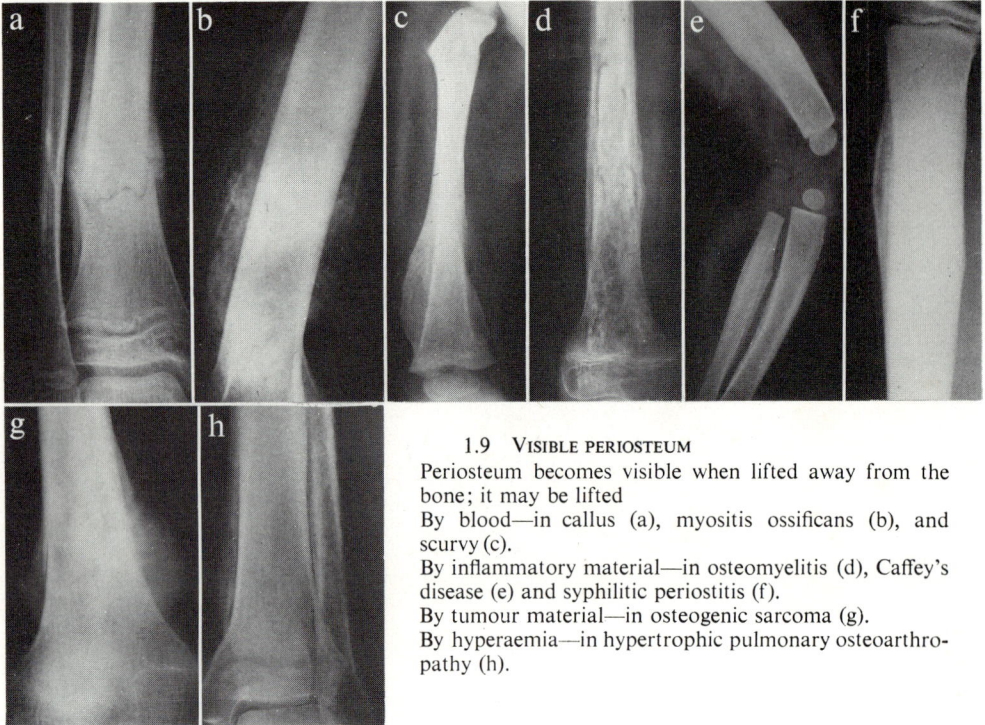

1.9 VISIBLE PERIOSTEUM
Periosteum becomes visible when lifted away from the bone; it may be lifted
By blood—in callus (a), myositis ossificans (b), and scurvy (c).
By inflammatory material—in osteomyelitis (d), Caffey's disease (e) and syphilitic periostitis (f).
By tumour material—in osteogenic sarcoma (g).
By hyperaemia—in hypertrophic pulmonary osteoarthropathy (h).

A single rarefied area — This may be due to one of the following conditions:
Inflammation, for example a Brodie's abscess, which has a sclerosed margin and is often lobulated.

Solitary cyst, which has a well-defined but not sclerosed margin and is situated on the shaft side of an epiphyseal line.

Other cysts occur in association with osteoarthritic joints; they are usually small and situated in the subchondral area. Similar small cysts have been described in adults with no osteoarthritis; from their contents these have been called 'bone ganglia'.   In sarcoidosis also multiple bone cysts may occur, especially in the fingers.
Benign tumour: a chondroma usually shows specks of calcification and occurs in short bones; a giant-cell tumour is often trabeculated and at the very end of a long bone; both have a clearly defined edge.
Malignant tumour: an osteolytic sarcoma has no well-defined edge.
Multiple rarefied areas — these may be due to one of the following:
Fibrous dysplasia: cysts occur in one or several bones (page 69).
Storage diseases: Gaucher's disease is a familial primary lipoidosis with reticulum cell hyperplasia; the spleen is huge and the liver often enlarged; the cells are also found in bone marrow where x-rays show osteolytic areas.
The secondary lipoidoses constitute a group of disorders which may be stages of a single disease process called histiocytic granulomatosis or histiocytosis 'X'. The group includes: (1) Hand-Schüller-Christian disease: there are multiple deposits in the bones, especially the skull, vertebrae and femora (showing as sharply defined translucent areas on x-ray), in the pituitary gland (causing diabetes insipidus), in the orbit (causing exophthalmos), in the skin and many other soft tissues.   (2) Letterer-Siwe disease: this is probably an acute form of (1). It occurs in infants and is rapidly fatal.   (3) Eosinophilic granuloma of bone: the deposits may be single or multiple, but are not numerous and recovery is usual, with or without treatment. Collapse of a vertebra containing such a deposit is thought to be responsible for Calvé's disease.

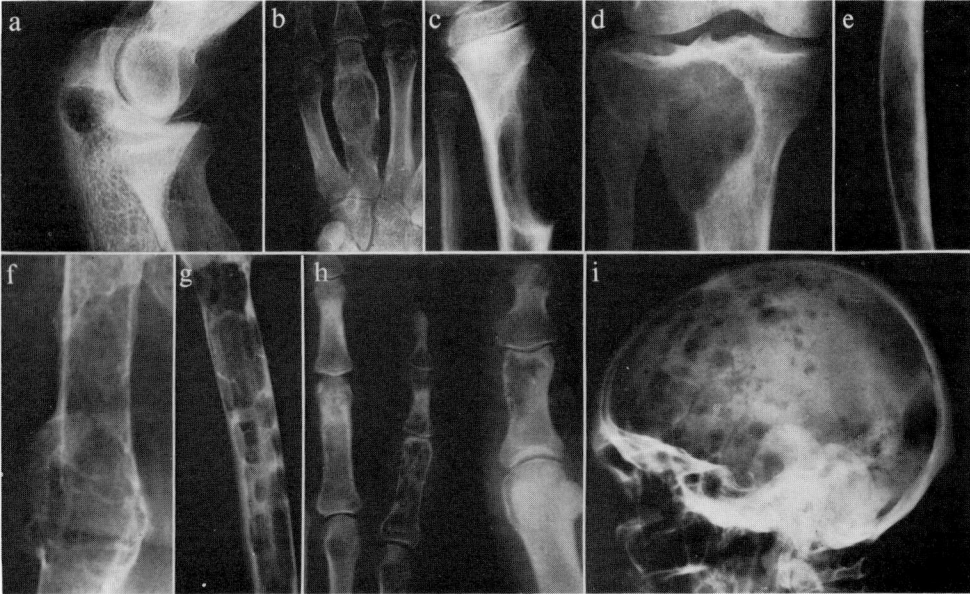

1.10 EXAMPLES OF RARE AREAS OF BONE
Single: Brodie's abscess (a), tuberculous dactylitis (b), solitary cyst (c), giant-cell tumour (d), eosinophilic granuloma (e).
Multiple: Hand-Schüller-Christian disease (f), hydatid disease (g), sarcoidosis in the hand and foot (h), secondary deposits (i).

Malignant disease: In leukaemia the bones may show ill-defined areas of rarefaction; there is also anaemia, enlargement of the spleen, liver and lymph nodes, and often haemorrhages in the skin or gut. In secondary carcinoma and myelomatosis multiple areas of bone rarefaction also occur (*see* Chapter 8).

A single area of increased density — This may be due to one of the following conditions.

Aseptic necrosis, which may follow trauma or occur without obvious cause.

Septic necrosis: a sequestrum is dense, probably because of avascularity.

Tumours: increased calcification may occur in a benign tumour (for example, chondroma) or in part of an osteogenic sarcoma. In some cases of anaemia or leukaemia the medullary cavity is obliterated by new dense bone (osteomyelosclerosis).

Multiple areas of increased density — These may be due to one of the following:

Engelmann's disease: in this rare condition sclerosis occurs, often symmetrically in the long bones, and sometimes in the skull (**page 69**).

Tumours: with prostatic carcinoma patchy secondary deposits of sclerosis may occur and in the pelvis the appearance may be confused with Paget's disease. Secondary deposits from breast carcinoma are usually osteolytic, but may occasionally be osteoblastic and dense.

Poisoning: widespread increase in bone density, often concentrated in the metaphyses, occurs in lead, bismuth, or phosphorus poisoning and in fluorosis.

X-RAY OF A JOINT

Position — The joint may be dislocated, subluxed or in a position of deformity.

Joint space — In chronic inflammation (for example, rheumatoid arthritis) the space is uniformly decreased. In osteoarthritis the decrease occurs chiefly where pressure is transmitted, and there may be lipping or osteophytes at the edges.

The joint space is increased in some varieties of osteochondritis (for example, Perthes' disease) and occasionally when a joint is distended with fluid.   Loose bodies may be visible within the joint space, and occasionally menisci are calcified.

Joint line — In chronic arthritis the articular surfaces are irregularly eroded.   In osteochondritis dissecans a crater is seen on one convex surface.

Suggestions for further reading

Ansell, B. M. (1972).   'Hypermobility of Joints.'   In *Modern Trends in Orthopaedics—6*, Ed. by A. Graham Apley.   London; Butterworths

Baldursson, H. *et al.* (1969).   'Tumoral Calcinosis with Hyperphosphatemia.'   *J. Bone Jt Surg.* **51A**, 913

Beighton, P. (1969).   'Orthopaedic Aspects of Ehlers–Danlos Syndrome.'   *J. Bone Jt Surg.* **51B**, 444

Cheyne, C. (1971).   'Histiocytosis X.'   *J. Bone Jt Surg.* **53B**, 366

Hoppenfeld, S. (1976).   *Physical Examination of the Spine and Extremities.*   New York; Appleton Century Crofts

Lloyd-Roberts, G. C. *et al.* (1970).   'Arthrogryposis Multiplex Congenita.'   *J. Bone Jt Surg.* **52B**, 494

Murray, R. O. and Jacobson, H. G. (1977).   *The Radiology of Skeletal Disorders.*   2nd Edn.   Edinburgh; Churchill Livingstone

Wynne-Davies, R. (1970).   'Acetabular Dysplasia and Familial Joint Laxity.'   *J. Bone Jt Surg.* **52B**, 704

CHAPTER 2

INFLAMMATION OF BONE AND JOINT

PERIOSTITIS

Following acute osteomyelitis new subperiosteal bone is laid down. The term
' periostitis ' is then best avoided, for all the bony components are involved. There
are 2 varieties of true periostitis, both chronic.

FOLLOWING INJURY — A haematoma following trauma may ossify, leaving bone which
is thickened on the surface (the knobbly shins of a footballer is an example). X-rays,
however, show that the deep aspects of the cortex and the medulla are normal.

CHRONIC FROM THE START (SYPHILITIC PERIOSTITIS) — Spirochaetes carried by the bloodstream may be deposited in bone. Cellular infiltration is succeeded by fibrosis. Subsequently, because of obliterative endarteritis the bone locally becomes avascular, with
characteristically dense sclerosis.

2.1 SYPHILIS
(a, b, c) congenital—
with diffuse periostitis
of many bones;
(d) acquired periostitis
of the femur.

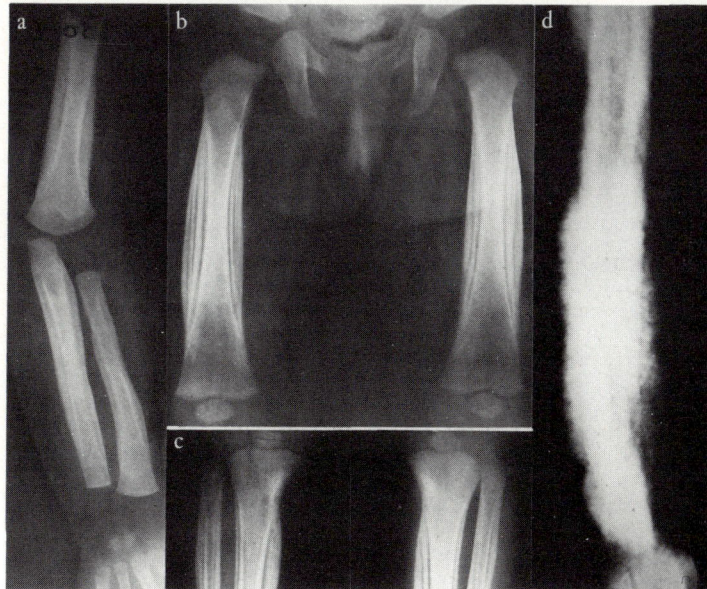

Diffuse periostitis — This sometimes occurs in congenital syphilis; it is usually bilateral
and often painless. Many bones may be involved and the appearance then is not unlike
that in Caffey's disease. Occasionally only the metaphyses are involved.

Localized disease (*gummatous osteoperiostitis*) — This occurs in congenital or acquired
syphilis. Subcutaneous bones chiefly are affected and there may be more than one lump

15

on a bone. Each lump is smooth, hard and sometimes tender; x-rays show considerable density. Later the centre may necrose and the overlying skin break down, leaving a punched-out ulcer with a yellow slough covering bare bone. When this process affects the tibia the thickening on the anterior border makes the bone appear bent (sabre tibia, page 10).

DIFFERENTIAL DIAGNOSIS

Periostitis must be differentiated from:

EWING'S TUMOUR (page 94) — New periosteal bone is laid down in layers parallel to the shaft. The clinical and radiological features usually subside rapidly with radiotherapy, but diagnostic biopsy may be necessary.

OSTEOID OSTEOMA (page 86) — A localized area of cortical thickening is present. Unless a clear area (the nidus) can be seen on x-ray, biopsy may be necessary.

HYPERTROPHIC PULMONARY OSTEOARTHROPATHY — Ninety per cent of patients with this condition have chronic intra-thoracic disease, usually bronchial carcinoma. The ends of the long bones (including the hands and feet) are symmetrically affected by irregular but widespread thickening (Fig. 1.9, page 12), but without alteration in the rest of the bone. Clubbing of the fingers is common and some patients complain of burning pain in the feet, which may be relieved by section of the vagus nerve.

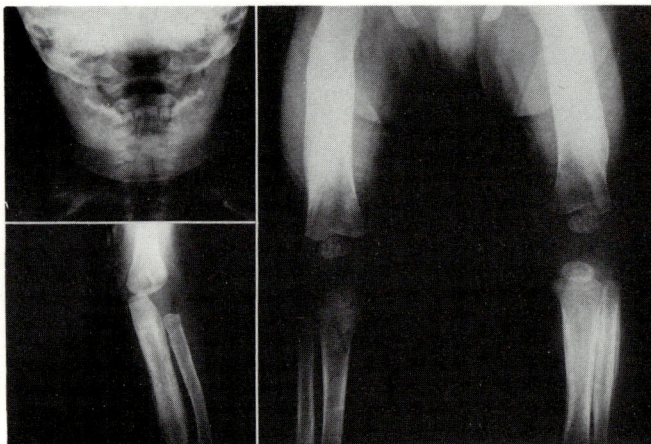

2.2 CAFFEY'S DISEASE Infantile cortical hyperostosis may be due to infection. The appearance of the long bones is not unlike that of congenital syphilis; the mandibular enlargement, however, is characteristic.

INFANTILE CORTICAL HYPEROSTOSIS (Caffey's disease) — In this rare disease, which may be due to a virus infection, subperiosteal new bone is laid down over a wide area of many bones. An infant under 6 months old develops swellings, which may be tender, on the mandibles, long bones and sometimes the scapulae. Often there is fever. The condition should not be confused with osteomyelitis, which is never so widespread, nor with scurvy, which occurs in older infants and is associated with anaemia and bleeding disorders. Caffey's disease recovers spontaneously and the x-ray appearance of the bones returns to normal.

OLD RICKETS — As in syphilis the tibia may be bent, but both tibiae are affected, the bend is in the lower quarter, and the bone is not thick.

PAGET'S DISEASE (page 74) — The bone is thick but, unlike a sabre tibia, the posterior border also is bent.

ACUTE OSTEOMYELITIS

The causal organisms are usually staphylococci, though in young children strepto-coccal infection is not uncommon. Occasionally pneumococci, haemophilus or brucellosis may be responsible; and patients with sickle-cell anaemia are prone to develop salmonella bone infections.

The bloodstream is invaded usually from a minor skin abrasion, rarely from a boil. In children the organisms settle in the metaphysis at the growing end of a long bone, possibly because: (*a*) more blood flows to the growing end; (*b*) the rapidly growing cells are unduly susceptible; (*c*) the delicate vessels have been injured and the haema-toma is a suitable medium for bacterial growth; or (*d*) the hairpin arrangement of capillaries has slowed down the rate of blood flow. In young infants the very end of the bone may be involved, and in adults the mid-shaft may be attacked.

Bone may be infected directly from a wound, but usually this does not present as acute osteomyelitis, because the path of infection also provides a route for drainage.

2.3 ACUTE OSTEOMYELITIS

In young infants infection may settle near the very end of the bone; joint infection and growth disturbance easily follow. In children, metaphyseal infection is usual; the growth disc acts as a barrier to spread.

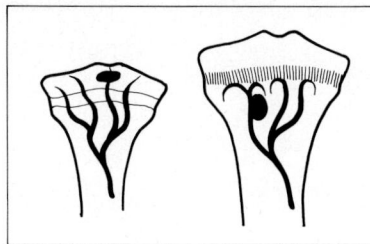

PATHOLOGY

SUPPURATION — Pus forms within the medulla and, being in a confined space under tension, forces its way along the Volkmann canals to the surface of the bone. It then spreads subperiosteally, both around the bone and along the shaft to re-enter the bone at another level, or burst out into the soft tissues. The growth disc and joint capsule are rarely penetrated, except in young infants.

NECROSIS — Bone dies when its blood supply is cut off by infective thrombosis, by rising tension within a rigid bony cavity, or by the stripping up of the periosteum. Dead bone becomes dense, and pieces may separate as sequestra which act as foreign-body irritants, causing persistent discharge through a sinus until they escape or are removed.

NEW BONE FORMATION — New bone forms from the deep layer of the periosteum. If bone formation is extensive, it constitutes an encasing involucrum which may contain holes (cloacae); ultimately the bone often appears widened.

CLINICAL FEATURES

A history of a preceding skin lesion, an injury, or a sore throat may be obtained. A few days later there is rapid onset of fever and malaise and of pain. The pain is localized, unrelieved by rest and often severe. The patient, usually a child, is ill and toxaemic, with a rapid pulse and high fever. There is leucocytosis and a positive blood culture.

The dramatic illness just described is by no means invariable. In children the constitutional disturbance may be misleadingly mild, perhaps because of antibiotics given for some predisposing condition. The local signs are as follows:

LOOK — The limb is held still. It looks normal at first but later swelling and redness may appear.

FEEL — If the child allows the limb to be touched, localized 'finger-tip' tenderness is felt over a metaphysis, and later warmth and oedema.

MOVE — The child may not permit movement of the limb. Usually the neighbouring joint, though irritated, has at least a few degrees of painless movement.

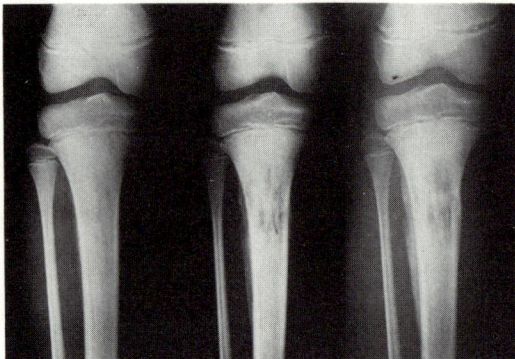

2.4 ACUTE OSTEOMYELITIS
The first x-ray, two days after symptoms began, is normal—it always is; metaphyseal mottling and periosteal changes were not obvious until the second film taken 14 days later; eventually much of the shaft was involved.

X-RAY — For the first 10 days x-rays show no abnormality. Later there is patchy rarefaction of the metaphysis, and periostitis which shows as a thin line parallel to the shaft. Later still, as healing occurs, there is sclerosis and new periosteal bone; sometimes sequestra are seen, which are very dense and separated from the surrounding bone.

DIFFERENTIAL DIAGNOSIS

In acute suppurative arthritis tenderness is diffuse, and all movement at the joint is abolished by muscle spasm.

In acute rheumatism the pain tends to flit from one joint to another, and there may be carditis, rheumatic nodules or erythema marginatum.

Patients with sickle-cell disease may, during a crisis, present with features indistinguishable from acute osteomyelitis. Operation is somewhat hazardous and antibiotics are given first. But both conditions may co-exist, and diagnostic doubt is sometimes inevitable. Should drainage be indicated, the essential is to avoid hypoxia during and after the operation.

TREATMENT

ANTIBIOTICS — Blood and, if possible, aspiration material are sent immediately for culture, but the prompt administration of antibiotics is so vital that the result is not awaited. Because of the prevalence of penicillin-resistant organisms, Blockey and McAllister (1972) advise the following combination: (1) fusidic acid in aqueous suspension, 5 ml. daily for children aged 1–5 years, 10 ml. twice daily for older children; plus (2) erythromycin stearate 30 mg./kg. body weight daily in divided doses. Other regimes are available and are used if the sensitivity tests so indicate. Antibiotic treatment should continue for a minimum of three weeks (six for a severe attack or complications).

SPLINTAGE — A splint is desirable but should not conceal the affected area. Often bed rest, possibly combined with traction, is sufficient. With acute osteomyelitis of the upper femur, traction or splintage is needed to prevent hip dislocation.

DRAINAGE — If antibiotics are given early, drainage is often not necessary. If a subperiosteal abscess can be detected (overlying oedema is a useful sign), or if pyrexia and local tenderness persist for more than 24 hours after adequate antibiotics, the pus should be let out by aspiration or incision; it should be cultured and tested for sensitivity. Opinion is divided as to whether the medulla should be drained by drilling.

COMPLICATIONS AND SEQUELS

Nowadays, with antibiotics, the child nearly always recovers and the bone may return to normal. If treatment is delayed or the organism proves insensitive to antibiotics the following complications may occur.

SEPTICAEMIA — This occasionally proves fatal.

METASTATIC INFECTION — This may involve other bones, joints, serous cavities, the brain or lung.

SUPPURATIVE ARTHRITIS — This may occur (a) in very young children, in whom the growth disc is not an impenetrable barrier; (b) where the metaphysis is intracapsular, as in the upper femur; or (c) from metastatic infection.

ALTERED LENGTH OF BONE — In infants epiphyseal damage may lead to shortening, sometimes severe. In older children, however, the bone occasionally grows too long because metaphyseal hyperaemia has stimulated the growth disc.

CHRONIC OSTEOMYELITIS — This is much the commonest sequel (see below).

CHRONIC OSTEOMYELITIS AS THE SEQUEL TO ACUTE OSTEOMYELITIS

PATHOLOGY

An area of bone has been destroyed by the acute infection; cavities are therefore present and are surrounded by dense sclerosed bone. Bits of dead bone (sequestra) usually remain. They are imprisoned in fibrous tissue and sclerosed bone but may act as irritants, provoking the living tissue to produce sero-pus; this escapes through a sinus which tends to persist because the sequestra cannot escape. Bacteria also are imprisoned in fibrous tissue, where they often remain dormant for years, but at any time infection may flare.

CLINICAL VARIETIES

SINUS — A sinus may persist because of sequestra, foreign bodies, or because the organisms are resistant. As with all forms of truly chronic osteomyelitis, x-rays show areas of bone rarefaction surrounded by dense sclerosis, and sometimes sequestra.

Treatment is usually conservative because the discharge may be no more than a nuisance, and a dry dressing protects the clothing. Most antibiotics fail to penetrate the barrier of fibrous tissue plus bone sclerosis. Fucidin is an exception and, especially when combined with sequestrectomy, is sometimes successful.

The complete excision of diseased bone occasionally helps. Radical surgery should be combined with systemic antibiotics and local instillation of antibiotic solution using a continuous irrigation and suction technique.

FLARES (RECURRENT ACUTE OSTEOMYELITIS) — At any time, even as long as 50 years after apparent healing, the bacteria may escape from their fibrous prison and the wound flare. The patient becomes feverish but not very ill or toxic. There is local pain, redness and tenderness.

Treatment is usually unnecessary because the flare subsides after a few days' rest. The patient expects to be given antibiotics but their value is doubtful. Occasionally an abscess forms; if it discharges spontaneously there is immediate relief, but if it remains painful it should be incised.

SINUS WITH RECURRENT FLARES — Frequently-repeated flares and a constant smelly discharge may render the condition and even the limb itself an intolerable nuisance, in which case amputation may be preferable; but continuous antibiotic irrigation and treatment with hyperbaric oxygen should be tried first.

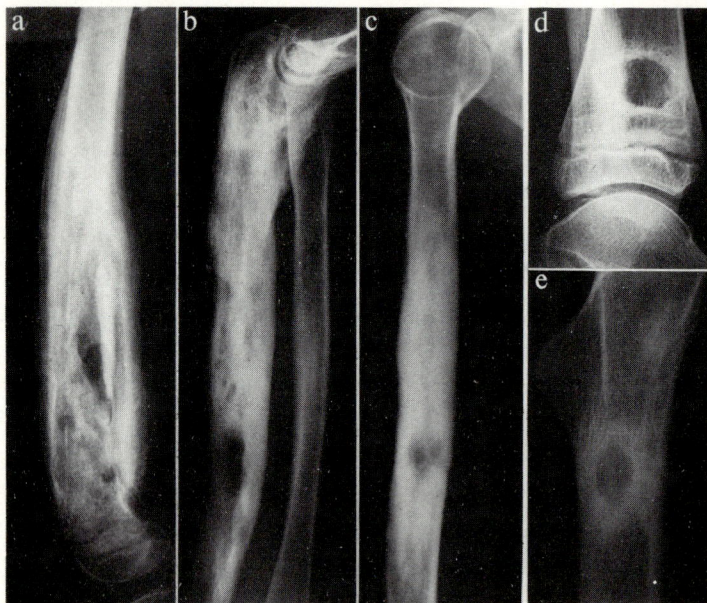

2.5 CHRONIC OSTEO-MYELITIS
(a) The periosteum is thick and a sequestrum visible; (b) shows characteristic altered architecture; (c) Salmonella osteomyelitis in a patient with sickle-cell disease; (d and e) Brodie's abscesses, with sclerosis surrounding a rare area.

CHRONIC OSTEOMYELITIS OF INSIDIOUS ONSET

Four varieties of chronic osteomyelitis appear to be chronic from the start:

BRODIE'S ABSCESS — A Brodie's abscess is usually small and situated in the metaphysis of a long bone, though it may be of any size and occur anywhere in the bone. Clinically it may remain silent for years, or present with recurrent attacks of pain. During an attack the bone is tender and there may be a little swelling. X-rays show a translucent area with a well-defined margin and a small area of surrounding sclerosis, beyond which the bone looks normal.

Treatment is operative. Under antibiotic cover the abscess is opened. Rarely it contains pus, but usually clear sterile fluid. The abscess wall is removed and the wound sutured.

TUBERCULOUS OSTEOMYELITIS (*see also* Chapter 4) — This is a chronic infection which as a rule remains clinically silent until it presents as: (*a*) a joint inflammation, from irritation or eruption into a nearby joint; (*b*) deformity, from collapse of soft bone, as in the spine; (*c*) swelling, possibly of the bone itself (as in dactylitis) or a cold abscess.

X-rays show an area of bone destruction with ill-defined margins and surrounding bone atrophy, in contrast with Brodie's abscess.

SPIROCHAETAL OSTEOMYELITIS — Syphilis of bone is a rare tertiary manifestation, producing localized or diffuse lesions. Localized gummata may occur in any part of the bone, but are usually subperiosteal in subcutaneous bones, and the overlying skin may break down. Diffuse periostitis may cause a sabre tibia (page 10). Diffuse osteomyelitis presents as an aching, tender bone, sometimes with sequestra and sinuses. In congenital syphilis, epiphysitis and dactylitis also occur.

In bone syphilis x-rays may show periosteal thickening and punched-out translucent areas in the midst of dense sclerosis. The lesions are often multiple. Serological tests are essential for diagnosis.

Treatment is directed to the underlying disease. Penicillin and iodides are given.

Yaws may produce bone lesions similar to those of syphilis. Several bones are usually affected. The main changes are periosteal new bone formation and areas of rarefaction in the cortex; sclerosis is less than in syphilis.

CHRONIC NON-SUPPURATIVE OSTEOMYELITIS (GARRÉ) — The bone is thickened and radiologically dense (sclerosing osteitis). The clinical features, x-ray appearance and response to treatment strongly resemble those of an osteoid osteoma (page 86).

ACUTE SUPPURATIVE ARTHRITIS

CAUSE AND PATHOLOGY

The causal organisms are usually staphylococci, occasionally streptococci and, rarely, other organisms. The joint is invaded through a penetrating wound, by eruption of a bone abscess, or by blood spread from a distant site. Infection spreads through the joint; the articular cartilage disintegrates and is removed by polymorphs. Pus may burst out of the joint to form abscesses and sinuses. Later, with healing, opposing surfaces may adhere (fibrous ankylosis); often, however, trabeculae grow across the joint (bony ankylosis).

CLINICAL FEATURES

There may have been a wound. Within a few days (sometimes only 48 hours) the patient rapidly becomes ill, with severe throbbing pain and swelling, a rapid pulse and high swinging fever. The white cell count is raised and blood culture positive.
Many of the local signs can be elicited only in superficial joints.

LOOK — The skin looks red, the joint is held flexed and it is fusiformly swollen.

FEEL — The skin feels hot, there is diffuse tenderness and fluctuation.

MOVE — All movements are grossly restricted and often completely abolished by pain and spasm.

X-RAY — For the first 2–3 weeks the appearance is normal, then the bone shows widespread patchy rarefaction, and the joint space may be narrowed. With healing, the bone recalcifies; the joint space may remain narrow and irregular, or be completely obliterated and crossed by trabeculae.

DIFFERENTIAL DIAGNOSIS

In acute osteomyelitis tenderness is pinpointed to bone, and a little joint movement is permitted.

In rheumatic fever the pain is less severe and is eased by large doses of salicylates; the general signs of rheumatism may be found.

In acute non-suppurative arthritis there is less general illness and the local signs are much less severe.

IMMEDIATE TREATMENT

ASPIRATION — Under anaesthesia the pus is aspirated as soon as possible and the fluid replaced by penicillin. Formal incision is advisable at the hip, or elsewhere if the pus is too thick to aspirate. The pus is cultured and the organisms tested for sensitivity.

ANTIBIOTICS — In addition to the penicillin instilled into the joint, intramuscular injections are started immediately. With deep joints which have been opened, systemic antibiotics should be combined with continuous irrigation using an antibiotic solution.

The injections are continued for several weeks, a more effective antibiotic being substituted if tests so indicate.

SPLINTAGE—The joint must be rested either on a splint or in a widely split plaster. At the hip, traction or splintage is imperative.

TREATMENT OF THE AFTERMATH

Once the patient's general condition is good and the joint is no longer painful or warm, further damage is unlikely.

If articular cartilage has been preserved, the aim is to regain movement. Gentle and gradually increasing active movements are encouraged (not passive and never forced). The patient is allowed up wearing a splint which is taken off for non-weight-bearing exercises. Gradually weight is taken and the splint is eventually discarded. At all stages the patient is carefully watched for signs of a flare.

If articular cartilage has been destroyed, the aim is to keep the joint immobile while ankylosis is awaited. Splintage in the optimum position (page 128) is therefore continuously maintained, usually by plaster, until ankylosis is sound. The patient is allowed up, and, when the bone has recalcified, to take weight.

GONOCOCCAL ARTHRITIS

The joint infection is probably blood-borne. Synovitis may be followed by a purulent effusion, containing gonococci; if treatment is delayed the articular cartilage may be destroyed. Frequently the onset is acute with a migrating synovitis or early arthritis; sometimes suppuration may follow. Occasionally there is a haemorrhagic vesico-pustular rash characteristic of gonococcal or meningococcal septicaemia.

CRYSTAL SYNOVITIS

GOUT — In this metabolic disorder the serum uric acid is abnormally high because of excessive production, inadequate excretion, or both. Crystals of sodium biurate may be deposited in bone (producing radiolucent ' cysts '), in cartilage (producing chalky tophi in the ears or fingers), in bursae (producing bursitis at the knee or elbow), or in joints.

The joints mainly affected are the toe joints (especially the metatarso-phalangeal joint of the hallux), the ankles, the finger joints and the wrists. Urate crystals are acutely irritating, and an attack of painful arthritis comes on rapidly. The skin overlying an affected joint is red, hot and dry; the joint is swollen and held still. In early attacks the x-ray is normal, but extensive bone deposits are revealed as punched-out translucent areas under the cartilage. Secondary osteoarthritis may develop.

The diagnosis is suggested by the family history, previous similar attacks, circumstantial evidence (attacks provoked by trauma, operations, or a drinking bout), x-ray appearance, and by hyperuricaemia; it should be remembered that the uric acid level is sometimes raised in non-gouty patients who are taking various drugs including aspirin. Confirmation requires the presence of tophi or identification of urate crystals in the joint fluid.

The acutely inflamed joint should be rested; aspiration helps relieve pain and permits identification of the crystals. Phenylbutazone (200 mg t.d.s.) or indomethacin (50 gm t.d.s.) is given until the acute attack subsides. Interval or prophylactic treatment, whether by uricosuric drugs or allopurinol, should be supervised by a physician.

2.6 GOUT
The chalky deposits are seen clinically as lumps (a, b) and radiologically as translucent areas (c).

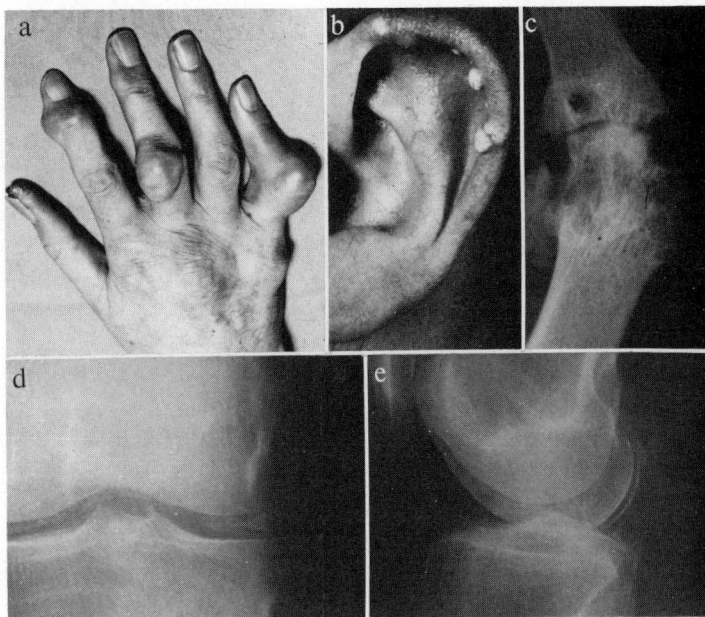

Pseudo-gout. There are no tophi, but the menisci and articular cartilage calcify (d, e).

Pseudo-gout — The term crystal-induced synovitis is used not only for gout (in which the crystals are of sodium bi-urate), but also for pseudo-gout (in which they are of calcium pyrophosphate). In pseudogout attacks of acute arthritis resembling gout may occur but, unlike gout, the shoulders, hips, knees and ankles are mostly affected. The acuteness of the inflammation may even suggest suppurative arthritis, but aspirated synovial fluid does not contain bacteria-laden pus cells; it contains crystals. The condition may be a complication of hyperparathyroidism, diabetes and renal failure. It is not uncommon in the elderly and is associated with chondro-calcinosis, i.e. calcification visible in hyaline and in fibro-cartilage. Secondary osteoarthritis may develop. Treatment is similar to that of acute gout, but no interval treatment is available.

CHRONIC ARTHRITIS

There are three main varieties of chronic arthritis, each important enough to merit a separate chapter.

RHEUMATOID ARTHRITIS (Chapter 3) — Usually many joints are affected, especially small joints. Muscle wasting is considerable and the patient is unwell. X-ray films of an affected joint show rarefaction of bone and uniform decrease of joint space.

TUBERCULOUS ARTHRITIS (Chapter 4) — Usually only one joint is affected, often a large one. Muscle wasting is marked and the patient is sometimes unwell. X-rays show rarefaction of the bones and an irregular joint space.

OSTEOARTHRITIS (Chapter 5) — Usually only one or perhaps two joints are affected. Unlike the other varieties, osteoarthritis is not inflammatory, so that muscle wasting is slight and the patient is fit in himself. X-rays show no bone rarefaction, and diminution of joint space occurs only where pressure is borne.

Suggestions for further reading

Bjelle, A. and Sundén, G. (1974). 'Pyrophosphate Arthropathy.' *J. Bone Jt Surg.* **56B**, 246

Blockey, N. J. and McAllister, T. A. (1972). 'Antibiotics in Acute Osteomyelitis in Children.' *J. Bone Jt Surg.* **54B**, 299

Clawson, D. K. and Dunn, A. W. (1967). 'Management of Common Bacterial Infections of Bones and Joints.' *J. Bone Jt Surg.* **49A,** 164

Currey, H. L. F. and Mason, R. M. (1969). 'Gout and Chondrocalcinosis.' In *Recent Advances in Orthopaedics*, Ed. by A. Graham Apley. London; Churchill

Mollan, R. A. B. and Piggot, J. (1977). 'Acute Osteomyelitis in Children.' *J. Bone Jt Surg.* **59B,** 2

Morrey, B. F. *et al.* (1976). 'Suppurative Arthritis of the Hip in Children.' *J. Bone. Jt Surg.* **58A,** 388

Paterson, D. C. (1970). 'Acute Suppurative Arthritis in Infancy and Childhood.' *J. Bone Jt Surg.* **52B,** 474

CHAPTER 3

RHEUMATOID ARTHRITIS

CAUSE

The cause of this common and crippling disease is not established.   It is sometimes familial, and it may be that any one of several precipitating factors can, in genetically predisposed individuals, initiate the disease; such factors may include infections, psychological trauma or joint injury.   Synovial changes, once initiated, may be sustained by an auto-immune process.   These changes are part of a general systemic illness better called 'rheumatoid disease' because of its widespread manifestations. This self-perpetuating process is much more likely to occur in those individuals with 'rheumatoid factor' in their circulation (seropositive).

PATHOLOGY

The characteristic pathological change is the rheumatoid nodule, in which an area of fibrinoid necrosis of collagen tissue is surrounded by a radially disposed palisade of fibroblasts.   Another but less common general feature is arteritis which may give rise to skin lesions and to neuropathies.

In a rheumatoid joint the synovial membrane, which is affected first, contains collections of lymphocytes and plasma cells.   The membrane becomes hyperaemic, swollen and proliferated; from its edges a pannus of inflammatory material spreads over the articular cartilage.   The pannus not only inflicts direct damage by adhering to and penetrating into the cartilage, it also acts as a mechanical barrier preventing absorption of nutrient synovial fluid; in fact the inflamed synovium behaves in an almost 'malignant' fashion.   Where cartilage destruction has occurred erosions may develop in the already rarefied bone.

The synovial hypertrophy and increased fluid production result in swelling of the joint; the capsule and ligaments become lax or stretched and, in some situations, tendons are dislodged.   These features, together with muscle spasm, tendon ruptures and muscle imbalance, lead to joint deformities which may progress to subluxation or even dislocation.

As healing occurs, inflammatory granulation tissue is gradually converted to fibrous tissue, with permanent restriction of movement.   Secondary osteoarthritis is liable to supervene in a joint with faulty mechanics and damaged cartilage. Rarely, bony ankylosis occurs between eroded articular surfaces.

The synovium of tendon sheaths also can hypertrophy.   Nodules may develop on the tendons themselves or the tendons may be eroded and rupture.   At the wrist, swelling may lead to median nerve compression.

SYMPTOMS

The onset is usually gradual with malaise, tiredness, loss of weight or generalized muscle pains.   Joint symptoms soon follow—pain, stiffness (especially after rest), swelling and deformity; these also are usually gradual in onset, affecting small joints first, especially the wrists, fingers and toes.   The tendency is for the disease to spread slowly and symmetrically up the limbs, involving the larger joints. Occasionally the onset and course are more rapid; and sometimes a single large joint is affected first. Remissions are common, but often are followed by further exacerbations, so that increasing stiffness and deformity occur and the disease may not burn itself out until many years have elapsed.

SIGNS

The disease is at least 3 times commoner in women, the highest incidence of onset being between the ages of 25 and 55. During periods of disease activity the patient is unwell, often with fever and loss of weight; the sedimentation rate is raised, anaemia is common, and occasionally lymph nodes are enlarged. These features subside during remissions, and the sedimentation rate is a useful index of activity.

The corresponding illness in children is called Still's disease. The joint changes are similar to those of adult rheumatoid disease but are usually preceded by more severe general illness; pyrexia and skin rashes are common and there may also be lymphadenopathy, splenomegaly and pericarditis.

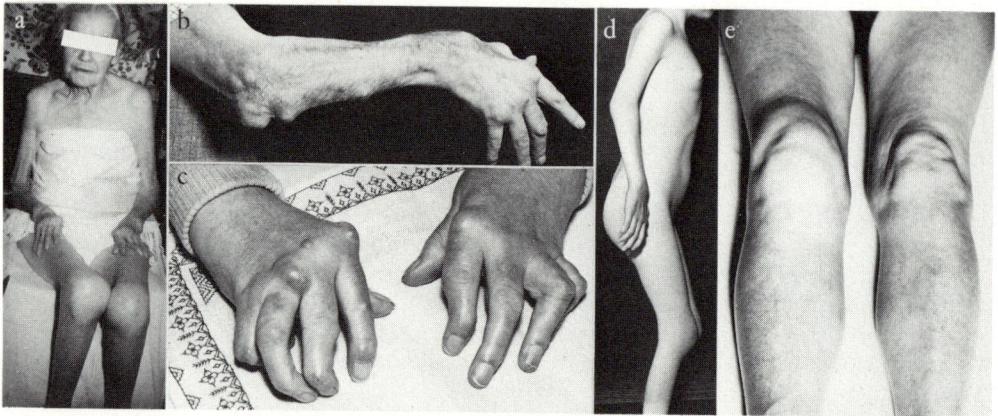

3.1 RHEUMATOID ARTHRITIS
(a) Widespread crippling deformities; (b) rheumatoid nodules; (c) the combination of deformities and nodules is pathognomonic; (d) Still's disease; (e) this patient presented with monarticular disease, but polyarthritis developed later — the term ' monopoly ' seems appropriate.

In most patients with rheumatoid arthritis the Rose-Waaler and latex serum tests for rheumatoid factor are positive; but some 25 per cent of patients are sero-negative and the prognosis in them is better. In sero-positive patients nodules may develop. These are hard, not tender, and vary from 3 mm to 3 cm in diameter; they may be palpable in subcutaneous tissues, bursae or tendons, and when present are diagnostic.

Cervical spine involvement is common and may be symptomless; but atlanto-axial or mid-cervical disease may lead to neurological damage, particularly if the patient is mis-handled under anaesthesia.

Although small joints (notably the metacarpo-phalangeal joints) are characteristically affected first, the disease may begin in a single large joint and remain confined to that joint for months or even years; eventually other joints also are involved. The signs in affected joints are as follows:

LOOK — The skin is shiny, atrophic, and sometimes almost translucent. The joint is swollen and looks fusiform; muscle wasting makes the swelling more obvious.

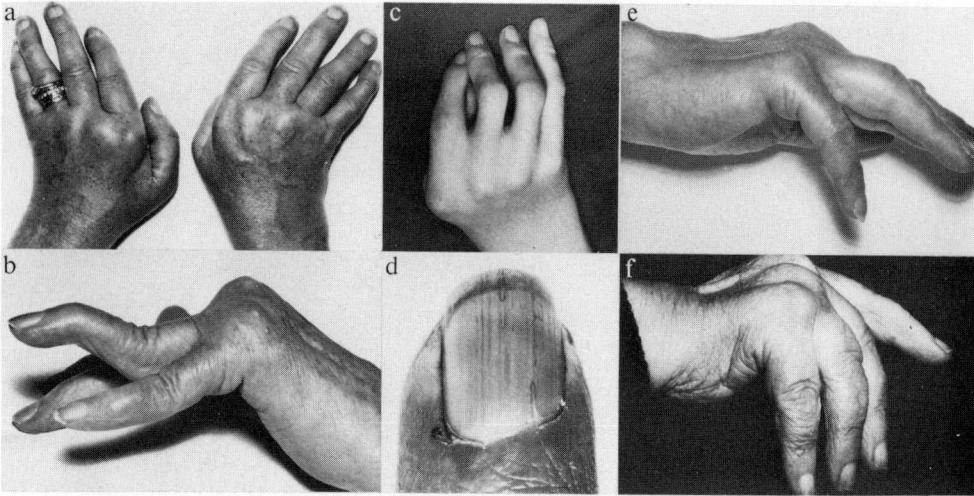

3.2 RHEUMATOID HANDS
(a) Ulnar drift; (b) swan-neck deformity; (c) boutonnière deformities; (d) 'nail-fold lesion' due to arteritis; (e) dropped finger; (f) three dropped fingers.

Deformity is a marked feature. At the hips fixed flexion is common, at the knees fixed flexion and backward subluxation, and at the wrists fixed flexion with forward subluxation; all these are largely due to muscle imbalance. The important hand deformities have more complex causes.

Ulnar drift is the most obvious feature of the metacarpo-phalangeal subluxation, which develops progressively. Contributory factors are: (1) the normal line of pull of the finger tendons is towards the ulnar side; (2) synovial swelling may 'shoulder' the extensor tendons ulnarward; (3) exuberant synovium may block the proximal excursion of the transverse fibres of the extensor expansion on the radial side, while on the ulnar side movement remains unimpeded, (4) the wrist may be unstable and radially deviated; and (5) in the resting posture of the hand gravity favours ulnar deviation.

Swan-neck deformity (hyperextension at the proximal finger joint and flexion at the distal) occurs if: (1) the action of flexor sublimus is impeded by synovial swelling or forward subluxation at the proximal finger joint; or (2) the sublimis tendon or the volar plate ruptures in front of the proximal interphalangeal joint.

Despite deformity normal flexion is at first possible; later it can be accomplished only if the proximal interphalangeal joint is prevented from hyperextending, and eventually the deformity becomes fixed and finger flexion is lost (Barton, 1976). Secondary articular changes rapidly develop.

Boutonnière deformity (flexion at the proximal finger joint and hyperextension at the distal) occurs when the middle slip of the extensor tendon is stretched by synovial swelling or undergoes attrition rupture.

Dropped fingers (one or more) follow rupture of extensor tendons, usually at the level of the wrist.

FEEL — During activity the skin feels moist and warm. There is diffuse tenderness, the synovium feels thick and fluid may be detectable.

MOVE — During a phase of activity movement is restricted by pain and spasm. With quiescence a reasonably good range may return; but often considerable stiffness remains and occasionally fibrous ankylosis may occur.

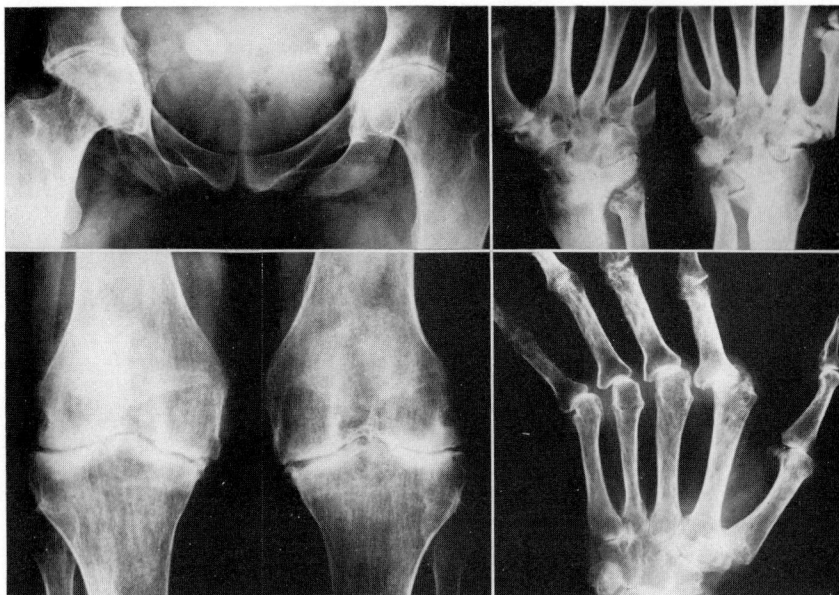

3.3 JOINT DAMAGE
With destruction of articular cartilage the joint space becomes irregular, and narrowed or obliterated. Many joints may be wrecked.

X-RAY — An early feature is diffuse rarefaction of bone; at the same time erosions may be
seen at the synovial attachments and in the subchondral bone. Later the joint space
becomes uniformly decreased and may completely disappear. Once the joint space has
narrowed secondary degenerative changes with sclerosis may develop. Occasionally
huge cysts (called 'geodes') are seen.

DIFFERENTIAL DIAGNOSIS

Chronic arthritis affecting many small joints is usually due to rheumatoid arthritis,
but a similar pattern and systemic disease also occur in psoriatic arthritis, systemic
lupus erythematosus and chronic gout. In purely degenerative conditions such as
primary generalized osteoarthritis (which also affects the fingers) there is no systemic
illness.

If the disease starts in proximal joints and bursae it mimics the syndrome of
' polymyalgia rheumatica ' whose other associations include the dangerous giant-cell
(cranial) arteritis. The sedimentation rate is very high. Steroids are effective in
relieving pain and suppressing the disorder.

When rheumatoid arthritis begins in one large joint the following conditions must
be considered. In the first three there is also systemic illness, but in all of them the
tests for rheumatoid factor are negative.

ANKYLOSING SPONDYLITIS — Occasionally this presents in one large joint, but the age
of onset (usually below 30), the predilection for males, the presence of low back stiffness
and x-ray changes in the sacro-iliac joints all help establish the diagnosis.

REITER'S DISEASE — In this syndrome bilateral joint disease (predominantly affecting the
legs) occurs. There is however also a history of urethritis or dysentery, and of con-
junctivitis. In treatment the drug of choice is phenylbutazone.

TUBERCULOUS SYNOVITIS — The patient may present with a warm, swollen joint, muscle
wasting, limited movement, a raised sedimentation rate and possibly rarefaction on

x-ray. The presumptive diagnosis is tuberculous synovitis, but the Rose–Waaler test may be positive or biopsy may show the condition to be rheumatoid in nature, and other joints may later become affected, even after an interval of many years.

VILLOUS SYNOVITIS — Despite gross swelling there is remarkably little wasting (page 265).

INTERMITTENT HYDROPS — This condition affects one or both knees in women. At intervals the joint swells rapidly, then slowly subsides. The cause is unknown, but occasionally rheumatoid arthritis develops later.

SYPHILITIC ARTHRITIS — In this rare condition one or more large joints become swollen, usually without pain. The synovium feels thick and lumpy (gummata). X-rays show bone erosion at the synovial attachments, and periostitis. Painless effusion into both knees also occurs in congenital syphilitics aged 5–15 years (Clutton's joints). Treponemal serology establishes the diagnosis.

GENERAL TREATMENT

If the patient is ill, or if weight-bearing joints are inflamed, a period of bed rest is advisable; but sustained flexion of the neck, back and hips must be avoided. The diet must be adequate and any anaemia dealt with. The pursuit and eradication of septic foci is traditional but has no specific action on rheumatoid disease. Adequate explanation and re-assuring pep talks are valuable and in severe cases it may be necessary to arrange for occupational retraining or domestic reorganization.

Drugs are always needed and are of three main types: (1) analgesic and anti-inflammatory drugs which should be tried first; (2) specific anti-rheumatoid drugs which are used if after many months analgesics prove inadequate; and (3) suppressant drugs which are withheld as long as possible and are only used in special circumstances. Many of the drugs used have serious side effects demanding precautionary regular blood counts and urine tests; a physician should control drug treatment. A scientifically based pecking order for drugs would be useful.

ANALGESIC AND ANTI-INFLAMMATORY DRUGS — Salicylates are traditional and often tried first, especially soluble aspirin (300 mg tablets, dose up to 4 g daily). Proprionic acid derivatives and fenamates are useful alternatives to aspirin and are claimed to have less gastrointestinal side affects.

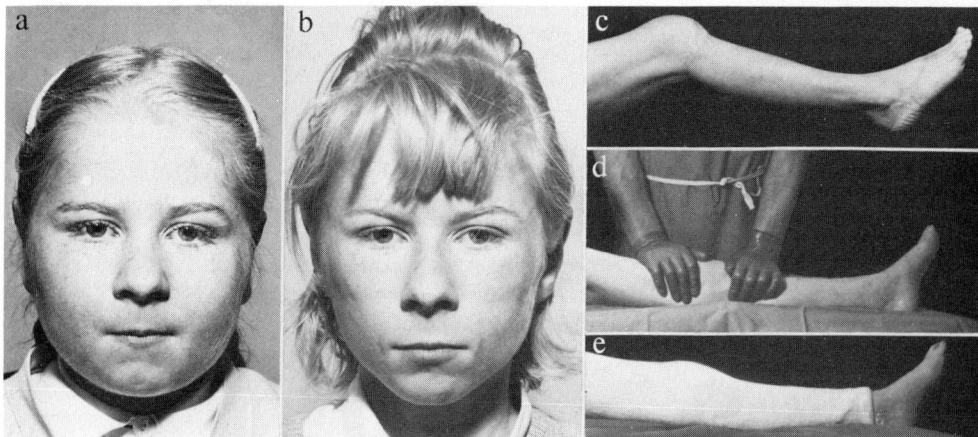

3.4 TWO ASPECTS OF TREATMENT
(a) This girl developed a 'moon-face' on prolonged steroids: contrast the appearance in (b) 2 years after stopping steroids. (c, d, e) Correction of fixed flexion by manipulation: two days later the plaster was bivalved for exercises.

Phenylbutazone is sometimes effective, but may cause blood dyscrasias, peptic ulceration or oedema (100 mg tablets, dose 300 mg daily).   Indomethacin is a useful alternative which shares only one risk (peptic ulceration) with phenylbutazone, but causes the additional risk of cerebral side effects, mainly headache (25 mg tablets, dose 50–100 mg daily).

SPECIFIC DRUGS — These may actually reduce the activity of rheumatoid arthritis.   Gold is usually given (after a small test dose) as weekly intramuscular injections of 50 mg of sodium aurothiomalate ('Myocrysin'), the urine being tested before each injection; complications include dermatitis, bone-marrow depression and nephrosis.   The alternative is penicillamine (125 mg of base daily, slowly increasing); but it shares many of the complications of Myocrysin and both drugs should be controlled by a physician.

SUPPRESSANT DRUGS — Steroids may reduce inflammation, but the destructive effects of the disease continue silently; it is a mistake to believe that, given early, they may stamp out the disease.   Although their administration commonly affords short-term relief, long-term relief is quite uncommon and complications are so frequent that these drugs should be withheld as long as possible.

Steroids are indicated when other drugs have failed, and when the disease is still active (they can have no possible effect upon deformities which are the legacy of 'burnt out' disease).   The chief indications are: (1) in fulminating disease; (2) to provide relief for perhaps 3 or 4 years when the risks are outweighed by the advantages (for example in women with young families, or in men at a critical stage of their careers); (3) to alleviate (by means of a single dose each night) disabling morning pain and stiffness.   Steroids must not be given to patients with tuberculosis, and are dangerous to those with psychosis, peptic ulcer, or generalized osteoporosis.

Prednisone and Prednisolone.   These are the most reliable steroids.   It is usual to start with one 5 mg tablet daily; the subsequent dosage is titrated against the patient's needs, but should not exceed 10 mg daily and every effort is made to keep the maintenance dose as low as possible.   Any patient on steroids should always carry a steroid card.   If he sustains a major injury the dose should be temporarily increased.   If anaesthesia is required 100 mg of hydrocortisone hemisuccinate should be given on the morning of operation, followed by 100 mg of hydrocortisone acetate post-operatively and again next morning; this precaution remains necessary for a considerable time even after steroids have been discontinued.

Complications include mental changes (euphoria or depression and insomnia); changes in appearance (moonface, deposition of fat, hirsutism, acne and pigmentation); altered electrolyte balance (increased water and sodium retention with hypopotassaemia); increased blood pressure; and decreased glucose tolerance.   In addition osteoporosis and pathological fractures may occur, the signs of acute inflammation may be suppressed, and wound healing is sometimes delayed.   After prolonged therapy the adrenal cortex may become even 'lazier' so that the patient is dependent upon the drug and suffers severely if it is withdrawn.

Azathioprine — This immuno-suppressive drug is useful when the disease is not controlled by an acceptable dose of prednisone or prednisolone.   The dose (2·5 mg/kg body weight/day) needs careful blood-count monitoring, because the drug is a marrow suppressant.

Hydrocortisone acetate — This is useful for intra-articular injection, which may be indicated when only two or three joints are painful; up to 100 mg may safely be injected into a large joint.   Repeated injections over a long period of time may, if they render the joint painless, lead to degenerative changes resembling those found in Charcot's disease.

LOCAL TREATMENT

SPLINTAGE AND PHYSIOTHERAPY — During the acute stage a joint may need splintage to relieve pain and prevent deformity.   Plastic or plaster splints are used from which the limb is lifted several times daily and put through a full passive range.   As the disease subsides active exercises are encouraged and the patient is mobilized with walking aids or in a warm pool. At an early stage the patient's daily activities are assessed so that provision can be made for handicaps at home, travelling and work. Local heat or steroid injections into joints may help at specific sites, but fixed deformity usually needs manipulation under anaesthesia.

OPERATIONS — Surgical treatment can be of considerable value and is being used with increasing frequency. The selection and timing of operations is difficult, but is facilitated by considering the disease in three stages:

(1) *Early* — In this stage synovial hypertrophy and muscle imbalance are the dominant features. Synovectomy is of great value in relieving pain and sometimes may even restore muscle balance. Destruction of articular cartilage is halted, sometimes for several years.

Synovectomy is most rewarding at the knee, the wrist, the elbow and above all at the metacarpo-phalangeal joints of the fingers; if ulnar drift has already begun, the dorsi-lateral capsule should be tightened by overlapping and the extensor indicis proprius re-routed to the radial side. Excision of proliferated tendon sheaths also is valuable,

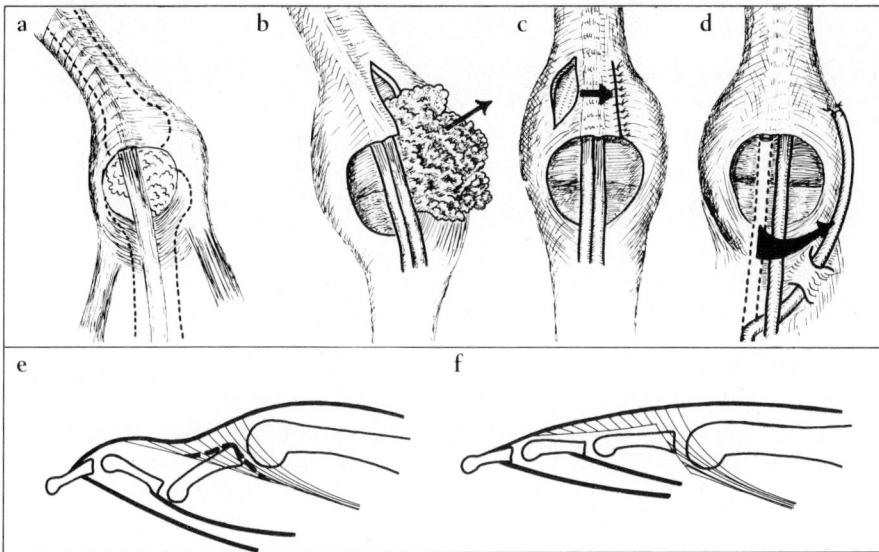

3.5 HAND OPERATIONS
(a) Synovial hypertrophy has ' shouldered ' the extensor tendon out of its groove: the resulting ulnar drift may be treated by synovectomy (b), followed by dividing the capsule on the ulnar side and reefing it on the radial side (c), and by rerouting the extensor indicis proprius (d). Swan-neck deformity (e). Littler's release (f) is useful before arthritis develops.

particularly at the back or front of the wrist; it should always accompany other repair procedures. Concurrent active disease, especially in sero-positive patients, must be energetically treated to promote the best surgical results.

(2) *Intermediate* — In this stage deformities are becoming fixed partly because muscle balance persists uncorrected and partly because of fibrosis. The knee and elbow for example become fixed flexed; and in the hand deformities may develop and deteriorate quite briskly to become fixed. ' Dropped fingers ', due to attrition ruptures of extensor tendons and trigger fingers are common.

Synovectomy may still be indicated, but now needs to be supplemented by other procedures. At the knee adherent menisci may need to be excised, adhesions divided and the fat pad mobilized.   In the hand, early swan-neck deformity can sometimes be corrected by lively splintage which pulls the proximal phalanges into correct alignment but, if the extensor expansion is fibrosed or the intrinsic muscles unbalanced, then Littler's release operation (excising the triangular portion of each side of the extensor expansion distal to the transverse fibres) is valuable.   Boutonnière can sometimes be corrected by repairing or tightening the middle slip of the extensor tendon.

Wherever tendon action is impeded by synovial hypertrophy or by thickening of the tendon sheath these should be dealt with.   Ruptured tendons should be repaired early; late repair fails and tendon transfer is then indicated.   Extensor tendon ruptures on the dorsum of the wrist may be caused by a sharp spike of bone projecting backwards from the ulna; excision of the lowest inch of the ulna at the time the tendon is repaired not only prevents further ruptures from occurring but also restores rotation of the forearm.

ARTHRODESIS   EXCISION   JOINT REPLACEMENT

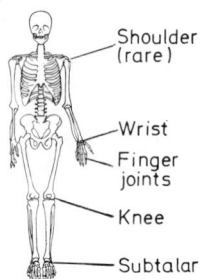 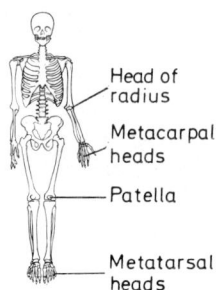 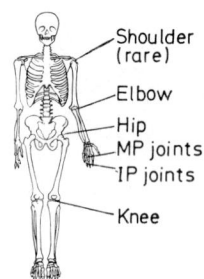

3.6   SALVAGE SURGERY
Sites where late operation may be useful.

(3) *Late* — The features of this stage—articular destruction, fibrosis, fixed deformity and often joint subluxation—cannot be reversed; but function can often be improved by 'salvage' procedures particularly arthroplasty and arthrodesis.

At the elbow, excision of the radial head combined with synovectomy and anterior transposition of the ulnar nerve is useful.   Joint replacement, though at first highly successful, may fail (because of loosening) after 2 or 3 years.

At the wrist, arthrodesis is the operation of choice and can usefully be combined with excision of the lower ulna to restore rotation.

In the fingers, the metacarpo-phalangeal joints should never be arthrodesed, but their function can sometimes be improved by excising the metacarpal heads or by replacement arthroplasty (page 131); extra-articular causes of stiffness or instability must be dealt with at the same time.   Interphalangeal joints should not be excised; but replacement is a distinct possibility; before considering arthrodesis (which is rarely indicated) serial manipulations and plasters are worth trying, the aim being to keep these joints slightly flexed.

In the spine, localized fusion should be considered if the atlas migrates upwards, or if it subluxes forward more than 4 mm; with neurological complications, operation is strongly indicated.

At the hip, total replacement (page 132) is often helpful, especially where both hips are stiff, or the knee on the same side is affected.   The possibility of post-operative infection is, however, greater than when replacement is performed for osteoarthritis.

At the knee, if only one is involved arthrodesis is a certain way of relieving pain; but the other knee may become affected and bilateral arthrodesis is unacceptably disabling.

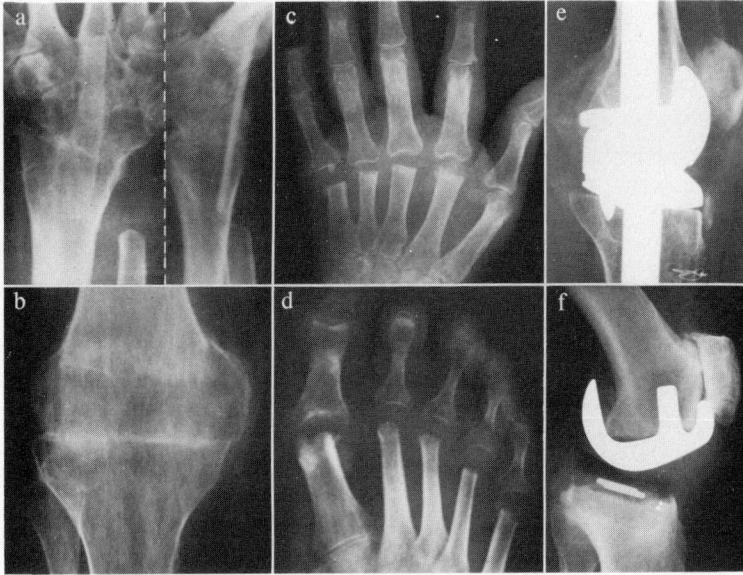

3.7 EXAMPLES OF SALVAGE SURGERY
(a, b) Arthrodesis; (c, d) excision; (e, f) arthroplasty.

Benjamin's double osteotomy (page 285) is a possibility, but joint replacement is increasingly popular. Before there is much joint destruction or instability, surface replacement is indicated; later a linked or hinged prosthesis may be needed (page 135).

In the foot, painful callosities associated with subluxed metatarso-phalangeal joints respond well to multiple arthroplasties; an ellipse of skin containing the callosities is first removed, then the metatarsal heads and proximal portions of the proximal phalanges are excised (Fowler's operation).

Suggestions for further reading

Barton, N. J. (1976). 'Editorial.' *The Hand*, **8**, 3

Copeman, W. S. C. (1969). *Textbook of the Rheumatic Diseases*, 4th Edn. Edinburgh; Livingstone

Cruess, R. L. and Mitchell, N. S. (1972). *Surgery of Rheumatoid Arthritis*. Oxford and Edinburgh; Blackwell

Flatt, A. E. (1974). *The Care of the Rheumatoid Hand*, 3rd Edn. St. Louis; Mosby

Lipscomb, P. R., Peterson, L. F. A. and Linscheid, R. L. 'Surgery for Rheumatoid Arthritis.' A series of instructional course lectures. *J. Bone Jt Surg*. (1968) **50A**, 575 (*et seq*.).

Macintosh, D. L. and Hunter, G. A. (1972). 'The Use of Hemiarthroplasty Prosthesis for Advanced Osteoarthritis and Rheumatoid Arthritis of the Knee.' *J. Bone Jt Surg*. **54B**, 245

Meijers, K. A. E. *et al*.' (1974). 'Dislocation of the Cervical Spine with Cord Compression in Rheumatoid Arthritis.' *J. Bone Jt Surg*. **56B**, 668

Mowat, A. G. *et al*. (1971). 'Polymyalgia Rheumatica.' *J. Bone Jt Surg*. **53B**, 701

Rana, N. A. *et al*. (1973). 'Atlanto-Axial Subluxation in Rheumatoid Arthritis.' *J. Bone Jt Surg*. **55B**, 458

CHAPTER 4

TUBERCULOSIS

GENERALIZED TUBERCULOSIS

CAUSE

The body is invaded by tubercle bacilli, human or bovine. Formerly, 85 per cent of cases were bovine in origin, but pasteurization and tuberculin-tested herds have reduced this figure to 25 per cent. The bacilli enter the body via the lung (droplet infection) or the gut (swallowing infected milk products) or, rarely, through the skin.

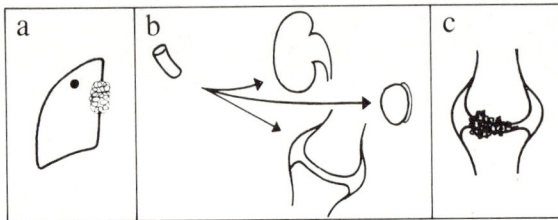

4.1 THE TUBERCULOUS PROCESS
The primary infection is usually arrested in the local lymph glands (a); secondary spread is by the blood stream (b); the term 'tertiary' can be used for the local destructive lesion (c).

PATHOLOGY

PRIMARY COMPLEX — The initial lesion in lung, pharynx or gut is a small one with lymphatic spread to regional glands; this combination is the primary complex. Usually the bacilli are fixed in the glands and no clinical illness results, but occasionally the response is excessive, with clinical enlargement of glands in the neck or abdomen.

Even though there is usually no clinical illness, the initial infection has two important sequels: (*a*) within glands which are apparently healed or even calcified, bacilli may

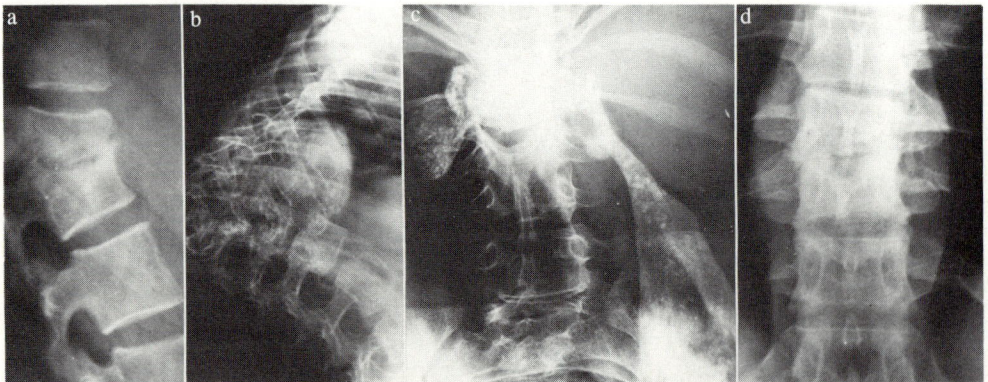

4.2 THE TUBERCULOUS PROCESS IN THE SPINE
Tuberculous osteomyelitis (a) leads to forward collapse (b). Pus is extruded forming abscesses (c, d).

34

survive for many years, so that a reservoir for potential reinfection exists; (b) the body has been sensitized to the toxin (a positive Heaf test being an index of sensitization), and should reinfection occur, the response is quite different, the lesion being a destructive one which spreads by contiguity.

SECONDARY SPREAD — If resistance to the original infection is low, widespread dissemination via the bloodstream may occur, giving rise to miliary tuberculosis or meningitis. More often blood spread occurs months or years later, perhaps because of lowered resistance. Bacilli escape from their lymphatic prison, and may be deposited in many tissues. Probably most of the bacilli are destroyed, but others survive giving rise to destructive lesions of which two or three often coexist.

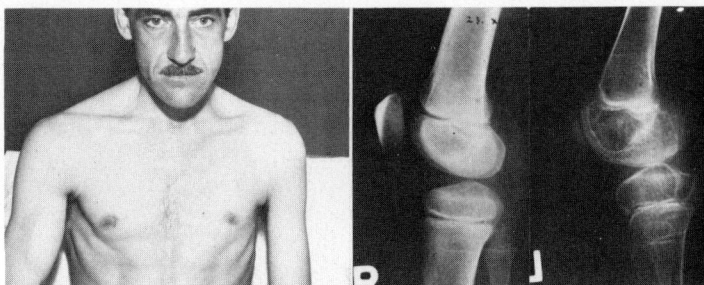

4.3 ACTIVE
            TUBERCULOSIS
A characteristic feature is wasting of muscle (note the left deltoid), and ' wasting ' of bone (note the rarefaction of the left knee).

TERTIARY LESION — The surgeon usually sees tuberculosis as a locally destructive lesion to which the term 'tertiary' may be applied. The bacilli, having gained a foothold in sensitized tissue, multiply. Giant-cell systems develop, grow and coalesce, destroying normal tissue and replacing it by caseous material. So long as this process is active, destruction and caseation continue to extend by direct contiguity, and the bone is slowly 'eaten away'. In addition the bone 'melts away', that is, it undergoes rarefaction, a consequence of the increased blood supply occurring in chronic inflammation. Because it is being eaten away and melted away the bone tends to collapse; caseous material and tuberculous pus are squeezed out forming a cold abscess which, if it reaches the surface, may discharge and leave a sinus. The muscles also 'melt away' and their wasting is a marked feature of joint tuberculosis.

CLINICAL FEATURES

Tuberculosis of a bone or joint is merely the local manifestation of a general disease; even though the bone or joint may be the presenting feature, a second focus (for example, in the lung or uro-genital tract) often co-exists. The general illness is gradual in onset, with a long history; the patient feels off colour and may complain of lassitude, poor appetite, loss of weight and night sweats. Often he looks thin and pale, though he may have a malar flush. Slight evening pyrexia is usual, the sedimentation rate raised and the Heaf test positive. Frequently the illness is mild; but in Asians who live in England it is often more acute, with greater systemic disturbance.

TREATMENT

Recumbency and a sanatorium life, once the cornerstones of general treatment, have been superseded by chemotherapy. Once drug treatment is stabilized and the patient reasonably fit he need not be in hospital. Until recently the standard regime (the doses are for adults) was: streptomycin (1 g by intramuscular injection daily);

INAH (iso-nicotinic acid hydrazide — 200 mg daily by mouth); and PAS (para-aminosalicylic acid — 16 g daily by mouth). Usually streptomycin was given only every other day after three months and was discontinued after six months; the other two drugs continued for at least a year. Nowadays rifampicin (450 mg daily in divided doses) is often substituted for PAS. Controlled trials in spinal tuberculosis have suggested that streptomycin can perhaps be omitted altogether, except in resistant cases; the cautious retain it for three months. Other drugs, such as ethambutol (25 mg/kg body weight daily, reducing), are also becoming available.

COMPLICATIONS

DISSEMINATION — The secondary spread of tuberculosis is via the bloodstream. Consequently, miliary tuberculosis or meningitis may occur — both used to be fatal before the introduction of chemotherapy.

AMYLOID DISEASE — Associated with chronic tissue destruction there is increased production of auto-antibodies which react with serum globulins and ground substance to produce an insoluble glycoprotein called amyloid. This is deposited in the ground substance of many tissues, particularly in the walls of arterioles. The main organs involved are the liver, spleen, kidneys, pancreas, adrenals and intestinal mucosa, but almost every tissue may be affected to some degree.

The disease occurs not only with tuberculosis but also with other chronic bone or joint infections, in leprosy, in malaria, and particularly in rheumatoid arthritis. The patient is pale, puffy, waxy, wasted and oedematous. The spleen, kidney and liver are enlarged. Proof of diagnosis may be obtained by the congo red test, liver puncture or gum biopsy. The only hope is eradication of the disease, when the amyloid process may be reversed.

JOINT TUBERCULOSIS

Joint tuberculosis is a local manifestation of a general disease. Nevertheless the disease as it affects any joint merits separate description and this is conveniently divided into three stages.

(1) *Active disease* — The disease has the upper hand and the patient may be ill in himself. There is local active inflammation as shown by warmth, muscle wasting and bone rarefaction. At first the disease is confined to the synovium or to the interior of the bone, the articular cartilage remaining normal; from this early disease restoration to normal is still possible. Later the articular cartilage may be damaged, giving a true arthritis, from which complete resolution is no longer possible.

(2) *Healing phase* — Gradually the patient gains the upper hand and masters the disease. Any general illness subsides. Locally the disease is arrested, pain and warmth disappear and the bones recalcify. If the disease was arrested before articular damage (early), healing may be by resolution to apparent normality; if articular cartilage has been damaged (late), healing is by fibrosis.

(3) *Aftermath* — Once a joint has suffered a true arthritis with erosion of articular cartilage the damage is permanent and the resulting fibrous joint is unsound; i.e., increasing deformity may occur and even after many years of quiescence, bacilli may be liberated from their fibrous prison, causing the infection to flare up again.

STAGE 1: ACTIVE DISEASE

PATHOLOGY

Bacilli carried in the bloodstream are deposited in bone or synovium. A bone focus (osteomyelitis) consists of an irregular abscess cavity in the metaphysis or epiphysis; sometimes the cavity extends through the epiphyseal plate. Synovial infection (synovitis) may be directly from the bloodstream or follow local extension from a bone focus. The synovial membrane becomes thick, grey and oedematous. The joint is irritated by the adjacent focus but, in this early stage, articular cartilage is undamaged.

From the bone or synovial focus the disease may extend or erupt into the interior of the joint. Once penetration has occurred, spread throughout the joint is rapid. A pannus of tuberculous granulation tissue spreads over the synovial membrane and

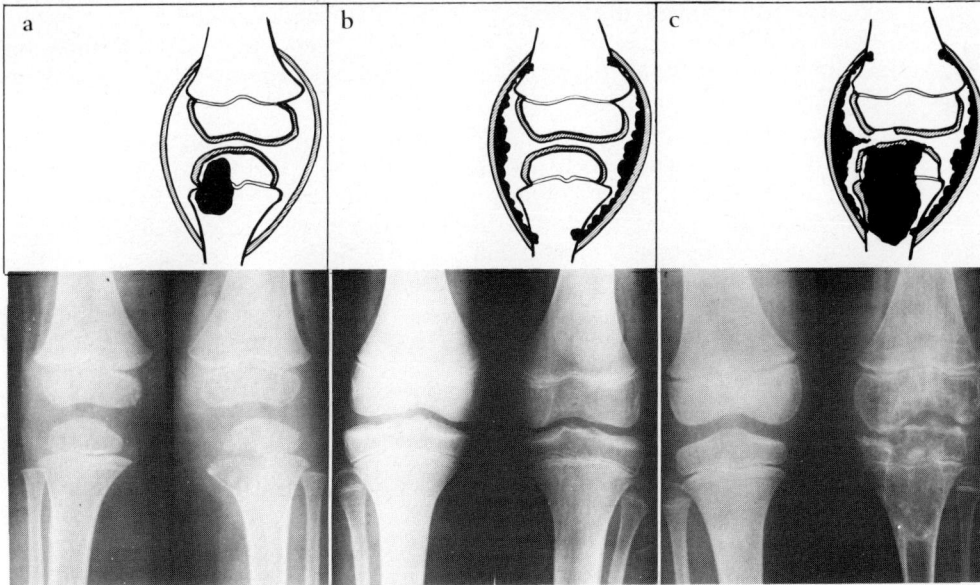

4.4 ACTIVE JOINT TUBERCULOSIS — THE THREE VARIETIES
Osteomyelitis (a) and synovitis (b) are 'early' and can heal by resolution. Arthritis (c) is 'late' and can heal only by fibrosis.

across the articular cartilage. Infection also extends in the subchondral bone, so that the articular cartilage is attacked on both sides. It is extensively eroded, but not completely absorbed, for this requires phagocytes as in a septic arthritis. The term 'tuberculous arthritis' is best reserved for the condition just described, in which articular destruction has taken place. If unchecked, the tuberculous caseation extends into the soft tissues as an abscess; this in turn may track to the surface forming a sinus.

SYMPTOMS

The cardinal symptoms of any joint disease are pain, limp, swelling, stiffness and deformity. All these are minimal in early tuberculosis. Pain is usually slight or absent, sometimes no more than a little ache after activity. Limp is the usual presenting symptom in the lower limb; like pain it is at first slight and increased by activity. Swelling is noticed only in superficial joints; it is not gross but is noticed by the patient because of muscle wasting. Stiffness and deformity, though present, are rarely complained of until articular cartilage has been attacked.

Once there is true arthritis with cartilaginous damage the cardinal symptoms become more severe. Pain is sometimes constant, or may take the form of 'night cries', the explanation of which is that during waking hours the joint is held immobile by muscle spasm and as this relaxes with sleep the damaged joint surfaces rub together, waking the patient. If the patient is able to walk a pronounced limp is present.   Swelling and wasting are marked, stiffness considerable and deformity (especially shortening) usually obvious.

SIGNS

LOOK — The joint is held in a position of deformity and is a little swollen.   Muscle wasting is marked and makes the joint swelling more apparent.

FEEL — The skin feels warm (not hot), and the joint contains some fluid (never a lot). It is sometimes possible to feel thickening of the synovial membrane and its attachments may be tender.   A bone focus may also be slightly tender.   With arthritis the joint feels thick, doughy and diffusely tender.   These signs can, of course, be elicited only in superficial joints.

MOVE — Movement in all directions is limited, though at first by only a few degrees; attempting to force any movement to its extreme is painful and may provoke spasm. The muscles are wasted and the patient may be unable to make them properly taut.   As arthritis supervenes all movements are grossly limited and may be virtually abolished; any attempt at movement is now painful and provokes immediate spasm.

X-RAY — Rarefaction is a constant and well-marked feature; the medulla looks like ground glass and the cortex like a thin line ('pencilling').   Sometimes the epiphyses are enlarged, probably (like the rarefaction) a result of long-continued hyperaemia.

With osteomyelitis, an irregular rarefied area is seen, often extending from metaphysis into epiphysis; with synovitis, bone may be eroded at the synovial attachments.

As long as the disease is in its early stages, the joint space remains normal in width and the joint line clean and unbroken.   Once arthritis has developed the joint space becomes abnormal, being narrowed if the destruction is mainly cartilaginous, or widened if much bone has been eroded; the joint line is irregular.

DIFFERENTIAL DIAGNOSIS

In the early stage tuberculosis must be distinguished from:

TRANSIENT SYNOVITIS — The cause is unknown.   A joint becomes slightly painful and swollen, there is a little warmth and wasting, limitation of extremes of movement and a normal x-ray picture.   In fact the joint is irritable and clinically indistinguishable from early tuberculosis.

Management — (1) The patient is put to bed for 3–6 weeks (if the hip is involved, skin traction is applied).   During this time, other evidence of tuberculosis is sought by x-ray examination of the chest, the Heaf test, and so on.   (2) If irritability has then disappeared, activity is gradually resumed under careful supervision.   (3) If irritability has persisted or returns with activity, biopsy of synovial membrane or of regional lymph nodes is performed.   The specimen is sent for section, culture and guinea-pig inoculation.   Drug treatment is started at once. (We used to 'wait and see' if a joint was tuberculous, hence it was called an 'observation' knee or hip; now we 'look and see'.)

CHRONIC SYNOVITIS — Occasionally a chronic synovitis presents with warmth, wasting, irritability and generalized rarefaction.   It is clinically indistinguishable from tuberculosis but a positive Rose–Waaler test or biopsy shows it to be rheumatoid in nature; and years later other joints may become involved.   It is therefore a monarticular variety of what is usually a polyarthritis.

Once a true arthritis is present diagnosis is usually easy, but the following conditions should be considered.

ACUTE ARTHRITIS — An arthritis due to pyogenic organisms is usually a dramatic condition.   The onset is rapid and the patient ill with a high swinging fever.   There is leucocytosis and a positive blood culture.

SUBACUTE ARTHRITIS — Occasionally, diseases such as amoebic dysentery, brucellosis or smallpox are complicated by arthritis. The history, clinical features and pathological investigations usually enable a diagnosis to be made.

HAEMORRHAGIC ARTHRITIS — The physical signs of blood in a joint may resemble those of tuberculous arthritis. If the bleeding has followed a single recent injury the history and absence of wasting are diagnostic. Following repeated bleeding, as in haemophilia, the clinical resemblance to tuberculosis is closer, but there is also a history of bleeding elsewhere.

TREATMENT

As long as a tuberculous joint remains active there are (in addition to general treatment) three principles governing local treatment:

REST — By this is meant local rest as distinct from recumbency. H. O. Thomas long ago said that the rest must be prolonged, uninterrupted, rigid and enforced. For the knee, his splint is still the best. A hip is most effectively rested on a double abduction frame, though for adults this is very cumbersome and often dispensed with. The shoulder may be rested in an abduction frame and the elbow in a plaster gutter, but for both these joints a simple sling is often used.

TRACTION — This overcomes spasm, prevents collapse of soft bone, and keeps inflamed surfaces apart. Skin traction is used for the knee, skin or skeletal traction for the hip, and gravity plus a sling for the upper limbs.

CLEARANCE OPERATIONS — Operations in active tuberculosis are not designed to excise all the locally diseased tissue; this is neither possible nor safe. The object is to evacuate dead material, thereby facilitating the drug attack and promoting more rapid healing. Once antibiotics and rest have been in progress for a few weeks, operation may be considered. A tuberculous osteomyelitis in an accessible site is best evacuated and the wound sutured; this may prevent it from bursting into the joint. Even with arthritis, excision of diseased synovium and gentle removal of tuberculosis débris and sequestra is often worth while if the disease is not settling rapidly; not only is healing more rapid but a useful range of movement may result.

LOCAL COMPLICATIONS

ABSCESS — An abscess forms when the bone or joint is perforated. Caseous material, often in large quantities, exudes along the soft-tissue planes. The abscess walls are thick and its contents creamy. A fluctuant swelling forms which, unlike a pyogenic abscess, is not hot (hence the term 'cold abscess').

The usual treatment of an abscess is aspiration, repeated when necessary. After a while the contents become too thick to flow through a needle and it is then best, under antibiotic cover, to incise the abscess, evacuate its contents and suture the skin.

SINUS — When an abscess becomes subcutaneous it is liable to perforate the skin and give rise to a sinus; often this is an index of poor resistance. The sinus track communicates with the joint and so may permit secondary infection.

In treatment, streptomycin instilled into the sinus is often successful. Given in this way, the drug is still absorbed, so care must be taken to avoid the total dosage being excessive.

STAGE 2: HEALING PHASE

PATHOLOGY

If the disease is arrested before articular cartilage has been damaged, healing by resolution may occur. Once there has been a true arthritis, however, although healing may occur, restoration to normal is impossible.   Tuberculous granulation tissue is slowly converted to fibrous tissue in which the bacilli are imprisoned. Opposing joint surfaces stick together giving a fibrous ankylosis which may be long (as in the hip or elbow) or short (as in the knee).   Bony ankylosis almost never occurs unless there has been secondary infection.

CLINICAL FEATURES

The patient is fit and the joint is no longer painful.   The local signs are as follows:

LOOK — The joint is not swollen, though some wasting is still present.   Any sinus will have dried up.

FEEL — The skin is no longer warm, and the joint no longer thick or tender.

MOVE — If early disease has healed by resolution movement slowly returns; if there has been articular destruction, stiffness remains.

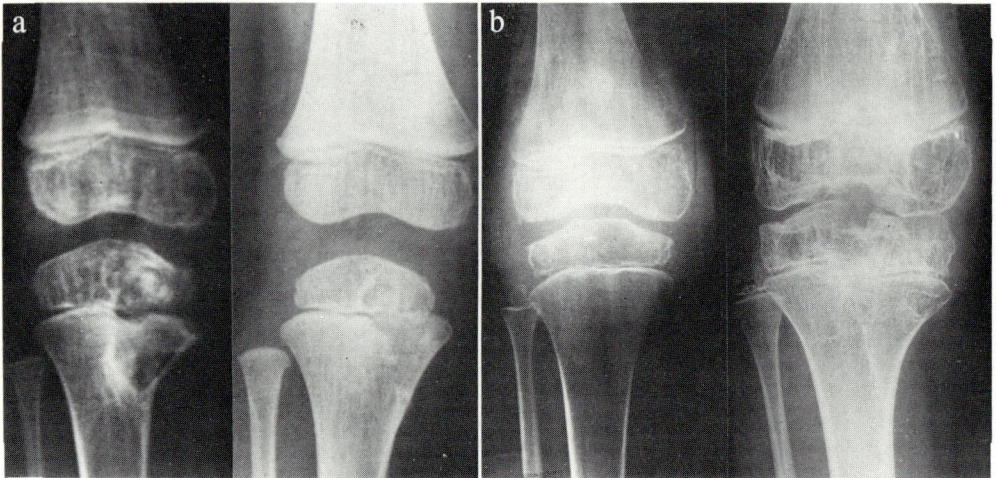

4.5   HEALING TUBERCULOSIS
(a) Osteomyelitis, and the same knee after healing — the joint has not been involved and recalcification has occurred; (b) synovitis in this case has progressed to arthritis.

X-RAY — The bones recalcify, but some permanent alteration of bone architecture nearly always remains.   An arthritis, even though recalcified, has a permanently altered joint space and an irregular joint line.

TREATMENT

As the disease heals, general treatment is gradually discontinued.   Local treatment depends upon whether the disease was arrested early or only arrested after it had progressed to a true arthritis.

IF ARRESTED EARLY — The aim is to restore movement, therefore splints are removed. The joint is, however, protected from stress, which is only gradually allowed.

Thus in the lower limb, the patient first lies in bed without splints but still on traction. The traction is then released for increasing periods and finally removed altogether.   He then gets up but avoids taking weight (using a patten and crutches for the hip and a weight-relieving caliper for the knee).   After a time he is allowed to take weight for gradually increasing periods until he is walking about normally.

During all this time he is continually observed.   If symptoms or signs increase, he goes back a stage; if there is steady progress he goes forward (Thomas' test of recovery). At no time is movement forced; it is only permitted to return of its own accord.

In the upper limb treatment is much simpler, for the splint or sling is merely dispensed with for increasing periods of time while the patient uses his arm.

IF ARRESTED LATE — The aim, once articular cartilage has been extensively destroyed, is to obtain the shortest possible fibrous ankylosis in the optimum position.   Movement is therefore prevented but stress is permitted so that the joint surfaces impinge more closely together.

In the lower limb traction is taken off and a caliper or plaster applied with the joint in the optimum position.   Weight bearing is started.   After some months a removable splint (of polythene, leather or metal) may be used and is taken off for bath or bed. Some form of splint may be needed permanently or until the joint is arthrodesed.

In the upper limb a somewhat longer fibrous ankylosis may be permitted and indeed is almost inevitable, because gravity exerts a constant traction force.   At the shoulder, even after arthritis, splintage is gradually discarded; a sling is used for a time and gradually left off.   If there is pain the joint is arthrodesed.   At the elbow, a moulded leather or polythene splint may be used permanently, but often a sling is sufficient and sometimes even this may be dispensed with.

STAGE 3: AFTERMATH

PATHOLOGY

A joint which has suffered a true arthritis heals by fibrosis (unless there has been secondary infection).   A fibrous joint is 'unsound' because (a) the fibrous tissue shrinks with time, giving increasing deformity; and (b) it may tear with stress, liberating bacilli and provoking a flare.

CLINICAL FEATURES

There is stiffness and, in the lower limb, a limp.   Pain may be felt at times, especially after the joint has been subjected to stress.   Deformity is usually present and may slowly increase with time.

LOOK — Scars from old sinuses are common.   The limb may be held in a deformed position, it may be short and is always thin.

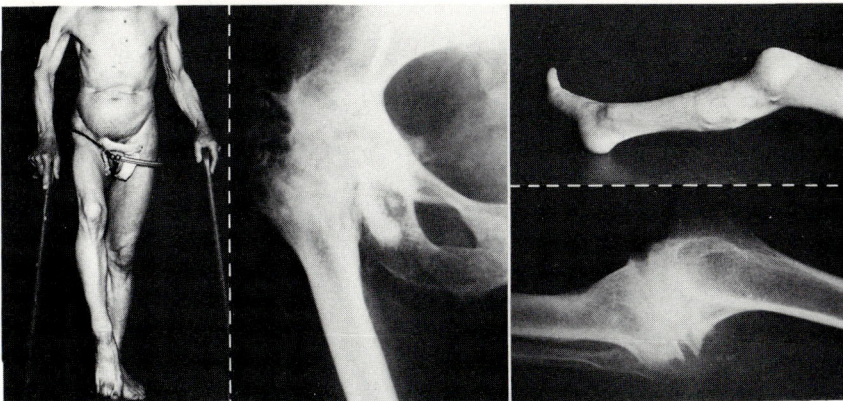

4.6   THE AFTERMATH OF TUBERCULOUS ARTHRITIS
Joint destruction and deformity: flexion and adduction at the hip; flexion, lateral rotation and backward subluxation (triple deformity) at the knee.

Deformity is due partly to bone destruction and partly to prolonged muscle spasm; the joint is pulled into characteristic positions.

FEEL — There is no warmth or tenderness unless there has been a recent flare.

MOVE — Movement is always considerably limited.   At the knee a short fibrous ankylosis often occurs so that only a few degrees of movement are present.   Elsewhere there may be up to half the normal range.

X-RAY — The bone is well calcified but its architecture is often faulty.   The joint space may scarcely be visible and the joint line is grossly irregular.   Abscesses in the vicinity of the joint may be calcified.

DIFFERENTIAL DIAGNOSIS

The aftermath of an old tuberculous joint is usually easy to diagnose.   There are, however, three other fairly common causes of a stiff, deformed or painful joint of long standing.

OLD SUPPURATIVE ARTHRITIS — The history is of a more acute illness and there is often bony ankylosis.

RHEUMATOID ARTHRITIS — Many joints are affected, commonly small joints, particularly in the hands.

OSTEOARTHRITIS — There are no scars, little wasting and the x-ray appearance is characteristic (page 48).

TREATMENT

In the absence of a flare, general treatment is not required; the only local treatment needed may be a removable splint and, in the lower limb, a raised shoe.

Operations — For deformity, especially at the hip, an osteotomy is valuable.

For unsoundness at any joint arthrodesis is the best treatment.   An extra-articular arthrodesis is possible at the hip or shoulder, but elsewhere it must be intra-articular. For deformity plus unsoundness at the hip it is convenient to combine extra-articular arthrodesis by means of an ischio-femoral graft with an osteotomy (Brittain's operation).

COMPLICATIONS

The most important complication of an old tuberculous arthritis is a flare.   This is a local reactivation of the disease, though it may be accompanied by a lighting-up of the general illness too.   A flare may occur if the patient's resistance drops, or if trauma liberates bacilli from their fibrous prison.   That is why a fibrous joint is an unsafe joint.

If an old tuberculous joint suffers trauma it is probably wise not to await a flare, but to put the joint at rest immediately and to institute drug treatment.   If a flare has actually occurred these measures are certainly necessary and it is best, once active inflammation subsides, to proceed with arthrodesis.

EXTRA-ARTICULAR TUBERCULOSIS

Tuberculosis of bone or synovium may, as already described, irritate a joint, or erupt into and infect it.   Tuberculosis may also, however, involve bone without affecting a joint and may attack the synovial lining of tendon sheaths or bursae.

TUBERCULOUS OSTEOMYELITIS

Within the bone an irregular area of destruction occurs and may be seen on x-ray. The infection being chronic is often not painful and may remain clinically silent until one of the following occurs.

SOFT BONE COLLAPSES — This occurs particularly in the spine where a diseased vertebral body collapses, infecting the one below and squashing caseous material into the soft tissues as an abscess (page 200).

A SWELLING APPEARS — In tuberculosis of flat bones (rib or skull) an abscess is the usual presenting feature; in tuberculous dactylitis a localized swelling or a sinus is usual (page 177).

SYNOVIAL TUBERCULOSIS

Infected synovium becomes thick, oedematous and villous. Excess fluid may be produced, giving a painless swelling and, where there is friction, particles of fibrin are moulded to resemble melon seeds. Synovial infection may affect tendon sheaths or bursae.

TENOSYNOVITIS — The commonest site for tenosynovitis is in front of the wrist (*see* Compound Palmar Ganglion, page 171), but the fingers or ankle region are sometimes affected. A painless swelling appears insidiously; it is fluctuant and often there is weakness and muscle wasting. Instillation of streptomycin is sometimes successful, or excision of the sheath may be necessary.

BURSITIS — The least rare sites for bursitis are the subdeltoid and gluteal bursae. A painless, cold, fluctuant swelling slowly develops, wasting is slight and the underlying joint normal. Treatment is by excision under drug cover.

Suggestions for further reading

Hodgson, A. R., Wong, W. and Yau, A. (1969). ' X-ray Appearances of Tuberculosis of the Spine. Springfield, Illinois; Charles C. Thomas

Robins, R. H. C. (1967). ' Tuberculosis of the Wrist and Hand.' *Br. J. Surg.* **54**, 211

Seddon, H. J. (1976). ' The Choice of Treatment in Pott's Disease.' *J. Bone Jt Surg.* **58B**, 395

Somerville, E. W., and Wilkinson, M. C. (1965). *Girdlestone's Tuberculosis of Bone and Joint.* 3rd Edn. London; Oxford University Press

Wilkinson, M. C. (1969). 'Tuberculosis of the Spine Treated by Chemotherapy and Operative Debridement.' *J. Bone Jt Surg.* **51A**, 1331

— (1969). 'Tuberculosis of the Hip and Knee Treated by Chemotherapy, Synovectomy and Debridement.' *J. Bone Jt Surg.* **51A**, 1343

CHAPTER 5

OSTEOARTHRITIS AND OSTEOCHONDRITIS

OSTEOARTHRITIS

Osteoarthritis* is a degenerative process involving the whole joint, but beginning in the articular cartilage. It takes years for osteoarthritis to become manifest, so that it is commoner after middle life. Biochemical changes in joints do occur with age, but the ageing process alone does not cause osteoarthritis. Something more needs to happen to articular cartilage before it degenerates; the essential feature is a discrepancy between the strength of the cartilage and the force to which it is subjected.

Articular cartilage distributes the stress passing across a joint; literally it spreads the load. If the load is too great cartilage gives way; but even with normal loads cartilage gives way if it has been weakened by damage or disease, or if it is unsupported by normal bone (Solomon, 1976).

CAUSES

From the above it is clear that there are two groups of causes: excessive load and defective cartilage. In an affected joint the causal factor may be difficult to find, but is worth seeking; it is reasonable to regard all osteoarthritis as secondary to a cause which diligence will discover. (Even so-called primary generalized osteoarthritis is probably secondary — *see* page 51).

EXCESSIVE LOAD — The total force crossing a joint may be excessive, or applied over too small an area, or both factors may be combined.

(1) *Total force too great* — It is not generally realized how great are the forces to which articular cartilage is subjected. Thus, in a normal hip the lever system is such that with each step a force of 4 to 6 times the body weight is transmitted; if the lever system is faulty, as in coxa valga, the force is greater still. Similarly with genu varum the force increases very considerably with each centimetre that the knee deviates from the centre of gravity of the body. Objects being carried (including surplus fat) obviously increase these forces still further.

(2) *Area too small* — With joint deformity the area available for load transmission is usually reduced. Obvious examples are congenital hip subluxation (in which part of the head is lateral to the acetabulum), and an old slipped upper femoral epiphysis.

(3) *Both factors combined* — In genu varum, congenital hip subluxation, and similar disorders, not only is the area for load transmission too small, but the actual force also is increased because of the faulty lever system.

DEFECTIVE CARTILAGE — The articular cartilage may be injured, affected by disease, or deprived of support by normal bone.

(1) *Damaged cartilage* — Articular cartilage may be damaged by a single major injury such as an osteochondral fracture. Repeated minor injury is equally damaging and

---

*There is still no universally acceptable alternative to this word, so it persists in spite of the misleading implication that the disease is inflammatory. The word 'osteoarthrosis' is in vogue, but is etymologically unjustified. The initials 'O.A.' could represent either term — they also stand for 'old age'.

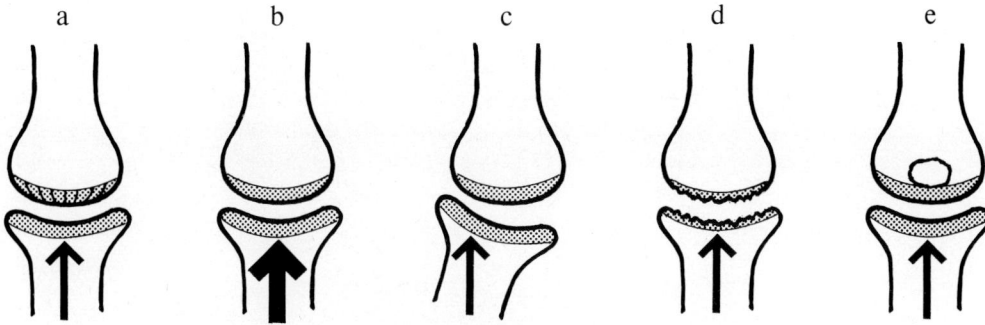

5.1 CAUSAL FACTORS IN OSTEOARTHRITIS
(a) In the normal joint cartilage distributes pressure over a wide area; (b) the load may be excessive or (c) applied over too small an area. (d) The cartilage may be weakened (by damage or disease), or (e) unsupported because of underlying bone necrosis.

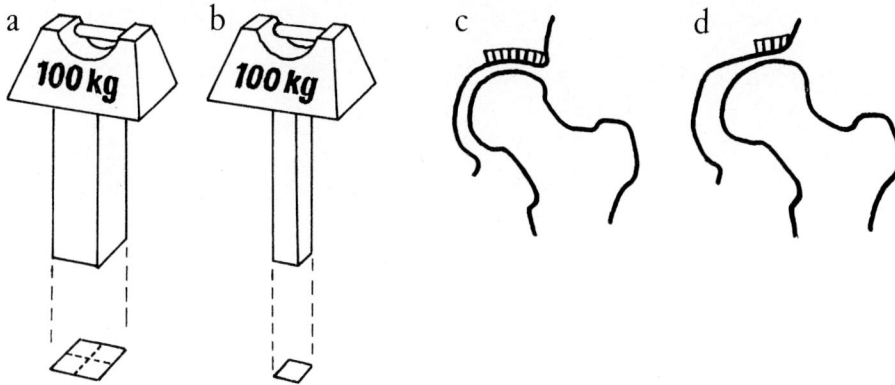

5.2 OSTEOARTHRITIS CAUSES
The area for load transmission must not be too small. (a) Assume the column is 1 cm square: the load is 100 kg/cm². (b) With a column 0·5 cm square the area is 0·25 cm², the load 400 kg/cm². (c) A normal hip; with subluxation (d) the line is half as long, so the load/cm² is 4 times as great.

occurs in a wide variety of conditions such as: recurrent subluxation of the patella; certain occupations or recreations (for example at the elbow with javelin throwing); undue joint laxity (congenital, following ligament injury, or when ligaments and capsule are insensitive to pain or position); and the repeated abrasive action of loose bodies or a torn meniscus.

In haemophilia (*see* page 53) repeated bleeding leads to synovitis; hydrolytic enzymes are liberated causing an inflammatory response which damages cartilage; further damage results from the accumulation of iron within individual cells. A similar effect may account for the joint degeneration in haemochromatosis.

(2) *Diseased cartilage* — The cartilage may be weakened by inflammatory or metabolic disorders.

Inflammatory disorders. Rheumatoid arthritis is the commonest inflammatory cause of weakened articular cartilage (*see* page 25), but unrecognized low-grade inflammation is probably not uncommon and the associated bone softening might explain the appearance in protrusio acetabulae (Otto pelvis). Much less frequent causes are septic and tuberculous arthritis.

5.3 OSTEOARTHRITIS
CAUSES
Excessive load. (a) Congenital hip subluxation; (b) varus knee. In both the load is excessive because the lever system is faulty and the load distributed over too small an area.

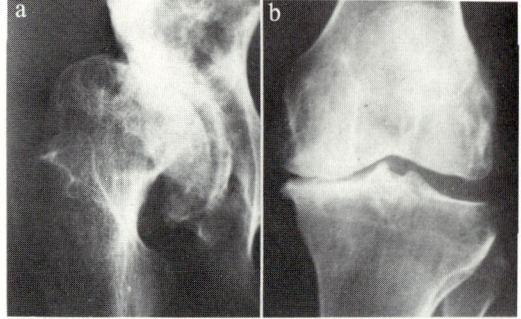

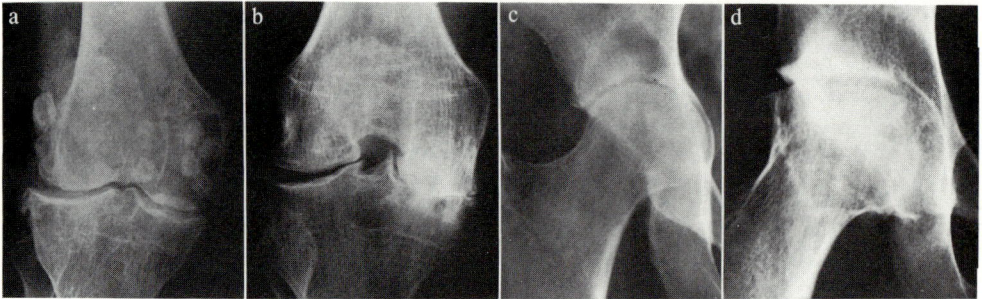

5.4 OSTEOARTHRITIS CAUSES
Defective cartilage. The cartilage may be damaged by (a) loose bodies, or (b) bleeding in haemophilia. It may be diseased as in (c) rheumatoid arthritis, or unsupported as in (d) avascular necrosis.

Metabolic disorders. Two metabolic disorders which weaken articular cartilage (gout and pseudo-gout) are described on pages 22 and 23. A much rarer example is *alkaptonuria* in which homogentisic acid is deposited in the urine which turns black on standing, and sometimes in cartilage which also looks black (hence the term ochronotic arthropathy); x-rays show calcified intervertebral discs and menisci.

(3) *Unsupported cartilage* — If subchondral bone is deprived of its blood supply it becomes necrotic (avascular necrosis). Obvious examples are caisson disease, hip fractures and dislocations.

'Idiopathic' avascular necrosis is the term applied to a less obvious but no less important group. Originally it was recognized as occurring chiefly in alcoholic middle-aged men, in whom high serum lipids and altered blood coagulability led to arterial infarcts. Many other conditions also predispose to arterial infarction and therefore to avascular necrosis; they include hyperuricaemia and sickle-cell anaemia. Of special importance is the high dose of steroids used for immuno-suppression after renal transplant, following which severe degenerative changes may develop rapidly.

PATHOLOGY

ARTICULAR CARTILAGE AND BONE — The earliest changes found in the cartilage are an increase in its water content and a decrease in the amount of proteoglycan. The cartilage looks irregular and pitted, and may feel soft. Microscopically it undergoes fibrillation and minute cartilage flakes ('detritus') are shed into the joint. This shedding process means that cartilage is being rubbed away; such wear is of course maximal where the load is greatest (the stress area) and here the cartilage becomes thin.

At non-stress areas cartilage is not rubbed away or thinned; nevertheless it is unhealthy, because it is undernourished. (Articular cartilage is nourished by imbibition of synovial fluid and of transudates from subchondral vessels, a process facilitated by intermittent compression; this pumping action is lacking at non-stress areas).

Trueta showed that the response to cartilage degeneration is often seen first in the non-stress area. Here the subchondral vessels hypertrophy, and invade the cartilage which calcifies and later ossifies (hence the osteophytes). The hyperaemia spreads into the bone beneath the stress area, but here pressure prevents the vessels from penetrating into the cartilage; the cartilage continues to be rubbed away and the exposed unprotected bone becomes dense and eburnated. Fatigue fractures occur in the subchondral trabeculae and cysts develop where pressure is greatest (Freeman 1972).

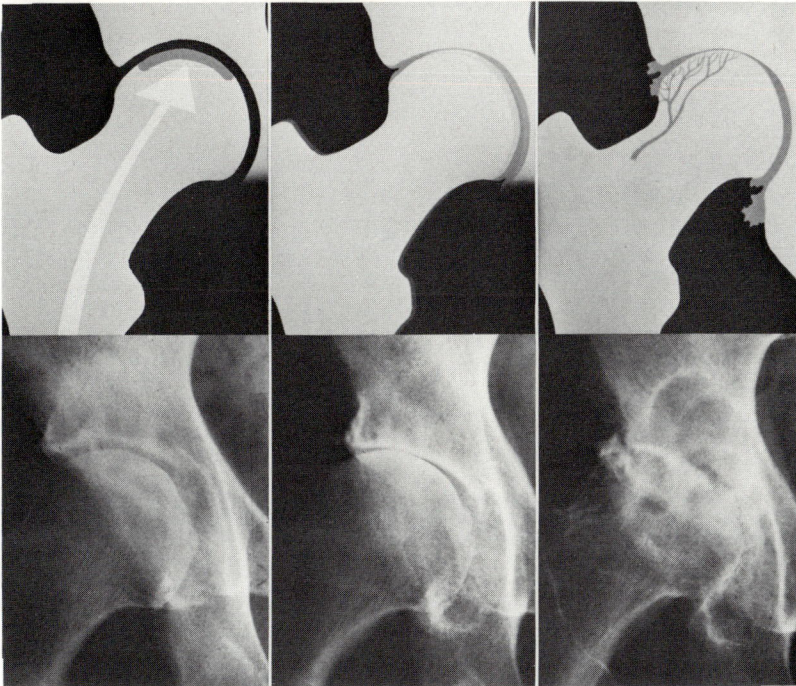

5.5 PATHOLOGY OF OSTEOARTHRITIS
Where stress is taken the cartilage is abraded and the joint space becomes narrower. The vascular reaction is followed by osteophyte formation. Cysts form at high spots of pressure.

SYNOVIAL MEMBRANE AND CAPSULE — The cartilaginous detritus is deposited on the synovial lining which first hypertrophies; flakes of cartilage then penetrate to the subsynovial layer and there may induce fibrosis. The fibrosis extends into the capsule which becomes thickened and inelastic; and, as the fibrous tissue matures, it shrinks, thus limiting movement.

The restriction of movement consequent upon fibrosis is a cardinal feature. At the hip, for example, full extension is required for normal walking; even slight restriction manifests itself early, for the capsule is abundantly supplied with pain fibres; consequently symptoms appear early. By contrast, at the elbow extremes of movement are rarely used; slight capsular shrinkage is unnoticed by the patient and he is not constantly injuring the capsule by attempts to stretch it. Weight-bearing certainly aggravates osteoarthritis. but the need to reach the extremes of range in everyday use is probably more important in determining which joints present with symptoms. Thus the ankle is rarely a clinical problem, but the carpo-metacarpal joint of the thumb often is.

The spine is not often affected by osteoarthritis, for again extremes of range are not constantly required. Lipping of the vertebrae (spondylosis) as a result of disc degeneration is common, but not degeneration of the intervertebral joints themselves.

5.6 PATHOLOGY OF OSTEOARTHRITIS

Capsular fibrosis soon limits extremes of movement: at the elbow the extreme position is rarely needed — symptoms are late and slight; at the hip the extreme position is needed — symptoms are early and severe.

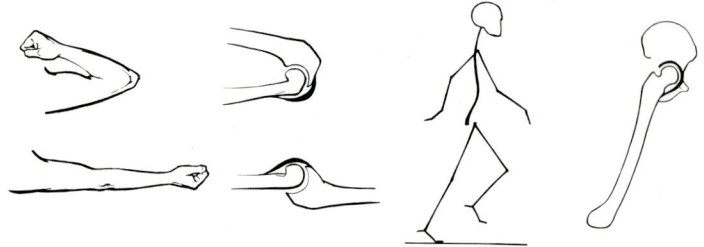

SYMPTOMS

PAIN — This is the leading symptom. In early osteoarthritis pain occurs after a night's rest and then wears off; later, after use, the joint aches again. As the disease progresses, pain becomes more severe and more constant, sometimes disturbing sleep. Three distinct varieties of pain have been described (Helal, 1965): capsular (on forcing extremes), muscular (following exertion), and venous (after standing, and at night).

STIFFNESS — This too is an important symptom. At first it is noticed only after the joint has been still for some time. Later it is constant and gradually increases.

DEFORMITY — Capsule shrinkage and muscle imbalance produce deformity. At the hip the patient may notice increasing shortness of the leg because of flexion and adduction deformity.

LIMP — This is common and due to pain or deformity.

GIVING WAY — This sometimes occurs, possibly because a synovial fringe has been nipped, or occasionally because an osteophyte has broken off to form a loose body.

SWELLING — Swelling is only noticeable at superficial joints such as the knee.

SIGNS

The patient is fit. One joint only is affected; occasionally two or even three may be involved, but this is not a true polyarticular disease like rheumatoid arthritis. The local signs in an affected joint are as follows:

LOOK — There are no scars and only slight wasting. Swelling may be due to fluid (in the knee) or to osteophytes (at the metatarso-phalangeal joint of the hallux). Deformity may be obvious—the hip may be held flexed, adducted and externally rotated.

FEEL — There is no warmth. In superficial joints localized tenderness is common, and fluid or osteophytes may be felt.

MOVE — Movement is always restricted, but is painless within the permitted range. The restriction is characteristically asymmetrical; some movements much more than others. Thus, at the hip, extension, abduction and internal rotation are far more limited than their opposites. Crepitus is common.

X-RAY — Usually the joint space is diminished asymmetrically (or eccentrically) — i.e. only at the pressure area; but if the underlying cause is a disease such as rheumatoid arthritis, the joint space is equally diminished in all areas. Beneath the pressure area

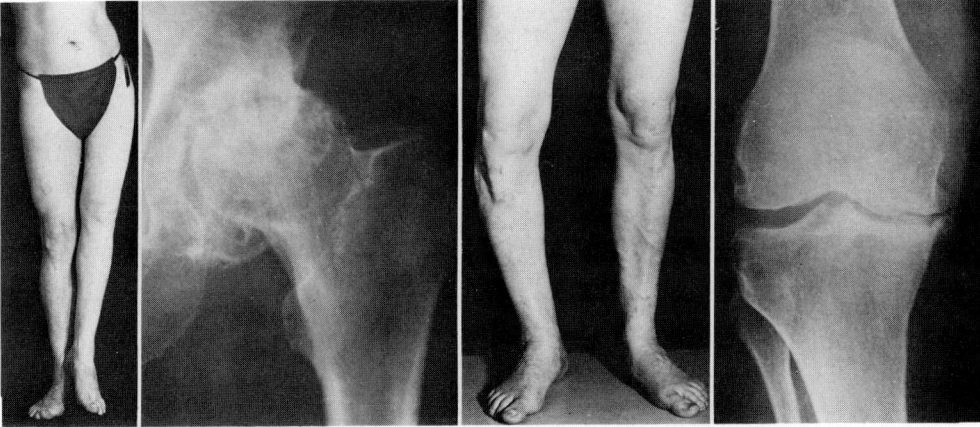

5.7 OSTEOARTHRITIS
Deformity and diminished joint space at the hip and the knee.

the bone becomes sclerosed and cysts sometimes develop. At the non-pressure areas there may be lipping and osteophytes.

TREATMENT

The theoretical list of possibilities includes:

Analgesics — Aspirin and codeine are invaluable; phenylbutazone occasionally helps where these have failed.

Warmth — A hot-water bottle, liniments, massage and radiant heat are all methods of applying superficial warmth; short-wave diathermy penetrates more deeply.

Diet — Obesity increases the load on the cartilage and may need treatment.

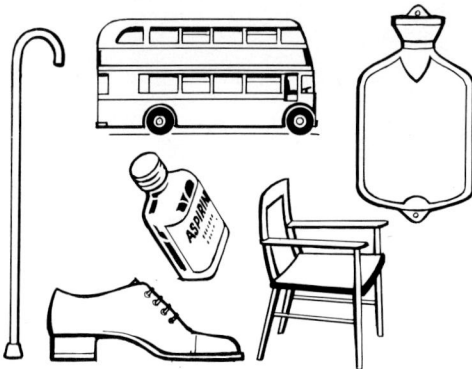

5.8 CONSERVATIVE
TREATMENT
Simple measures to relieve pain in osteoarthritis of the hip: analgesics, warmth, a raised heel and a stick; ' don't stand when you can sit, don't walk when you can ride '.

Modified activity — The patient may need to restrict his activities; exercise within the limits of pain, however, should be encouraged. At the hip a walking stick greatly reduces stress and (especially combined with a raised heel) permits walking without forcing hip extension.

Splintage — Rest may comfort a painful joint, but, unless splintage is intermittent or short-lasting, stiffness may increase.

Arthrodesis — This is the only certain way to abolish pain permanently; but the penalty of total stiffness is to increase the stresses on other joints.

Arthroplasty — Although theoretically more desirable, arthroplasty is less certain to relieve pain. The joint capsule (with its pain fibres) needs to be removed, or at least to be taken off stretch.

Osteotomy — Pain is often relieved because stress is now distributed more widely and because the capsule is no longer tight in positions of habitual use. Occasionally the joint undergoes remarkable ' biological regeneration '; again this may be due to better distribution of pressure, but the relief of venous congestion in the subchondral sinusoids may be a factor (Helal).

To choose from this list, the main question is: how bad is the pain? If the pain is mild treatment is conservative; if severe, it is surgical. Such over-simplification implies that we can measure pain: we cannot, but we can assess it by asking the patient how much it interferes with his work, hobbies and sleep. When no clear-cut decision is possible it is sometimes worth while trying to increase joint range by manipulating the joint under anaesthesia; hydrocortisone is injected to minimize the otherwise inevitable fibrosis.

5.9 OPERATIVE TREAT-
MENT
The three basic operations:
(a) arthrodesis, (b) arthroplasty and (c) osteotomy:

at the hip

at the knee.

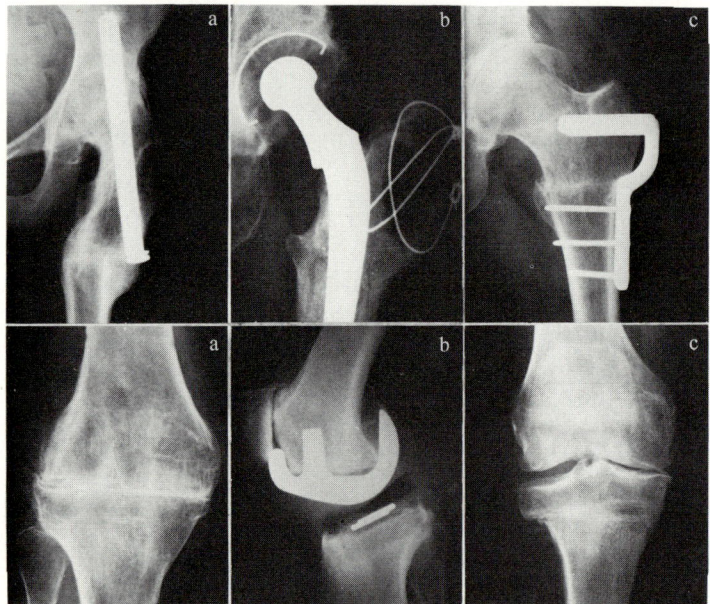

REGIONAL SURVEY OF OSTEOARTHRITIC JOINTS

Acromio-clavicular joint — Osteoarthritis is clinically rare, though often seen on x-ray. There is pain, tenderness and limitation of shoulder movement, especially adduction. Treatment is conservative; only very rarely is the lateral end of the clavicle excised.

Gleno-humeral joint (*see* page 155) — Osteoarthritis of the shoulder is much rarer than is commonly supposed, but cuff lesions are often diagnosed incorrectly as osteoarthritis.

Elbow (*see* page 164) — Osteoarthritis may follow severe injuries or loose bodies. Although limitation of movement occurs early, the patient rarely complains of it. For pain, the treatment is physiotherapy and a removable splint. Operation, other than for removal of loose bodies, is rarely needed, but joint replacement and arthrodesis are possibilities. An ulnar palsy is not uncommon and the nerve may need to be transposed.

Wrist (*see* page 170). — Osteoarthritis of the radio-carpal joint usually follows injury. A polythene splint with the wrist slightly dorsiflexed is usually sufficient treatment. Where osteoarthritis is associated with non-union of the scaphoid excision of the radial styloid process is useful. Only rarely is arthrodesis necessary.

Thumb (*see* page 191) — The carpo-metacarpal joint is a common site for osteoarthritis, but surgery is not often necessary.   Manipulation under anaesthesia combined with hydrocortisone injection is often valuable.   Arthrodesis gives excellent results but the wrist must be kept in plaster for 3 months after operation.   Excision arthroplasty allows the patient to return to work in 2–4 weeks and also gives very good results, but complete relief from pain is less certain than with arthrodesis.

Fingers — Heberden's nodes are associated with osteoarthritis of the terminal finger joints. Post-menopausal women are chiefly affected.   This common condition is sometimes called primary generalized osteoarthritis, but it is strongly familial and clearly genetic factors are involved.   Any pain soon disappears, but the ugly lumpiness is permanent.

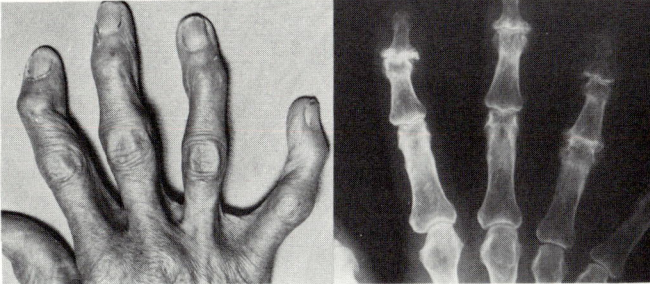

5.10 PRIMARY GENERA-
LIZED OSTEOARTHRITIS
The terminal interphalan-
geal joints are affected.

Cervical spine (*see* page 194) — Osteoarthritis of the facet joints usually accompanies disc degeneration and the disease is then called spondylosis.   Neck movements are limited and pain radiates from the neck to one or both upper limbs.   Physiotherapy, a collar, or occasionally manipulation (without anaesthetic) are useful.

5.11 EXAMPLES OF OSTEO-
ARTHRITIS AT OTHER SITES
(a) Elbow, at which symptoms are rare; (b) carpometacarpal thumb joint at which they are common.

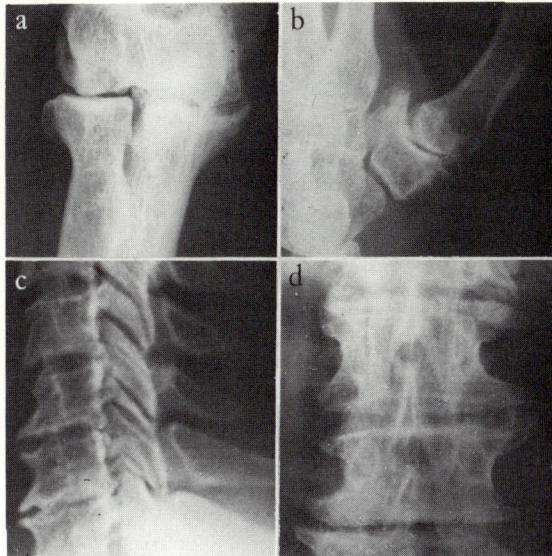

(c) and (d) Cervical and lumbar spondylosis are really the results of disc degeneration, but may be associated with osteoarthritis of the facet joints.

Lumbar spine (*see* page 221) — Osteoarthritis of the facet joints may follow spinal deformities, or be associated with degeneration of discs (spondylosis).   Physiotherapy and a corset are the usual methods of treatment, rarely spinal fusion is used.

Hip (*see* page 252) — Osteoarthritis of the hip is a common and important clinical problem. There is pain, often referred to the knee, stiffness and deformity.   In conservative treatment a raised heel and a walking stick are especially useful.   Arthroplasty (especially joint replacement) is often indicated, osteotomy less often and arthrodesis only rarely.

Knee (*see* page 283) — Osteoarthritis affects the patello-femoral section of the knee much more often than the femoro-tibial.   At the patello-femoral section, it is often a sequel to chondromalacia patellae; if conservative measures (physiotherapy, a removable splint, manipulation and injections) fail, the patella may be excised, or the tibial tubercle advanced.

Osteoarthritis of the femoro-tibial section may be treated by tibial osteotomy or by arthrodesis.   Arthroplasty is useful in bilateral disease.

Ankle (*see* page 293) — Although the ankle is a weight-bearing joint, extremes of movement are rarely required and osteoarthritis is therefore uncommon.   It may follow severe injury or a loose body.   If conservative measures fail, arthrodesis is the best operation.

Hallux (*see* page 305) — Osteoarthritis of the metatarso-phalangeal joint (hallux rigidus) is common.   A rockered sole usually relieves the pain.   The commonest operation is arthroplasty in which the metatarsal head or the proximal portion of the phalanx is excised.   The joint is sometimes arthrodesed.

NEUROPATHIC JOINTS (CHARCOT'S DISEASE)

CAUSE AND PATHOLOGY

A neuropathic joint is one in which the appreciation of pain and position sense from the capsule is lost.   Consequently there is no reflex safeguard against injuries and a rapid progressive degeneration occurs.   In some cases the changes appear to begin suddenly and to be initiated by a fracture into the joint.

The underlying neurological conditions include tabes, syringomyelia, myelomeningocele and peripheral neuritis, usually diabetic.   Leprosy and congenital indifference to pain are other possibilities.   A Charcot-like neuropathy has also been reported following frequently-repeated hydrocortisone injections into rheumatoid joints.

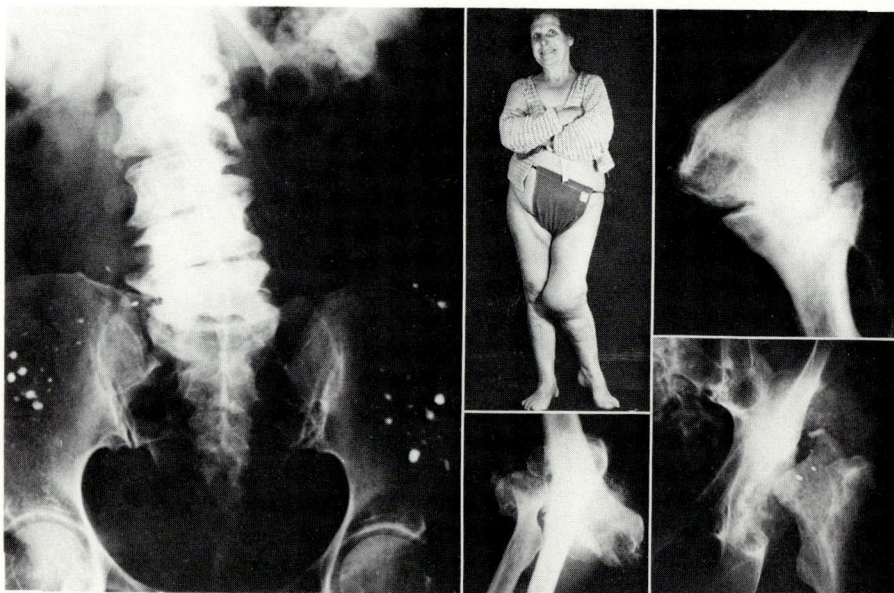

5.12   CHARCOT'S DISEASE
The vertebrae are distorted and dense, the buttocks show the radio-opaque remains of former injections: the knee, elbow and hip joints look grotesque.   Moral: ' If it's bizarre, do a W.R.'.   Note also the happy smile (though not all Charcot joints are tabetic, nor are they always painless).

GENERAL SYMPTOMS AND SIGNS

In tabes, adults over 45 are usually affected.   They often complain of lightning pains.   The pupils may be Argyll Robertson in type; knee and ankle jerks are often lost, and there is no pain on squeezing the tendo achillis.

In syringomyelia the condition often dates from early adult life.   Characteristically, there is dissociated sensation (loss of pain and temperature sense, but not of touch).   Scoliosis is common.

LOCAL SYMPTOMS AND SIGNS

The patient complains of weakness, instability, swelling and deformity of the affected joint.   The symptoms may progress surprisingly rapidly.   The appearance of an established Charcot's joint suggests that movement would be agonizing, and yet it is painless.   This paradox is diagnostic.

LOOK — Swelling is considerable and deformity gross.   The joint may be subluxed or even dislocated.

FEEL — There is no warmth or tenderness.   Fluid is greatly increased and bits of bone can be felt everywhere.

MOVE — Often the joint is flail, normal movements being increased and abnormal movements present.   These movements are painless.

X-RAY — The joint is subluxed or dislocated, gross bone erosion is obvious and there are irregular calcified masses in the capsule.

TREATMENT

The underlying condition may need treatment, but the affected joints cannot recover.   They should, if possible, be stabilized by external splintage (for instance, by a caliper).   Operation is not advised.

HAEMOPHILIA

Haemophilia is the commonest of a group of bleeding disorders due to genetically determined faults in the synthesis of certain clotting factors.   It is a recessive X-linked disorder due to a defect of factor 8 and affects some 3000 patients in Britain.   Patients with more than 40 per cent of the average value react normally to haemorrhage; levels of 20–40 per cent may cause trouble if the patient suffers prolonged bleeding at operation or after injury, patients with 5–20 per cent bleed excessively with less severe trauma, and below 5 per cent spontaneous bleeding may occur.   Less common is Christmas disease, due to a defect of factor 9.   Patients with either disease may present with any of the following orthopaedic problems.

ACUTE BLEEDING INTO A JOINT OR MUSCLE — With trivial injury a joint (usually a large joint) may rapidly fill with blood.   Pain, slight warmth, boggy swelling, tenderness and limited movement are the outstanding features.   The resemblance to a low grade inflammatory joint is striking, but the history is diagnostic.   The appropriate factor (' cryoprecipitate ' merely refers to a method of manufacture) should be given without delay; early factor replacement is the only method of controlling a bleed — external pressure is useless and has caused loss of a limb.   If the factor is not available, plasma (which must be very fresh) is given.   Aspiration is avoided unless distension is severe.   A removable splint is wise.

Acute bleeding into muscles (especially the forearm, calf or thigh) is less common.   A painful swelling appears with deformity of the appropriate joint.   Occasional complications are acute Volkmann's ischaemia and pressure on a peripheral nerve, but decompression is unwise and ineffective. The treatment is early factor replacement and splintage. Later, operation may be needed to correct fixed deformity.

Home treatment with factor concentrate is being developed; it is useful as emergency treatment, avoids delay, and may be all that is needed for minor bleeds.

JOINT DEGENERATION — This is the sequel to repeated bleeding. An affected joint shows wasting and fixed deformity not unlike a tuberculous or rheumatoid joint. X-rays show osteoporosis, joint space narrowing and, in the knee, a curiously square appearance of the intercondylar notch. Operative treatment (including osteotomy and joint replacement) is feasible, but must be covered by factor replacement; continued cover is needed throughout the period of healing and subsequent mobilization.

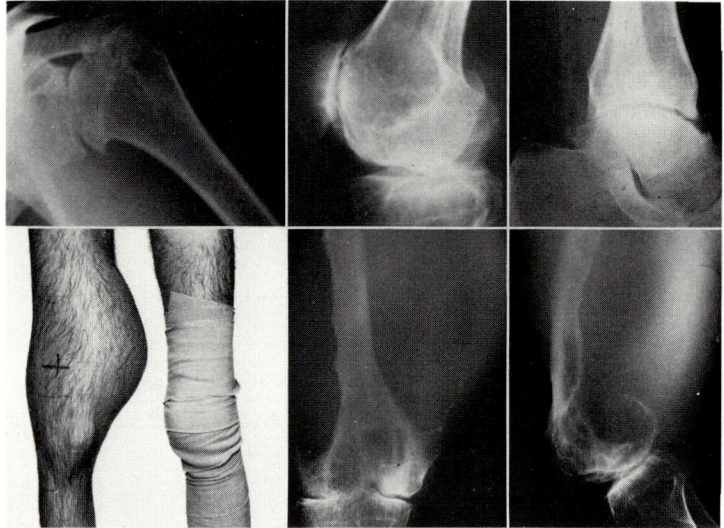

5.13 HAEMOPHILIA
Top row: Joint degeneration after repeated bleeding. Bottom row: A pseudo-tumour which was subsequently grafted.

PSEUDOTUMOURS AND CYSTS — These follow repeated local bleeding. The size of the bleed is critical; if absorption of the blood is not accomplished, there is increased fluid absorption by osmosis with pressure on the surrounding tissues, in which fragile capillaries allow further bleeding. A swelling appears which may slowly increase in size. Bone is eroded giving rise either to a cystic appearance resembling a giant cell tumour, or to extensive osteolysis. In addition to factor replacement, the tumour may need to be excised and weakened bone may need reinforcement by grafting.

FRACTURES — The bleeding which accompanies any fracture must first be controlled. The fracture is then treated on its merits; internal fixation (under factor replacement) is often used for unstable fractures. Union is not delayed.

OSTEOCHONDRITIS

This is a collection of entities which fall into three distinct and quite different groups.

'CRUSHING' OSTEOCHONDRITIS

CAUSE AND PATHOLOGY

From a study of serial x-rays and of experimental material it seems clear that the blood supply to a bone or part of it becomes inadequate. The resulting avascular bone looks dense on x-ray, stops growing, and may fragment with stress. At the hip (and possibly elsewhere) new blood vessels grow in and, by a process of 'creeping substitution', replace the dead bone; but the shape does not return to normal.

The problem is to know why this occurs only at certain sites and particular ages. Probably anatomical variation in the shape of the bones or in their vascular supply is important. Whatever the underlying abnormality trauma is a likely precipitating cause—a single definite injury, a series of minor injuries, or possibly damage to exposed vessels by the pressure of a synovial effusion.

As usual with a disease of doubtful aetiology constitutional, metabolic and endocrine disorders have all been incriminated; with so localized a process these notions seem far-fetched. Aseptic emboli also have been blamed; in middle life they are important as a cause of avascular necrosis (page 46), but there is no evidence that they play a part in the young age group affected by osteochondritis.

REGIONAL SURVEY OF 'CRUSHING' OSTEOCHONDRITIS

The first two varieties described affect the end of a bone, the next two the whole of a bone, and the last two affect the spine.

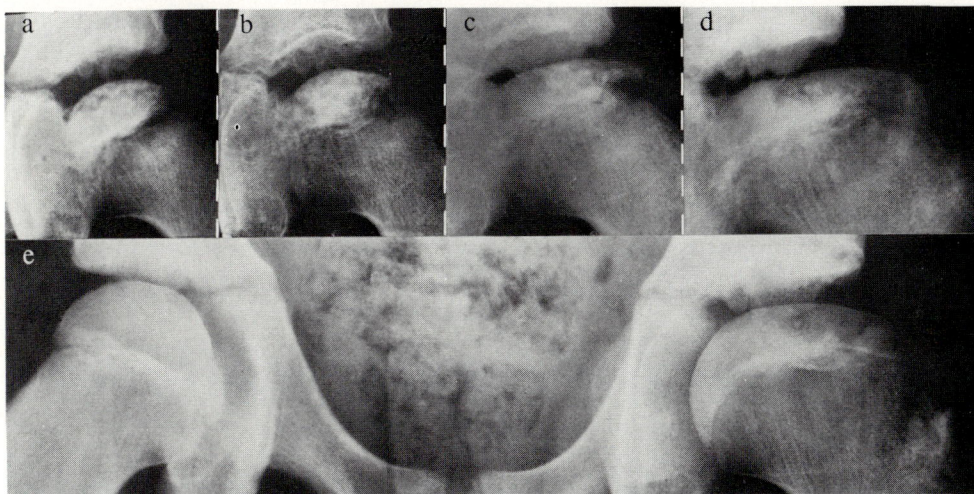

5.14 PATHOLOGY OF 'CRUSHING' OSTEOCHONDRITIS
This patient had Perthes' disease: (a, b, c, d) show the serial changes over a period of 4 years; at 5 years from onset (e) the density of the femoral head has returned to normal, but it remains flatter than the other side.

Hip (Perthes' disease, page 243) — The changes occur in children aged 5–10. The hip joint is temporarily irritable, with slight ache and limp. Later there are few signs except perhaps loss of abduction in flexion. X-rays show the femoral head flat, dense and fragmented, and the joint space increased. The gross x-ray changes are in marked contrast with the paucity of clinical signs. While the hip is irritable traction is needed; later, relief from weight-bearing, osteotomy or 'supervised neglect' are the possibilities.

Metatarsal (Freiberg's disease, page 308) — The patient presents between the ages of 15 and 25 years with metatarsalgia. The second metatarsal head feels thick and tender, and the neighbouring joint is irritable. X-rays show a flat metatarsal head, thick neck and increased joint space. If a protective pad fails to give relief, the metatarsal head is excised.

Navicular (Köhler's disease, page 299) — A child aged between 3 and 5 years presents with pain, limp, tarsal swelling and tenderness. The bony nucleus is squashed, fragmented and dense. Complete recovery occurs if the foot is temporarily rested.

Lunate (Kienböck's disease, page 170) — This presents in young adults, sometimes following injury. The wrist becomes painful, stiffish and locally tender. The lunate bone looks

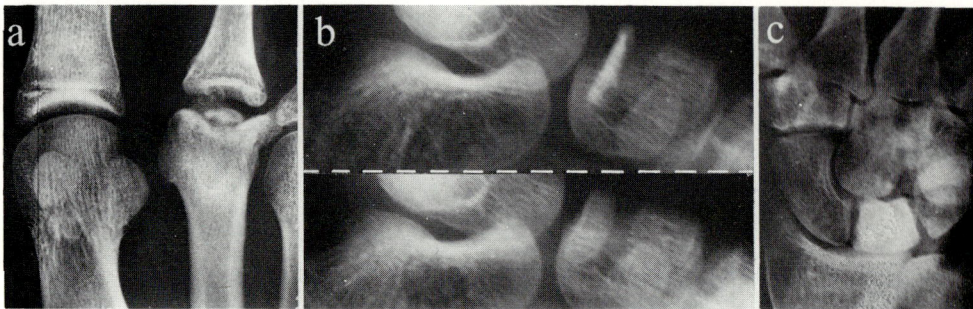

5.15   EXAMPLES OF ' CRUSHING ' OSTEOCHONDRITIS
(a) Freiberg's disease of the second metatarsal; (b) Köhler's disease of the navicular, compared with the normal side below; (c) Kienböck's disease of the lunate.

squashed, dense and fragmented.   Later, osteoarthritis develops.   Splintage often helps but arthrodesis may prove necessary.

Thoracic spine (Scheuermann's disease, page 212) — The plate-like upper and lower epiphyses of several adjacent vertebrae (usually thoracic 6–10) appear fragmented, the bodies become wedge-shaped, and the disc spaces narrow.   Adolescents present with a smooth rigid kyphosis and pain.   Treatment consists of palliation or a brace.

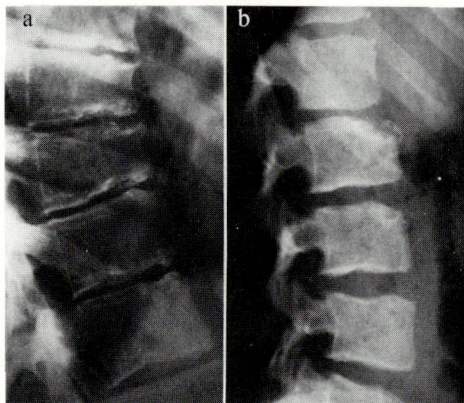

5.16   OSTEOCHONDRITIS
(a)   Thoracic (Scheuermann's disease); note the irregular growth discs; (b) lumbar — the front corner is affected and the vertebra bigger from back to front.

Lumbar spine — Only the front of the plate-like epiphysis is affected, and usually only one or two vertebrae.   The front corner of the vertebrae looks eroded, the disc space below narrowed and the body below expanded.   Adolescents complain of pain and stiffness after exercise. Once tuberculosis is excluded, no treatment is necessary; spontaneous clinical recovery occurs.

'SPLITTING' OSTEOCHONDRITIS (DISSECANS)

CAUSE AND PATHOLOGY

Only convex surfaces are affected, and trauma is the likely cause, probably an osteochondral fracture or a stress fracture.   A fragment splits off and non-union may then follow, perhaps because the fragment is avascular.

First a line of demarcation appears on the articular surface.   On x-ray it looks as if an ovoid segment is becoming separated.   It may revascularize and return to normal; or become partly detached and then break off completely.   The resulting crater and the trauma caused by the loose body are likely to cause osteoarthritis.

Occasionally several joints are affected in several members of a family, implying a genetic or constitutional factor.

REGIONAL SURVEY OF 'SPLITTING' OSTEOCHONDRITIS

The knee is much the commonest joint to be affected, then the elbow, and rarely the ankle or other joints. The condition usually starts in adolescence but may not present until a loose body causes locking or osteoarthritis develops.

Knee (femoral condyle, see page 283) — The patient aged 15–20 may present with vague ache or swelling and a tender medial femoral condyle (rarely lateral). At this stage x-rays show a line of demarcation and recovery may occur if the knee is kept in plaster for 3 months.

Later there may also be giving way or locking. Operation is then necessary. If the fragment is loose it may be fixed back into position, or excised.

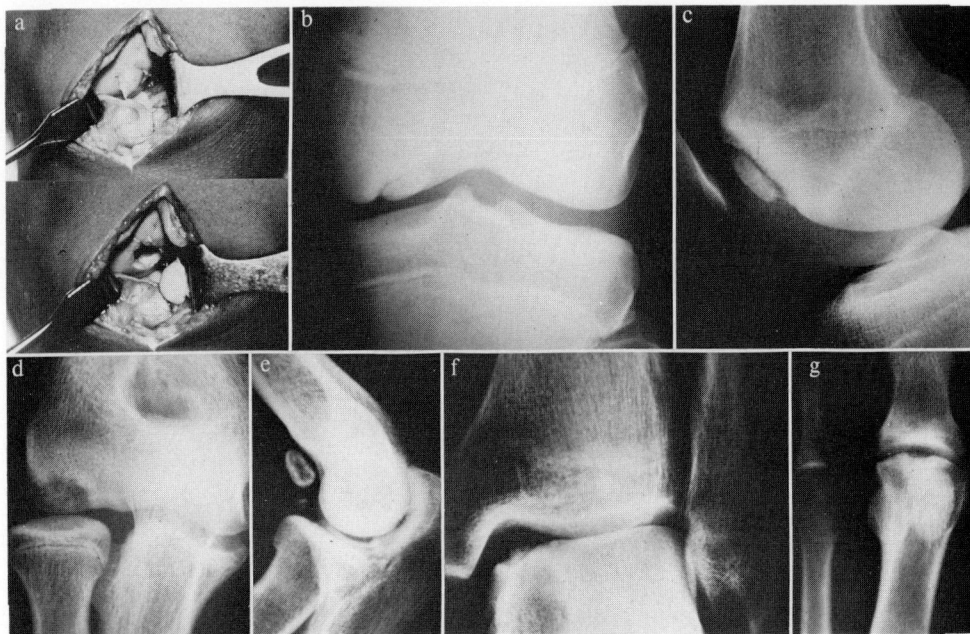

5.17 'SPLITTING' OSTEOCHONDRITIS
(a) The fragment becomes separated and may break away. The knee (b, c) and elbow (d, e) are the commonest sites; but the process may affect any convex articular surface such as the talus (f) or the first metatarsal head (g).

Elbow (capitulum, see page 166) — 'Splitting' osteochondritis of the elbow rarely presents until the loose body has separated to give locking, or still later with osteoarthritis. X-rays show an irregular cyst-like appearance in the capitulum, a large radial head and a loose body which may, however, be apparent only in the lateral view. Later, loose bodies may need to be removed.

Ankle (talus) — The patient may complain of locking from a loose body, or pain, swelling and stiffness from osteoarthritis. If seen early, the fragment, which separates from one corner of the upper surface of the talus, may be excised.

Other sites — Osteochondritis dissecans has also been described in the hip (where it may be a sequel to Perthes' disease), and in the first metatarsal head (where it may lead to hallux rigidus), in the head of the talus, and in metacarpo-phalangeal joints.

'PULLING' OSTEOCHONDRITIS (TRACTION)

CAUSE AND PATHOLOGY

Following excessive strain on a powerful tendon, the apophysis to which it is attached becomes fragmented and irregular in appearance. The x-ray changes are not easy to demonstrate convincingly because a normal apophysis often looks irregular shortly before it fuses with the parent bone.

REGIONAL SURVEY OF 'PULLING' OSTEOCHONDRITIS

The knee is much the commonest site; occasionally the heel is affected.

Knee (Osgood-Schlatter's disease, see page 275) — Children aged between 10 and 15 are affected. The tibial tubercle is swollen and tender, and extension of the knee against resistance sometimes hurts. X-rays show irregular fragmentation of the apophysis into which the patellar ligament is inserted. The disease may be bilateral.

5.18 ' PULLING ' OSTEO-
            CHONDRITIS
This is really a traction lesion, but dignified by eponyms: (a) Schlatter's disease, (b) Johansson-Larsen's disease.

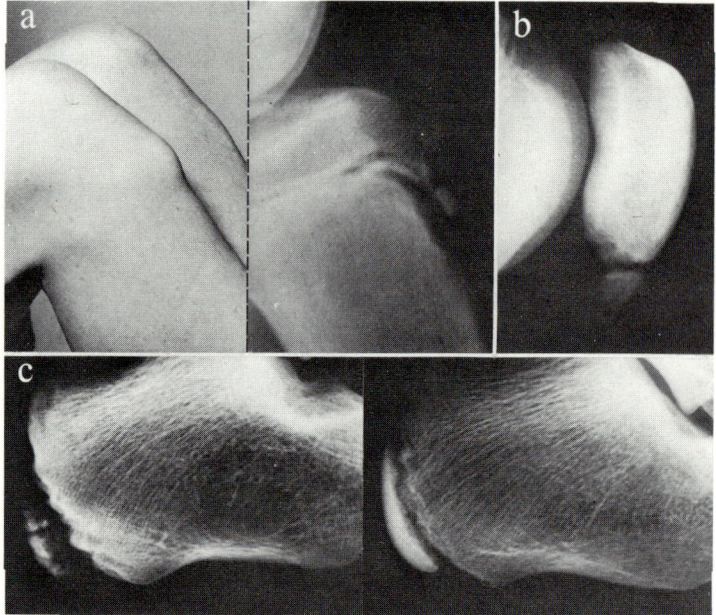

(c) Sever's disease, compared with the normal on the right.

Spontaneous recovery usually occurs and it is necessary only to curtail the child's activities, especially cycling and soccer. If pain persists, a straight plaster tube is worn for 2 months. A separate bony fragment on the deep surface of the patellar tendon may cause persistent pain which is relieved by excision.

Rarely, similar changes affect the lower pole of the patella (Johansson-Larsen's disease).

Heel (Sever's disease, see page 294) — This presents in a child aged about 10 with a painful, tender heel. X-rays show increased density and sometimes fragmentation of the apophysis into which the tendo achillis is inserted. Quite often the unaffected heel shows identical changes. The only treatment is to see that the child avoids wearing flat-heeled shoes.

Suggestions for further reading

Aichroth, P. (1971). 'Osteochondritis Dissecans of the Knee.' *J. Bone Jt Surg.*
    53B, 440 and 448
Chung, S. M. K. and Ralston, E. L. (1969). 'Necrosis of the Femoral Head
    Associated with Sickle-Cell Anaemia and its Variants.' *J. Bone Jt Surg.*
    51A, 33
Freeman, M. A. R. (1972). 'The Pathogenesis of Primary Osteoarthrosis: An
    Hypothesis.' In *Modern Trends in Orthopaedics—6*, Ed. by A. Graham
    Apley. London; Butterworths
Harrington, K. D. *et al.* (1971). 'Avascular Necrosis of Bone after Renal
    Transplantation.' *J. Bone Jt Surg.* **53A**, 203

Helal, B. (1965). 'The Pain in Primary Osteoarthritis of the Knee.' *Postgrad. Med. J.* **41,** 172

Johnson, J. T. H. (1967). 'Neuropathic Fractures and Joint Injuries.' *J. Bone Jt Surg.* **49A,** 1, 1

Laskar, F. H. *et al.* (1970). 'Ochronotic Arthropathy.' *J. Bone Jt Surg.* **52B,** 653

Smillie, I. S. (1961). *Osteochondritis Dissecans.* Edinburgh; Livingstone

Solomon, L. (1976). 'Patterns of Osteoarthritis of the Hip.' *J. Bone Jt Surg.* **58B,** 176

CHAPTER 6

DYSPLASIAS, DYSTROPHIES AND MALFORMATIONS*

Bone dysplasia is taken to mean a generalized disorder of bone (and cartilage); achondroplasia and osteogenesis imperfecta are typical examples.

Malformation syndromes may involve bone, but not necessarily; the term implies structural defects in more than one system or area. Examples are the nail–patella syndrome and Marfan's syndrome.

Conditions grouped under the heading localized malformations were formerly termed 'congenital'. This word implies a deformity which is present at birth and due to developmental error. Since some localized malformations are not apparent at birth the word 'congenital' is best avoided.

GENETIC CONSIDERATIONS

If there are genetic factors associated with a disorder then, in the simplest possible terms, there are three groups to consider:

(1) *Chromosome anomalies* — The defects, whether of chromosome number or of structure, can be seen under a simple light microscope and involve large groups of genes. Damage to the individual is severe and most abort, are stillborn, or die during the first year of life with multiple congenital defects. The great majority of cases are sporadic (non-familial).

(2) *Single gene disorders* — This group have the familiar dominant, recessive and X-linked modes of inheritance. *Dominance* indicates that only one gene of a pair is abnormal and the disorder typically affects both sexes and all generations, perhaps up to 50 per cent of near relatives being affected. There tends to be a wide variation of expression, from the very mild to very severe (e.g. osteogenesis imperfecta). *Recessive inheritance* indicates that both genes of a pair are abnormal and the disorder thus appears in the children of apparently unaffected parents (who have only one abnormal gene each). Up to one in four sibs may be affected and the range of expression is not so variable as in dominant inheritance. *X-linked inheritance* means that the gene concerned is on the X chromosome, of which females have two and males only one. Thus an X-linked disorder can *never* pass from father to son, the father inevitably passing his X chromosome only to his daughters. X-linked recessive disorders affect males only. X-linked dominant disorders are more common in females than males.

(3) *Multifactorial inheritance* means that multiple genes together with environmental factors are acting. Inheritance is complex and it is probable that most common congenital malformations (spina bifida, congenital dislocation of the hip, clubfoot) belong to this group.

The sporadic case, where this is the first appearance in a family of a particular abnormality, may be: (*a*) Non-genetic—perhaps due to some accident in the intra-uterine environment (e.g. thalidomide deformities). (*b*) A new mutation of a disorder of dominant inheritance (this will become apparent in the next generation).

* I am happy to acknowledge considerable help in the preparation of this chapter (especially the genetic aspects) from Ruth Wynne-Davies, F.R.C.S. Further details are available in her book *Heritable Disorders in Orthopaedic Practice*.

(*c*) The first appearance of a homozygote in a disorder of recessive inheritance. It may be possible to detect some biochemical abnormality in the parents.

Many of the rare disorders described in this chapter are of single gene inheritance, and two generalizations may be made:

(1) Disorders which are typically confined to one limb (Ollier's disease, dysplasia epiphysealis hemimelica, melorheostosis) tend to be non-genetic.

(2) Known enzyme disorders (e.g. homocystinuria) tend to be of recessive inheritance.

ACHONDROPLASIA

This disease is of autosomal dominant inheritance, but since most individuals do not marry and have children, cases are usually sporadic. Cartilage cells produced by the epiphyses fail to line up properly and undergo degeneration.

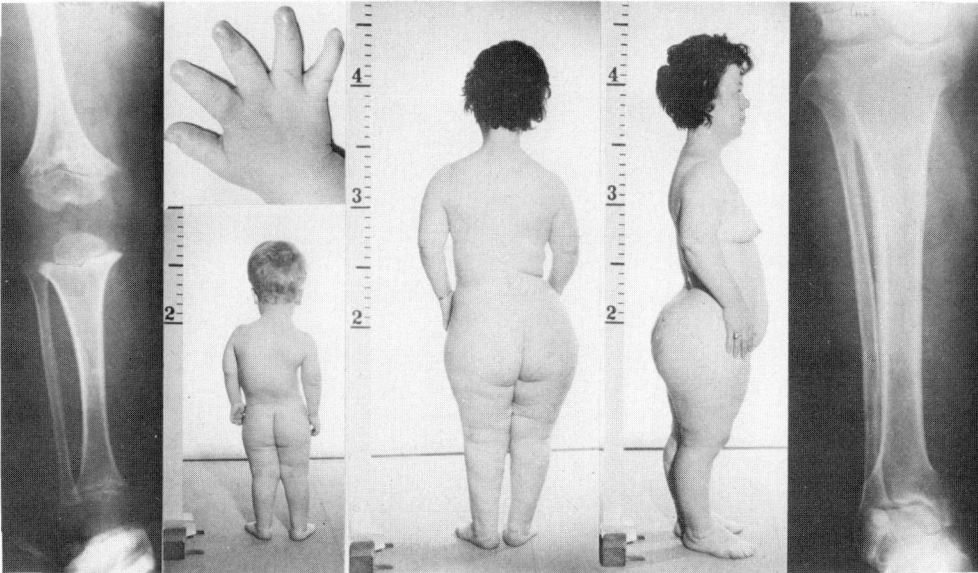

6.1 ACHONDROPLASIA
This boy and his mother show the typical features of the classical disease, although their slight scoliosis is uncommon. The child's epiphyses have V-shaped notches. If his mother had them also, her present x-rays clearly show that they did not distort growth.

CLINICAL FEATURES

If the child survives the first year he becomes a short-limbed dwarf with normal intelligence and often with excellent muscles. The skull is large and brachycephalic, with bulging vault and forehead, and a flat nose. The limbs are grossly short, notably the proximal segments, so that the hands do not reach the buttocks and the patient may be able to kiss his toes while keeping his knees straight. The fingers are short, stubby and unusually equal in length. The trunk, though not very short, may have a thoracic kyphosis and a lumbar lordosis, producing the prominent buttocks which, together with the other features described, account for the popularity of achondroplasiacs as circus dwarfs.

The vertebral pedicles are short and, in the lumbar spine, too close together; consequently the spinal canal is narrow (spinal stenosis), and disc prolapse (which is common) has exceptionally severe effects (a feature noted also in dachshunds, who are of course achondroplasiac).

X-RAYS

These show relative thickness and shortness of the pipe bones. The metaphyses at the knee are splayed out peripherally and may contain a central notch into which the central part of the epiphysis dips. The skull as a whole is large but its base is too short. The pelvis is too small for normal delivery.

6.2 SPONDYLO-EPIPHYSEAL
DYSPLASIA
Usual variety.

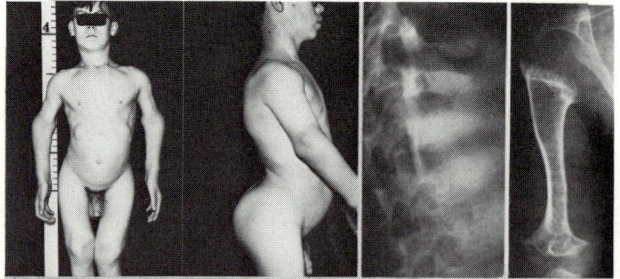

Pseudo-achondroplasiac type.

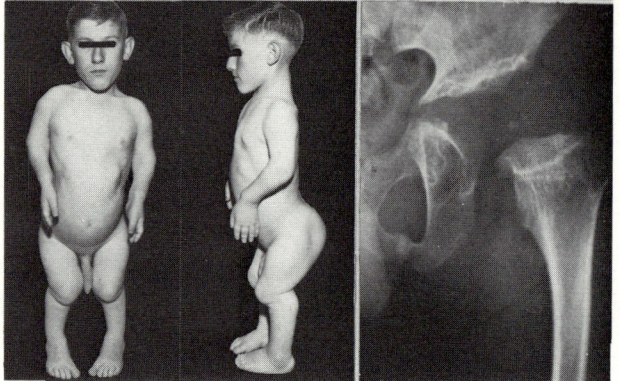

DIAGNOSIS

The 'classical' disorder described above must be differentiated from its variants, and from other causes of short-limbed dwarfism.

In *hypochondroplasia* dwarfism is less marked and the skull is normal.

In *diastrophic dwarfism* other deformities are associated, notably club foot (a very stiff and intractable variety), joint contractures, cauliflower ear, and scoliosis.

In *chondro-ectodermal dysplasia* (Ellis–van Creveld syndrome) dwarfism is associated with cardiac disorders, polydactyly and hypoplastic nails and teeth. The limb shortness, unlike that in achondroplasia, affects distal segments more than proximal.

In *spondylo-epiphyseal dysplasia* dwarfism is associated with grossly distorted large proximal joints, a normal skull and irregular platyspondyly. The term covers a group of disorders, including one which is X-linked and therefore affects only males. In most the trunk (unlike that in achondroplasia) is disproportionately short; but one variety is short-limbed and is called pseudo-achondroplasia, although the distorted joints preclude the supple agility of classical achondroplasia.

OSTEOGENESIS IMPERFECTA (Brittle bones)

The process of bone manufacture is faulty and stops short at the 'woven bone' stage. Consequently the bones bend too easily and break too easily. There are two distinct varieties: (1) Congenita (of sporadic or of recessive inheritance): multiple fractures occur before, during or soon after birth. (2) Tarda (of autosomal dominant inheritance): this is less severe, and the patient likely to survive into adult life. The tendency to fracture diminishes after puberty.

CLINICAL FEATURES

As well as short stature and limb deformities, the clinical features may include: a broad skull (with Wormian bones visible on x-ray), blue sclera, otosclerosis (although deafness does not come on until adult life), scoliosis, ligament laxity and a tendency to bruise easily. The limb deformities result from the bending of soft bone combined with mal-union of fractures. Coxa vara, bowing of the femur and tibia, knock knees, plano-valgus feet, and dislocation of the radial head are all fairly common.

The appearance depends upon the variety. In the congenita type dwarfism and deformities are severe; the limbs are bent and the spine scoliotic, but deafness and blue sclerae are not marked features. In the tarda variety deformity is much less; the spine and limbs are often straight, but the sclerae are blue and deafness is common in middle life.

The shafts of the long bones are bent and slender: the ends, however, appear large and are sometimes cystic. A tri-radiate pelvis and biconcave vertebral bodies are other sequels of the bone softening; osteoporosis is marked.

COMPLICATIONS AND TREATMENT

The fractures are frequently greenstick in type and unite rapidly with routine treatment. Very occasionally a tremendous periosteal reaction develops; the appearance of this 'hyperplastic callus' mimics that of a bone sarcoma.

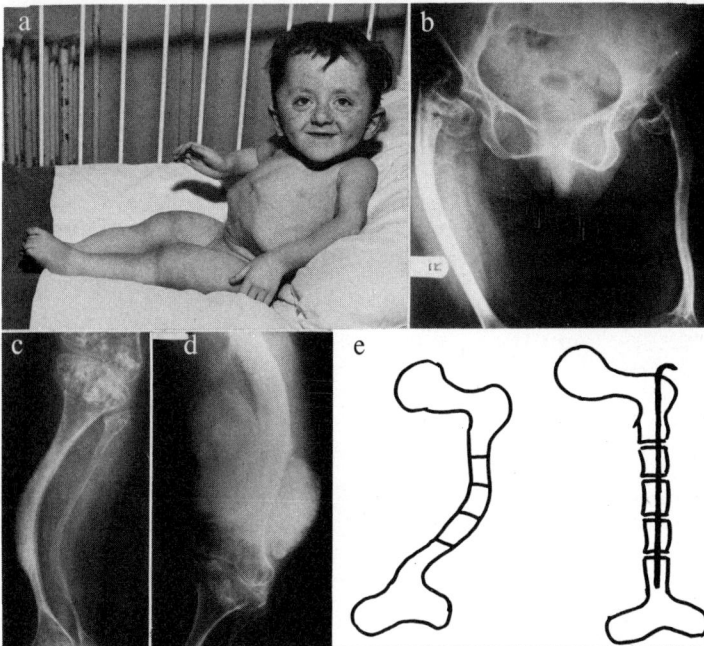

6.3 BRITTLE BONES
(a) The patient may look like Humpty Dumpty (who probably had brittle bones); (b, c) the bones develop characteristic deformities; (d) hyperplastic callus—a rare complication; (e) the 'kebab' procedure for straightening a bent bone.

No general treatment is known. To prevent mal-union of fractures intramedullary nailing is useful; and, where severe deformity has already occurred, the shaft can be divided into segments and held straight with an intramedullary nail (the 'kebab' treatment).

MUCOPOLYSACCHARIDE DISORDERS

This group is characterized by inborn errors of mucopolysaccharide (MPS) metabolism. They differ from each other in mode of inheritance, type of MPS found in the urine, and in their clinical features. Dwarfism (when present) is 'proportionate', i.e. shared by trunk and limbs. Among the least rare are the following.

MORQUIO–BRAILSFORD DISEASE — Development is apparently normal for the first year or two; thereafter dwarfism becomes progressively obvious. The spine is kyphotic and the manubriosternal angle is 90 degrees (a pathognomonic feature). The vertebrae are too flat (platyspondyly) with a narrow tongue of bone projecting forwards. The hips are grossly distorted and genu valgum or varum often severe. Ligamentous laxity is marked, but the skull and mentality are both normal. Keratan sulphate is found in the urine.

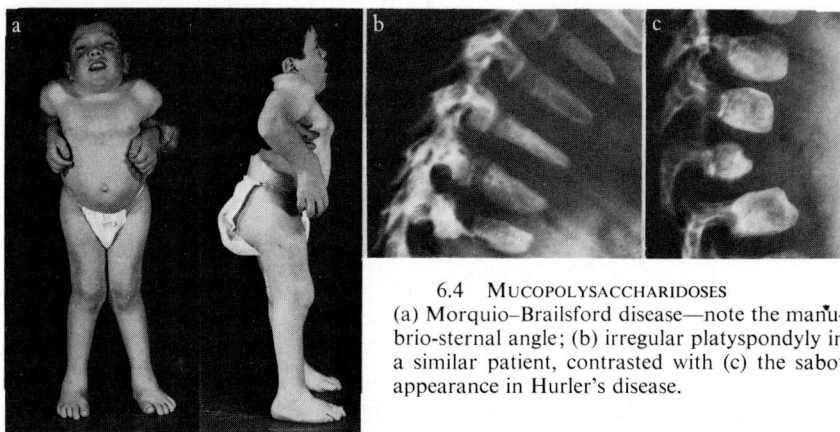

6.4 MUCOPOLYSACCHARIDOSES
(a) Morquio–Brailsford disease—note the manubrio-sternal angle; (b) irregular platyspondyly in a similar patient, contrasted with (c) the sabot appearance in Hurler's disease.

HURLER'S DISEASE — The synonym 'gargoylism' is justified by coarse skin, bloated lips and eyelids, wide-set eyes and corneal opacities. Mental retardation is noted early. The limb deformities may resemble those in Morquio-Brailsford disease. There is, however, no platyspondyly or 'tonguing', although the lower part of a vertebra may protrude forwards. There is no ligament laxity; indeed these children are stiff-jointed. Dermatan sulphate and heparan sulphate are found in the urine. Cardiopulmonary complications are common, so that, in contrast to Morquio–Brailsford disease, they rarely survive into adult life.

HUNTER'S DISEASE differs slightly from Hurler's and is less severe. It is of X-linked recessive inheritance and therefore all patients are male.

MULTIPLE EXOSTOSES (Diaphyseal aclasis)

In this disorder of autosomal dominant inheritance there is failure of bone remodelling: as tubular bones grow in length, the excess metaphyseal bone is not absorbed but forms irregular exostoses. It has been suggested that the affected bones 'squander their growth potential'; cells destined for growth in length escape laterally from the juxta-epiphyseal region to form metaphyseal excrescences—certainly affected tubular bones are diminished in length.

CLINICAL FEATURES

The skull and spine are normal, although often the patient is slightly short. Multiple lumps are found on the upper humerus, the lower end of the radius and ulna, around the knee, above the ankle, and occasionally on flat bones. No lumps grow on the epiphyses, and only rarely does an exostosis migrate with growth as far as the middle third of the shaft. In contrast with dyschondroplasia the fingers have only tiny knobs, or none at all. Bowing of the radius, and valgus deformity at the knees and ankles, are not uncommon; some deformities may be produced by an exostosis from one bone pressing on its neighbour. X-rays show irregular metaphyses, with sessile or pedunculated exostoses projecting from the surface.

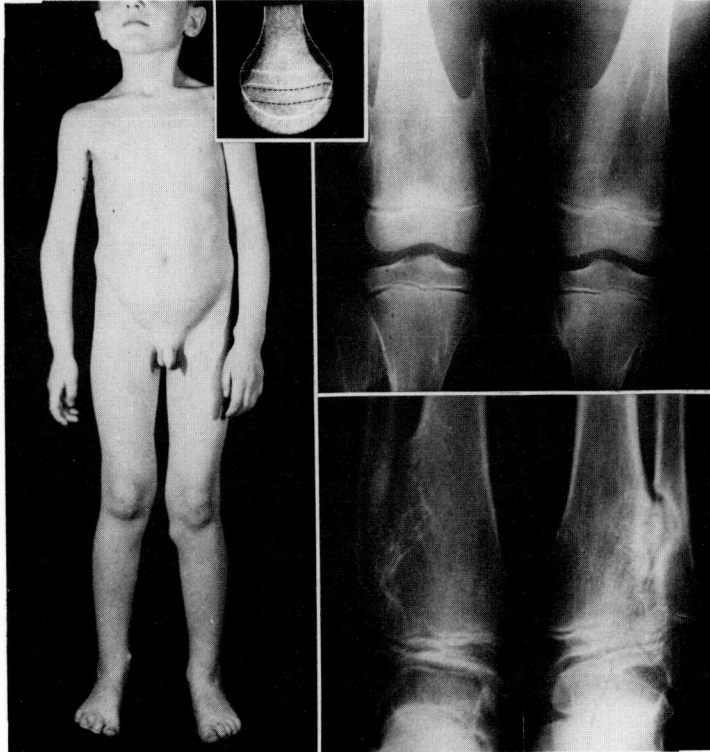

6.5 MULTIPLE EXOSTOSES One member of a family with diaphyseal aclasis; the inset illustrates failure of bone remodelling.

TREATMENT AND COMPLICATIONS

A lump may interfere with tendon action and need removal. The lumps stop growing when the parent bone does, except occasionally in the pelvis, scapula, upper humerus or ribs, where one may continue to grow. Malignant change is said to occur in 5 per cent of patients.

MULTIPLE CHONDROMAS (Dyschondroplasia, Ollier's disease)

This rare disease is not familial. Ossification of cartilage at the growth discs is faulty, islands of cartilage remaining unossified within the shaft.

CLINICAL FEATURES

Typically the disorder is unilateral; indeed only one limb or even one bone may be involved. An affected limb is short and, because the metaphysis contains irregularly distributed islands of cartilage, there is deformity. Common deformities are valgus

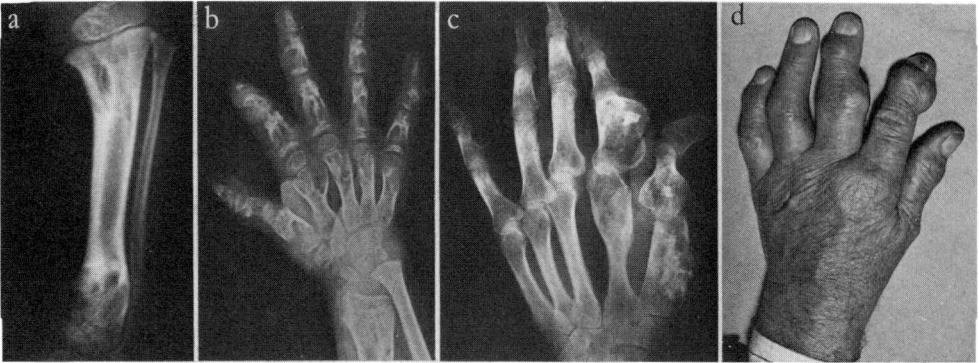

6.6 OLLIER'S DISEASE
(a), (b) In this child the left arm and leg were severely affected. (c), (d) Two adult patients.

at the knee and ankle, and relative shortening of the ulna so that the radius is curved and sometimes dislocated. The fingers or toes frequently contain multiple enchondromata, which are characteristic of the disease and may be so numerous that the hand is crippled. Malignant change in 1 per cent of the chondromata has been reported. A rare variety of dyschondroplasia is associated with multiple haemangiomata (Maffucci's disease).

X-rays show large translucent islands or columns of cartilage in the metaphysis. As the child grows these islands develop irregular dense spots. The shaft, although often curved, is usually of normal structure. The epiphyses may be mottled or streaky. The fingers nearly always show multiple chondromata with stippled calcification. Even when the disease is clinically unilateral, the other side may show radiographic abnormalities.

MARBLE BONES (Osteopetrosis, Albers–Schönberg disease)

In this familial disease the bones are excessively dense and structureless on x-ray. Two forms are described: (*a*) tarda, a mild version, of recessive inheritance; and (*b*) congenita, the severe form. In this severe variety aplastic anaemia is common because there is little true medulla; cranial nerves may be compressed by narrowing of

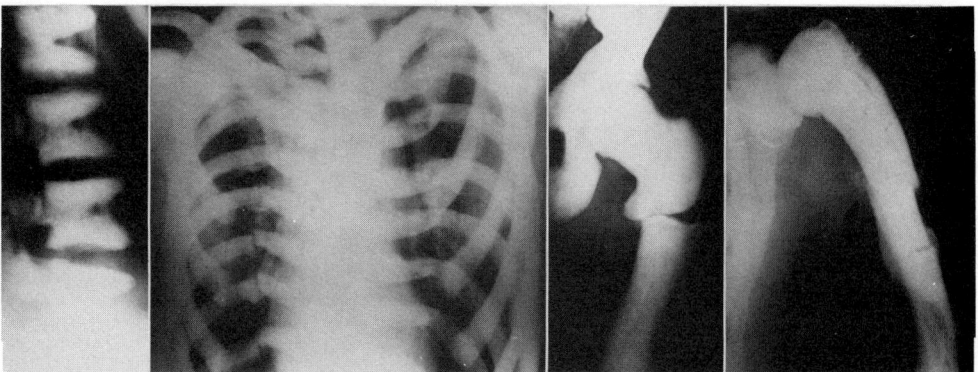

6.7 MARBLE BONES
Despite the remarkable density the bones break easily; but, as in this humerus, union occurs without special difficulty.

the foramina, the pituitary fossa encroached upon to cause insufficiency, and dental caries may lead to osteomyelitis of the jaw. Although hard the bones (like marble) are brittle, and fracture easily.

CANDLE BONES, SPOTTED BONES AND STRIPED BONES

Candle bones (melorheostosis, Leri's disease) is not familial. The patient presents with pain and stiffness, usually confined to one limb. X-rays show irregular patches of sclerosis, usually distributed in linear fashion through the limb; the appearance is reminiscent of the wax which congeals on the side of a burning candle. Scleroderma and joint contractures may be associated.

In spotted bones (osteopoikilosis) numerous white spots are seen in the x-rays of many bones; there may also be whitish spots in the skin (disseminated lenticular dermatofibrosis).

In striped bones (osteopathia striata) x-rays show lines of increased density parallel to the shafts of long bones, but radiating like a fan in the pelvis. The condition is symptomless.

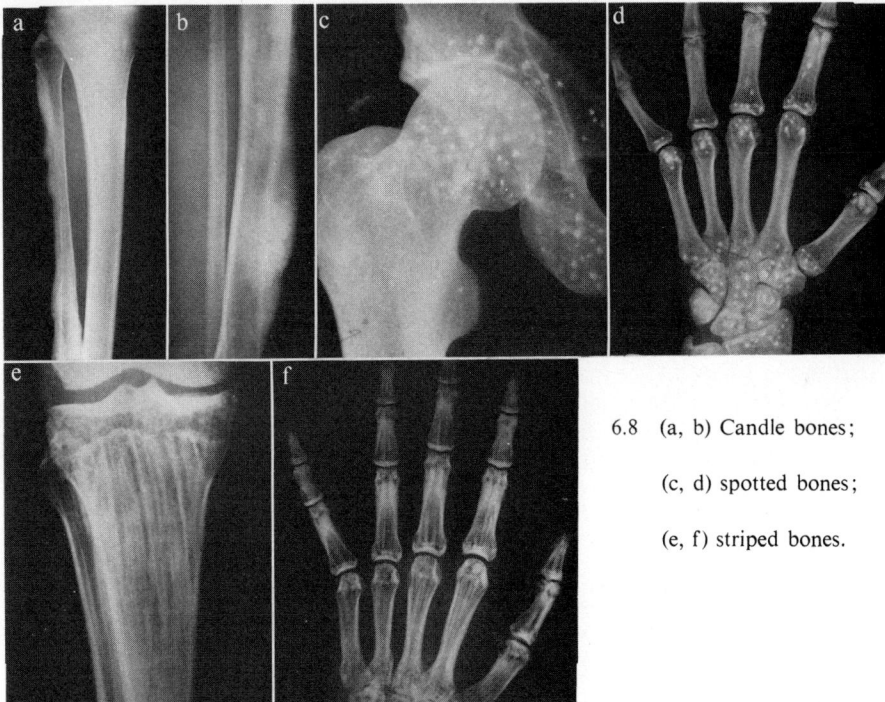

6.8 (a, b) Candle bones;

(c, d) spotted bones;

(e, f) striped bones.

CLEIDO-CRANIAL DYSOSTOSIS

In this condition of autosomal dominant inheritance there is faulty development of membrane bones, chiefly the clavicles and skull. The patient is somewhat short, with a large head, flat-looking face and drooping shoulders. The skull is brachycephalic, the teeth appear late and develop poorly. Because the clavicles are partly absent, the patient can bring his shoulders together in front of the chest. Spinal curvature and widening of the symphysis pubis are not uncommon. The radius may be short and the elbows valgus. The hands are curious in that the index finger is often too long, while the terminal phalanx of the thumb (or other fingers) is too short. The mentality is normal.

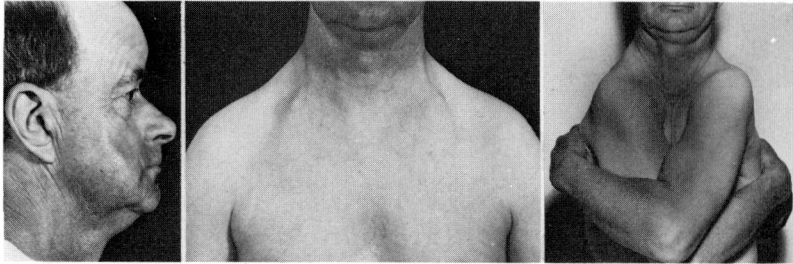

6.9 CLEIDO-CRANIAL DYSOSTOSIS
The squashed face, sloping shoulders and trick movement are unmistakable.

X-rays show that a part of each clavicle is absent, usually the outer half, sometimes the middle third, and, rarely, the inner quarter. Wormian bones occur in the skull, the pubis usually shows deficient ossification, and sometimes there is coxa vara.

EPIPHYSEAL DYSPLASIAS

Dysplasia epiphysealis multiplex is the least rare of this group, some of which are familial. The face, skull and spine are normal. Many major epiphyses are affected. On x-ray they appear late and close early; they are ill-formed, irregular and mottled. In time their architecture becomes normal but not their shape, so that deformity and stiffness result. In one large series there was a strong familial incidence and only the lower limbs were affected.

Dysplasia epiphysealis punctata may be a variation of multiplex, but a severe one, with epiphyseal mottling obvious at birth. Conradi's disease (chondrodysplasia calcificans congenita), in which mental retardation, dwarfism, congenital heart disease and cataracts occur, also has epiphyseal mottling visible from birth, but the mottling disappears with growth.

Dysplasia epiphysealis hemimelica affects epiphyses, usually of the ankle but sometimes also of the knee. One limb only is involved and usually only half the epiphysis (medial or lateral); in the affected area osteochondromatous lumps develop. The child presents because of the lump or because of stiffness. Treatment consists of removing the excessive epiphyseal material.

METAPHYSEAL DYSPLASIAS

Familial metaphyseal dysplasia (Pyle's disease) is of autosomal recessive inheritance. There is failure of modelling in the metaphyses of the long bones; they are too wide and lack the normal elegant contours.

Cranio-metaphyseal dysplasia has limb changes like a mild version of Pyle's disease, but in addition has marked skull changes—a curiously prominent forehead and a squashed-looking nose.

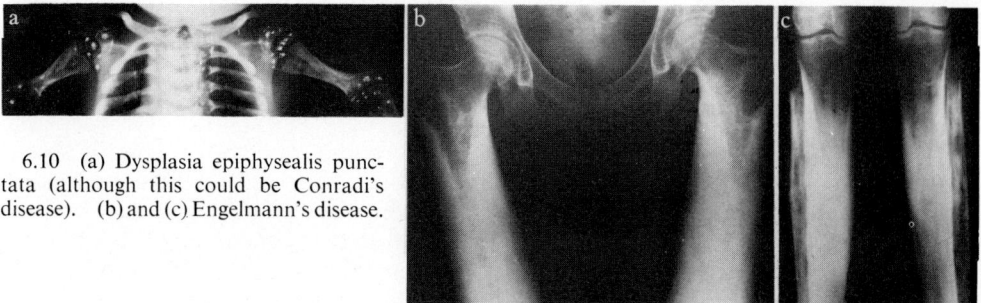

6.10 (a) Dysplasia epiphysealis punctata (although this could be Conradi's disease). (b) and (c) Engelmann's disease.

Metaphyseal dysostosis is of autosomal dominant inheritance. The metaphyses are an odd shape and may look irregularly cystic. The mild version is called Schmid's disease; in the severe type (Jansen's disease) dwarfing is severe and deafness may occur.

DIAPHYSEAL DYSPLASIAS

Progressive diaphyseal dysplasia (Camurati's or Engelmann's disease) is characterized by fusiform widening and sclerosis of the shafts of the long bones and sometimes also of the skull. Often the femur, tibia and forearm bones are symmetrically affected. Cortical thickening is both superficial (causing widening) and deep (sometimes causing medullary obliteration); the bone ends are normal. The patient presents with painful limbs, weakness or a peculiar gait.

Cranio-diaphyseal dysplasia is characterized by expansion of the long bone shafts coupled with gross bony thickening of the skull and face, so that the term leontiasis ossea is sometimes used.

FIBROUS DYSPLASIAS (Fibrocystic disease)

Fibrous dysplasia is probably a developmental defect. The process may affect one bone (monostotic), one limb (monomelic) or many bones (polyostotic). A solitary bone cyst may usefully be considered as one variety of fibrous dysplasia; it is also the commonest. In all varieties the cellular fibrous tissue in the medullary spaces of the

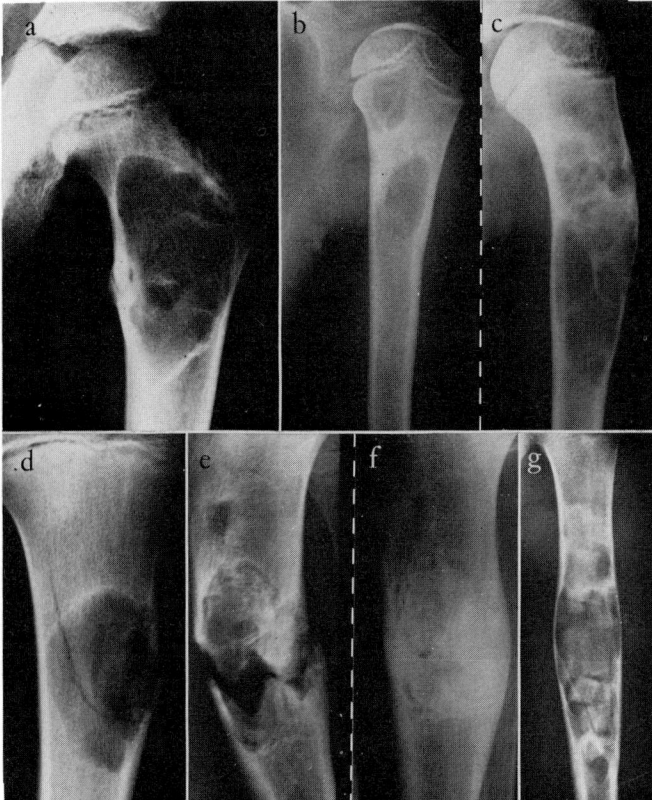

6.11 SOLITARY CYST
(a) Cyst in typical site; (b, c) cyst extending with growth;

(d) fine crack through cyst; (e, f) more severe fracture, followed by healing; (g) cyst which had fractured twice, and healed only after chip grafts were inserted.

bone proliferates, destroying trabeculae; the bone may be expanded and the cortex eroded. The resulting cavities contain fluid or fibrous tissue, the walls contain giant cells.

CLINICAL VARIETIES

SOLITARY CYST — This usually occurs in the upper humerus, femur, or tibia, but other bones may be affected. Solitary cysts are seen in children up to the age of puberty and after that become increasingly rare. Clinically a cyst presents with local ache, or as a pathological fracture.

X-rays show a translucent area on the shaft side of the growth disc. The cortex may be thinned and the bone expanded. The cyst is rounded and has a clear cut edge but no surrounding sclerosis (for differential diagnosis *see* page 12).

Because cysts are hardly ever seen in adults, it is presumed that many disappear spontaneously. A fracture through a cyst often results in the cyst becoming obliterated. If the cyst is troublesome or increasing in size it should be evacuated, the wall scraped and the cavity filled with bone chips.

MONOSTOTIC FIBROUS DYSPLASIA — This rare condition occurs chiefly in adolescents and may remain symptomless until the bone breaks. In part of one bone the lamellar pattern is replaced by irregular cysts and fibrous bands which may be calcified (the x-ray appearance is often a mixture of 'bubbles and stripes'). When the affected area is in the metaphysis and abuts against part of the epiphysis, the bone grows bent. Osteotomy is then required. If the bone is straight, radiotherapy may be tried; but, where feasible, excision of the affected area and grafting is better.

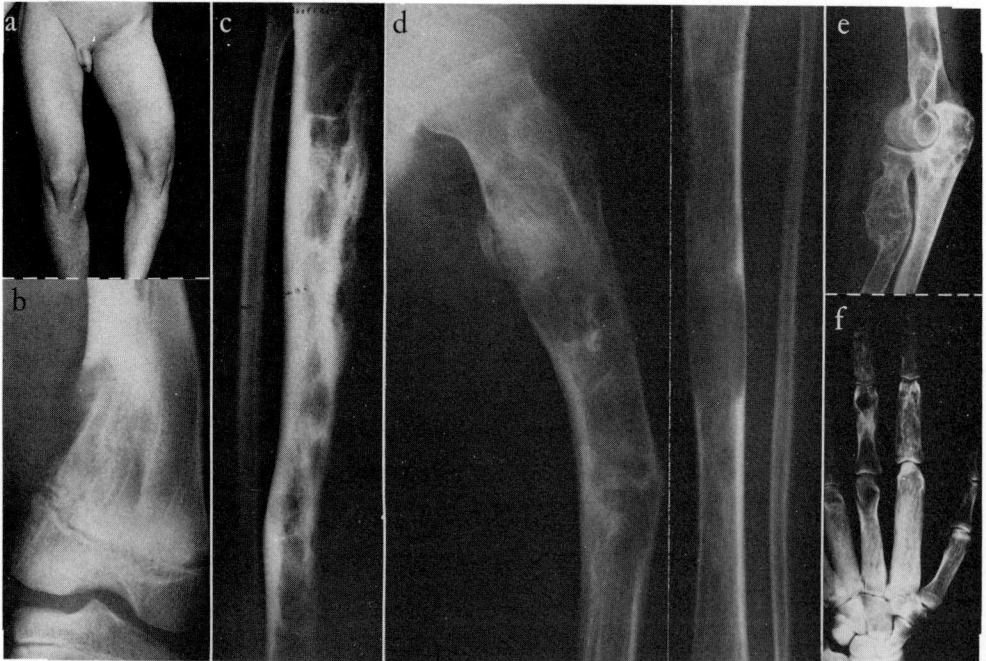

6.12 FIBROUS DYSPLASIA
(a, b) Monostotic, and affecting only part of the bone; (c) affecting the whole of one bone; (d, e, f) are examples of polyostotic fibrous dysplasia, with several bones affected.

POLYOSTOTIC FIBROUS DYSPLASIA — The major long bones are chiefly affected, often only in one limb, sometimes in one half of the body; sometimes lesions are scattered throughout the skeleton.

Patients may present with bone enlargement, deformity, pain or a fracture. X-rays show cystic areas and patches or streaks of calcification in the shafts (not the epiphyses) of long bones; the cortex may be thinned and the bone ballooned. The short bones often show a uniform ground-glass appearance; the skull may be irregularly thickened with numerous dense spots. In contrast to hyperparathyroidism the bones are not markedly osteoporotic.

Albright's disease is a combination of polyostotic fibrous dysplasia with skin pigmentation; when it occurs in girls sexual precocity is likely.

MALFORMATION SYNDROMES

NAIL–PATELLA SYNDROME (Osteo-onychodysplasia)

A dominant autosomal gene is responsible for this curious familial disorder. The nails are hypoplastic and the patellae unduly small or absent. The radial head may be subluxed laterally and bony excrescences ('horns') develop on the lateral aspect of the ilium. Congenital nephropathy may be associated.

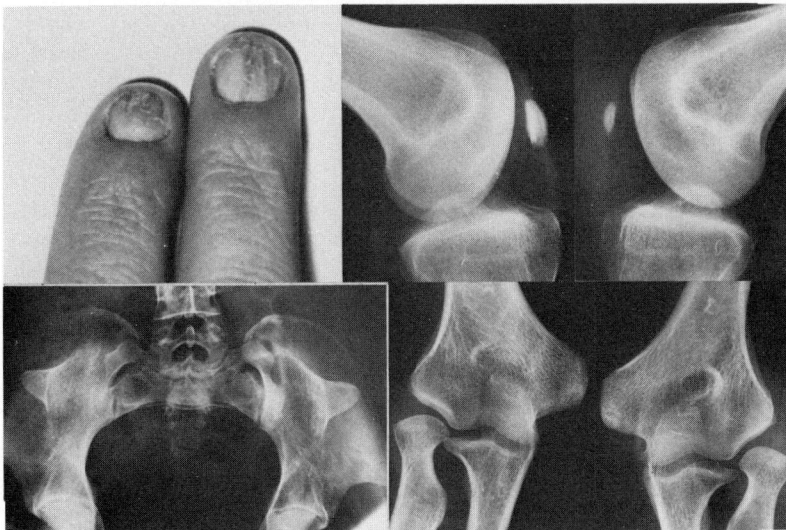

6.13 THE NAIL-PATELLA SYNDROME
The dystrophic nails, minute patellae, pelvic 'horns' and subluxed radii combine to make an unmistakable picture.

MARFAN'S SYNDROME

In this disorder of autosomal dominant inheritance there is a defect in elastin or collagen, or both. Ocular lens dislocation and aortic aneurysms are often the presenting features. The patients are tall, with a long lower body segment and often with chest deformities. Despite the absence of vertebral anomalies scoliosis is common. The limbs are unduly long, especially the distal segments, so that the term arachnodactyly (spider fingers) has been used. Generalized joint laxity is usual, but often the finger and toe joints have contractures. Other features include a high arched palate and hernias.

HOMOCYSTINURIA — This metabolic disorder of autosomal recessive inheritance resembles Marfan's disease in general build and proneness to lens dislocation.   But osteoporosis and widening of epiphyses and metaphyses occur only in homocystinuria (the osteoporotic vertebrae may be flat or biconcave); scoliosis and arachnodactyly, however, are less frequent.   Moreover, mental defect is much commoner in homocystinuria and stickiness of platelets increases the risk of post-operative thrombosis.   The diagnostic feature is of course the presence of homocystine in the urine.

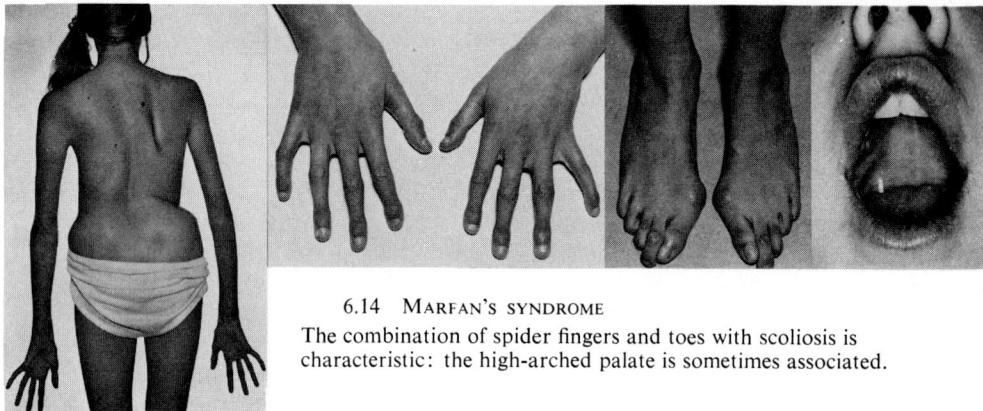

6.14   MARFAN'S SYNDROME
The combination of spider fingers and toes with scoliosis is characteristic: the high-arched palate is sometimes associated.

ACROCEPHALO-SYNDACTYLY (Apert's syndrome)

In this disease of dominant inheritance the head is peculiar in shape, with a high broad forehead ('tower-shaped'), a flattened occiput, bulging eyes and a prominent jaw. Unless premature fusion of the cranial sutures can be prevented eye changes and mental retardation occur.   The associated syndactyly of fingers and toes is of an unusual type; the three 'inboard' digits are joined together.

The combination of Apert's syndrome with polydactyly of the toes is called *Carpenter's syndrome.*

CHROMOSOME ANOMALIES

These include numerical anomalies (e.g. too few chromosomes, as in Turner's syndrome; or too many, as in Down's syndrome); and structural anomalies such as translocation of a group of genes.   Chromosome anomalies are always associated with multiple defects and usually with mental retardation.

LOCALIZED MALFORMATIONS

Most localized malformations (e.g. spina bifida, congenital hip dislocation and talipes) are more suitably discussed in their appropriate regional chapters.   Some general observations and a few special groups are conveniently considered here.

GENERAL OBSERVATIONS

Congenital limb anomalies include extra bones, absent bones and fusions.   Complete absence of a limb is called amelia, almost complete absence (a mere stub remaining) phocomelia, and partial absence ectromelia; defects may be transverse or axial.   In the hands and feet brachydactyly, syndactyly, polydactyly and symphalangism are among the many possibilities.   When genetic factors are present at all, the inheritance is dominant. Detailed elaboration of terminology interests the philologist more than the surgeon.

Absent radius — Although sometimes an isolated phenomenon (page 169) absence (or dysplasia) of the radius may be associated with pancytopenia; this condition (Fanconi's anaemia) leads to early death. In another syndrome with radial absence the blood cells are normal but there is a deficiency of platelets.

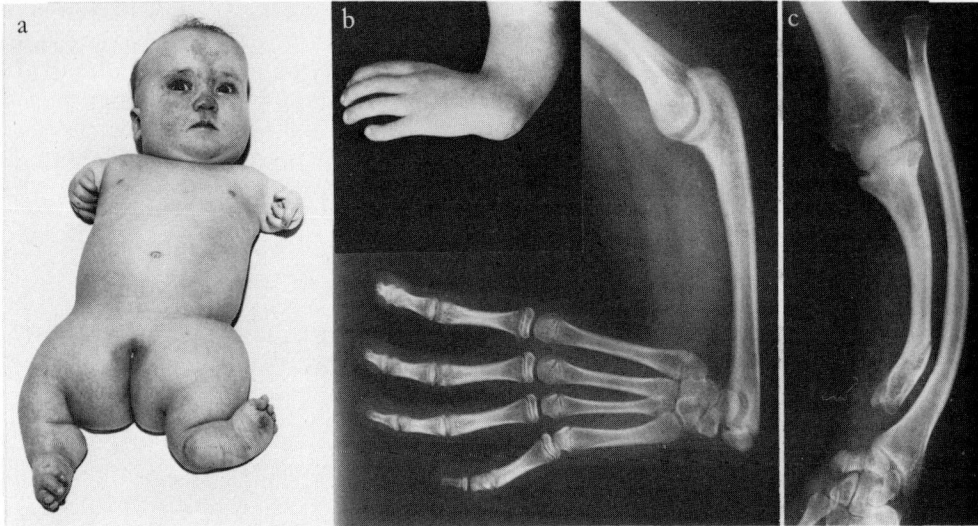

6.15 LOCALIZED MALFORMATIONS (1)
(a) Phocomelia in a thalidomide baby, (b) absent radius (radial club hand), (c) the radius is normal in length, the ulna dysplastic and short — hence the dislocation.

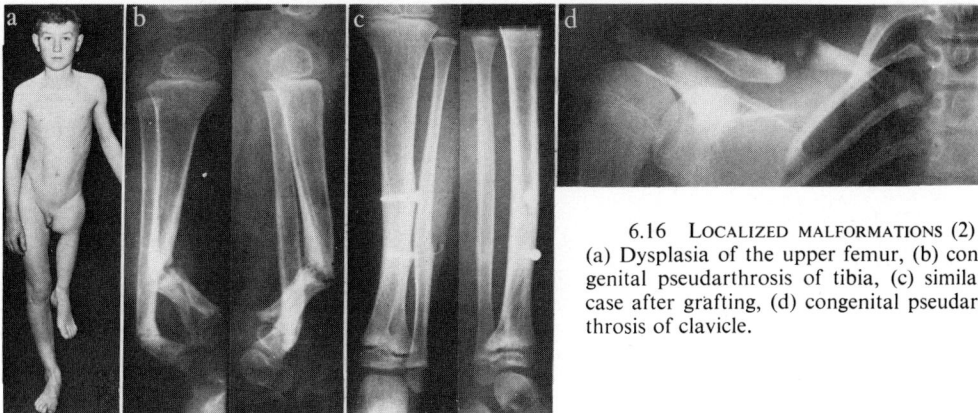

6.16 LOCALIZED MALFORMATIONS (2)
(a) Dysplasia of the upper femur, (b) congenital pseudarthrosis of tibia, (c) similar case after grafting, (d) congenital pseudarthrosis of clavicle.

Dysplasia of the upper femur — In its most benign form shortening is less than 3 in. and treatment no different from that for leg inequality in poliomyelitis (page 140). But if the dysplasia is combined with coxa vara, shortening may be too severe for practicable leg lengthening; an artificial extension may be feasible but amputation often permits greater prosthetic elegance. If the entire upper third of the femur is missing the situation is still worse; but the 'absent' part may in fact be cartilaginous, in which case bone grafting can provide hip stability and therefore more satisfactory limb-fitting. If the upper third (or even more) is truly absent the only prospect for even mediocre prosthetic fitting is to perform one of several heroic operations described by van Nes (1966): e.g. femoral osteotomies to make the foot point backwards so that its muscles activate the 'knee' of a prosthesis.

Congenital pseudarthrosis of the tibia — As usual, the term 'congenital' is ambiguous for the fracture is not necessarily present at birth; the unbroken tibia may contain an area of neurofibromatosis, or of fibrous dysplasia, or may simply be bowed forwards. Fracture below the mid-shaft occurs within the first two years of life; if treated by conservative methods non-union is inevitable. McFarland's technique is reasonably successful: a graft is inserted from healthy bone above to healthy bone below, by-passing the angulated abnormal area. An alternative is dual onlay grafting. It should be noted that, whereas anterior bowing (tibial kyphosis) is dangerous, posterior bowing is said to be innocuous, and to correct itself without fracture.

Other anomalies of the leg — Absence of the tibia usually demands amputation. Absence of the whole or part of the fibula may be associated with tibial bowing, with leg shortening or with absence of the fourth or fifth rays of the foot. Leg lengthening is exceedingly difficult, and if osteotomy seems inappropriate amputation (preferably Syme's) is needed.

Congenital pseudarthrosis of the clavicle is probably due to pressure by the subclavian artery on the developing clavicle. In every reported unilateral case the right side has been affected — except in one patient with dextrocardia. The child is brought up with a painless lump. Treatment, if required, is by excision or grafting.

PAGET'S DISEASE (Osteitis deformans)

The cause of this common disease (3 per cent of people over 40) is unknown, although the curious geographic distribution (for example the notable rarity in Norway and Japan) should provide a clue. It is characterized by high rates of bone formation and resorption; the plasma alkaline phosphatase and hydroxyproline are high and there is increased excretion of hydroxyproline in the urine.

In the so-called vascular stage, the spaces left by bone absorption fill with vascular fibrous tissue. On both sides of the cortex new osteoid tissue forms, but it is not converted to mature bone; hence, although thick, the bone is soft and bends. Moreover, the new lamellae are not regularly arranged so that later (in the so-called sclerotic stage) even though the lamellae calcify and become thick and sclerosed, the bone is easily broken.

CLINICAL FEATURES

Paget's disease affects men and women equally. Only occasionally does it present in patients of under 50, but from that age onwards it becomes increasingly common. The disease may for many years remain localized to part or the whole of one bone, the pelvis and tibia being the commonest sites, the femur, skull, spine and clavicle the next commonest.

When only a single bone is affected it becomes painful and bent. The pain is a dull constant ache which is worse at night but rarely becomes severe unless fracture occurs or sarcoma supervenes. Diagnosis is easy; the bone looks bent, feels thick, and the skin over it is unduly warm; hence the term 'osteitis deformans'.

The patient with generalized Paget's disease may have few complaints, but a wide variety of distressing symptoms can occur: headache, deafness, deformities, stiffness, limb pain and sometimes fractures and heart failure. The skull enlarges so that bigger hats are required. Otosclerosis may produce deafness and occasionally pressure on the optic nerve produces blindness. There is considerable kyphosis so that the patient becomes shorter and apelike, with bent legs and his arms hanging in

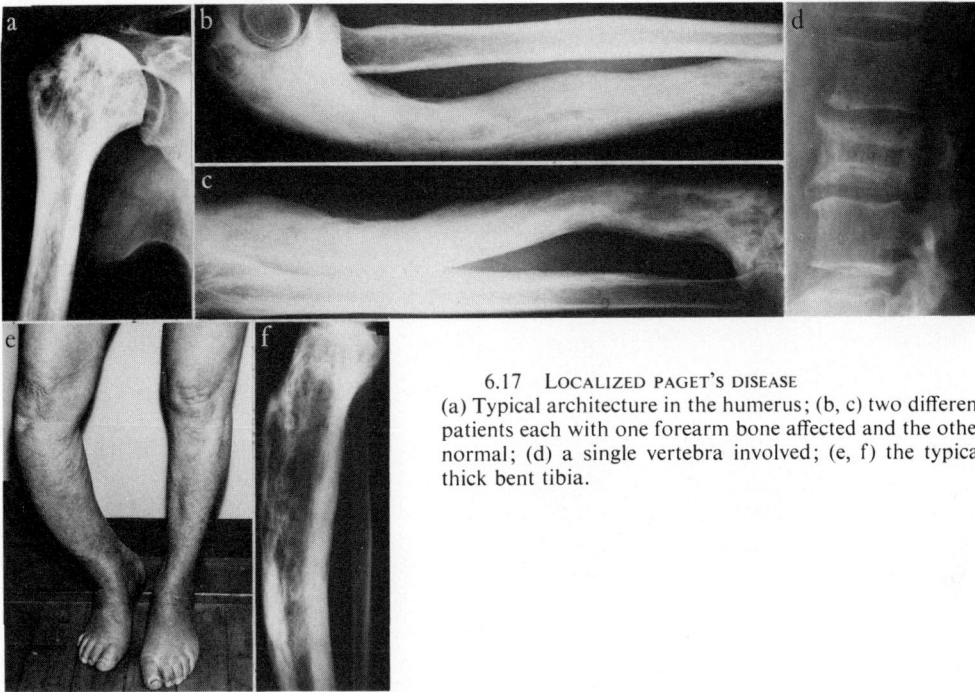

6.17 LOCALIZED PAGET'S DISEASE
(a) Typical architecture in the humerus; (b, c) two different patients each with one forearm bone affected and the other normal; (d) a single vertebra involved; (e, f) the typical thick bent tibia.

front of him. Backache and root pain are common. There is slight coxa vara, and considerable anterolateral bowing of the legs. When the disease extends up to a joint surface, that joint is usually stiffish and deformed.

X-rays show that the bone as a whole is thick and bent; its density in the vascular stage is decreased and in the sclerotic stage increased. The trabeculae are coarse and widely separated, giving a streaky or honeycomb appearance. In the vascular stage, areas of porosis shaped like a candle flame are seen in the cortex. Later, the thick cortex often shows, on its convex aspect, fine subperiosteal cracks probably resulting from stress; the junction of cortex and medulla is indistinct.

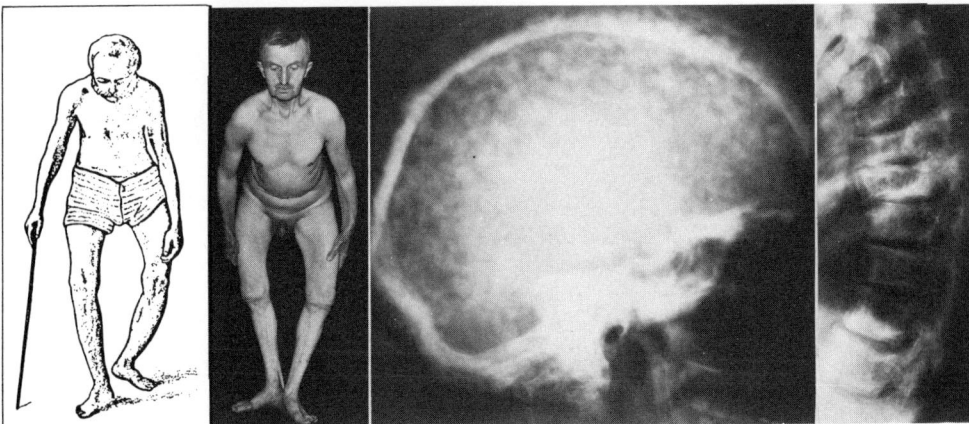

6.18 GENERALIZED PAGET'S DISEASE
Paget's original case compared with a modern photograph. The skull and spine are characteristic.

COMPLICATIONS

The most important general complication is high output cardiac failure. The possibility of deafness and occasionally of optic atrophy has already been mentioned.

The chief local complications are sarcoma and fracture. Paget's disease is one of the few causes of bone sarcoma occurring in an elderly patient, but the frequency is uncertain, published figures varying between 1 and 11 per cent. Sarcoma may be the presenting symptom; it should certainly be suspected if a previously diseased bone becomes more painful, swollen and tender.

Fractures are common in Paget's disease, especially in the femur. In the femoral neck they are often vertical, elsewhere the fracture line is usually partly transverse and partly oblique, like the line of section of a felled tree.

In spite of all these complications most patients with Paget's disease come to terms with the condition and live to a ripe old age.

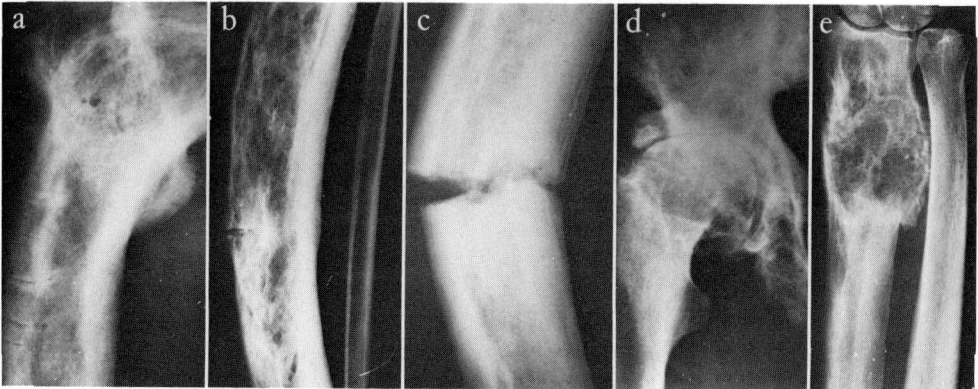

6.19 COMPLICATIONS OF PAGET'S DISEASE
(a) Fine cracks (micro-fractures) on the convex aspect, often associated with pain; (b) incomplete fracture; (c) the characteristic line of a complete fracture; (d) secondary osteoarthritis; (e) sarcoma.

TREATMENT

Until recently treatment was necessarily symptomatic, but now drugs which suppress bone turnover are becoming available, notably calcitonin, diphosphonates, glucagon and mithramycin; they are more likely to be effective when the disease is active and bone turnover is high. Persistent pain is the usual indication, but drugs have also been used in the hope of slowing or even reversing the process in the relatively young.

Calcitonin is the most widely used drug. It inhibits osteoclastic activity and lowers the levels of the serum alkaline phosphatase and the urinary hydroxyproline. 50–100 I.U. are injected, daily for three to six months, then three times a week for a further six months; but if no pain relief occurs within six weeks of beginning, further treatment is probably not worthwhile. Salmon calcitonin is 40 times more potent than porcine and is less likely to give allergic reactions, though a preliminary scratch test is advisable. Diphosphonates can be given orally, but are not yet generally available. Combinations of calcitonin and diphosphonates may prove useful.

Fractures occurring in Paget's disease sometimes unite slowly if they occur during the sclerotic stage. Because of this, and also because the patients are usually elderly, internal fixation is frequently employed. The operation must be performed with great care for there is a risk of splitting the sclerotic bone. No matter whether external splintage or internal fixation is used, advantage should be taken of the fracture to straighten the bone.

Suggestions for further reading

Aegerter, F and Kirkpatrick, J. A. (1975). *Orthopaedic Diseases.* 4th Edn. Philadelphia; Saunders

Bailey, J. A. (1970). 'Orthopaedic Aspects of Achondroplasia'. *J. Bone Jt Surg.* **52A**, 1285

Barry, H. C. (1969). *Paget's Disease of Bone.* Edinburgh and London; Livingstone

Brenton, D. P. *et al.* (1972). 'Homocystinuria and Marfan's Syndrome'. *J. Bone Jt Surg.* **54B**, 277

Fixsen, J. A. and Lloyd-Roberts, G. C. (1974). 'The Natural History and Early Treatment of Proximal Femoral Dysplasia.' *J. Bone Jt Surg.* **56B**, 86

Hardinge, K. (1972). 'Congenital Anterior Bowing of the Tibia.' *Ann. R. Coll. Surg. Engl.* **51**, 17

Henry, A. (1969). 'Monostotic Fibrous Dysplasia.' *J. Bone Jt Surg.* **51B**, 300

Hoover, G. H. *et al.* (1970). 'The Hand and Apert's Syndrome.' *J. Bone Jt Surg.* **52A**, 878

King, J. D. and Bobechko, W. P. (1971). 'Osteogenesis Imperfecta.' *J. Bone Jt Surg.* **53B**, 72

Lloyd-Roberts, G. C. (1971). *Orthopaedics in Infancy and Childhood.* London; Butterworths

Lloyd-Roberts, G. C., Apley, A. G. and Owen, R. (1975). 'Reflections upon the Aetiology of Congenital Pseudarthrosis of the Clavicle.' *J. Bone Jt Surg.* **57B**, 24

Russell, R. G. G. and Smith, R. (1973). 'Diphosphonates.' *J. Bone Jt Surg.* **55B**, 66

Wynne-Davies, R. (1973). *Heritable Disorders in Orthopaedic Practice.* Oxford; Blackwell

Wynne-Davies, R. and Fairbank, T. J. (1976). *Fairbank's Atlas of General Affections of the Skeleton.* Edinburgh; Churchill Livingstone

CHAPTER 7

NUTRITIONAL, METABOLIC AND ENDOCRINE DISORDERS

RICKETS AND OSTEOMALACIA

Vitamin D deficiency causes rickets in children and osteomalacia in adults. The causes of deficiency are: inadequate diet; insufficient sunshine (usually combined with inadequate diet); malabsorption (in coeliac disease, steatorrhoea, obstructive jaundice and other disorders); and a defect of vitamin D metabolism. Whatever its cause, vitamin D deficiency leads to reduced absorption of calcium and phosphorus. Compensatory hyperparathyroidism helps to restore the serum calcium to normal and contributes to the low serum phosphorus. The serum alkaline phosphatase is high and the plasma 25-hydroxycholecalciferol is low. The disorder is rare in Britain, though less so in immigrants.

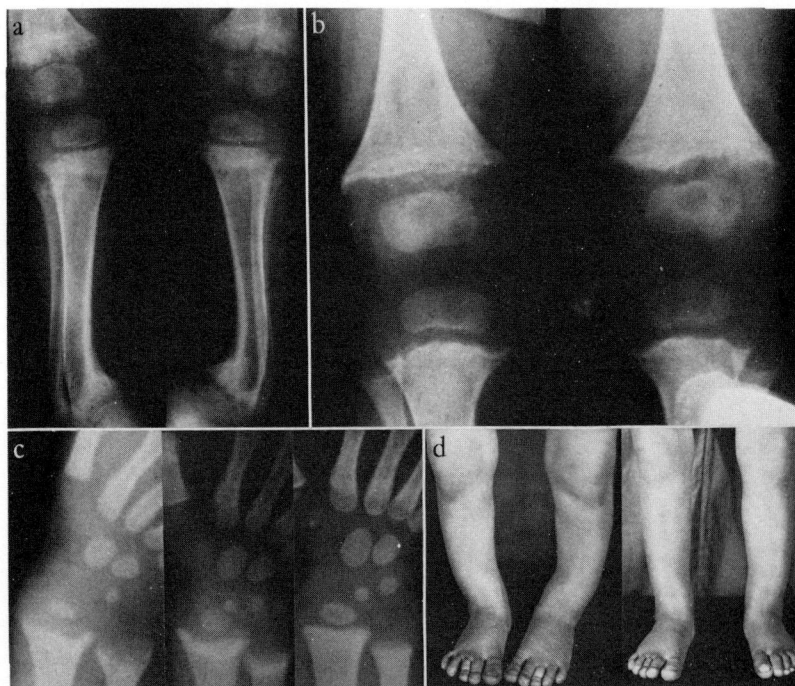

7.1 RICKETS
(a, b) Florid disease; (c) series showing the response to treatment; (d) before and after osteotomy for the neglected case.

CLINICAL FEATURES

CHILDREN — The infant with rickets is fretful, restless, and liable to bronchitis and diarrhoea; in the first few months tetany or convulsions may occur. Thereafter secondary bone changes are evident; enlargement of bone ends; bending of long bones (coxa vara, bowed femora, knock knees and bow legs); bossing of the skull (' hot-cross-bun head '); and enlargement of the costo-chondral junctions (' rickety rosary '). Dentition is delayed, bone pain not uncommon, and the muscles are flabby. X-rays show general decalcification, epiphyses which appear late, growth discs which are too deep and metaphyses which are too wide.

ADULTS — The adult with osteomalacia may feel unwell with back ache, bone pain and tenderness, and muscle weakness. Predisposing factors include pregnancy, prolonged anticonvulsant therapy and a previous gastrectomy. X-rays show general decalcification and also Looser's zones (pseudo-fractures). These begin as compression stress fractures, often symmetrical, especially in the scapulae, ribs, pubis and femoral neck; they are incomplete fractures which heal with callus lacking in calcium, hence their translucence. Diagnosis can be confirmed by iliac crest biopsy which shows excessive uncalcified osteoid.

TREATMENT

Vitamin D must be given (orally or parenterally), any underlying cause dealt with, and an adequate intake of calcium ensured. Deformity in children may improve; otherwise osteotomy is indicated.

RENAL (Uraemic) OSTEODYSTROPHY

By definition the patient has chronic renal disease. The skeletal consequences are: (a) Rickets or osteomalacia, because the diseased kidney fails to complete the metabolism of vitamin D; (b) osteosclerosis (and sometimes soft-tissue calcification) because the reduced renal excretion leads to a raised serum phosphorus; and (c) osteitis fibrosa, because the combination of high serum phosphorus and low vitamin D results in low serum calcium, which stimulates excessive secretion of parathormone.

Most patients present with renal symptoms. The children are stunted, pasty-faced and with rachitic deformities. X-rays show a mixture of changes: the growth discs are often wide as in rickets, but the bone density is often increased (osteosclerosis); in addition the cystic changes of osteitis fibrosa may occasionally be present and

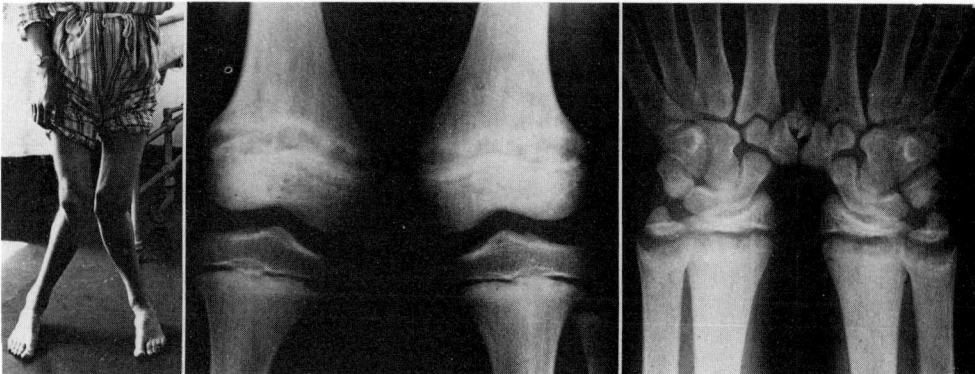

7.2 RENAL OSTEODYSTROPHY
Gross knock knee in an adolescent is suspicious; the wide irregular growth discs are almost diagnostic. The wrists usually show the changes particularly well.

sometimes the epiphyses (especially of the lower radius and upper femur) look as if they are slipping off the shafts.

The renal condition must of course be treated. With evidence of rickets or osteomalacia vitamin D is given; minute doses of 1.25 dihydroxycholecalciferol are said to be effective. Hyperphosphataemia is treated with aluminium hydroxide; and occasionally the hyperparathyroidism requires operative treatment.

HYPOPHOSPHATAEMIA

Impaired renal tubular reabsorption results in a low serum phosphorus level; the serum calcium is normal but the alkaline phosphatase level may be raised. Three forms of the disease are described, the first two occurring in children.

Familial hypophosphataemia is a genetic disorder of sex-linked dominant inheritance. The children present with rickets-like deformities, are short in stature and easily fatigued.

Cystinosis is of autosomal recessive inheritance. Cystine is deposited in the kidney (among other tissues) and renal failure may supervene. The clinical picture again is of a stunted child with rachitic deformities.

Wilson's disease is one of a group of disorders which present in adults with bone pain and muscle weakness; others include hereditary tyrosinaemia and excessive intake of aluminium hydroxide antacids.

TREATMENT

Massive doses of vitamin D used to be given (familial hypophosphataemia was formerly called ' vitamin-resistant rickets ', a term which should be abandoned). Nowadays only small doses of vitamin D are given, but combined with high doses of oral phosphorus; careful monitoring of dosage is essential. Adults may require calcium supplements.

HYPOPHOSPHATASIA

In this disease of autosomal dominant inheritance the enzyme alkaline phosphatase is lacking. Consequently, even though the supply of vitamin D may be adequate, calcium is not deposited in bone. In the severe neo-natal form the infant dies in the first year. Milder forms present with rachitic deformities in childhood or recurrent fractures in adults. No specific treatment is available but spontaneous improvement commonly occurs.

NOTE — *Hyperphosphatasia* is a very rare recessively inherited disorder which presents clinically as juvenile Paget's disease.

HYPERPARATHYROIDISM

Parathormone is chiefly concerned with the homeostasis of calcium. The hormone decreases excretion of calcium and increases that of phosphorus. Excess parathormone from an adenoma (which may be part of multiple endocrine adenomas) or from hyperplasia (occasionally familial) causes hypercalcaemia. Bone changes are uncommon (10–20 per cent) and sometimes called osteitis fibrosa.

The patients, usually middle-aged women, present with fatigue, lethargy and occasionally bone pain (the bones may bend or break). Kidney stones, pancreatitis or peptic ulceration may occur. Occasionally gout or pseudogout may follow the hyperuricaemia which often accompanies hyperparathyroidism.

X-rays show a mixture of cystic changes, erosions, coarsening of the trabecular pattern, osteoporosis and occasionally patchy sclerosis. The skull looks granular

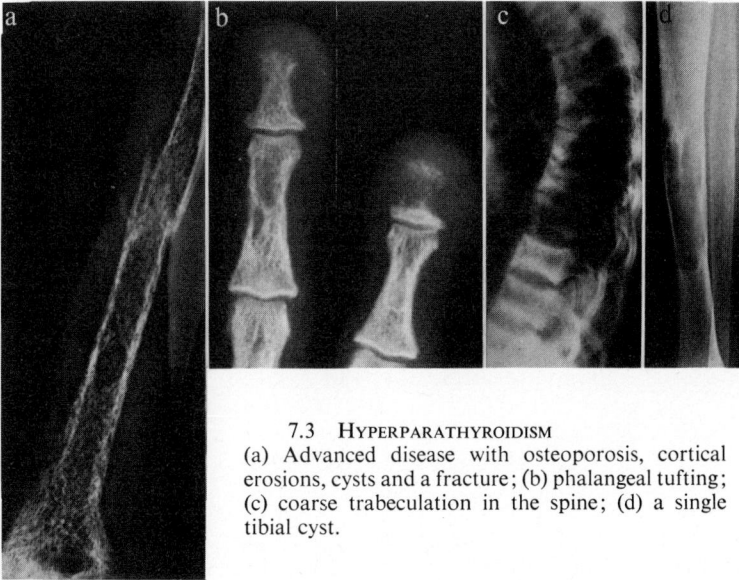

7.3 HYPERPARATHYROIDISM
(a) Advanced disease with osteoporosis, cortical erosions, cysts and a fracture; (b) phalangeal tufting; (c) coarse trabeculation in the spine; (d) a single tibial cyst.

and fuzzy ('pepper-pot skull'); in the spine the vertical trabeculae alone may be visible. The long bones show sub-periosteal erosions and multiple cysts (the so-called 'brown tumours' look cystic on x-ray). The hands show characteristic changes; scalloping of the middle phalanges, and 'tufting' of the terminal phalanges, that is disappearance of the outline with only longitudinal trabeculae remaining.

Following removal of the adenoma or part of the hyperplastic tissue, the bone changes regress.

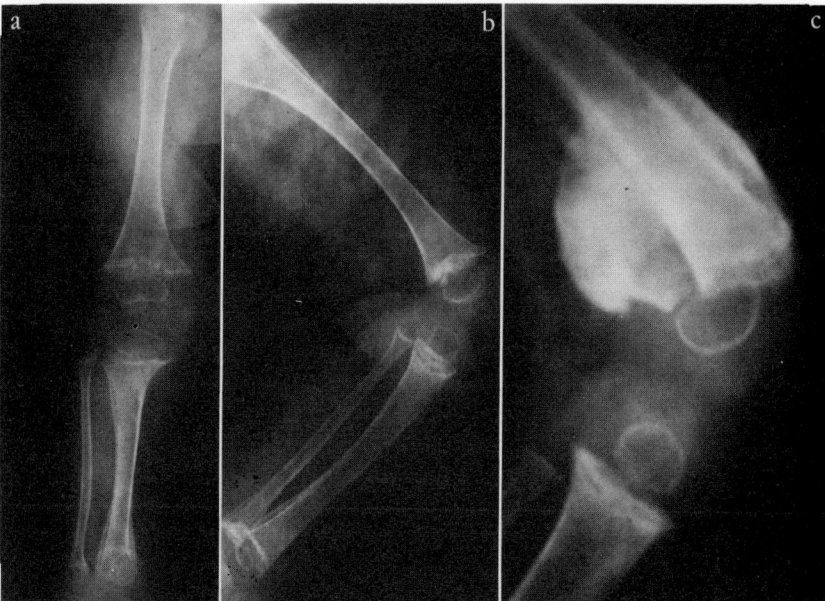

7.4 SCURVY
(a, b) The ring sign, the corner sign, and small subperiosteal haemorrhages; (c) the femoral epiphysis has displaced, and the subperiosteal haemorrhage has calcified.

INFANTILE SCURVY (Barlow's disease)

The diet is deficient in vitamin C. Cartilage calcifies but does not form normal osteoid tissue.

The infant is a poor specimen, irritable, pale, undernourished, anaemic and, in severe cases, with spongy gums. Subperiosteal haemorrhages occur with pain, swelling and extreme tenderness. Rickets may coexist. Fractures and epiphyseal separations may occur and they heal slowly.

On x-ray there may be general rarefaction, but this is most marked in the epiphyses which become almost translucent, though their periphery remains distinct (ring sign); the metaphysis looks normal, but a band of translucency extends just deep to it, and if this band involves the cortex the metaphyseal edge looks curiously unsupported (corner sign); calcification in subperiosteal haemorrhages may also be visible.

Treatment consists in giving large doses of vitamin C in concentrated form.

HYPERVITAMINOSIS

Hypervitaminosis A occurs in children following excessive dosage; in adults it occurs only in explorers who eat Polar bear livers. There may be bone pain, and headache and vomiting due to raised intra-cranial pressure. X-ray shows increased density in the submetaphyseal region and subperiosteal calcification.

Hypervitaminosis D occurs if too much vitamin D is given. It exerts a parathormone-like effect so that, as in the underlying rickets, calcium is withdrawn from bones; but metastatic calcification occurs. In treatment the dose of vitamin D must be properly regulated and the infant given a low calcium diet but plentiful fluids.

OSTEOPOROSIS

Reduction of bone density (osteopenia) occurs in a variety of conditions including osteoporosis and osteomalacia. The characteristic feature of osteoporosis is that the bone, though reduced in quantity per unit volume, is otherwise normal; bone resorption has outstripped bone formation. Ageing is accompanied by gradually increasing osteoporosis, a normal process sometimes accelerated by inactivity and diminished food intake. Osteoporosis is also liable to develop soon after the menopause, perhaps because of endocrine involution. In younger patients it may occur following paralysis or immobilization, with rheumatoid arthritis, liver disease, Cushing's disease or brittle bones; and occasionally idiopathically.

CLINICAL FEATURES

The patients, usually women, do not complain of osteoporosis, which is symptomless, but of the complications resulting from weakened bone. Fractures occur with little force, especially in the spine, lower radius and femoral neck. Backache is common and loss of height with thoracic kyphosis an early feature.

The widespread osteoporosis is readily seen in x-rays of the spine, where the soft vertebral bodies are indented by the discs and become biconcave. One or more vertebrae may be wedged because of fractures.

TREATMENT

Post-menopausal bone loss can possibly be prevented by oestrogen therapy, providing this begins fairly soon after the menopause. Apart from this osteoporosis cannot be prevented. Treatment aims at diminishing further bone loss and managing

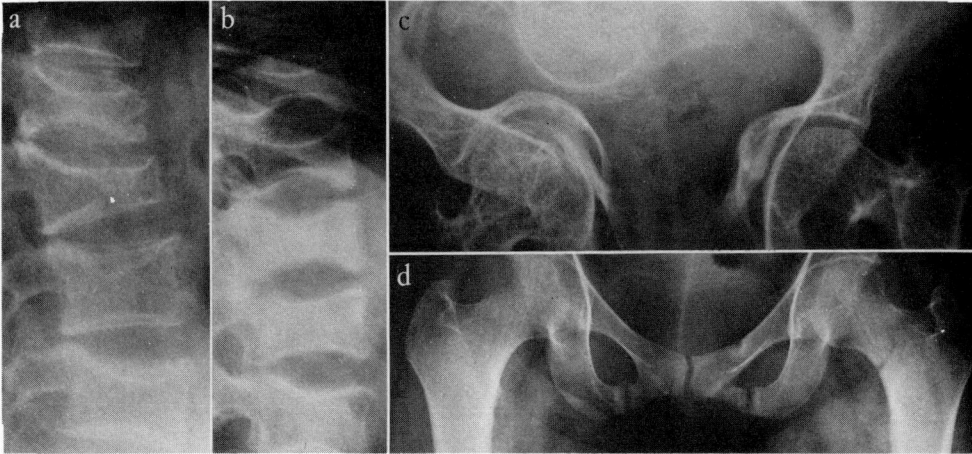

7.5 OSTEOPOROSIS AND OSTEOMALACIA
(a) Senile osteoporosis with fracture; (b) ballooned discs and biconcave vertebrae;
(c) in this brittle-bone patient the bone softening has resulted in a triradiate pelvis;
and (d) osteomalacia with Looser's zones in the pubis and left femoral neck.

the complications. It is important to ensure that the ageing are kept active and that their diet contains enough proteins, minerals and vitamins. Improvement has been reported with fluoride therapy supplemented by calcium and vitamin D. Fractures should be treated by methods which minimize or avoid immobilization of the patient. It is important to remember that these patients (unlike those with osteomalacia) are not ill, nor affected by muscle weakness or generalized pain. The distinction is especially important in the elderly where both conditions may co-exist, and because osteomalacia can be corrected by vitamin D.

Osteomalacia	Osteoporosis
Common in ageing women	
Prone to pathological fracture	
Decreased bone density	
Ill	Not ill
Generalized chronic ache	Pain only after fracture
Muscles weak	Muscles normal
Looser's zones	No Looser's zones
Alkaline phosphatase increased	Normal
Serum phosphorus decreased	Normal
Sedimentation rate raised	Sedimentation rate normal
Usually responds to vitamin D	No response to vitamin D

JUVENILE OSTEOPOROSIS

Very occasionally a young patient with backache is x-rayed and found to have osteoporosis—despite normal blood chemistry. The temptation to administer potentially dangerous drugs should be resisted, for the condition recovers spontaneously.

Suggestions for further reading

Dent, C. E. and Watson, L. (1966). 'Osteoporosis', Supplement to *Postgrad. med. J.*, October, 1966

Mankin, H. J. (1974). 'Rickets, Osteomalacia, and Renal Osteodystrophy.' *J. Bone Jt Surg.* **56A,** 101 (Part I), **56A,** 352 (Part II)

Nordin, B. E. C. (1971). 'Clinical Significance and Pathogenesis of Osteoporosis.' *Br. med. J.*, **1,** 571

Paterson, C. R. (1974). *Metabolic disorders of Bone.* Oxford; Blackwell

CHAPTER 8

TUMOURS

CLASSIFICATION

The World Health Organization (1972) has proposed a classification of bone tumours, of which the following is an abstract:

Bone-forming tumours — including osteoma, osteoblastoma and osteosarcoma.

Cartilage-forming tumours — including chondroma, chondroblastoma, and chondrosarcoma.

Giant-cell tumours — which form a group on their own.

Marrow tumours — including Ewing's tumour and myeloma.

Vascular tumours — including haemangioma, glomus tumours and angiosarcomas.

Other connective tissue tumours — including lipoma, liposarcoma and fibrosarcoma.

Other tumours — including chondroma, adamantinoma, neurilemmoma and neurofibroma.

For completeness they add a further group of 'tumour-like lesions', such as bone cysts, fibrous dysplasia and eosinophilic granuloma which in this book are described elsewhere. In the present chapter benign tumours of bone are described first, doubtful ones next, then malignant bone tumours; the final section deals with soft tissue tumours and lumps.

BENIGN OR MALIGNANT?

A benign tumour remains local; from a malignant tumour cells may migrate to distant sites and grow parasitically.

Nearly all benign bone tumours occur in adolescents or in young adults, and stop growing when bone growth is complete. Their benign character is displayed on x-ray by their clearly defined edges.

All the primary malignant bone tumours (except the very rare parosteal fibrosarcoma) are highly malignant and usually fatal. They occur in young people, are painful, and have no definite margin on x-ray.

It should be clearly understood that all primary bone tumours, whether benign or malignant are rare; this is in contrast with secondary deposits in bone which, especially over the age of 50, are relatively common.

OSTEOMA

CANCELLOUS OSTEOMA (exostosis) — Strictly speaking this is a minor disorder of growth rather than a true tumour. It consists of a conical lump of bone with a cap of cartilage; it arises by a broad base from the metaphysis of a normal bone and points away from the growing end. It stops enlarging when bone growth ceases and does not invade or metastasize.

An adolescent presents with a painless lump at the growing end of a long bone, the knee being a favourite site. Although the lump is bony hard, it may be covered by a bursa. Occasionally the lump interferes with tendon action. On x-ray the medulla and

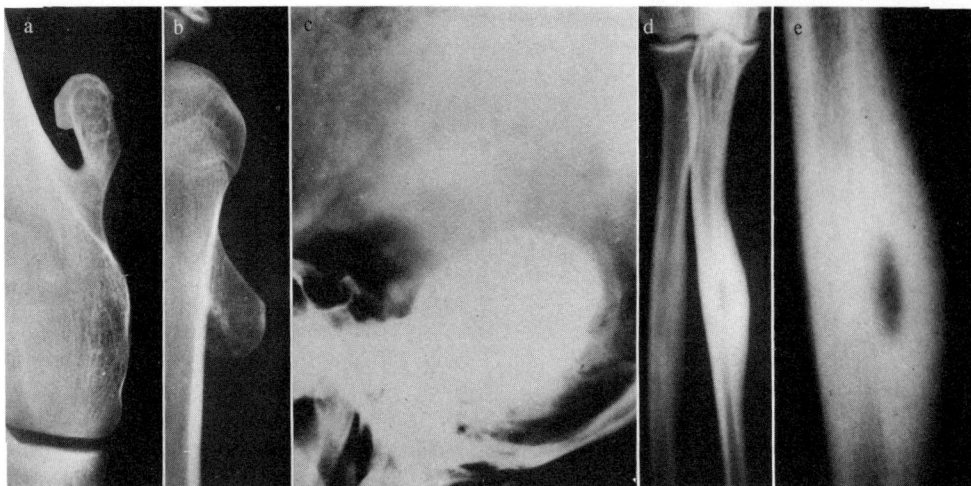

8.1 VARIETIES OF OSTEOMA
(a, b) Cancellous osteoma (simple exostosis), pointing away from the growth disc;
(c) compact (ivory) osteoma, made of excessively dense bone; (d) osteoid osteoma;
(e) enlarged view of the same case to show the translucent nidus.

cortex of the tumour are continuous with the parent bone via a broad base at the meta-physis.

The diagnosis is from diaphyseal aclasis in which the metaphyses look irregular and there are multiple exostoses.   If a cancellous osteoma is troublesome it is excised.

COMPACT OSTEOMA (ivory exostosis) — This rare tumour is said to arise from precartila-ginous cells of the epiosteum.   Microscopically only normal bone cells are seen.   Macro-scopically the tumour is a squat sessile knob of ivory-hard bone.   It does not metastasize.

An adolescent or a young adult presents with a lump.   The commonest site is the outer surface of the skull, where the only symptom is of a hard, painless lump.   The tumour may occasionally occur on the inner surface of the skull (and then give rise to focal epilepsy), or may grow into the paranasal sinuses.   On x-ray a sessile plaque of exceedingly dense bone with a well-circumscribed edge is seen.

The tumour is best excised.   It is so hard that a small area of surrounding normal bone must be excised with the tumour.

OSTEOID OSTEOMA — Microscopically the tumour consists of osteoid tissue with trabeculae of newly formed bone, in a vascular connective tissue groundwork.   It is small, usually less than 1 cm in size, round or oval in shape, and is encased in dense bone.

Osteoid osteoma is most commonly seen in patients aged 10–25 years.   Any bone except the skull may be affected and the spine is not uncommon, but over half the cases occur in the femur or tibia.   The only symptom is pain, which is sometimes severe and is not relieved by rest.   Often the pain continues for many months, and until the x-ray appearances were fully described, many patients were judged to be hysterical, especially as salicylates are sometimes effective in relieving pain.

The important x-ray feature is a small radiolucent area, the so-called 'nidus'.   In medullary lesions there may be slight surrounding sclerosis, but in the cortex thickening and sclerosis are often so dense that the nidus (which may itself contain a radio-opaque centre) can be seen only in tomograms.

It is sometimes difficult to distinguish an osteoid osteoma from a small Brodie's abscess without biopsy.   Ewing's tumour and chronic periostitis must also be excluded (*see* page 10).   Rarely, regional osteoporosis occurs with an osteoid osteoma and the x-ray appearance then resembles joint tuberculosis.

Excision of the affected area cures the pain and the tumour does not recur.

BENIGN OSTEOBLASTOMA — This rare vascular tumour, sometimes called a giant osteoid osteoma, usually affects adults.   It occurs in the spine (often with scoliosis) or the major limb bones. Pain and tenderness are features.   X-ray shows a well-demarcated osteolytic lesion which may extend to both sides of a growth disc and sometimes contains flecks of calcification.   Treatment consists of excision or curettage and bone grafting.

CHONDROMA

SHORT BONE CHONDROMA — This, the commonest variety, arises from precartilaginous cells and consists only of normal cartilage.   The tumour is well encapsulated, often lobulated, and never becomes malignant.   It occurs in one of the short pipe bones—a metacarpal, metatarsal or proximal phalanx.

The patient, aged 10–20 years, presents with a swelling or, more commonly, with a fracture after trivial injury.   X-ray shows a well-defined rare area often with characteristic specks of calcification.   *Enchondroma* is the term used when the tumour is entirely within the medulla; the cortex is ballooned and thin, but remains intact until a fracture occurs.   An *ecchondroma* is similar but protrudes well beyond the confines of the bone.

The differential diagnosis is from a solitary cyst (which has no calcification), and from dyschondroplasia (in which the chondromas are multiple).   The tumour with its lining capsule should be excised and a bone graft or chips inserted.

LONG BONE CHONDROMA — A true chondroma may rarely involve a long bone.   The patient, a teenager or young adult, may complain of a constant ache.   X-ray shows a rare area usually well-defined and with a mottled appearance due to irregular calcification. Malignancy may supervene and the tumour is therefore best excised.

8.2   CHONDROMA
AND OSTEO-
CHONDROMA
(a)   enchondroma;   (b) ecchondroma; (c) benign chondroblastoma;

(d, e) osteochondromata.

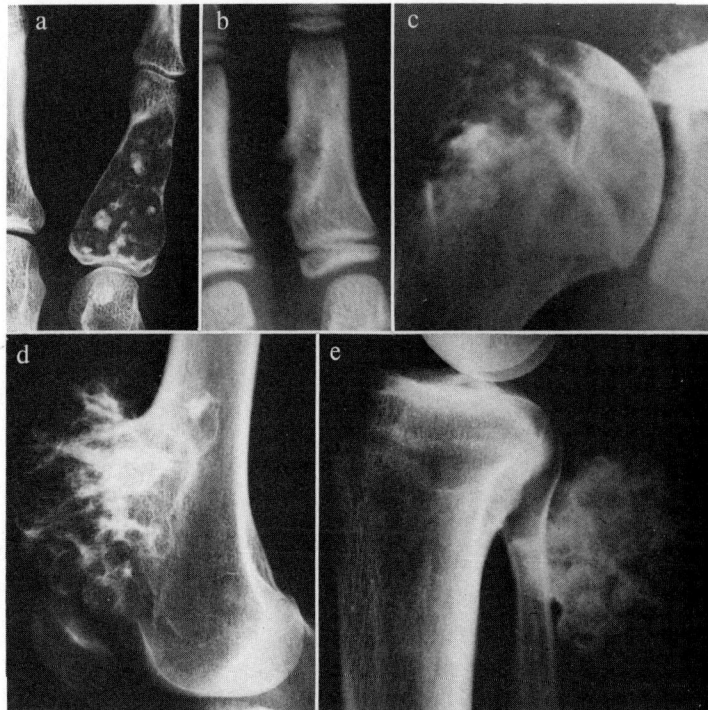

FLAT BONE CHONDROMA — It is almost impossible to make a confident clinical diagnosis of chondroma in a flat bone; usually the tumour proves to be a benign chondroblastoma or an osteochondroma (*see* below).   The tumour should, if possible, be excised.

BENIGN CHONDROBLASTOMA — This is a rare tumour in which the cells, instead of being normal chondrocytes are immature chondroblasts.   The tumour starts in the epiphysis, usually of the proximal humerus or femur, though the pelvis or other bones can be affected.   Males are more commonly affected, especially in their 'teens or twenties, and the presenting symptom is a constant ache gradually increasing in severity.   X-ray shows a well-defined area of rarefaction eccentrically placed in the epiphysis, with no reaction in the surrounding bone.   Malignant change does not occur, and simple curettage is the best treatment.

OSTEOCHONDROMA

The tumour arises from precartilaginous cells.   On section, areas of normal bone and cartilage cells are seen.   Macroscopically, a big, lobulated, cauliflower-like mass arises from a wide base and is covered by a cap of cartilage.

The patient is usually aged 10–25 years.   He presents with a large lump which is painless, although occasionally there may be slight ache or interference with the action of a tendon.   The commonest site is the growing end of a long bone, especially around the knee.   Occasionally an osteochondroma arises from the pelvis or scapula.   If the lump is growing from the inner aspect of the pelvis, intra-pelvic pressure may develop.   The lump is large, sessile, lobulated, attached to bone but not to skin or muscle, and is not tender.

On x-ray the tumour can be seen to arise from within the medulla of the parent bone.   It has a broad base, is large and lobulated.   There is irregular calcification.   The cartilage cap is invisible on x-ray and no clearly defined separation into cortex and medulla is seen.

It is thought that in 1–2 per cent of cases, the tumour becomes malignant in adult life; it then becomes larger, painful and the outline on x-ray becomes more fluffy. The tumour should therefore be excised.   Excision may be technically difficult because of the anatomical site.

OTHER BENIGN TUMOURS

ANEURYSMAL BONE CYST — This tumour-like lesion contains cavities filled with blood.   It chiefly occurs in the spine and the metaphysis of long bones.   It is an expanding lesion thinning and destroying the cortex.   Because of its rarefied appearance on x-ray it can resemble a giant-cell tumour, but it usually occurs at a younger age and is benign. Curettage gives good results.

HAEMANGIOMA — When this rare tumour occurs in the spine it is a source of persistent backache.   X-rays show vertical striations which can be distinguished from Paget's disease by the lack of bone expansion.   In the skull and pelvis the so-called ' sun burst ' or ' soap bubble ' appearance with radiating spicules is typical and may suggest malignancy, but there is no associated cortical or medullary destruction.   In the pipe bones a haemangioma may cause elongation of the bone; usually it presents as a pathological fracture.   X-ray shows a shaggy trabeculated tumour expanding the bone.   At operation these tumours bleed profusely, and radiotherapy is a wiser method of treatment.

FIBROUS TUMOURS — *Fibrous cortical defect* is a benign 'tumour' of children.   It is discovered accidentally on x-ray, which shows a gap in the cortex of a long bone metaphysis; the margin is well-defined, sometimes scalloped and often sclerosed.   Most of these

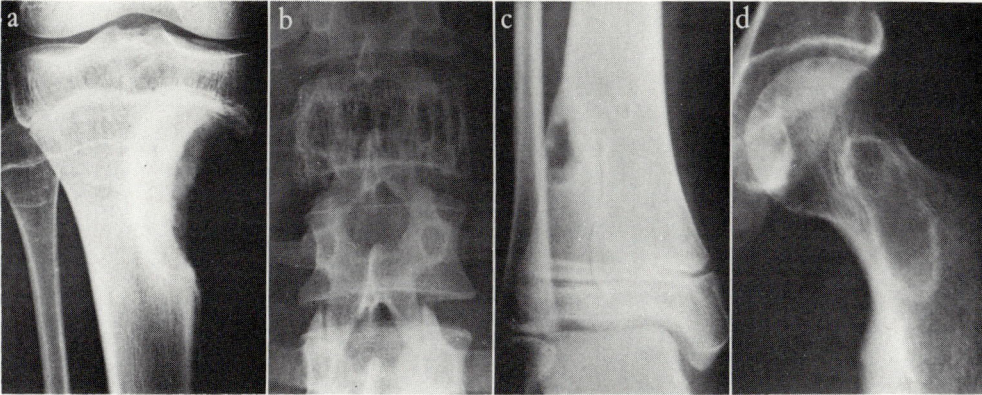

8.3 OTHER BENIGN TUMOURS
(a) Aneurysmal bone cyst; (b) haemangioma of vertebra; (c) fibrous cortical defect
(if large, this is sometimes called a non-ossifying fibroma); (d) chondromyxoid
fibroma.

defects heal spontaneously, but it seems likely that some may grow, so that pathological
fracture is a possibility; these larger varieties are seen in adolescents and are called *non-ossifying fibromas*.

Chondromyxoid fibroma is entirely different. It presents as a chronic ache in patients
aged 10 to 30; the lower limb is usually involved. X-rays show a round or oval rare area
often eccentrically placed in the metaphysis, but occasionally crossing the growth disc.
Malignant change has been recorded and though curettage may prove adequate, where
feasible the tumour should be resected.

GIANT-CELL TUMOUR

PATHOLOGY

The adjective 'benign' was formerly used but is misleading: only about one-third
remain truly benign; one-third become locally invasive, and one-third metastasize.

Most giant-cell tumours consist of a stroma of spindle cells containing large num-
bers of multinucleated giant cells in a vascular framework. Some have fewer giant
cells each of which has only a few nuclei; these are thought to be more malignant.
Grading on a cellular basis is used but is not prognostically reliable.

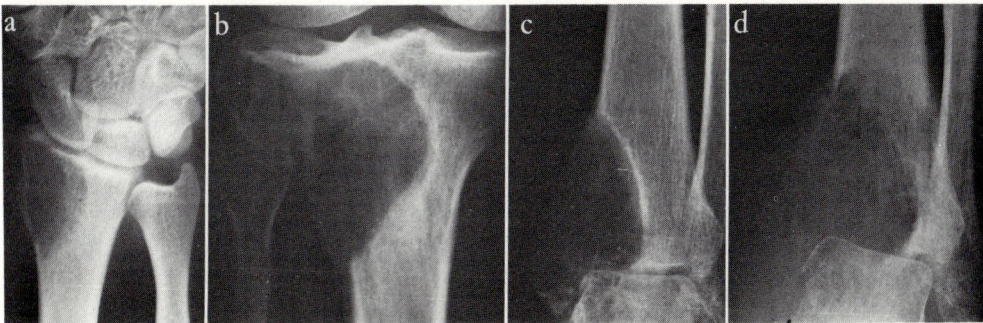

8.4 GIANT-CELL TUMOURS
(a, b, c) In each of these the tumour abuts against the joint margin, and is asymmetrically placed — these are characteristic features; in (d) malignant change has supervened and the junction of the tumour with the rest of the bone is no longer well
defined.

Macroscopically the tumour is large and asymmetrically placed at the end of a bone.   It looks reddish-brown, oozes blood and often contains patches of fat.

CLINICAL FEATURES

The tumour usually occurs between the ages of 20 and 40.   It is nearly always situated at the very end of a long bone.   Possibly, however, it originates in the metaphysis but grows so rapidly that by the time it is seen clinically, it abuts against the joint.   The usual presenting symptom is vague discomfort, sometimes with slight swelling.   A history of trauma is not uncommon and pathological fracture occurs in 10–15 per cent of cases.

On examination, there is a vague swelling of the end of a long bone.   (Egg-shell crackling is rare nowadays because of early diagnosis.)   The neighbouring joint is often irritated.

X-rays show a rarefied area situated asymmetrically at the end of a long bone abutting against the articular surface.   Often there are trabeculae and a 'soap-bubble' appearance.   So long as the tumour is benign there is a sharp, clearly-defined line of junction with the rest of the bone.   The cortex is very thin and sometimes ballooned, but is intact unless a fracture has occurred.

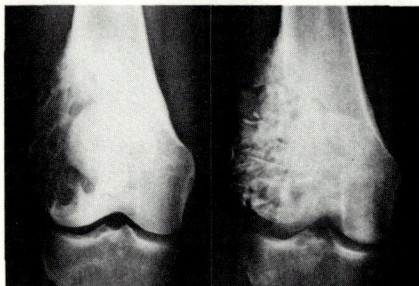

8.5   GIANT-CELL TUMOUR
Treatment by excision and bone grafts.

TREATMENT

Wide excision is the treatment of choice where the site permits.   Radical radiotherapy (5000–6000 r in 5–6 weeks) produces reasonably good results and is used where excision would severely impair function.   Sometimes excision and radiotherapy are combined.   If malignancy has already supervened the alternatives are radiotherapy or amputation.

CHORDOMA

This rare tumour arises from notochordal remnants.   The usual site is the sacrococcygeal spine but the cervical spine can be affected.   The tumour has been called 'benign' because metastasis is rare; but it is locally malignant, growing to a large size and invading surrounding structures.   It may present as a lump, or with pain from nerve involvement, or with pelvic obstruction.   The usual x-ray appearance is a large osteolytic area in the mid-line, occasionally containing flecks of calcification.   If excision is not feasible radiotherapy should be tried.

OSTEOSARCOMA

PATHOLOGY

Osteosarcoma (formerly called osteogenic sarcoma) implies a primary tumour arising from bone and producing bone.

Primitive spindle cells with numerous mitoses are characteristic. Their products may be predominantly fibroblasts (when the tumour looks like a 'fibrosarcoma'), chondroblasts (when it looks like a 'chondrosarcoma') or mucoid cells (when it looks like a 'myxosarcoma'). But these are all variants of one tumour. In addition there are bone cells of two main varieties: osteoblasts which lay down bone, and giant-cell osteoclasts which destroy bone.

The macroscopic appearance is enormously variable, but the tumour is a big one situated in the metaphysis. If bone destruction predominates, the tumour is very soft and vascular (osteolytic); if there is a fair amount of bone formation, it is more grey and gritty (osteoblastic).

The tumour extends within the medulla, destroying bone. The cortex is eroded and sooner or later perforated. The periosteum is not at first penetrated but is pushed away from the shaft. New bone may be laid down along the Haversian canals (sun-ray spicules) and at the angles of periosteal elevation (Codman's triangle). Eventually the periosteum is penetrated and soft tissues are then rapidly infiltrated. The tumour metastasizes via the bloodstream, chiefly to the lungs but also to other bones, commonly the skull and femur.

CLINICAL FEATURES

The incidence of osteogenic sarcoma is highest between the ages of 10 and 20 years and thereafter falls rapidly. (An older group is considered on page 93). The commonest site is at the metaphysis of a long bone, especially around the knee.

A history of trauma is present in more than half the cases but is thought to have no aetiological significance; it merely draws attention to the underlying disorder. Pain is usually the first symptom; it is constant, worse at night and gradually becomes severe. Sometimes the patient presents with a lump. A pathological fracture is rare.

On examination a lump (usually large) can nearly always be seen or felt. The overlying skin may be shiny with prominent veins. The lump feels tender and lacks a

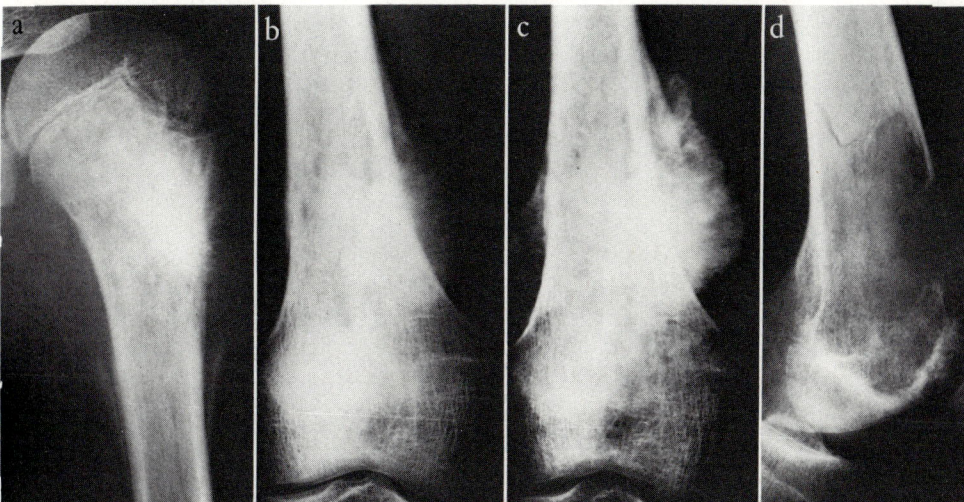

8.6 OSTEOSARCOMA
(a) Characteristic appearance with sun-ray spicules and Codman's triangle; (b) another case before, and (c) after radiotherapy; (d) predominantly osteolytic tumour.

definite edge.   It is attached to bone and often to muscles.   If growing rapidly it feels warm and it may pulsate.

The x-ray appearances are very variable but show a combination of bone destruction and bone formation.   The medulla contains an area of rarefaction, sometimes with patchy sclerosis; the tumour has an ill-defined junction with the rest of the shaft.   The cortex is somewhere perforated.   The periosteum may show sun-ray spicules and Codman's triangle; these are not common but when they do occur are characteristic.   An adjacent soft tissue mass, containing spicules of new bone, may be seen.

DIFFERENTIAL DIAGNOSIS

A painful lump near the end of a long bone in a young person must be presumed to be a sarcoma until the contrary is proved, if necessary with the aid of biopsy. Other conditions which must be considered are as follows:

(*a*) Post-traumatic swellings such as callus and myositis ossificans, which may be differentiated on x-ray.

(*b*) Infective conditions such as osteomyelitis, or syphilis of bone; in every case a white cell count and tests for syphilis are essential.

(*c*) Benign tumours which are characterized both clinically and on x-ray by a well defined edge.   The chest should always be x-rayed to exclude secondary deposits, and a biopsy must be performed.

TREATMENT

The formerly appalling prognosis has markedly improved with combined therapy, though precise figures are not yet available.   The fundamentals are simple: amputation for the primary, chemotherapy for mini-secondaries, radiotherapy in reserve.

Amputation is the mainstay of treatment, with biopsy an essential preliminary.   Formerly very high amputations were needed (e.g. above knee for even a low tibial tumour); effective chemotherapy protects against stump recurrence, and amputation through the affected bone (providing it ensures complete removal of the primary tumour) is now sufficient.

Chemotherapy aims to destroy undetectably minute (micro-, nano-, or pico-) metastases.   It must begin soon after amputation, certainly within 10 days.   The drugs are highly toxic, so must be given in centres equipped to deal with bone marrow, renal and cardiac complications.   Various protocols are under trial.   In Britain the drugs used are Doxorubicin, Vincristine and Methotrexate, a folic acid antagonist.   Huge doses of Methotrexate are used; a few hours later the patient's normal cellular activity is 'rescued' by Citrovorum factor.   Vincristine, Methotrexate and Citrovorum factor are administered at 21-day intervals, or alternating with Doxorubicin.   This regime may have debilitating side-effects and requires hospital admission for a day or two every three weeks, for at least a year.   Unsuspected secondaries may be revealed by bone scanning.   If the patient survives for 30 months a cure may reasonably be claimed.

Radiotherapy is used to control tumours at surgically inaccessible sites, such as the pelvis and jaw.

Other Methods include: (*a*) resection of solitary (or even multiple) pulmonary metastases when rendered 'static' by chemotherapy; (*b*) excision of stump recurrences, also combined with chemotherapy; (*c*) immunotherapeutic techniques are being tried (a portion of the excised tumour is implanted into a sarcoma survivor, removed after 14 days, and 'sensitized' lymphocytes from it infused into the patient).

OLDER BONE SARCOMAS

LATE OSTEOSARCOMA

Osteosarcoma is essentially a disease of young people, but a similar tumour can arise in older people as a result of malignant change in previously abnormal bone. An example is Paget's disease, although some cases of malignancy in Paget's disease are not osteosarcoma but fibrosarcoma (*see below*).

CHONDROSARCOMA

So-called 'primary chondrosarcoma' is merely a confusing name for an osteo-sarcoma in which cartilage cells predominate: the term should be abandoned because these tumours behave like any other osteosarcoma. But a true chondrosarcoma can occur, as a metaplastic change in a pre-existing osteochondroma or long-bone chondroma (the term 'secondary chondrosarcoma' may be used).

This true chondrosarcoma affects people aged 35–55. They complain of a constant ache or of recent increase in size of a previously stationary lump. The x-ray appearances are very variable, the key feature being a change in the pre-existing 'benign' tumour. The possibilities of surgical treatment are radical local excision with prosthetic replacement of the adjacent joint, or amputation. The prospects for survival are reasonable, but where neither method is practicable radiotherapy may be tried.

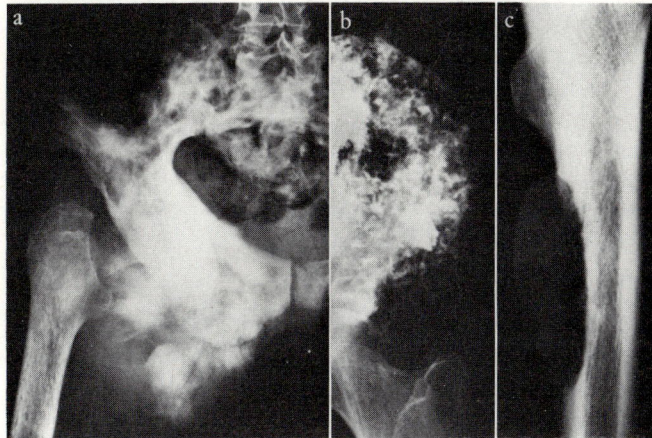

8.7 OLDER SARCOMAS (a) Osteosarcoma in Paget's disease; (b) malignant change in osteochondroma; (c) parosteal sarcoma.

FIBROSARCOMA OF BONE

The phrase 'of bone' is here added to distinguish this tumour from parosteal fibro-sarcoma described below. Fibrosarcoma of bone may arise in previously abnormal bone. (Paget's disease and irradiated giant-cell tumours are examples.)

The patients are aged over 30 (often over 50) and present with pain or a patho-logical fracture. X-rays show an osteolytic lesion which may be completely surrounded by reactive subperiosteal new bone. Treatment is by amputation or radiotherapy; the survival rate is better than that for osteosarcoma.

PAROSTEAL FIBROSARCOMA

This rare tumour does not arise from bone cells but from the fibrous layer of the periosteum. Microscopically, fibroblasts dominate the picture, macroscopically the tumour is firm, grey and encapsulated.

The patient is aged over 30.   He presents with constant ache, or a lump which is growing and which feels like hard rubber.   X-ray shows cortical erosion and sometimes the faint outline of the tumour.   Amputation gives a high cure rate, but if the site is unsuitable local excision followed by radiotherapy carries a reasonably good prognosis.

EWING'S TUMOUR (Reticulocytoma)

PATHOLOGY

The tumour arises from reticulum cells lining the marrow spaces.   Microscopically, sheets of small dark polyhedral cells with no regular arrangement and no ground substance are seen.   Macroscopically, the tumour is lobulated and often fairly large. It may look grey (like brain), or red (like red-currant jelly) if haemorrhage has occurred into it.

Local spread is similar to that of osteogenic sarcoma.   The periosteum appears to resist the tumour and may lay down layers like an onion.   Distal spread is (a) via the blood to the lungs and also often to other bones; (b) via the lymphatics.

CLINICAL FEATURES

The tumour occurs most commonly between the ages of 10 and 20 years (rarely 5 to 30).   A long bone is usually affected, especially the tibia.   The tumour is situated anywhere in the bone.

Pain and a limp are the chief presenting symptoms; the pain is throbbing, worse at night and often severe; a history of trauma is common.   The patient is sometimes ill and may be pyrexial.   The lump is warm, tender, has an ill-defined edge and is attached to bone and to soft tissues.   The pain, swelling and pyrexia may all fluctuate from time to time.

The x-ray appearances vary widely.   Sometimes a rarefied area can be seen in the medulla and often the cortex is perforated.   'Onion-layers' of visible periosteum are said to be characteristic.

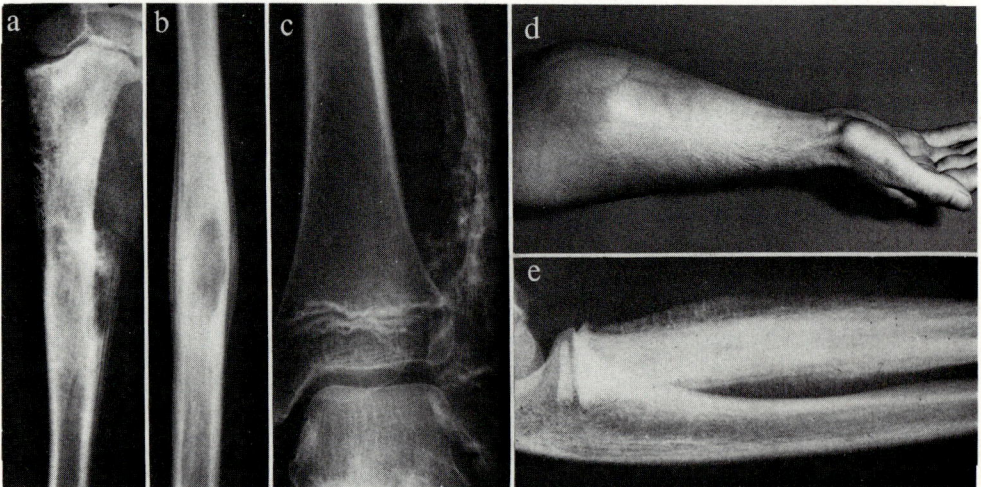

8.8   EWING'S TUMOUR
(a) Of the humerus; (b) of the mid-shaft of the fibula; (c) of the lower fibula; (d, e) secondary adrenal neuroblastoma mimicking Ewing's tumour.

DIFFERENTIAL DIAGNOSIS

Blood examination is important to exclude staphylococcal osteomyelitis (which Ewing's tumour may closely resemble) and to exclude syphilis.

Biopsy is essential to exclude other tumours affecting bone, notably adrenal neuroblastoma and reticulum-cell sarcoma; both these conditions, as well as Ewing's tumour are sometimes called 'round cell sarcomas of bone' but there are important differences.

Adrenal neuroblastoma metastasizes to bone and the deposits strongly resemble Ewing's tumour. Histologically, however, the round-cells of neuroblastoma are arranged in characteristic rosettes. In 60 per cent of neuroblastomas the urine contains the catecholamine derivative vanillylmandelic acid.

Reticulum-cell sarcoma in bone is sometimes a solitary lesion; in which case (after biopsy has established the diagnosis) radiotherapy may effect a cure. If, however, there is generalized involvement of the reticulo-endothelial system (malignant lymphoma) the prognosis is poor and treatment is by chemotherapy.

TREATMENT

Where feasible Ewing's tumour is treated by a local sterilizing dose of radiotherapy followed by actinomycin or cyclophosphamide; but the many possible variations are the subject of a world-wide trial. Surgery is not used unless, after radiotherapy, an unhealed pathological fracture causes symptoms warranting amputation.

MULTIPLE MYELOMA

PATHOLOGY

The tumours are said to arise from plasma cells of the bone marrow. The typical microscopic picture is of plasmacytes with a large eccentric nucleus containing a spoke-like arrangement of chromatin. The tumours are found wherever red marrow occurs; that is, in the trunk bones, skull and root bones. They are usually multiple from the start; they are small, and grey or purple in colour. They look like multiple secondaries, but no primary tumour is ever found.

CLINICAL FEATURES

The patient, aged 45–65, presents with weakness, bone pain or a pathological fracture. The bone pain is constant and backache in particular is common, sometimes with root pain and occasionally paraplegia. Anaemia, cachexia and chronic nephritis all contribute to the general ill-health.

X-rays may show nothing more than overall reduction in density; more often there are multiple punched out defects with no marginal new bone around them. These make it difficult to exclude those cases of multiple secondary deposits in which no primary can be found.

Investigations of importance in establishing a diagnosis are: urinalysis, which in over half the cases shows Bence–Jones protein; electrophoretic analysis of plasma and urine, which shows a characteristic pattern; and sternal marrow puncture, which reveals the typical myeloma cells. Often an unusually high sedimentation rate (over 100) alerts suspicion and prompts the surgeon to undertake these investigations.

TREATMENT

Radiotherapy and chemotherapy relieve pain and pressure effects for a time, and may prolong survival. Pathological fractures in the limbs are best treated by internal fixation. Spinal fractures are treated with a brace, unrelieved cord pressure may need decompression.

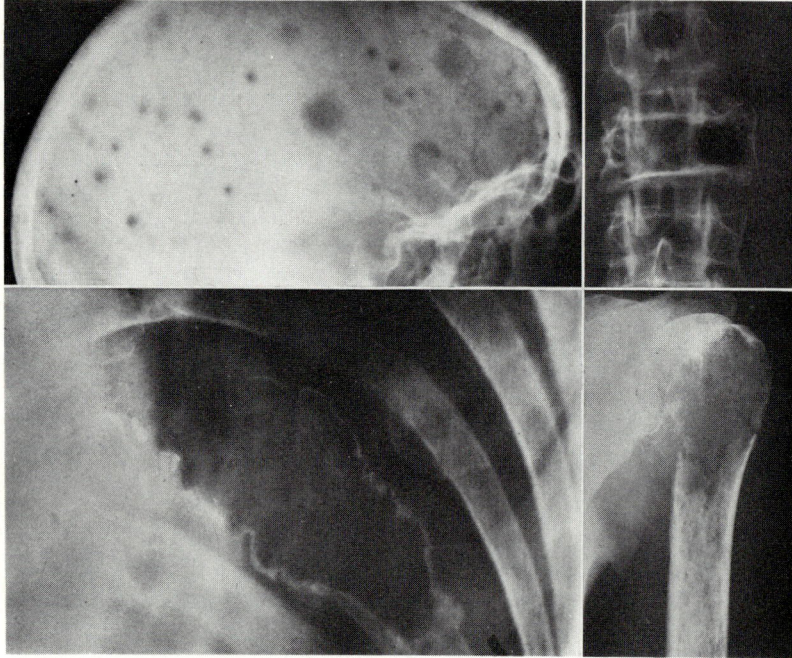

8.9 MYELOMATOSIS
In the skull and spine the appearance resembles that of secondary carcinoma; the rib and humerus are more characteristic of myelomatosis.

PLASMACYTOMA

This is the name often applied to a solitary myeloma. The patient presents with pain, a lump or a pathological fracture. X-ray shows a multilocular expanding osteolytic lesion in a red marrow area. Years may elapse before multiplicity becomes apparent. Treatment is by radiotherapy.

SECONDARY CARCINOMA OF BONE

PATHOLOGY

In two-thirds of cases, secondary bone deposits arise from carcinoma of the breast or prostate, because these are the most common primary tumours. In a further one-sixth of cases, the deposits arise from other carcinomas (of thyroid gland, kidney, bronchus, genitalia, bladder, gastro-intestinal tract). In the remaining one-sixth, no primary tumour is found.

The macroscopic and microscopic appearances correspond to those of the primary tumour.

There are three possible routes whereby the deposit may travel from the primary tumour to the bone.

(a) Most bone secondaries arise from tissue whose veins do not drain via the portal system into the liver. The cells travel via the vena cava and heart to the lung (where carcinoma cells can always be found microscopically in cases of bone deposits). In the lung, clumps of cells multiply, then probably penetrate capillaries to enter the systemic circulation and so reach bone.

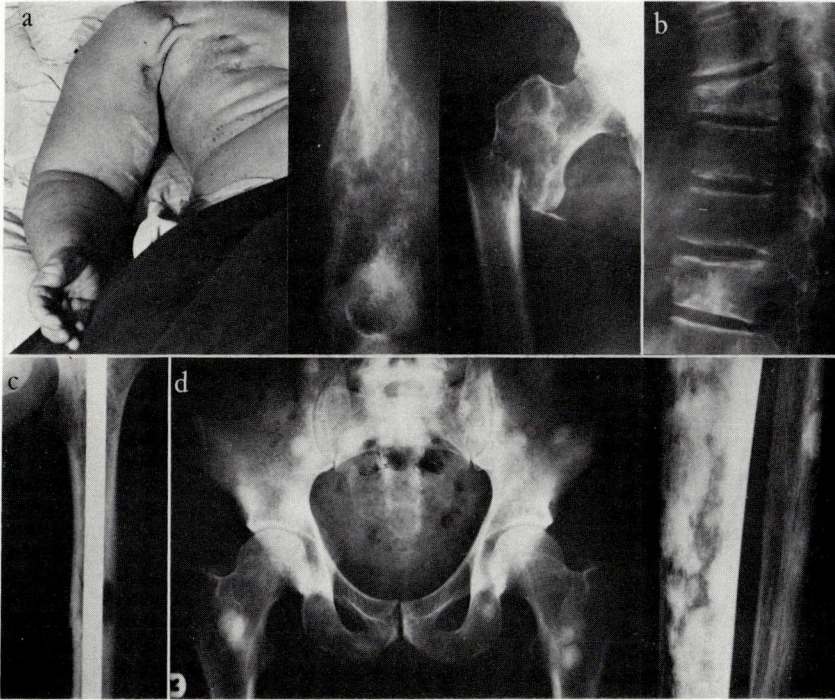

8.10 SECONDARY DEPOSITS
(a) This patient presents an all-too familiar picture; (b) spinal secondaries; (c) osteo-lytic deposits are liable to fracture and invite internal fixation; (d) osteoblastic deposits in the pelvis and tibia, from prostatic carcinoma.

(*b*) There is also a direct connection between the pelvic plexus of veins and the vertebral veins, which explains why pelvic primaries are especially liable to give deposits in the pelvic bones and spine.

(*c*) Tumours of the rectum and of some other epithelial tissues may invade bone directly.

The above theories fail to explain why the muscles, heart and spleen enjoy immunity from secondary deposits.

CLINICAL FEATURES

The patient is usually aged 50–70 years and secondary deposits are found chiefly where red bone marrow is plentiful, namely, in the trunk bones (vertebrae, skull, pelvis, ribs) and 'root' bones (upper ends of the humerus and femur).

The primary tumour may be obvious but sometimes even a meticulous search fails to reveal it. The neck, breasts, axillae, lungs, abdomen and genitalia should be examined, and rectal or vaginal examination is usually necessary. Investigations which may be required include x-rays of the chest and urogenital tract, blood count, sedimentation rate, electrophoresis and estimation of the serum phosphatases.

The secondary deposit usually presents either with local ache or as a pathological fracture. Some deposits, however, are clinically silent, being revealed only by x-ray. Many fail to show even on x-ray but can be revealed by bone scanning using radio-active isotopes.

X-RAY APPEARANCES

OSTEOLYTIC DEPOSITS — These are much the commoner variety and 90 per cent of breast secondaries are of this type. One or more rare areas are seen in the medulla. Later the cortex appears mottled and may be destroyed so that the bone collapses. There is little or no periosteal reaction.

OSTEOBLASTIC DEPOSITS — Deposits from carcinoma of breast or bowel are occasionally osteoblastic, but much the commonest are prostatic secondaries, probably because the cells contain much phosphatase (serum acid phosphatase is increased). A single vertebral body may look too dense. More often the pelvis shows mottled increase of density; and this latter must be distinguished from Paget's disease, in which the alkaline phosphatase (not the acid) is increased. Lymphoma deposits also may resemble prostatic metastases.

TREATMENT

By the time a patient has developed secondary deposits the prognosis, as far as life is concerned, is almost hopeless. Occasionally, radical treatment (by combined surgery and radiotherapy) of a solitary secondary deposit and of its parent primary may be rewarding and even apparently curative. This applies particularly to hypernephroma and thyroid tumours; but in the great majority of cases, and certainly in those with multiple secondaries, treatment is entirely symptomatic. For that reason elaborate witch-hunts to discover the source of an occult primary tumour are to be deprecated; the search may be diagnostically satisfying, but is therapeutically valueless and psychologically harmful.

Most patients with secondary deposits can, however, be made comfortable for a time by one or more of the following measures.

(1) DRUGS — Ordinary analgesics should be tried first; later larger doses or more powerful drugs become necessary. Although a fatal outcome is inevitable it may be long delayed, so that caution must be exercised in using habit-forming drugs until the condition is advanced.

The pain of secondary deposits from the breast or prostate can often be relieved by drugs which control the hormone environment; moreover, these drugs sometimes delay the advance of the condition and relief may last for several years. For prostatic secondaries stilboestrol is the most effective drug. With secondary deposits from the breast androgenic drugs are usually best in pre-menopausal patients, and oestrogens in those past the menopause.

Cytotoxic drugs, which damage cells in proportion to their mitotic activity, are often valuable. They include alkylating agents such as the nitrogen mustards, and anti-metabolites such as various folic acid antagonists; actinomycin D possibly comes into this second category.

(2) IRRADIATION — Deep x-ray therapy and other forms of irradiation are exceedingly valuable. A primary tumour may shrink in size and become painless, the pain from secondary deposits also is usually relieved at least for a time, and paraplegia due to spinal deposits sometimes recovers. Moreover, irradiation can usefully be combined with other forms of treatment.

(3) OPERATIVE TREATMENT — A fungating tumour is usually best excised, although occasionally it can be controlled by radiotherapy. Intractable pain from secondary deposits may occasionally require surgical methods for its relief; these include division of sensory nerves, nerve roots, nerve tracts in the spinal cord, and the intrathecal injection of alcohol. In addition, the hormone environment of secondary breast deposits can sometimes be controlled by oöphorectomy combined with adrenalectomy, or by hypophyseal ablation.

(4) THE TREATMENT OF FRACTURES — A patient with secondary deposits often does not present until pathological fracture occurs. In treating these fractures it is important not to be too timid. An over-cautious conservative approach often means a painful lingering death. It is better to accept the small risk of operative methods with internal fixation; if the bone is too weak for effective plating it may first be plugged with acrylic cement. The pain of the fracture is immediately relieved and the patient usually able to get up and about. If operation is followed by radiotherapy the fracture often unites satisfactorily; moreover, the use of internal fixation enables the patient to be taken to the radiotherapy department without discomfort. Vertebral fractures through secondary deposits are treated by radiotherapy and a spinal support.

Prophylactic internal fixation is a neglected but valuable technique; if x-rays suggest the possibility of subsequent fracture, fixation is well worth considering.

SOFT TISSUE TUMOURS AND LUMPS

The vital question (as with bone tumours) is whether the tumour is benign or malignant. When doubt exists a biopsy is essential and the features of a lump which arouse suspicion are: pain, especially in a previously painless lump; recent or rapid increase of size; an indefinite edge; and attachment to surrounding structures. The regional lymph nodes should be palpated and, since malignant soft-tissue tumours almost invariably metastasize to the lungs, the chest should be x-rayed. The account which follows is intended only as a summary of those soft-tissue tumours likely to be encountered in orthopaedics.

FATTY TUMOURS —A *lipoma*, one of the commonest of all tumours, may occur almost anywhere, the subcutaneous layer being a favourite site. It consists of lobules of fat with a surrounding capsule which may become tethered to surrounding structures. The patient, usually aged over 50, complains of a painless swelling. The lump is soft and almost fluctuant; the well-defined edge and lobulated surface distinguish it from a chronic abscess. Fat is notably radiotranslucent, a feature which betrays the occasional subperiosteal lipoma. Lipomata may be multiple.

Liposarcoma is exceedingly rare but should be suspected if a previously existing lipoma (especially in the buttock or thigh) grows rapidly or becomes painful.

FIBROUS TUMOURS — *Fibromas* are widely distributed and not uncommon. They consist of masses of fibrous tissue often arranged in whorls. A hard fibroma is usually round and has a well-defined edge. A soft fibroma contains many blood vessels, is often diffuse and its edges may be ill-defined; differentiation from a fibrosarcoma is difficult and indeed the risk of a soft fibroma becoming malignant is sufficient to justify early excision-biopsy. Recurrence of any fibroma after excision (Paget's recurring fibroid) is suspicious.

8.11 LIPOMAS
(a) Subcutaneous, (b) intramuscular, (c) subperiosteal.

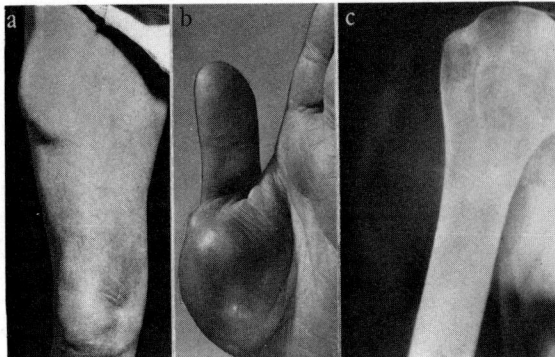

Fibrosarcoma, the commonest malignant soft tissue tumour, is composed of spindle cells with elongated nuclei. The tumour appears to be encapsulated but the capsule is not effective in preventing penetration of surrounding tissues. The lack of a definite edge and attachment to surrounding structures are the main clinical features. Treatment is wide excision or amputation, combined with radiotherapy.

SYNOVIAL TUMOURS — *Hyperplasia* of the synovium such as that occurring in villous synovitis (page 265) is probably inflammatory in origin and should not be confused with neoplasia. A true synovioma may occur wherever synovial membrane is found—in joints, tendon sheaths or bursae; foam cells with a high cholesterol content are a prominent microscopic feature and the term xanthoma is often applied. The patient complains of a lump, or of interference with tendon action. The lump is round or oval, firm, well-defined, and becomes less mobile when the appropriate tendons are tautened. A fairly common site is the back or front of the hand. When the tumour is growing within a joint the diagnosis is unlikely to be made until mechanical interference with joint action leads to surgical exploration. The treatment is local excision.

A malignant synovioma is rare. The patient presents with a rapidly growing swelling. The lack of a well-defined edge may be apparent if a tendon sheath is involved; but in a joint (the knee is the commonest site) the swelling may become very large before its malignant character is obvious. On x-ray the combination of bone defects and a soft-tissue 'snowstorm' is characteristic. With a combination of radiotherapy, chemotherapy and excision (or amputation) about half the patients survive.

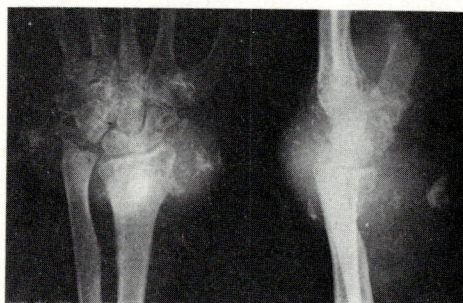

8.12 MALIGNANT
SYNOVIOMA
Note the 'snow-storm' appearance.

BLOOD VESSEL TUMOURS — A *haemangioma* may be capillary or cavernous. The capillary variety is commoner and the congenital skin naevus ('birth mark') its most familiar example. A cavernous haemangioma may be deep or superficial; because it consists of a sponge-like collection of blood spaces it feels soft and can be emptied by pressure. Haemangiomata may calcify, and sometimes there is associated hypertrophy of an affected limb.

Aneurysms may be (*a*) congenital (for example cerebral); (*b*) the sequel to disease (nowadays arterio-sclerosis is a much commoner cause than syphilis); or (*c*) traumatic (in half of these the accompanying vein also is damaged causing an arterio-venous fistula). The cardinal sign is a pulsating lump. The lump is in the course of an artery and can be reduced by proximal pressure. The pulsation is expansile not transmitted; it is visible, palpable and audible. Distally the pulse may be diminished in volume and the tissues poorly nourished. An aneurysm which has been present since childhood may cause overgrowth of a limb.

The diagnosis of an aneurysm is easy—providing the possibility is borne in mind; the consequence of failure may be alarming or disastrous. The nurse who ostentatiously sprinkles sawdust on the floor when a house surgeon is about to incise an 'abscess' has observed pulsation which he has missed.

NERVE TUMOURS — A *neuroma* is not a true tumour but an overgrowth of connective tissue following trauma. In an amputation stump the lump is round and may be tender. On a plantar digital nerve it may be too small to feel, but causes pain and localized tenderness (Morton's metatarsalgia, page 308). A *schwannoma* is a tumour arising from schwann cells occurring within a nerve and forming a round well-defined lump which causes little numbness or weakness. Its removal without damaging the nerve is difficult. A *neurilemmoma* is clinically similar but grows from the nerve sheath and is easier to remove.

A *neuro-fibroma* contains whorls of cellular fibrous tissue and arises from the interstitial tissue of a peripheral nerve. The lump is in the line of a nerve and can be moved only from side to side across the nerve; it may be soft or firm and is sometimes tender.

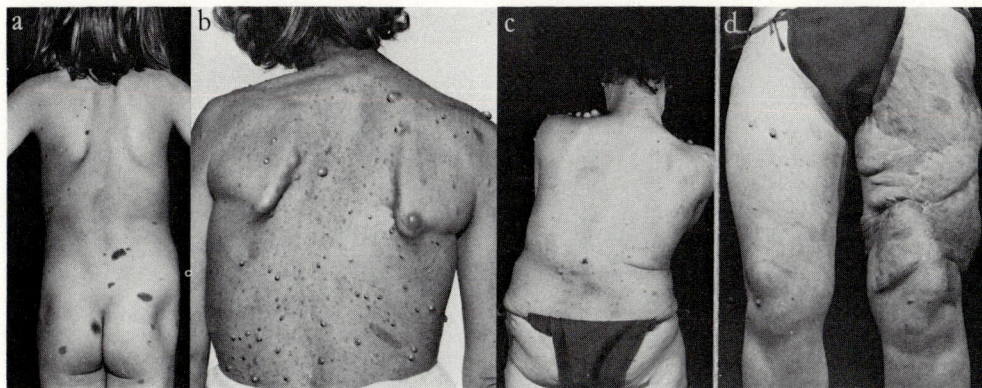

8.13 NEUROFIBROMATOSIS
(a) Café-au-lait spots, (b) molluscum fibrosum with slight scoliosis; (c) and (d) a patient with scoliosis and elephantiasis.

Paraesthesia is not uncommon. Sometimes a nerve root is involved and compression of the spinal cord or cauda equina may occur.

Multiple neurofibromatosis (von Recklinghausen's disease) is of autosomal dominant inheritance. The neurofibromas are associated with café-au-lait spots and sometimes with skin nodules (molluscum fibrosum). Scoliosis develops in 30 per cent of patients, and occasionally hypertrophy of one limb. The nerve tumours themselves may be palpable or may cause symptoms when situated in a confined space such as the spinal canal. Occasionally x-ray reveals pressure erosion of bone, and rarely one of the tumours undergoes malignant change. Neurofibromatosis has other curious skeletal associations including disturbance of bone growth, anomalies of bone architecture and pseudarthrosis of the tibia (page 174).

OTHER TUMOURS — A *ganglion* (page 171) is probably not a true tumour. Ganglia occur chiefly in the hand or foot, occasionally round the knee. The lump may be soft and fluctuant, or so tensely cystic as to feel almost bony. It is well-defined and, except in the fingers, not usually tender. Occasionally a ganglion presses on a nerve or penetrates between its fibres causing paraesthesia and weakness. Ganglion cyst of bone is the term applied to a well-defined rare area in bone (near a joint) which histologically resembles a ganglion.

A *rhabdomyoma* (tumour of a striped muscle) is rare and should not be confused with the lump which follows muscle rupture. Both are in the line of a muscle, can be moved across but not along it, and harden with muscle action; the muscle rupture however has a depression distal to the lump and the lump is not getting bigger. If a tumour is suspected early exploration is advisable because malignant change is not uncommon; not infrequently the swelling proves to be normal muscle fibres in an anomalous situation.   A *rhabdomyosarcoma* is very rare.   It occurs mainly in the buttock, thigh or leg.   The patient presents with ache and a rapidly growing ill-defined mass attached to and moving with the affected muscle.

A *glomus tumour* is rare but very painful.   It consists of mixed neural, vascular and muscle elements.   The overlying skin is often bluish, but the tumour, which is subcutaneous, is often minute in size and never bigger than a pea.   The characteristic features are pain, sensitivity to cold and exquisite tenderness.   Any part of the body may be affected, especially the fingers and toes; sometimes it occurs beneath the nail and it may erode the bone.   The treatment is excision.

Suggestions for further reading

Campbell, C. J., Cohen, J. and Enneking, W. F. (1975). ' New Therapies for Osteogenic Sarcoma.' *J. Bone Jt Surg.* **57A,** 143

Carroll, R. E. *et al* (1972).   'Glomus Tumours of the Hand.' *J. Bone Jt Surg.* **54A,** 691

Clough, J. R. and Price, C. H. G. (1968).   'Aneurysmal Bone Cysts.' *J. Bone Jt Surg.* **50B,** 116

Eyre-Brook, A. L. and Price, C. H. G. (1969).   'Fibrosarcoma of Bone.' *J. Bone Jt Surg.* **51B,** 20

Friedman, B. *et al.* (1971).   'Round-Cell Sarcomas of Bone.' *J. Bone Jt Surg.* **53,** 1118

Geschickter, C. F. and Copeland, M. M. (1949).   *Tumours of Bone.*   3rd ed. Philadelphia; Lippincott

McGrath, P. J. (1972).   'Giant-cell Tumour of Bone.' *J. Bone Jt Surg.* **54B,** 216

Price, C. H. G. and Goldie, W. (1969).   'Paget's Sarcoma of Bone.' *J. Bone Jt Surg.* **51B,** 205

Schajowicz, F. *et al.* (1972).   *Histological Typing of Bone Tumours.*   Geneva; World Health Organization

Sweetnam, R. (1976).   ' Surgical Treatment of Osteogenic Sarcoma.' *Proc. Roy. Soc. Med.* **69,** 547.

Takigawa, K. (1971).   'Chondroma of the Bones of the Hand.' *J. Bone Jt Surg.* **53A,** 1591

Willis, R. A. (1966).   *Pathology of Tumours.*   4th ed.   London; Butterworths

CHAPTER 9

PARALYTIC DISORDERS

In this chapter three disorders are discussed: spina bifida, cerebral palsy and polio-myelitis. Despite obvious differences they have one fundamental feature in common—namely, muscle weakness or paralysis.

WEAK OR PARALYSED MUSCLES

ASSESSMENT

In assessment it is important to examine not only individual muscles but also functional groups. Grading muscle power is most valuable in the floppy type of paralysis associated with spina bifida and poliomyelitis; in cerebral palsy it is useful but more difficult because spasticity obscures the undoubted weakness. Muscle charting pin-points the site and severity of paralysis; repetition enables progress to be recorded. The following grades are standard:

    0   total paralysis
    1   barely detectable contracture
    2   not enough power to act against gravity
    3   strong enough to act against gravity
    4   still stronger but less than normal
    5   full power

EFFECTS

(1) *Instability* — This occurs when the muscles which control opposing movements at a joint are both equally weak (the term 'balanced paralysis' is convenient). The joint is then floppy or flail.

(2) *Deformity* — This occurs when one group of muscles overpowers its antagonist—unbalanced paralysis. At first it can be overcome passively, but later the deformity becomes fixed. It must be appreciated that the action of some muscles is aided by gravity (e.g. ankle plantarflexors); consequently, in assessment, G must not be overlooked as it is often worth at least 1 point.

(3) *Shortening* — A paralysed limb fails to grow normally. Consequently paralysis which is predominantly unilateral and which arises in childhood causes limb inequality.

PRINCIPLES OF TREATMENT

(1) *Assessment of the whole patient* — This is an essential prerequisite of definitive treatment, especially if operation is contemplated. Has the patient the mental capacity to co-operate or to utilize any local improvement? Will a 'better' position lead to improved function? And is the situation complicated by skin anaesthesia, making splintage hazardous?

(2) *Instability* — Floppy joints often need to be stabilized. In the leg stability is an obvious essential for walking; but even in the arm it may be important to stabilize proximal joints in order to allow use of a normal hand. Stability can be achieved by splintage or by arthrodesis. Some examples of splintage for instability are shown in Fig. 9.2.

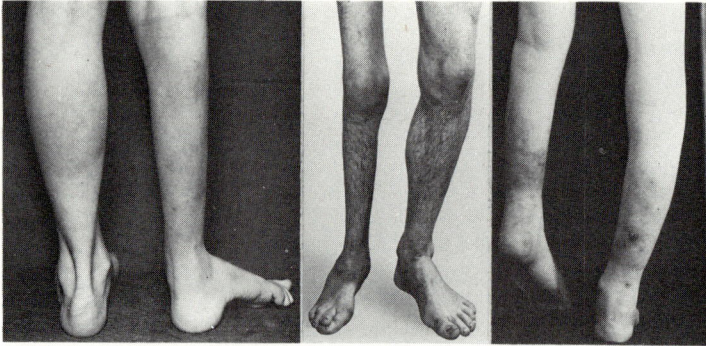

9.1 SOME EFFECTS OF PARALYSIS
Deformity, wasting, shortening and trophic changes.

(3) *Deformity* — Sometimes the establishment of deformity can be postponed (though rarely prevented) by passive stretching combined with intermittent splintage. It is often better to divide shortened tendons. Of necessity they belong to acting muscles, and the possibility of re-routing them more usefully must always be considered.

Tendon transplants are useful not only in treating deformity, but also in restoring a valuable action at the expense of one less important (*see* Fig. 9.3). The prerequisites for successful tendon transplant are: (*a*) any fixed deformity must first have been corrected; (*b*) the transplant must have enough power and excursion for its new task; (*c*) the new line should be as direct as possible; (*d*) it should be fixed under tension and if possible to bone. It is a great advantage if the transplant is synergic with the muscle being replaced. It should be remembered that the strength of a muscle will drop at least one point in the grading system when transposed.

Once deformity has become fixed tendon surgery alone is not enough: bone carpentry is needed. Thus, fixed varus deformity of the foot may be treated by subtalar fusion (which provides stability) combined with excising a laterally-based wedge of bone to make the foot plantigrade. Even then deformity is likely to recur unless the deforming tendon is divided or re-attached.

(4) *Shortening* — This is of importance only in the legs, where inequality of more than 1 inch needs treatment (*see* page 140).

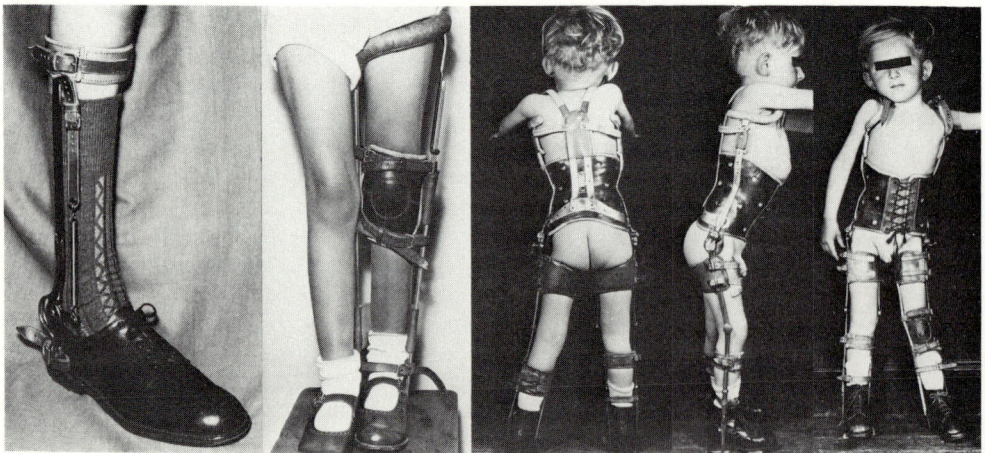

9.2 EQUIPMENT FOR STABILIZATION
The paralysed patient may need equipment, sometimes very extensive.

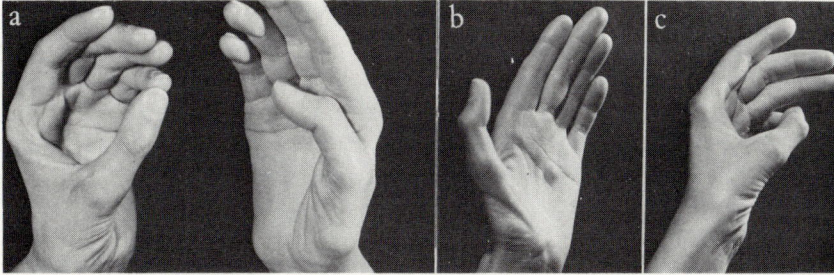

9.3 TENDON TRANSPLANTS
(a) In both hands the opponens pollicis was paralysed; in the left hand a sublimis transplant has restored opposition; (b) and (c) show the transplant in action.

SPINA BIFIDA

The incidence of spina bifida in Great Britain is approximately 3 per 1,000 live births. Formerly many of these babies soon died because of infection or hydrocephalus; early operation has increased the survival rate and highlighted the enormous surgical and social problems.

The cause is unknown, but there is a great geographic variation in frequency, even between different localities in Great Britain. The incidence is higher in certain races, in first-born children and in poor families. The familial incidence has made prophylaxis feasible. If one parent, or a previous child has a neural tube defect, there is a 5 per cent risk to the next child. Estimation of alpha-fetoprotein in the amniotic fluid (obtained by amniocentesis) shows if the fetus is affected and whether termination of pregnancy should be considered.

The term spina bifida simply means that the two halves of the neural arch have failed to fuse. Through the defect the membranes or cord may protrude; the cord itself may be undeveloped (dysplastic). The simplest classification is into closed lesions in which the skin is intact, and open lesions (aperta) in which it is not.

CLOSED SPINA BIFIDA

PATHOLOGY

Any of the following may be associated with closed spina bifida: dermal cysts; lipoma of the cauda equina; diastematomyelia (in which the cord is bifurcated by bone projecting backwards from the vertebral body); partial or complete absence of the sacrum; and, finally, meningocele. Meningocele is very rare and is merely a spinal hernia containing no neural elements, so that neurological lesions are said not to occur.

CLINICAL FEATURES

Although the skin is intact it is almost never normal. Some mid-line anomaly suggests the diagnosis, so that the term 'occulta' (meaning 'secret') is best avoided. The possible lesions range from a tiny dimple or excess of 'down', to a large pigmented naevus or a veritable 'faun's tail'. A bulge deep to the skin is suggestive of an associated lesion.

X-rays show the gap in the neural arch; widening of the spinal canal is common and the bony spur of diastematomyelia should be sought.

TREATMENT

The most important indications for treatment are neurological deficit, disturbance of bladder function, and weakness, numbness or trophic changes in one or both legs. These features may develop during growth, either because the cord is tethered at the defect, or because its distal portion is bulky and too immobile to escape damage when the patient moves his back. The state of affairs is best revealed by a cisternal air myelogram.

Should operation be needed it is best done by a neurosurgeon. Tethering bands or adhesions are divided and the cord mobilized; lipomata, dermoid cysts or bony spurs are excised.

OPEN SPINA BIFIDA

PATHOLOGY

Much the commonest open lesion is a myelomeningocele of the lumbar or lumbo-sacral region (60 per cent of all open spina bifidas). Through the bony defect protrudes a meningeal sac containing nerve roots and cord remnants which may be adherent to it. The sac is exposed with no skin cover. Hydrocephalus may be present at birth; with a communicating hydrocephalus the intracranial pressure may not be elevated until leakage from the spinal lesion is arrested by surgical closure.

CLINICAL FEATURES

The newborn baby has a translucent cystic lump in the mid-line of the back. The baby's posture may suggest paralysis and sometimes indicates its neurological level. Associated deformities are common, especially hip dislocation, genu recurvatum, talipes and claw toes. Such deformities may be due to intra-uterine paralysis or they may develop later because of unbalanced paralysis; sometimes they are primary, i.e. independent of the paralysis.

Muscle charting (page 103) should be performed within 24 hours of birth. Sharrard has shown convincingly that this is perfectly practicable; he suggests that the untreated child may, within a few days, become increasingly paralysed as enlargement of the meningeal sac exerts traction on adherent nerve roots.

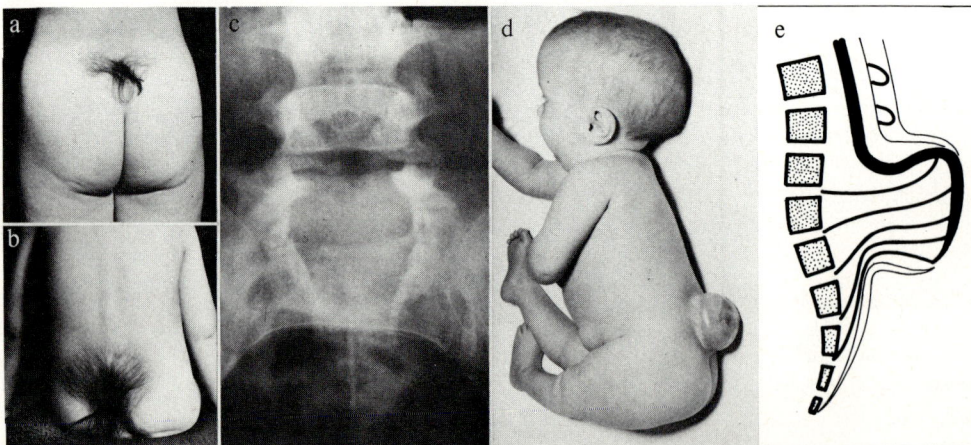

9.4 SPINA BIFIDA (1)
(a, b) Examples of the hairy patches which suggest a bony defect such as that in (c). (d, e) Myelomeningocele: the diagram shows the neural plaque on the surface, and also why traction lesions of the nerve roots develop with growth.

TREATMENT

Selection of patients for operation is ethically controversial. Most centres avoid urgent operation if the neurological lesion is high, the skull is enlarged, or spinal deformities are severe. In the remainder (about half) the skin lesion is closed early.

For subsequent management team-work is essential. The ideal is a combined clinic at which neurosurgery, orthopaedics, urology and paediatrics are all represented; but the key figure is the physiotherapist. As the child grows help is likely to be needed from the splint maker, the social worker and possibly the psychotherapist. But above all, the child will need parental understanding and ceaseless devotion. Treatment must begin so early that parents have little time to reflect upon the ethics or the magnitude of the problem.

Early management

(1) *Skin closure* should, in those patients with good prognostic signs, be performed within 48 hours. The neural plaque is carefully preserved and the skin widely undercut to facilitate closure. Only in this way can drying and ulceration be prevented.

(2) *Hydrocephalus* is the next priority. Usually it develops within a few days; treatment must not be delayed or brain damage follows. A ventriculo-caval shunt containing a valve (e.g. Spitz–Holter) is inserted. As the baby grows the shunt may need to be replaced.

(3) *Deformities* must be kept under control. The orthopaedic surgeon is usually not called upon for three weeks, and then only if the child is thriving, the back healed, and a shunt (if needed) working. At this stage muscle charting is repeated and a programme of stretching and strapping begun: stretching to keep deformity at a minimum; elastic strapping (or simple splints) to hold correction.

Two features dominate orthopaedic management; the bones are somewhat fragile (spontaneous fractures are common and frequently unite with excessive callus); and the skin is anaesthetic. Consequently manipulations must not be too forcible, and splintage should be intermittent. The skin must be protected from localized pressure and watched with extravagant vigilance—'a sore which takes a day to form may take a month to heal'.

(4) *Urinary problems* develop in 90 per cent of cases. Intravenous pyelography is used to detect any upper urinary tract dilatation, and is repeated at intervals. Males can usually be fitted with a penile appliance but in females urinary diversion is needed.

LEVELS		EARLY MANAGEMENT – TIMING	
HIP	KNEE	AGE	PROCEDURE
		1 DAY	Close skin defect
Flexion	L1	1 WEEK	Ventriculo-caval shunt
Adduction	L2 L3 — Extension		
Abduction	L4 L5 — Flexion	1 MONTH	Stretch and strap
Extension	S1 S2	6 MONTHS TO 3 YEARS	Orthopaedic operations
		WHENEVER NEEDED	Urogenital operations

9.5 SPINA BIFIDA (2)
The diagram shows the root levels concerned with hip and knee movements. The table is a simple guide to the timing of operations.

Subsequent management of paralysis and deformity

The guiding principles are:

(1) For the first 6–12 months deformities are treated by stretching and strapping (*see above*). Forcible overcorrection followed by plaster is forbidden: this combination, useful in other varieties of paralysis, is disastrous with spina bifida; the bones may break and the skin will ulcerate.

(2) Open methods of correcting deformity are best, but should be delayed until the child is several months old. Then short tendons are the main problem: they should be divided and, where appropriate, transplanted. Only when balance has been restored should any residual deformity be corrected by osteotomy.

(3) Splints alone are never used to obtain correction; they may be used to maintain it but even then only intermittently; their action is reinforced by frequently repeated stretching.

REGIONAL SURVEY

SPINE — Apart from the posterior defect which constitutes spina bifida, many other vertebral anomalies can occur, such as unsegmented bars, hemi-vertebrae and fused ribs, resulting in scoliosis, lordosis or kyphosis. Neonatal kyphosis may be so severe that spinal osteotomy is needed if the skin defect is to be closed.

Even moderate kyphosis or kyphos may later cause persistent skin ulceration; treatment consists in excising the kyphotic vertebrae and fixing the two halves of the spine together— a procedure less alarming than it sounds because the cord is already non-functioning. Many patients with high neurological lesions develop progressive lordoscoliosis aged 5 or 6. Bracing at best slows deterioration. When the child is old enough (about 10) operative correction and stabilization is often needed using a combination of Dwyer and Harrington instrumentation.

HIP — The aim is to secure hips straight enough to enable the child to stand in calipers, and flexible enough for him to sit. If the neurological level of the lesion is above L1, all muscle groups are equally paralysed (balanced); the hips are flail and no treatment other than splintage is needed. With a lesion from S1 downwards there may be pure flexion deformity; this can be corrected by elongation of the psoas tendon combined with detachment of the flexors from the ilium (Soutter).

Usually the lesion is between these two levels and the commonest hip problem is dislocation: 50 per cent of spina bifida children have subluxed or dislocated hips by the age of two. Some may be coincidental congenital dislocations, but most result from unbalanced paralysis; if the flexors and adductors can overpower the extensors and abductors, dislocation is almost inevitable. In infancy reduction (closed or open) is usually possible, perhaps aided by adductor tenotomy; but, because post-operative splintage

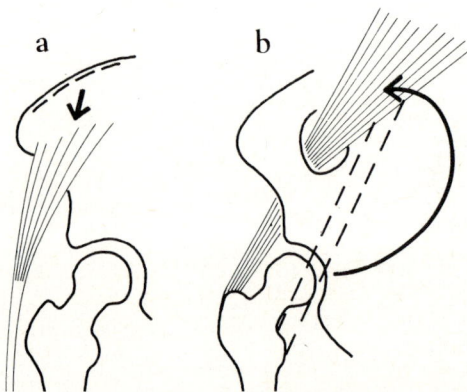

9.6 SPINA BIFIDA (3)
Two procedures for hip deformity.
(a) Soutter's muscle slide, (b) Sharrard's ilio-psoas transfer.

must be minimized, it is important to improve muscle balance. This is achieved by transplanting the psoas tendon from the lesser to the greater trochanter; flexor power is reduced and extensor-abductor power may be increased. Sharrard advocates threading the detached psoas through a large hole in the ilium, while Mustard prefers moving the tendon across the front of the bone.

In older children it may be difficult or impossible to reduce a dislocation. The possibilities then are varus osteotomy of the upper femur, or innominate osteotomy; often it is best not to intervene.

KNEE — Unlike the hip, the knee usually presents no problem, because the aim is simple— a straight knee suitable for straight calipers. Occasionally recurvatum develops and cautious elongation of the quadriceps may be called for. In older children fixed flexion may follow prolonged sitting. If stretching and splintage fail, one or more of the hamstrings may be lengthened, divided or re-inserted into the femur or patella. Not uncommonly the knees are straight and will not bend, making sitting difficult; extensive soft tissue release may be needed if subcutaneous tenotomy proves inadequate.

FOOT — The aim is a plantigrade foot with plantar skin strong enough not to break down easily. The floppy foot of balanced paralysis needs no surgery; accurately fitting footwear with strong external bracing is adequate. The same is true of any deformity which can be corrected passively; though in every case the patient and parents must be taught an elaborate ritual of skin care; pressure sores must, at all costs, be prevented.

Fixed deformities are common and varied. Tendon operations are often helpful and are best performed at or before the age of 6 months: pre-operative electrical testing may help in deciding if the short tendon is paralysed but contracted (in which case simple division is satisfactory), or is active but unopposed (in which case transplant is better). The common equino-varus deformity often requires extensive postero-medial release, also at the age of 6 months.

Vertical talus is not uncommon, with a rigid boat-shaped foot and possibly skin ulceration. Operative reduction is important and preferable to astragalectomy; it is performed at the age of 3 years or over. Still older children may need bone carpentry to restore a plantigrade foot. Should claw toes prove troublesome, flexor-extensor transplant is suitable for the outer 4 toes, and tenodesis of the long flexor (anchoring it to the proximal phalanx) for the hallux.

CEREBRAL PALSY

The term 'cerebral palsy' includes a group of disorders which result from non-progressive cerebral dysfunction, originating before the central nervous system has matured. It is not due to a single or specific type of brain damage although perinatal anoxia is almost certainly the commonest causal factor; others include trauma (to the brain or its vessels), kernicterus (with or without Rhesus incompatibility), and infection (perinatal or in early infancy).

GENERAL FEATURES

The incidence is from 0·5 to 2 per 1,000 live births, so that, as with spina bifida, the social and medical problems are immense. A history of difficult labour or early kernicterus may suggest the diagnosis, but at birth the disease is rarely recognized. Early symptoms include difficulty in sucking and swallowing, with dribbling at the mouth; the mother may notice that the baby feels stiff or wriggles awkwardly. Gradually it becomes apparent that the milestones are delayed (the normal child usually holds up its head at three months, sits up at six months and begins walking at about one year).

Intelligence is often impaired, but not as often as formerly supposed. Accurate assessment is important, for severe mental defect precludes useful treatment. The

I.Q. is often assessed too low because spasticity has hampered learning, and because of speech and hearing difficulties. The children are often emotionally unstable and may suffer from fits; skin sensation is usually normal.

LIMB SIGNS

The characteristic deformities take months or years to develop. They result from muscle inco-ordination and muscle imbalance, both the product of the upper motor neurone damage. Five main varieties of cerebral palsy are recognized, but mixed types are not uncommon.

SPASTIC PALSY — This is the commonest variety and the only one with which the orthopaedic surgeon is likely to be concerned. The muscles feel rigid, and resist stretching, and there is inability to relax; but stiffness takes time to develop, and the severely spastic child may have been a floppy infant. Tendon reflexes are increased and the plantar responses extensor. Some muscles, however, may feel flaccid and it must be realized that paresis of voluntary muscle is always an important feature. Imbalance gives rise to the characteristic deformities: adduction and internal rotation of the shoulder, flexion of the elbow, pronation of the forearm, flexion of the wrist, adduction of the thumb; flexion and adduction of the hips, flexion of the knee, and equinus of the foot.

In nearly one-third of cases the arm and leg on one side are affected (hemiplegia); in nearly one-third both legs are much more severely affected than the arms (diplegia); and in nearly one-third all four limbs are involved (quadriplegia). Monoplegia and triplegia are rare.

ATHETOSIS — This type is more common than was formerly supposed. Typically the limbs wave about with continual, irregular, worm-like movements which are purposeless. Usually the movements are uncontrollable, but sometimes the patient tries to keep the limb still by voluntarily contracting all the muscles of a particular joint. The condition may then be confused with the spastic type of cerebral palsy.

Often the face, tongue and speech muscles share in the athetoid movements and it is hard to resist incorrectly calling the children mental defectives.

ATAXIA — This type is relatively rare. There is an irregular intention tremor and inco-ordination, but no spasticity, flaccidity or athetosis.

RIGIDITY — This was formerly confused with the spastic type, but the muscles are in a constant state of increased tone and, on examination, do not ' give ' like spastic muscles.

ATONY — Atonic cerebral palsy may be part of the floppy baby syndrome due to anoxia and cerebral damage.

CONSERVATIVE TREATMENT

MENTAL TRAINING — It is important to decide early whether the child is educable, for if not, treatment is useless. But it is easy to underestimate mental ability; the child should be given the benefit of the doubt. A calm atmosphere in the home, but with adequate and affectionate stimulation, helps to make the most of the child's abilities. Education should start young, and special schools can provide suitable equipment as well as competition with similarly afflicted children. Speech therapy is important.

PHYSICAL TRAINING — There is no agreed technique of physical education. The aim is to teach new patterns of posture and movement. This is obviously easier if faulty habits, say, of walking, have not first to be unlearnt. Enthusiasm, gentleness and patience are the keynotes of success; when instructed, an intelligent mother with plenty of time is often the best physiotherapist.

Temporary splints are often necessary to prevent deformity or to maintain a correction obtained by manipulation. Splints should be taken off daily and the joints put through their full range of movement.

9.7 CEREBRAL PALSY (1)
(a) Scissors stance, (b) an older patient
able to stand better with calipers.

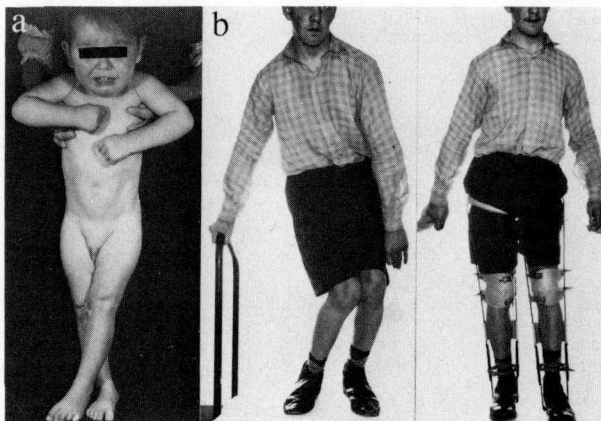

OPERATIVE TREATMENT

Operations have a definite, if limited, place in treatment. Hemiplegics respond best, partly because their mentality is usually normal. With diplegia or quadriplegia the results are often disappointing and surgery should certainly be avoided in patients with low intelligence and in those with athetosis or rigidity. Careful selection of patients is imperative, for the child who has struggled to learn to get about may, despite theoretically attractive operations, be unable to do so if he is off his feet for a few weeks.

The main task is to prevent or correct deformity, thereby improving posture and reducing the weight of splintage which the weak muscles have to carry around. The principles described on page 103 apply, but timing is difficult because spasticity hampers accurate muscle charting. If it can be established that deformity is progressing in spite of adequate conservative treatment, tendon surgery is worth while even in young children (aged two to ten). Thereafter it usually needs to be combined with bone carpentry and joint stabilization.

REGIONAL SURVEY

UPPER LIMB — Operative treatment is delayed longer than in the lower limb and is rarely indicated before the age of 12. Even then it is almost exclusively confined to the forearm, wrist and thumb.

For the pronated forearm, release of pronator teres is a possibility, or the tendon can be re-routed round the back of the forearm in the hope that it may act as a supinator. The combination of forearm pronation with wrist palmarflexion can sometimes be improved by transplanting flexor carpi ulnaris into one of the wrist extensors. If the fingers work better when held extended the best operation is wrist arthrodesis in slight dorsiflexion; when flexion deformity is severe the lower radius can usefully be tapered and embedded into the carpal bones.

The chief hand deformities are clenched fingers and thumb-in-palm. Finger function can be improved by elongating the flexor tendons, but it is important first to ensure that deformity can be overcome by steady pressure, for if there is joint contracture operation is useless. The thumb-in-palm deformity (flexion–adduction contracture) is very disabling and best treated by Matev's procedure (1972): first the flexor pollicis longus is elongated; then through a palmar incision all the thenar muscles are released; and finally abduction and extension are reinforced by shortening the appropriate tendons or by tendon transplants.

SPINE — Significant scoliosis develops in 12 per cent of cerebral palsy patients, but correction and stabilization are rarely needed.

LOWER LIMB — Although it is customary to consider each deformity individually Burke Evans (1971) has emphasized the inter-relationship between the various posture problems, especially lumbar lordosis, hip flexion, knee flexion and ankle equinus; this must be constantly borne in mind when surgery is being planned.

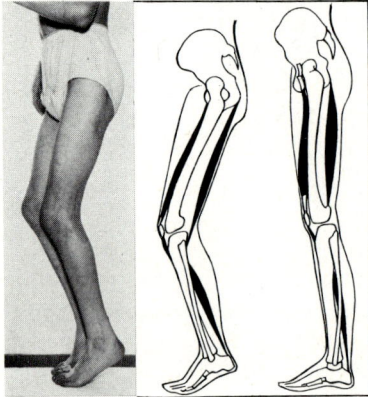

9.8   CEREBRAL PALSY (2)
Showing how the various flexion deformities in the lower limb can benefit from Egger's operation.

At the hip adductor overaction or contracture may be treated by tenotomy; this can be combined with obturator neurectomy, or the adductor origin can be transplanted to the ischial tuberosity.   Flexion deformity can be helped by dividing the psoas tendon, and medial rotation by dividing the front half of gluteus medius.   These operations may prevent the hip from dislocating—a constant danger.   If dislocation has already occurred they may be combined with varus osteotomy of the upper femur.   A long-standing dislocation may be irreducible; if discomfort makes operation imperative the femoral head can be excised.

At the knee flexion contracture can be treated by Egger's operation: the medial hamstrings are re-inserted into the femoral condyle, the biceps tendon is elongated and, if necessary the patellar retinaculae are divided.   Probably this combined procedure should be reserved for severe cases; for mild deformity releasing the hamstrings from the ischium is adequate.

In the foot equinus deformity is common; it may indeed be useful in a limb with flexed hip and knee.   But if correction is needed, elongation of the tendo achillis is probably best combined with gastrocnemius slide operation.   Tendo achillis elongation is combined with division of the peronei if there is also valgus deformity, or with division of tibialis posterior for varus deformity.   (Alternatively the tibialis posterior may be transplanted through the interosseus membrane to the front of the foot.)   But when these combined deformities are fixed, bone carpentry is needed: either calcaneal osteotomy or, more often, subtalar fusion.   Flexion deformity of the hallux or other toes is best treated by arthrodesis.

ANTERIOR POLIOMYELITIS

With the advent of successful immunization poliomyelitis has become a rare disease, but it has not disappeared, and the victims of earlier epidemics continue to pose challenging problems.

The surgeon is rarely called in before the convalescent stage; by then the patient is no longer ill or in pain.   Some anterior horn cells will have been destroyed by the virus; others, merely damaged by oedema, survive, and the muscles they supply can regain their lost power. Vigorous physiotherapy is needed to hasten recovery; consequently splintage must be kept to a minimum. Because of the associated trophic changes hydrotherapy also is useful. Operative treatment should not be considered before the definitive stage.

CLINICAL FEATURES (in the definitive stage)

The patient, except for residual paralysis, is fit; although, if the trunk muscles were involved, he may have respiratory difficulty and he may have scoliosis. An affected limb often looks bluish, wasted and deformed; if the disease occurred in childhood there may also be shortening. There are frequently extensive chilblains and the skin feels cold. When a badly paralysed limb is picked up it has a floppy feel which, in the presence of normal sensation, is characteristic.

TREATMENT

Further recovery is, by definition, impossible; further physiotherapy is useless. Severe trophic changes may need sympathectomy; and leg shortening is treated as described on page 140. The two remaining problems are deformity due to unbalanced paralysis, and instability from balanced paralysis (page 103); their management is described in the section which follows, but the importance of muscle charting is self-evident.

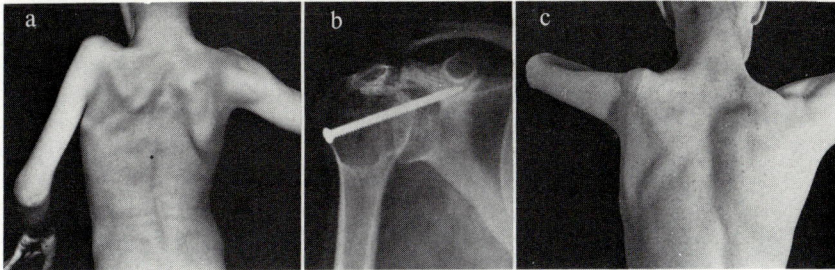

9.9 POLIOMYELITIS
(a) This patient had paralysis of the left deltoid; after arthrodesis (b) he could lift his arm (c) by using his scapular muscles.

REGIONAL SURVEY

UPPER LIMB — Providing the scapular muscles are strong abduction at the shoulder can be restored (Fig. 9.9) by arthrodesing the gleno-humeral joint (60 degrees abducted and 30 degrees flexed). Contracted adductors may need division, but a strong pectoralis major can, if needed, be used to provide elbow flexion; it is detached from its insertion and sutured to the biceps tendon. Proximal advancement of the forearm flexors is a less effective way of restoring elbow flexion.

Arthrodesis of the wrist is sometimes useful; deformity can be corrected and any active wrist muscle re-routed more usefully. In the thumb, weakness of opposition can be overcome by a sublimis transplant (Fig. 9.3); the tendon (usually of annularis) is wound round that of flexor carpi ulnaris (which acts as a pulley), threaded across the palm and fixed to the distal end of the first metacarpal.

TRUNK — Unbalanced paralysis causes scoliosis, frequently a long thoraco-lumbar curve which may involve the lumbo-sacral junction, causing pelvic obliquity. Operative treatment is often needed, the most effective being a combination of Dwyer's anterior fusion with posterior Harrington rod instrumentation.

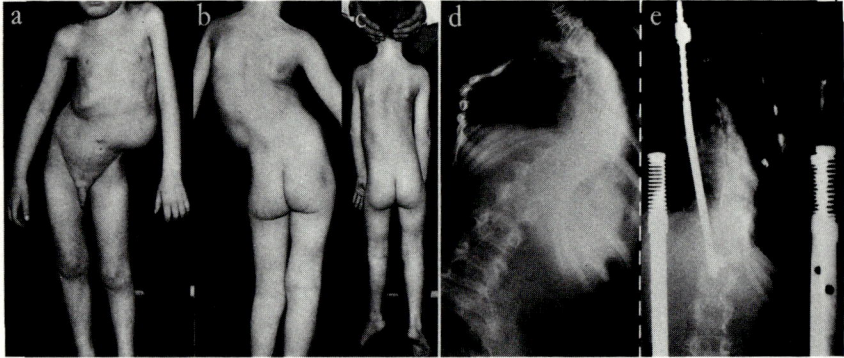

9.10 PARALYTIC SCOLIOSIS
The floppy curve (a, b) is at first telescopic (c). Later it becomes fixed (d) and may need correction and fusion (e).

LOWER LIMB — *At the hip* balanced paralysis causes instability; the resulting Trendelenburg gait cannot be avoided except by arthrodesis, which is rarely advisable. Unbalanced paralysis causes deformities similar to those in spina bifida and cerebral palsy. Fixed flexion can be treated by Soutter's muscle slide operation, or by transplanting psoas to the great trochanter. For fixed adduction with pelvic obliquity, the fascia lata and ilio-tibial band may need division.

At the knee instability is dangerous. The patient is liable to fall and needs a caliper—unless he has (or can be given) slight fixed plantarflexion of the foot; then weight-bearing thrusts the knee into hyperextension, imparting stability. Overaction of the extensors leads to genu recurvatum; only rarely is this severe enough to need operation (plication of the posterior knee capsule, tunnelling the semitendinosus and gracilis tendons through the tibia and through the femoral condyles, and criss-crossing the biceps tendon and ilio-tibial tract across the back of the knee). Fixed flexion with flexors stronger than extensors is commoner and must be corrected; the possibilities are hamstring division or hamstring to quadriceps transplant; but if fixed flexion remains, supracondylar osteotomy is needed.

In the foot instability can be controlled by a below-knee caliper, and foot-drop by a toe-raising spring. Often there is imbalance causing varus, valgus or calcaneo-cavus deformity: unless tendon re-routing can restore balance it is wise to stabilize operatively.

For varus or valgus the simplest procedure (Grice) is to slot bone grafts into vertical grooves on each side of the sinus tarsi; alternatively a triple arthrodesis (Dunn) of sub-talar and mid-tarsal joints is performed, relying on bone carpentry to correct deformity. With associated foot drop Lambrinudi's modification is valuable; triple arthrodesis is performed but the fully plantarflexed talus is slotted into the navicular with the forefoot in only slight equinus; foot drop is corrected because the talus cannot plantarflex further, and slight equinus helps to stabilize the knee. With calcaneocavus deformity Elmslie's operation is useful: triple arthrodesis is performed in the calcaneus position, but corrected at a second stage by posterior wedge excision combined with tenodesis using half of the tendo achillis. The associated claw toes are corrected by arthrodesing the interphalangeal joints in the straight position and re-inserting the long extensor tendons into the metatarsal necks.

Suggestions for further reading

Burke Evans, E. (1971). 'Hip Flexion Deformity in Spastic Cerebral Palsy.'
J. Bone Jt Surg. **53A.** 1465 (Editorial)

Lloyd-Roberts, G. C. (1971). *Orthopaedics in Infancy and Childhood.* London; Butterworths

Menelaus, M. B. (1971). *The Orthopaedic Management of Spina Bifida Cystica.* Edinburgh; Livingstone

Merle d'Aubigné, R. and Dubousset, J. (1971). 'Surgical Correction of Large Length Discrepancies in the Lower Extremities of Children and Adults.' *J. Bone Jt Surg.* **53A,** 411

Sharrard, W. J. W. (1969). 'The Orthopaedic Surgery of Cerebral Palsy and Spina Bifida.' In *Recent Advances in Orthopaedics*, Ed. by A. Graham Apley. London; Churchill

Sharrard, W. J. W. (1971). *Paediatric Orthopaedics and Fractures.* Oxford and Edinburgh; Blackwell

Tohen, A. *et al.* (1969). 'Extra-articular Subtalar Arthrodesis.' *J. Bone Jt Surg.* **51B,** 45

Walker, G. F. (1968). 'The Orthopaedics of Myelomeningocele in Infancy.' *Br. J. hosp. Med.,* July, 900

CHAPTER 10

PERIPHERAL NERVE LESIONS

GENERAL CONSIDERATIONS

CLASSIFICATION

NEUROTMESIS (complete division) — Although 'neurotmesis' means 'nerve cutting', the term is applied not only to a nerve which has been cut across but also to one which is so severely scarred that it cannot regenerate spontaneously. Neurotmesis may be caused therefore by open wounds, traction injuries, compression, or intraneural injections.

AXONOTMESIS (incomplete division) — Axonotmesis is incomplete in the sense that only the axons are divided; the endoneural tubes are undamaged. It occurs with closed fractures, dislocations and pressure injuries. Clinically it is at first indistinguishable from neurotmesis, but spontaneous recovery is likely.

NEURAPRAXIA (physiological interruption) — The axons are intact; the only lesion is degeneration of the myelin sheaths. The larger motor fibres are mainly affected, the smaller sensory fibres less so; hence motor loss may at first be total but sensory loss is rare (though subjective tingling is common). Spontaneous recovery is the rule.

PATHOLOGY

THE NERVE — The space between the cut ends fills with blood clot, the clot organizes and Schwann cells from each stump grow into it. Distally, the axons degenerate and are removed by phagocytes. The Schwann cells of the endoneural tubes multiply and, if the tube is not soon occupied by a growing axon, this multiplication narrows it.

Proximally, degeneration also occurs, but only for about 1 cm. Within a few days the cut axons proliferate and streams of axoplasm grow towards the gap. If obstructed by clot they form a bulky lump (neuroma). Otherwise they enter the Schwann tubes (not necessarily the correct ones) and grow along them. The advancing axon is followed by advancing myelinization. Eventually, the axon joins an end organ which enlarges unless it has in the meantime become too degenerate. The nerve fibre has 'matured' when the myelinated axon is connected to an end organ.

Experimentally the axons grow at a speed of 4 mm a day, but there is delay in starting, in crossing the gap, and in connecting with the end organ. In practice, the speed of recovery is 1–1·5 mm a day.

OTHER STRUCTURES — Denervated muscles waste, and the joints they control are liable to become deformed and stiff. The skin and nails may undergo trophic changes. The brain may 'forget' the pattern of muscle behaviour.

SYMPTOMS

There are no general symptoms. Local symptoms are numbness and weakness. With some partial lesions (particularly of the median nerve and the medial popliteal nerve) there may be pain and increased sweating (see Irritation Syndrome, page 119).

SIGNS

LOOK — There may be a scar of the causal wound. Anaesthetic skin looks smooth and shiny, the affected fingers are thin and tapering and their nails abnormal. Trophic ulcers may be present, especially in the foot. Muscle wasting is apparent and the attitude of a paralysed limb is characteristic.

FEEL — The anaesthetic skin feels smooth, cool and dry. A nerve bulb may be palpable and may be tender. Where sensory nerve damage exists, the patient himself will point to the anaesthetic areas; however, it is useful for the surgeon to map out the area of loss and to chart the quality of sensation in four grades, from total sensory loss up to 2-point discrimination.

MOVE — The patient cannot perform certain movements, though passive range may be full. Muscle tone and power are lost, and bulk diminished. In testing individual muscles, errors may occur, especially in the hand, because of anomalous innervation, trick movements, or supplementary movements. To assess recovery, power may usefully be charted in five grades (*see* page 103).

X-RAY — The bones may decalcify.

DIAGNOSIS

With a suspected nerve injury, the following questions arise.

Is a nerve lesion present? — A quick test for each nerve, in which a distal area of skin or a distally supplied muscle is examined, is useful.

At what level is the lesion? — Usually this is obvious from the injury; if it is not, individual muscles whose branches arise at successive levels must be tested. Special investigations are occasionally useful (*see* below).

What type of lesion is present? — Clinical examination may suggest a neurotmesis; a palpable neuroma confirms it. Partial division is liable to produce hyperaesthesia or excess sweating. With neurapraxia, paralysis is not total and recovery begins early. Special investigations may again be helpful.

Is the lesion recovering? — The muscle supplied nearest to and below the level of the lesion is tested.

SPECIAL INVESTIGATIONS

Nerve blocking — A small quantity of local anaesthetic may be injected into the injured nerve. If this is followed by greater sensory or motor loss the lesion is partial. Similarly, by injecting undamaged nerves, overlap can be recognized.

Electrical tests — Precise information of the nature, level and extent of recovery in nerve lesions can be obtained by: (1) the assessment of strength-duration curves in muscle; (2) electromyographic study of voluntary action potentials; and (3) the measurement of motor and sensory conduction velocities at varying levels.

TREATMENT

NERVE REPAIR — A divided nerve needs to be repaired. Difficulties arise in deciding whether the division is complete (neurotmesis) and in knowing when to operate. Nerve exploration with a view to repair is indicated when (*a*) the nerve is known to be divided because the lesion was seen at the wound toilet operation; (*b*) the nerve is presumed to be divided because recovery of the highest supplied muscle has not occurred in the calculated time, or because a palpable neuroma has developed; and (*c*) occasionally for diagnostic purposes.

It should be noted that some nerves, such as the brachial plexus and the posterior interosseus nerve, are hardly ever worth exploring, because they cannot be adequately sutured.

CARE OF PARALYSED PARTS — While recovery is awaited, the skin should be guarded against burns and the circulation assisted by massage. The joints should be moved through their full range twice daily to prevent stiffness. Splints may be necessary and 'lively splints' are the best; they hold the paralysed muscle in its shortened position by means of a spring which is weak enough to allow the unparalysed muscles to work against it. Electrical stimulation of paralysed muscles may help to preserve their mobility and bulk, but is not as useful as was formerly thought.

SECONDARY OPERATION — Even if recovery of the nerve cannot occur, the function of the limb may be improved by splints or operations. For example, tendon transplants are useful for an irrecoverable radial nerve injury; in the foot, stabilization may be helpful; occasionally a high sciatic nerve lesion may necessitate below-knee amputation.

TIMING OF NERVE EXPLORATION

Not too soon — Primary suture is justified when the wound is clean, the surgeon experienced and the operating conditions ideal. It is certainly indicated if a nerve has been accidentally divided during an operation, and probably wise whenever a digital nerve has been damaged. But it has disadvantages:

(*a*) A wound toilet operation should not entail unnecessary stripping of tissue; therefore adequate nerve mobilization is unsafe.

(*b*) It is impossible at this early stage to judge how much of the nerve has been damaged and needs to be pared away.

(*c*) The sheath is too thin to suture properly and takes 3 weeks to thicken.

Not too late — Excessive delay has the following disadvantages:

(*a*) The Schwann cells which bridge the gap and guide the growing axons attain their peak of activity at 3 weeks from injury; their activity then declines slowly.

(*b*) The Schwann tubes gradually become too narrow.

(*c*) The motor end-plates degenerate after a few months.

(*d*) The muscles atrophy and undergo interstitial fibrosis.

(*e*) The brain 'forgets' how to work the muscles.

The ideal time — Nerve repair should be performed as soon as practicable after 3 weeks from injury. However, it may be necessary to postpone repair because the wound is unhealed. It may also be wise to postpone repair if the nature of the lesion is uncertain; with closed fractures for example, 4 out of 5 nerve lesions recover spontaneously and it is worth waiting until the highest supplied muscle should have recovered.

If repair is delayed by as much as 18 months, then no worth-while motor recovery will occur, though sensory recovery is still possible; but it is better to explore too soon even if the nerve is found intact.

TECHNIQUE OF OPERATION

Tourniquet — If a tourniquet is necessary it should be a pneumatic one and it must be released and bleeding stopped before the wound is closed.

Exposure — A long incision is essential, and the nerve must be widely exposed well above and below the lesion, before the lesion itself is cleared. The nerve must be handled gently with rubber loops or with non-toothed forceps holding only the sheath. To obtain adequate mobilization branches may be stripped up.

Magnification — A loupe or a simple watchmaker's headpiece are of considerable value; but if fascicular repair or grafting is to be attempted an operating microscope is essential.

Resection — With complete division, the fibrous tissue of the proximal end is pared away with a razor blade until axons pout from the stump; similarly at the distal end until the empty tubes are seen. When the lesion is in continuity it is sometimes difficult to know whether resection is necessary or not; if the nerve looks and feels normal or only slightly thick, resection is not advised; if there is a soft fusiform neuroma resection is again inadvisable; if the neuroma is hard, it should be resected. A lateral neuroma usually needs resection; the cut ends are best joined by a graft, but can be sutured directly leaving the undamaged part of the nerve as a loop.

Suture — The sheath only is sutured, using atraumatic needles with fine silk ('virgin silk' is best) or wire. There must be no tension at the suture line, so that gaps must be bridged by mobilization of the nerve and, if necessary, transposition. Flexion of the appropriate joint also helps but it should not be too acute, nor should the process of straightening begin until at least 3 weeks after operation.

After-care — After closure of the wound, the limb is splinted for 3–6 weeks to relieve the suture line from tension. Physiotherapy is then started and is designed to keep the skin, muscles and joints in good condition.

NERVE GRAFTS — In nerve repair there is a critical resection length above which it is useless to try to bridge a gap. The length varies from 7 to 10 cm according to the individual nerve. With greater gaps, autogenous nerve grafts are possible and sometimes successful. If two major nerves (such as the ulnar and median) are irreparable by suture, a pedicle graft from the ulnar nerve may be used to bridge the gap in the median. Alternatively, in certain cases, cutaneous nerves can be spared for use as grafts. These include the lateral cutaneous nerve of the thigh, the saphenous, the sural, and the medial cutaneous nerves of the forearm. Because their diameter is small, several strips may be used (cable graft). Nerve grafts should aim at being 15 per cent too long.

BONE SHORTENING — This is a theoretical possibility to bridge a large gap; it is permissible only when there is established non-union of a fracture, and then but rarely.

PROGNOSIS

The following factors influence prognosis.

TYPE OF LESION — Neurapraxia always recovers fully; axonotmesis usually recovers well; neurotmesis carries the worst prognosis.

LEVEL OF LESION — The higher the lesion the worse the prognosis.

TYPE OF NERVE — Purely motor or purely sensory nerves recover better than mixed nerves, because there is less likelihood of axonal confusion.

SIZE OF GAP — Above the critical resection length suture is not successful.

AGE — In children the prognosis is better than in adults.

DELAY IN SUTURE — This is a most important adverse factor. After a few months, recovery following suture becomes progressively less likely.

ASSOCIATED LESIONS — Damage to vessels, tendons and other structures makes it more difficult to obtain recovery of a useful limb even if the nerve itself recovers.

IRRITATION SYNDROME (Causalgia)

This occurs only with an incomplete division or with an apparently intact nerve; it does not follow complete division. Usually there has been an open fracture or a gunshot wound, often with sepsis. The median nerve and the medial popliteal nerve are most often affected.

There is spontaneous and persistent burning pain which spreads beyond the territory of the affected nerve. It is severe and made worse by physical stimuli or emotional stress. The skin is shiny, moist and warm, with marked hyperaesthesia. Joints are stiff, muscles are wasted. If time and sedatives fail to bring relief, local anaesthetic injections or sympathectomy may help.

LESIONS OF INDIVIDUAL PERIPHERAL NERVES

BRACHIAL PLEXUS: BIRTH INJURIES

UPPER ARM TYPE (ERB'S PALSY)

A traction injury during difficult labour damages the plexus just proximal to Erb's point.   The nerves involved are C.5 and C.6; sometimes C.7 is slightly affected.

CLINICAL FEATURES

The mother notices that one arm is not being used.   The abductors and external rotators of the shoulder and the forearm supinators are paralysed.   The arm is therefore held to the side, internally rotated and pronated.   If recovery does not occur, contractures develop and x-rays show that the acromion and coracoid processes are elongated and droop downwards.

TREATMENT

Most cases (75 per cent) recover without treatment, but it is traditional to hold the arm abducted, externally rotated and supinated either on a splint or by tying the wrist behind the neck to the opposite axilla.   If contracture threatens, splintage and daily stretching are important.

If fixed deformities have been allowed to develop, they may require operative correction; for example, by osteotomy of the neck of the humerus for fixed internal rotation, or division of soft tissues for fixed adduction and pronation.

LOWER ARM TYPE (KLUMPKE)

This rare lesion follows breech delivery with the arm above the head.   The nerves damaged are C.8 and Th.1, especially Th.1.

CLINICAL FEATURES

The intrinsic muscles of the hand and the finger flexors are paralysed.   There may be some sensory loss in the ulnar forearm and hand and sometimes a Horner's syndrome.

TREATMENT

The fingers are kept supple in the hope of recovery, which is a slender one.   Splints and operations are useless.

BRACHIAL PLEXUS: LATER LESIONS

The commonest causes are gunshot wounds and motorcycle accidents, the latter causing traction which may avulse the roots.   Shoulder dislocation may give a partial paralysis, but it usually recovers.   Fractures of the clavicle rarely damage the plexus, and only do so if caused by a direct blow.   A cervical rib may compress the lower trunk.

CLINICAL FEATURES

In the whole-arm type, all the arm, forearm and hand muscles and some scapular muscles are paralysed.   Most of the limb is numb.   With injury at the level of the roots there is often a Horner's syndrome and sometimes associated cord damage; at the level of the trunks, the rhomboid muscles and serratus anterior muscle escape; and at the level of the cords the supraspinatus muscle escapes.   The closer the lesion

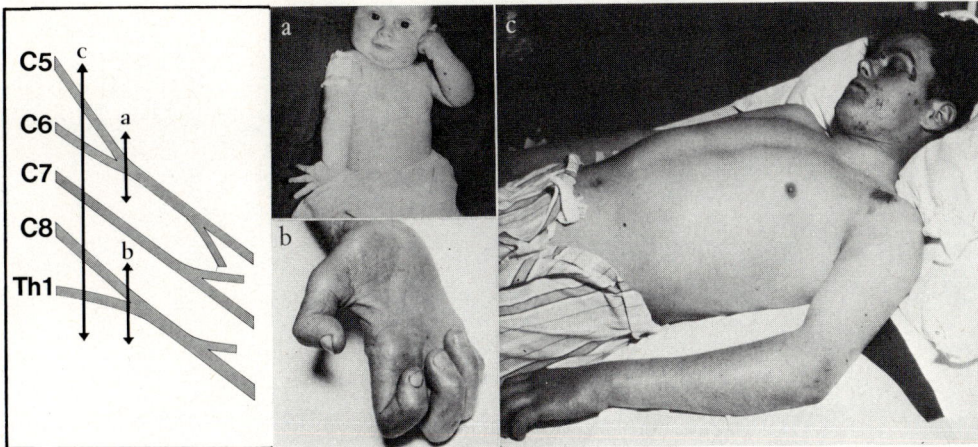

10.1 BRACHIAL PLEXUS
Site of the lesions and clinical appearance of brachial plexus injuries: (a) Erb's
palsy; (b) Klumpke type; (c) tell-tale abrasions on the face and shoulder show how
this motor-cyclist pulled his entire plexus apart.

to the cord, the worse is the outlook; bad prognostic signs include considerable
pain, a tilted cervical spine in the AP view, and a fracture of the appropriate transverse process. Prognostic aids include myelography, electromyography and skin
testing with histamine injections.

In the upper-arm type, the nerves involved are C.5 and C.6. As in Erb's palsy
the shoulder abductors and external rotators and the forearm supinators are paralysed.
Sensory loss involves the outer aspect of the arm and forearm.

The lower-arm type is rare. Wrist and finger flexors are weak, and the intrinsic
hand muscles are paralysed so that a claw hand develops. Sensation is lost in the
ulnar forearm and hand. There may be an associated Horner's syndrome.

TREATMENT

Suture is not possible in any brachial plexus lesion, because the nerves cannot be
mobilized to bridge a gap without tension. Operation is only justified for diagnosis
and prognosis and but seldom on these grounds.

The limb should be maintained in good condition because, with incomplete lesions,
a useful amount of recovery sometimes occurs after 2–3 years.

When the lower trunk is not involved, the hand remains useful. It is then sometimes worthwhile arthrodesing the shoulder so that the arm can be abducted by the
scapular muscles. The latissimus dorsi can be used to restore elbow flexion. Wrist
and finger extension can, in suitable patients, be restored by means of a Robert
Jones transplant (see page 124).

MEDIAN NERVE

Gunshot wounds or fractures may give high lesions. Cuts in front of the wrist may
divide the nerve. Dislocations of the carpal lunate often cause temporary nerve
compression. Compression beneath the carpal tunnel is common (page 179).

CLINICAL FEATURES

In low lesions the thenar eminence is wasted and the opponens pollicis muscle
paralysed (this should be tested by feeling the muscle as contraction is attempted,

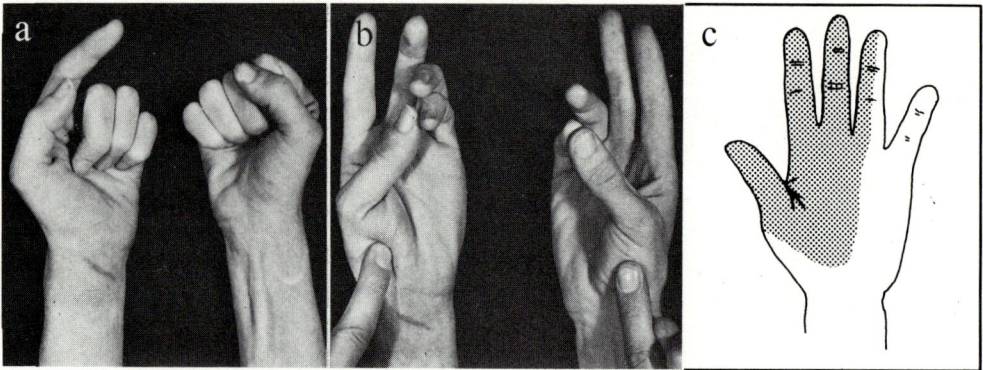

10.2 CUT MEDIAN NERVE
(a) The pointing index when trying to clench the hand; (b) opponens wasting; (c) sensory loss.

because opposition can be faked by a trick movement). Sensation is lost over the radial $3\frac{1}{2}$ digits, and this causes clumsiness, so that the patient cannot pick up a pin.

In high lesions the front of the forearm also is wasted; the thumb, index and middle finger flexors, the radial wrist flexor, and the forearm pronator muscles are all paralysed. Often the hand is held with the ulnar fingers flexed, and the index straight (pointing index). The middle finger may be flexed because its deep flexor, though paralysed, is joined to the unparalysed ulnar half of flexor profundus. Trophic changes are common.

TREATMENT

Suture should always be attempted in median nerve lesions. Extensive mobilization may be necessary; thus for lesions just above the wrist it may be necessary to extend the incision to above the elbow and to divide the bicipital fascia. Incomplete, but useful recovery is common.

While recovery is awaited wrist dorsiflexion should be prevented.

If no recovery occurs the disability is severe because of sensory loss and loss of pincer action. If sensation recovers, but not opposition, a sublimis-opponens tendon transplant may help.

ULNAR NERVE

An open wound may injure the nerve at any level. At the elbow, fracture of the medial epicondyle often causes damage, usually temporary. Fracture of the lateral condyle, if ununited, leads to a cubitus valgus with delayed ulnar palsy. Osteoarthritis of the elbow may cause ulnar palsy from friction neuritis. At the wrist, cuts with glass are common and a deep carpal ganglion may compress the nerve especially at the exit of the piso-hamate tunnel. Bilateral ulnar nerve lesion is rare in England, but occurs in leprosy.

CLINICAL FEATURES

In low lesions (wrist) the hand is clawed, the ring and little fingers being hyperextended at the metacarpo-phalangeal joints and flexed at the interphalangeal joints. Wasting of the intrinsic muscles is especially obvious in the first cleft which, on being pinched, feels much too thin. The little finger cannot be abducted actively against resistance, nor the middle finger waggled sideways. Sensation is lost over the ulnar $1\frac{1}{2}$ fingers.

In high lesions (elbow) although the hand is clawed the terminal interphalangeal joints of the two ulnar fingers are not flexed because half of the profundus muscle also is paralysed (loss of active flexion of the terminal joint of the fifth finger is a useful test).   Otherwise sensory and motor loss is the same as in low lesions.   In lesions well above the elbow, the flexor carpi ulnaris muscle also is paralysed.

TREATMENT

Exploration and suture of a divided ulnar nerve is well worthwhile and anterior transposition permits a gap to be bridged.   Transposition is also advised when a

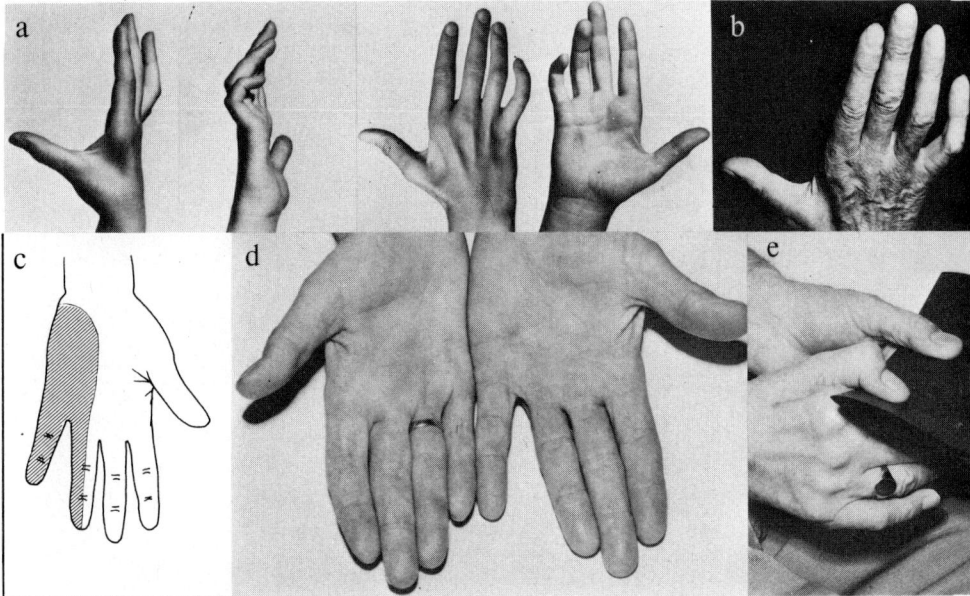

10.3   ULNAR NERVE LESIONS
(a) Low ulnar palsy: intrinsic muscle wasting; knuckle joints of ring and little fingers hyperextended (paralysed lumbricals), interphalangeal joints flexed (paralysed interossei). (b) High ulnar palsy: profundus action is lost, so the terminal interphalangeal joints are not flexed (ulnar paradox). (c) Sensory loss. (d) When the little fingers are pushed apart weakness of abductor digiti minimi is self-evident. (e) Froment's sign.

deformed or degenerate elbow has caused the lesion; not only is the palsy prevented from advancing further, but some degree of recovery usually occurs.   Some lesions at the elbow are due to compression of the nerve by a fibrous band at the proximal end of the flexor carpi ulnaris muscle.   Division of this band is not always sufficient and transposition is preferable.

While recovery is awaited, the skin should be guarded against burns.   Lively splints keep the hand supple and useful.

If recovery does not occur, the hand still has reasonable function.   Bunnell's operation (sublimis-extensor tendon transplant) is sometimes used but Zancolli's operation is probably better; through four longitudinal palmar incisions the volar capsule of the metacarpo-phalangeal joints is shortened by proximal advancement of a distally-based flap.

RADIAL NERVE

Open wounds may injure the nerve at any level. At the elbow, fractures may cause damage which is usually temporary. In the axilla a crutch palsy may occur; this always recovers.

CLINICAL FEATURES

In low lesions (posterior interosseus nerve) the posterior forearm looks flat and the patient can extend neither the interphalangeal joint of the thumb nor the meta-carpo-phalangeal joints of the fingers and thumb. There is no detectable sensory loss.

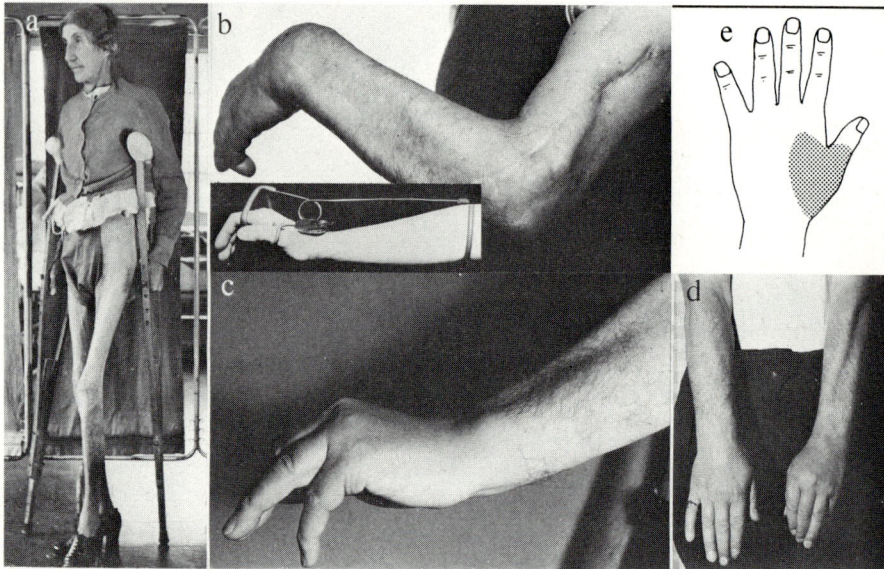

10.4 RADIAL NERVE LESIONS
(a) Crutches should not be thrust high into the axilla, or palsy may follow; (b) complete division with drop wrist (Inset — Brian Thomas splint); (c) this patient demonstrates the inability to extend the fingers at the knuckle joints, but he can straighten the interphalangeal joints with his intrinsic muscles; (d) wasting; (e) sensory loss.

In high lesions (around the elbow) the radial wrist extensors and the supinator muscle also are paralysed (the patient can still supinate the flexed elbow with his biceps muscle).

In very high lesions (axilla) the triceps muscle also may be paralysed. There is a small area of sensory loss on the dorsum of the first cleft.

TREATMENT

Suture below the elbow is rarely possible, because the nerve cannot be sufficiently mobilized. At or above the elbow suture may be worthwhile.

While recovery is awaited, a Brian Thomas splint is worn; this is a 'lively' splint holding the metacarpo-phalangeal joints straight and the thumb straight and abducted, while still permitting active use of the hand.

If recovery does not occur, the disability can be almost completely overcome by tendon transplants, of which the commonest is the Robert Jones transplant: the pronator teres tendon is transplanted to the radial extensors of the wrist; the palmaris longus tendon to extensor pollicis longus; the flexor carpi radialis tendon to the short extensor and long abductor of the thumb; the flexor carpi ulnaris tendon to the finger extensors and possibly to the long extensor of the thumb.

NOTE — Tourniquet palsy is more common in the upper than in the lower limb. It usually affects only or predominantly the motor fibres. Spontaneous recovery is usual.

LUMBO-SACRAL PLEXUS

The plexus as a whole is not liable to injury.

Individual roots may be compressed by an extradural tumour or a prolapsed intervertebral disc.

Pressure on L.5 root may cause weak gluteal muscles, weak foot dorsiflexors and altered sensation over the front of the leg and dorsum of the foot.

Pressure on S.1 root may cause weak gluteal muscles, weak foot plantarflexors and altered sensation along the sole of the foot.

Individual nerves (other than the sciatic) may be affected.

The lateral cutaneous nerve (L.2 and 3) may be compressed within fibres of the inguinal ligament, causing local tenderness and hyperaesthesia or numbness over the outer thigh. This is known as meralgia paraesthetica and is an example of a tunnel syndrome. If severe, the condition may be relieved by freeing the nerve or if necessary dividing it.

The femoral nerve (L.2, 3, 4) may be injured by a gunshot wound. This is rarely seen, because associated femoral artery damage often proves fatal. There is quadriceps paralysis and numbness of the anterior thigh and medial aspects of the leg.

SCIATIC NERVE

Division of the main sciatic nerve is rare except in gunshot wounds. Traction lesions may occur with traumatic hip dislocations and with vertical force fractures of the pelvis.

CLINICAL FEATURES

The calf and leg are thin and the patient walks with a drop foot; all muscles below the knee are paralysed. Because the quadriceps muscle is supplied by the anterior crural nerve it functions normally, but knee flexion is weak because the hamstring supply has been damaged. Sensation is absent below the knee (except on the medial side of the leg) and trophic ulcers often develop on the sole.

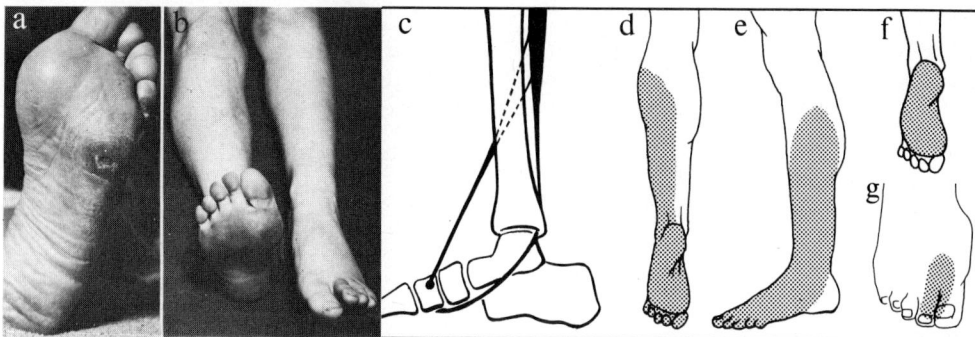

10.5   SCIATIC NERVE
Two problems in sciatic lesions are: (a) sensory loss, which may lead to trophic ulcer; and (b) foot drop, which can be treated with a toe-raising spring, or by transplanting tibialis posterior to the front (c). The remaining diagrams show the area of sensory loss following division of (d) complete sciatic nerve, (e) lateral popliteal nerve, (f) posterior tibial nerve, and (g) anterior tibial nerve.

TREATMENT

Suture should be performed if possible.

While recovery is awaited, below-knee irons and a toe-raising spring are worn. Great care is taken with socks, shoes and foot toilet to try to avoid trophic ulcers.

If recovery fails and sores develop, a below-knee amputation may be necessary.

ROOT COMPRESSION

The commonest cause of pain along the distribution of the sciatic nerve is root compression by a prolapsed intervertebral disc (*see* page 216).

LATERAL POPLITEAL NERVE

The main nerve may be damaged at the level of the neck of the fibula by traction when the knee is forced into gross varus, by pressure from a splint, from lying with the leg externally rotated, by skin traction, by an intraneural ganglion or by wounds. The musculocutaneous and anterior tibial branches are rarely injured except by gunshot wounds.

CLINICAL FEATURES

With a high lesion (the main lateral popliteal nerve), the outer side of the leg is wasted and the patient cannot dorsiflex or evert the foot and toes. He has a foot drop and therefore walks with a high stepping gait. Sensation is lost over the front and outer half of the leg and the dorsum of the foot and toes.

A low lesion involving only the musculocutaneous branch causes paralysis of the peroneal muscles with wasting; on dorsiflexion the foot is pulled into varus. Sensation is lost over the outer side of the leg, foot and toes.

A lesion involving only the anterior tibial branch causes paralysis of the tibialis anticus muscle and the long toe extensors. The front of the leg is wasted and the patient cannot dorsiflex his foot without everting it. Sensation is lost only in the first cleft.

TREATMENT

Where possible the nerve is sutured.

While recovery is awaited a toe-raising spring may be worn if necessary, and the skin must be guarded against ulceration.

If recovery does not occur, any disability can be minimized by tendon transplants (for example, detaching tibialis posterior, threading it through the interosseous membrane and attaching it in front), or foot stabilization. For foot drop following a stroke, an electrical device to stimulate the peroneal nerve is being tried.*

MEDIAL POPLITEAL NERVE

The nerve is rarely injured except in open wounds. A tarsal tunnel syndrome, in which the posterior tibial nerve is compressed in its fibro-osseous tunnel, has been described.

CLINICAL FEATURES

With a complete lesion of the main medial popliteal nerve, the calf is thin and the heel valgus. The patient cannot plantarflex his ankle. The intrinsic muscles of the

---

*A heel switch transmitter worn inside the shoe triggers an external stimulator (powered by a battery worn at the belt) to transmit radio-impulses through the skin in synchrony with the swing phase of gait. The receiver is implanted in the leg and connected to an electrode which activates the peroneal nerve.

foot are paralysed so that the toes are clawed. Sensation is absent over the sole (where there may be a trophic ulcer) and part of the calf.

A lesion of the posterior tibial branch alone causes much less wasting of the calf and weakness of plantarflexion. The toes are clawed from intrinsic muscle paralysis. Sensation is lost over the sole of the foot, but the sural supply remains.

Unlike the lateral popliteal nerve, the medial popliteal or the posterior tibial nerve may suffer from the irritation syndrome, especially when incomplete division is associated with sepsis. There is considerable pain, the skin is warm, wet and shiny and the joints are stiff.

TREATMENT

A complete lesion should be sutured if possible.

While recovery of a high lesion is awaited, a side-iron is worn which fits into a square socket in the heel of the shoe; this prevents the foot dorsiflexing too far. A lesion confined to the posterior tibial branch needs no splintage. Care is taken to avoid ulcers on the sole.

Occasionally an irritation syndrome is so severe as to warrant below-knee amputation.

Suggestions for further reading

' Aids to the Examination of the Peripheral Nervous System ' (1976). *M.R.C. Memorandum No. 45*, H.M.S.O.

Editorial (1972). 'Brachial Plexus Birth Injuries.' *Br. med. J.* **1,** 324

— (1972). 'Causalgia.' *Lancet* **1,** 1170

Omer, G. E. (1968). 'Evaluation and Reconstruction of the Forearm and Hand after Traumatic Tendon Nerve Injuries.' *J. Bone Jt Surg.* **50A,** 1454

Seddon, Sir H. J. (1975). *Surgical Disorders of the Peripheral Nerves.* 2nd Edn. Edinburgh and London; Churchill Livingstone

CHAPTER 11

FUNDAMENTALS OF ORTHOPAEDIC OPERATIONS

ARTHRODESIS

Surgical ablation of movement at a joint is called arthrodesis. With the rising success of total joint replacements the need for arthrodesis is declining. Its chief indications are pain and instability. An 'unsound joint' (i.e. a joint which, following inflammation, is painful or is becoming increasingly deformed) is often best treated by arthrodesis. The disadvantages are self-evident, but stiffness may be a small price to pay for permanent relief of pain.

TECHNIQUE

Ideally both joint surfaces should be denuded of articular cartilage, which usually demands preliminary dislocation. The rawed bone ends are shaped to fit and held in the required position (by internal fixation, external splintage or both) until soundly united.

The optimum positions for arthrodesis (and ankylosis) are as follows.

SHOULDER — 60 degrees of abduction, 30 degrees in front of the coronal plane and rotated so that the hand may reach the mouth.

ELBOW — 90 degrees of flexion for a clerk, straighter for a labourer. The radio-ulnar joint may be in the mid-position or more pronated for writing.

WRIST — A few degrees of dorsiflexion.

FINGERS — 20 degrees of flexion.

HIP — 20 degrees of flexion (to permit sitting), 10 degrees of abduction (more if there is shortening) and 5 degrees of external rotation.

KNEE — The straight position is best if there is any shortening; a few degrees of flexion causes the leg to stick out less but makes arthrodesis harder to achieve.

ANKLE — 90 degrees (slight equinus for women who wear higher heels).

SUBTALAR — Neutral (neither varus nor valgus).

TOES — In the fully straight position.

REGIONAL SURVEY OF ARTHRODESIS

SHOULDER — When performed for abductor muscle paralysis the joint surfaces are rawed and fixed by a screw. For the aftermath of tuberculosis, extra-articular arthrodesis can be used; the outer clavicle and acromion are osteotomized and hinged into a bed chiselled out of the humeral head. In either case the shoulder is held in plaster for three to six months.

ELBOW — Arthrodesis is rarely required because even an unsound elbow can be adequately protected by a sling or a removable polythene splint.

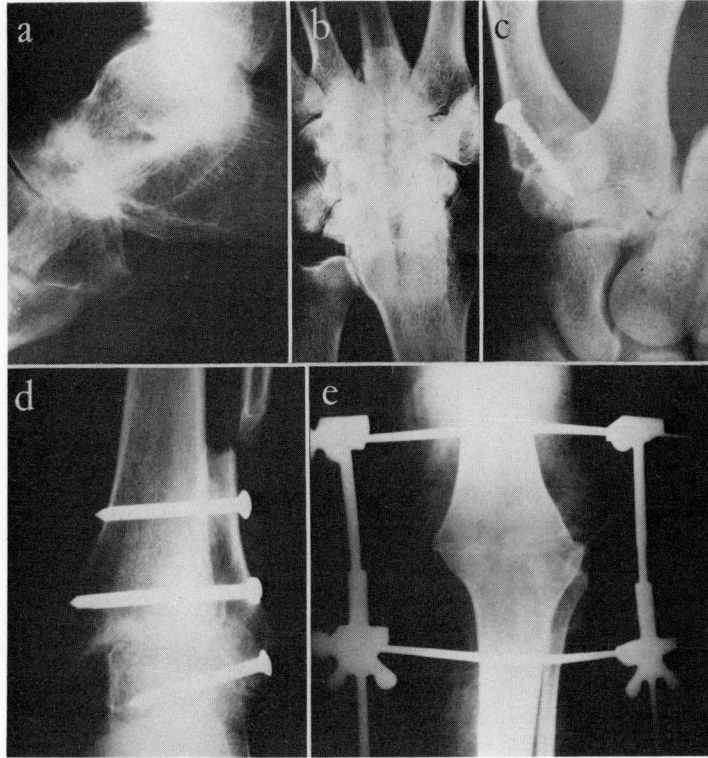

11.1 ARTHRODESIS—
VARIOUS TECHNIQUES
In all cases the joint surfaces are first denuded of
cartilage:
in subtalar mid-tarsal fusion (a), no other measures
are needed; at the wrist
(b), bone grafts are added;
at the carpo-metacarpal
joint of the thumb (c), a
screw may be inserted;

at the ankle (d), the fibula
can be screwed on as a
graft; at the knee (e),
Charnley's compression
clamps are applied.

WRIST — Arthrodesis may be required for arthritis or for paralysis. Through a posterior incision articular cartilage is removed from the proximal row of the carpus and from the lower radius. A strong bone graft is slotted into a trough extended from the radius to the second and third metacarpals. The joint is packed with cancellous chips, and the wrist held dorsiflexed in plaster.

THUMB — For painful osteoarthritis of the carpo-metacarpal joint the surfaces are rawed and the bones fixed with a screw or graft.

FINGERS — Arthrodesis of the terminal joint may be required for flailness due to a cut profundus tendon. The cartilage is removed and the joint held by a screw or wire.

SPINE — In the spine the term fusion is preferred to arthrodesis. The operation may be done from front or back. Anterior techniques are gaining in popularity, especially for spinal tuberculosis and for cervical disc lesions. The essential is to fix one or more bone grafts into cancellous bone; the grafts extend from a healthy vertebra above the lesion to a healthy one below it. Fixation is by ingenious carpentry, sometimes reinforced by internal fixation or external splintage.

In most techniques for posterior fusion a large area of bone is rawed (decorticated) and bone grafts or chips applied. In the lower lumbar spine inter-transverse fusion is popular; and for scoliosis it is usual to denude the facet joints, insert small grafts, and reinforce fixation with Harrington rods.

HIP — Arthrodesis is rarely employed nowadays except in treating the aftermath of an inflammatory arthritis such as tuberculosis. Some of the techniques are illustrated in Fig. 11.2.

KNEE — Arthrodesis is indicated after tuberculosis or for severe osteoarthritis. The patella, synovium and diseased tissues are excised (if the operation is for tuberculosis)

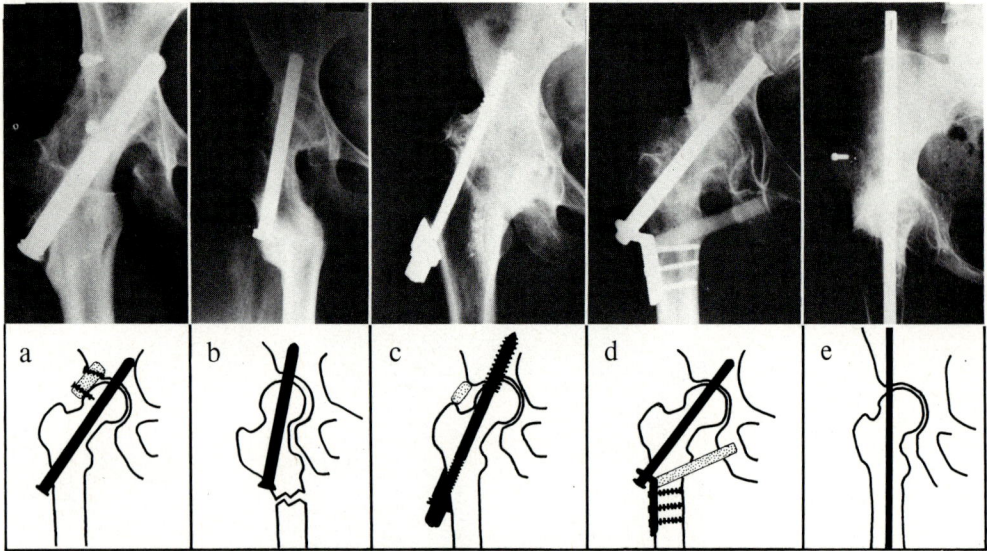

11.2 SOME TECHNIQUES FOR ARTHRODESIS OF THE HIP
(a) Watson-Jones; (b) Pyrford; (c) Charnley; (d) Norwich; (e) Transfixion. With
(a) and (c) a long hip spica is used; with (b) a short hip spica after six weeks' traction;
with (d) and (e) plaster can often be dispensed with.

and the bone ends sawn across. They are held together with the knee straight by parallel Steinmann pins inserted in the femur and tibia. The pins are connected at their outer ends by compression clamps (Charnley's technique).

ANKLE — Arthrodesis may be required for old tuberculosis, for osteoarthritis or for instability. The joint is rawed and held by compression clamps, or by a tibial graft inserted into a socket in the talus, or by using the lower fibula as an onlay graft and screwing it to tibia and talus.

SUBTALAR — Arthrodesis of the subtalar and midtarsal joints is used for degenerative changes following inflammation, injury, for failed correction of club foot, or to stabilize a paralysed foot. The joints are exposed from the outer side, dislocated, rawed and replaced in the plantigrade position (if the operation is for paralytic drop foot the talus is sometimes left in the equinus position, and the midtarsal joint dorsiflexed). For gross plano-valgus deformity the Grice–Green procedure is valuable. The sinus tarsi is approached from the lateral side and with a chisel two channels are cut; into these are jammed tibial grafts of trapezoid shape which fix the talus to the os calcis in such a way as to correct the valgus.

HALLUX — Arthrodesis may be used in treating rigidus or valgus if the interphalangeal joint is sufficiently hypermobile. The metatarso-phalangeal joint is rawed and fixed by a wire, screw or clamps.

OTHER TOES — Arthrodesis is often necessary for hammer toes or for claw toes. Cartilage and bone are removed until the bone ends fit together with the toe straight. It is then held by a collodion splint or wire.

ARTHROPLASTY

Arthroplasty, the surgical re-fashioning of a joint, is designed to relieve pain, or to restore movement, or both. The main varieties are:

(1) *Gap arthroplasty*, in which one articular bone end is excised (e.g. Girdlestone's or Keller's operations); or a whole bone is excised (e.g. the carpal trapezium).

(2) *Interposition arthroplasty*, in which a metal barrier is interposed after re-shaping one bone end (as in Platt's operation at the knee); or after re-shaping both bone ends (as in cup arthroplasty of the hip).

(3) *Partial joint replacement*, in which one articular bone end is replaced by a prosthesis (e.g. Moore's prosthesis for the upper femur, Neer's for the upper humerus and McIntosh's hemiprosthesis for the upper tibia).

11.3 ARTHROPLASTY—THE FOUR VARIETIES
(a) Gap arthroplasty, (b) interposition arthroplasty, (c) partial joint replacement, (d) total joint replacement.

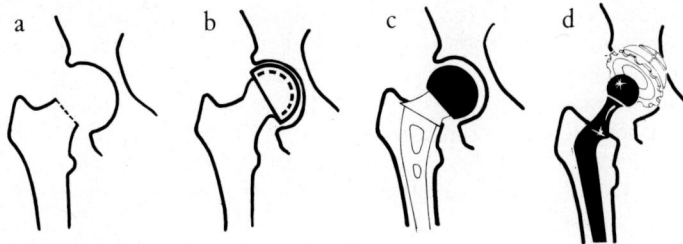

(4) *Total joint replacement*, in which both articular bone ends are replaced.   At the hip total replacement has proved brilliantly successful; most patients enjoy total pain relief and excellent movement.   Elsewhere (e.g. at the knee, elbow and finger joints) the successes are less spectacular and less regularly achieved.

REGIONAL SURVEY OF ARTHROPLASTY

SHOULDER — For some severe injuries Neer advises replacing the head of the humerus by a metal prosthesis with a stem extending into the shaft.   Total replacement joints have been developed by Reeves, Kessel and Lettin but it is too soon to assess their value.

ELBOW — Excision of the radial head (plus synovectomy) is useful in rheumatoid arthritis.   Total replacement gives excellent short-term results, but after 2 or 3 years loosening is not uncommon.

WRIST — Excision of the trapezium is useful in treating osteoarthritis of the carpo-metacarpal thumb joint.

FINGERS — At the metacarpo-phalangeal joints excision arthroplasty often relieves pain; it may, however, weaken the grip and it shortens the palm (the hand looks like a cretin's), so that total replacement is often preferred because of improved appearance and enhanced stability.   A variety of implants (hinged, linked, metal-to-metal, metal-to-polyethylene, polyethylene-to-polyethylene) is available both for metacarpo-phalangeal and for inter-phalangeal joints, and for use with or without cement.   There are, however, many

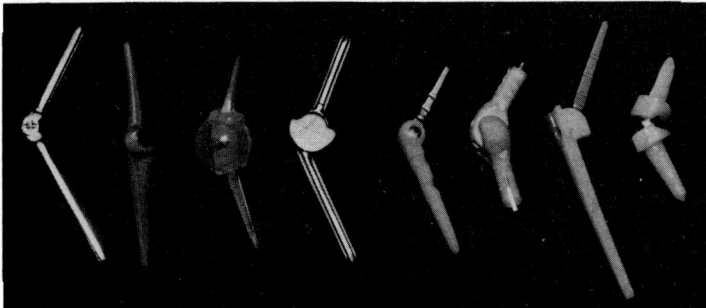

11.4 FINGER JOINT PROSTHESES
A sample of those available.   Reading from left to right: Flatt, Swanson, Calnan-Nicolle, Devas, St. Georg, Mathis, Schultz, I.C.L.H.

extra-articular causes of small joint stiffness in rheumatoid arthritis and unless these are dealt with implant surgery is not successful.

HIP — Every variety of arthroplasty has been used.

(1) Excision arthroplasty (Girdlestone) usually relieves much of the pain, but leaves considerable shortening and instability; nowadays it is rarely used except as a salvage operation when other methods fail.

(2) Interposition arthroplasty (Smith–Petersen) was formerly popular but is now usually reserved for patients in whom osteotomy is unsuitable and who are considered too young for total replacement. The acetabulum and femoral head are denuded of cartilage, reamed smooth and a hemispherical metal cup (or mould) interposed. After prolonged rehabilitation moderately successful results are often achieved.

(3) Partial replacement arthroplasty (e.g. Moore's operation) was, in most hands, a little more successful than cup arthroplasty (the past tense implies that it also has been largely superseded in treating osteoarthritis). The femoral head is removed and a long-stemmed metal prosthesis fitted into the upper femur.

(4) Total replacement at the hip is sufficiently important to merit a separate heading (see below).

KNEE — Patellectomy (a form of excision arthroplasty) is valuable when osteoarthritis is limited to the patello-femoral joint; some instability often results.

Interposition arthroplasty (Platt) is almost never done, but partial replacement is still used occasionally. In McIntosh's operation a portion of one or both tibial condyles is removed and replaced by a metal disc upon whose upper surface the femoral condyle can glide smoothly.

Total knee replacement is now an established procedure (page 135).

ANKLE — Several models of prosthetic ankle, mostly polyethylene-on-metal, are available, but the indications are few.

HALLUX — Keller's operation (excision of the proximal part of the proximal phalanx) and Mayo's operation (excision of the first metatarsal head) are extensively used in the treatment of hallux rigidus and hallux valgus. Silastic implants are occasionally used to fill the gap left by bone excision.

TOTAL HIP REPLACEMENT

Replacement arthroplasty of the hip is so popular that arthritic patients clamour for operation and surgeons continually devise new methods and new refinements of old models. The prostheses designed by the three great British pioneers are shown in Fig. 11.5. Most of the numerous others now available are based on similar principles.

INDICATIONS

These are difficult to define but can be considered under the following headings:

(1) *Pain* especially if severe enough to interfere with sleep or work.

(2) *Stiffness* especially of both hips, but even of one hip if associated with ipsilateral knee stiffness, back stiffness or sexual problems.

(3) *Age* is important. Below the age of (say) 55, osteotomy or arthrodesis should be considered. Replacement is indicated however if these have already failed or if any of the following special circumstances prevail: (*a*) The expectation of life is short (e.g. with patients who are necessarily having steroid therapy). (*b*) The quality of life is poor (e.g. the young woman with advanced osteoarthritis of both hips hoping to have children and to bring them up). (*c*) The amount of activity is limited (e.g. the patient with widespread rheumatoid arthritis has a built-in limitation of activity which will prevent excessive wear or stress of the prosthesis).

ESSENTIALS OF TECHNIQUE

The approach must adequately display the upper femur and the entire acetabulum. The synovium is then removed and (except in Charnley's operation) the entire capsule also. Next, the femoral head is removed, the upper shaft reamed and cancellous bone scraped away. The acetabulum is now deepened, shaped to fit the acetabular prosthesis and holes gouged or drilled in it to augment subsequent fixation.

The acetabular prosthesis is now fixed in position with cement (methyl methacrylate); the powdered polymer is mixed with the liquid monomer but not inserted until a skin has formed. After a trial of reduction the femoral component also is cemented in position. The joint is now reduced, its mobility and stability tested and the wound closed in layers with suction drainage.

Note — The important exception is Ring's prosthesis in which no cement is used. Hence the femoral scraping and acetabular holes are not needed. The acetabulum has a long threaded extension for fixation.

11.5 TOTAL HIP REPLACEMENT (1)
The three original models—all British: (a) Charnley, metal-on-plastic + cement; (b) McKee: metal-on-metal + cement; (c) Ring: metal-on-metal, no cement. With McKee's model a plastic acetabulum is nowadays often preferred.

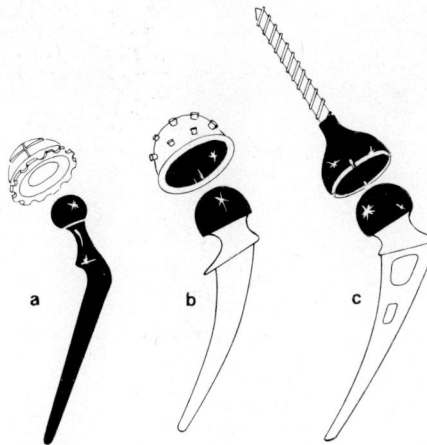

COMPLICATIONS

Hip replacements are usually performed on patients who are somewhat elderly; some are rheumatoid and may be having steroid therapy. Consequently the general complication rate is by no means trivial; deep vein thrombosis in particular is common.

The remaining complications are more likely to occur with this particular operation, or are peculiar to it. Factors which may contribute to their development include previous hip operations, severe deformity (e.g. protrusio acetabuli), an insufficiently sterile operating environment, and lack of experience or expertise on the part of the surgeon or his team.

Operative complications

(1) *Exposure:* an inappropriate or inaccurately placed incision may lead to major nerve damage, either by direct injury or by forcible retraction.

(2) *Acetabulum:* unless the new acetabulum is positioned with meticulous accuracy the hip may subsequently dislocate.

(3) *Femur:* while reaming the femur or driving home the prosthesis the femoral shaft may be penetrated or fractured. Great care is needed if the medullary canal is narrow or the bone osteoporotic.

(4) *Cement:* if the cement is inserted too soon after mixing, especially into the femur, absorption of the monomer may cause a considerable drop in blood pressure.

Post-operative complications

(1) *Dislocation (see above)* — This is most likely to occur soon after operation. Reduction is not difficult and traction or a hip spica usually allows the hip to stabilize; but re-operation may be needed for gross errors.

(2) *Infection* — The large bulk of foreign material restricts the access of the body's normal defence mechanism; consequently even slight wound contamination may be serious. Organisms may multiply in the post-operative haematoma to cause early infection; this may smoulder unrecognized only to flare later, or bacteria from a distant site may, even after years, settle in the hip.

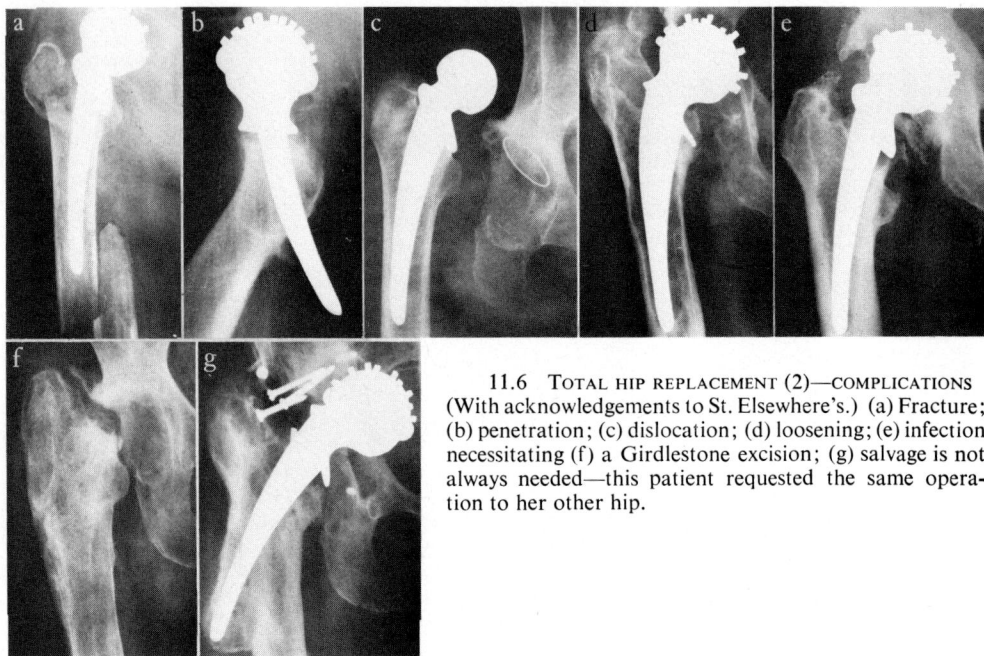

11.6 TOTAL HIP REPLACEMENT (2)—COMPLICATIONS (With acknowledgements to St. Elsewhere's.) (a) Fracture; (b) penetration; (c) dislocation; (d) loosening; (e) infection necessitating (f) a Girdlestone excision; (g) salvage is not always needed—this patient requested the same operation to her other hip.

Prophylaxis is the key. The wound should not be open for too long, the tissues should be handled gently and haematoma formation minimized. The asepsis required is of an even higher order than with other surgical procedures. Special operating enclosures are on trial; powerful filtration and careful aerodynamic design (e.g. laminar air-flow) minimize the chances of contamination. The instillation of antibiotics such as polymyxin is a further wise precaution.

Early wound infection sometimes responds to antibiotics. Later infection does so less often and may need operative 'débridement' followed by the continuous instillation of antibiotic solution combined with continuous drainage for two or three weeks. If all else fails the prosthesis and cement may have to be removed, a procedure euphemistically called 'conversion to a Girdlestone operation'.

(3) *Loosening* — Infection or major trauma may cause loosening; but even without either, torque forces may be great enough to break the bond between cement

and bone; hence the importance of low friction at the artificial joint interface and the increasing popularity of metal-on-plastic joints. Metal sensitivity, especially to cobalt, is another cause of loosening and another reason for preferring metal-on-plastic joints. If loosening causes sufficient pain the operation needs ' revision '.

(4) *Peri-articular calcification* — Masses of calcified deposits occasionally develop round the new joint and lead to considerable stiffness. The cause is unknown. Usually the patient's disposition is blamed, perhaps rightly, for if the second hip is operated on or the first is revised, the same complication is apt to occur.

(5) *Long-term effects* — Between two moving surfaces friction, however slight, is inevitable; one or other surface wears. With metal-to-metal joints the abraded particles form a sludge; but absorption also occurs, for metallic traces can be detected in, for example, hair and nails. With plastic-to-metal joints the abraded particles are of plastic, whose fate is uncertain. No harmful absorption effects from metal or plastic have been found in human subjects over periods of more than 15 years. Nevertheless the longer term effects are still unknown, and it seems wiser not to put younger patients at risk unless this is justified by the severity of the disability.

TOTAL KNEE REPLACEMENT

Knee replacement is less satisfactory than hip replacement because: (*a*) stability is dependent on the integrity of ligaments not, as in the hip, on the intrinsic shape; (*b*) complications are more frequent because the joint is so superficial; and (*c*) failure is more disastrous because the only salvage procedure is arthrodesis, a greater handicap than a Girdlestone hip arthroplasty.

The indication for replacement is therefore pain, which is both severe and known to arise in the tibio-femoral joint (patello-femoral pain may persist after replacement). Movement is rarely increased and the improvement in function is modest. The huge variety of prostheses (some 200) is an eloquent statement that many problems remain unsolved. The available prostheses can be grouped as follows:

(1) *Hinged Joints* (e.g. Walldius, Shiers, McKee, Stanmore) are used when the joint is destroyed, stability lost and the patient fairly decrepit. The term ' hinge ' implies constraint, and while hinges provide stability they lack rotation which the muscles impose; consequently they are liable to loosen, to break, or to erode the tibial or femoral shafts, unless inactivity severely limits their use.

(2) *Surface Replacements* (e.g. Gunston, Freeman, Geomedic, Denham) constitute the largest group. Though variations are great (some have two components, others four) all have two important features in common: (*a*) they prevent contact between worn surfaces; and (*b*) they regain stability by ' jacking the joint apart ', thereby restoring tension to the ligaments. Ligaments are rarely destroyed, even in rheumatoid arthritis; much more often they are lax because of bone and cartilage destruction.

(3) *Linked Joints* (e.g. Attenborough, Sheehan) provide stability yet permit rotation. They are relatively new and it is not known if they will stand the test of time. More bone is removed than with surface replacement, making salvage (if needed) more difficult. Their main indication at present is considerable deformity and instability.

NOTE — Patellar resurfacing can be combined with other procedures; it is still largely experimental.

a   b   c   d   e   f   g

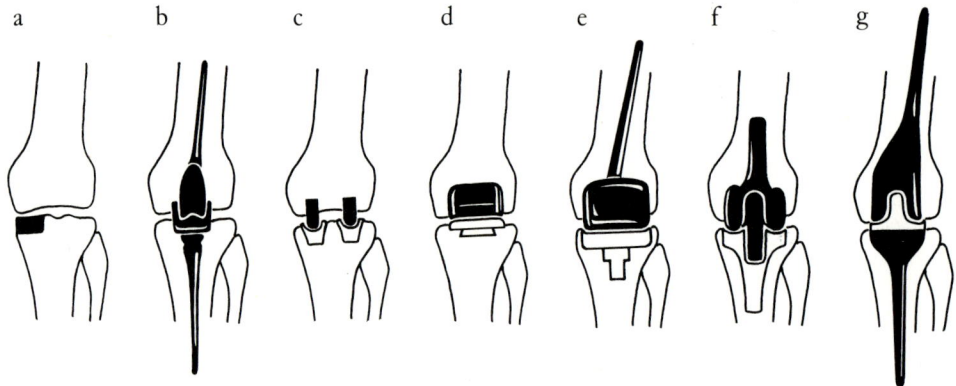

11.7 KNEE REPLACEMENT

(a) MacIntosh, (b) Stanmore, (c) Gunston, (d) Freeman, (e) Denham, (f) Attenborough and (g) Sheehan.

(a) is a hemi-arthroplasty, (b) is a hinged prosthesis, (c), (d) and (e) are largely surface replacements, (f) and (g) are linked prostheses.

COMPLICATIONS

(1) *Infection.* The methods for preventing and treating infection are similar to those used in hip replacement. If the prosthesis has to be removed, arthrodesis should be attempted; hence the advantage of non-bulky prostheses.

(2) *Loosening.* This results from faulty prosthetic design or inaccurate bone removal. It is important: (a) to overcome deformity (the knee should finally be 2° or 3° valgus, no more and no less); (b) to promote stability (by tailoring the bone cuts so that the collateral ligaments are reasonably tight in full extension); (c) to permit rotation (otherwise cemented prostheses are liable to loosen). A loose prosthesis can be re-cemented, but unless the cause is dealt with loosening will recur.

OSTEOTOMY

Osteotomy may be used to correct deformity (e.g. bow legs), to relieve pain (e.g. in osteoarthritis of the hip or knee), or to increase apparent leg length (e.g. with a short adducted hip).

There are three essential stages of the operation:

(1) BONE DIVISION — This should be performed as near as possible to the site of deformity. The bone may be divided transversely or obliquely according to the deformity which is to be corrected. It may be useful to divide only seven-eighths of the bone circumference with a chisel or saw and to break the remaining eighth by hand. Sometimes bone is divided in two places and the wedge between is excised; if so, the base of the wedge is on the convex side of the deformity.

(2) CORRECTION OF DEFORMITY — The aim is to obtain a complete correction, because deformity is more liable to recur if correction is only partial. The cut surfaces should be in close apposition when correction is complete.

(3) SPLINTAGE — If large areas of bone are in contact, plaster splintage is usually sufficient. Often, however, internal fixation is used, and sometimes compression. The correction must be held until the bone ends are completely united.

REGIONAL SURVEY OF OSTEOTOMIES

SCAPULA — Stamm has described an oblique osteotomy of the neck of the scapula which is valuable in treating a painful arc of shoulder movement (page 153).

UPPER HUMERUS — Occasionally osteotomy is required if the shoulder has become fixed in adduction or internal rotation because of disease or unbalanced paralysis.

LOWER HUMERUS — Varus deformity at the elbow from mal-union of a supracondylar fracture may be corrected by removing a wedge of bone from the outer side of the humerus just above the elbow (the radial nerve must be identified and avoided).

SPINE — In ankylosing spondylitis severe kyphosis may be associated with stiffness of the lumbar and cervical spine, so that the patient may be unable to see in front of him. By removing a wedge of bone from two adjacent laminae in the lumbar spine, a compensatory lordosis is produced.

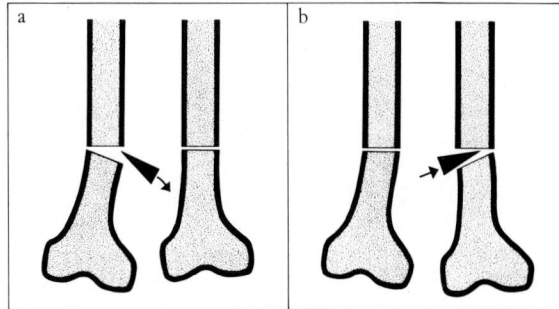

11.8 OSTEOTOMY
A bent bone may be straightened (a) by removing a wedge; or (b) by inserting one. (a) is easier but makes the bone shorter.

HIP — Osteotomy is an important method of treating a wide variety of hip disorders. The pelvis may be osteotomized (Salter, Chiari), or the upper femur divided, usually in the subtrochanteric region. The indications and techniques are described under the appropriate headings (congenital dislocation of hip, page 236; congenital subluxation of hip, page 239; tuberculosis, page 243; pseudocoxalgia, page 245; slipped epiphysis, page 249; osteoarthritis, page 254; and un-united femoral neck fracture, page 424).

SHAFT OF FEMUR — Osteotomy is occasionally required for congenital deformities, or those resulting from rickets, fibrous dysplasia or mal-union.

LOWER FEMUR — Genu valgum may be corrected by a supracondylar osteotomy, the correction being held in plaster. Similarly, a supracondylar osteotomy may be used to correct fixed flexion after inflammatory disease, or genu recurvatum after unbalanced paralysis. For genu varum (bow legs) tibial osteotomy is often preferred.

UPPER TIBIA — Osteotomy may be required for bow legs, angulation and rotation both being corrected. Great care is necessary to avoid damaging the bifurcation of the popliteal artery. Osteotomy is also valuable for osteoarthritis of the knee.

SHAFT OF TIBIA — Osteotomy may be indicated for old rickets or painful Paget's disease.

LOWER TIBIA — If mal-united, a Pott's fracture-dislocation may lead to osteoarthritis of the ankle. This can sometimes be prevented by an osteotomy three-quarters of an inch above the joint, the distal portion being angulated so as to bring the lower surface of the tibia horizontal.

FOOT — Osteotomies are used for talipes equinovarus deformity, claw foot and other deformities. Usually a wedge of bone is removed from the convex side of the deformity, the object always being to make the foot plantigrade.

TOES — Osteotomy of the first metatarsal is sometimes useful to correct hallux valgus in a young patient.

BONE GRAFTS

Bone grafts are used to impart stability, or to fill a gap: these functions may be termed 'splintage' and 'linkage' (Perkins, 1961). For splintage (e.g. for un-united fracture or in arthrodesis) strong cortical slab grafts are required; for linkage (e.g. after evacuating a bone cyst) cancellous chip grafts are needed. In many situations (e.g. non-union with a gap) both types should be used.

VARIETIES

Autografts are taken from the patient himself. Sources include (*a*) the posterior ilium, where many cancellous chip grafts and some cortical bone are available; (*b*) the upper tibia, from which strong cortical slabs and a small amount of cancellous bone can be obtained.

The great advantage of autografts is that they 'take' (i.e. become incorporated) more rapidly and more certainly than any other kind of graft. The only disadvantage is the obvious one: a further operative procedure is involved, with the possibility of haematoma formation, infection, pain, or even fracture.

Allografts (homografts) are taken from a genetically dissimilar human. Sources include (*a*) the fresh corpse of a reasonably young person without transmissible disease; (*b*) ribs removed during thoracic operations. The bone may be deep frozen, freeze-dried, stored in antiseptic solution, or boiled on removal, stored sterile and re-boiled before use.

The advantages are that ample supplies are available and the grafts can be pre-fabricated to fit the host site. The disadvantages are slow incorporation, a small risk of implanting transmissible disease and, most important, the possibility of immunological rejection. The various methods of preparation and storage aim to reduce this danger, but they correspondingly reduce the 'vitality' of the graft. Nevertheless remarkable results have been reported (Imamaliev, 1969) in which articular bone ends from fresh cadavers have, after storage at low temperatures, been transplanted successfully.

Xenografts (heterografts) are taken from non-human species. Calf bone, for example, can be de-natured, suitably cut and shaped, pre-packed and sterilized by irradiation.

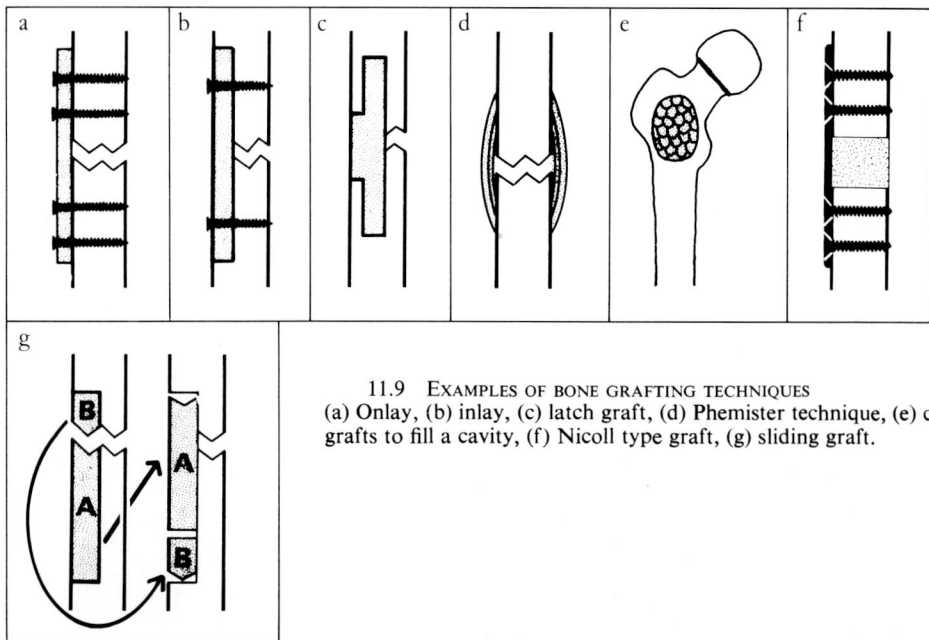

11.9 EXAMPLES OF BONE GRAFTING TECHNIQUES
(a) Onlay, (b) inlay, (c) latch graft, (d) Phemister technique, (e) chip grafts to fill a cavity, (f) Nicoll type graft, (g) sliding graft.

The advantages are the unlimited supply and the possibility of prefabrication to any desired shape.   But, although they are probably non-antigenic, these grafts have very limited osteogenic power and they are not much used.

TECHNIQUES
Some of the techniques used in bone grafts are shown in Fig. 11.9.   Whenever grafts are used for splintage firm fixation is important; even when accurate carpentry provides a snug fit, reinforcement by metal or plaster or both is desirable.

METAL IN BONE SURGERY

Metal is used extensively in surgery because it is strong, relatively inert in the body and easily sterilized; thus it is ideal for surgical instruments.   In orthopaedics it has other important uses: for skeletal traction (page 317); for internal fixation of fractures (page 319); and for joint arthroplasty (page 131).

CHOICE OF METAL
Stainless steels are fairly easy to machine, but lose their stainless quality if the surface is scratched.   Type 316 steel has been superseded by 316L whose minute carbon content (less than 0.03 per cent) is a safeguard against corrosion.

Cobalt base alloys (Vitallium, Vinertia, Stellite and others) may be cast or wrought. They are more difficult to manufacture and less versatile than steels, but not liable to corrosion.   Consequently cobalt alloys are ideal for plates and screws but have no advantage over stainless steel for metal-on-plastic prostheses.

Titanium alloys are easy to manufacture and probably equal to steel in versatility and strength.   They are well tolerated in the body and may become increasingly popular; but with metal-on-metal prostheses sludge forms readily.

DISADVANTAGES OF METAL
INFECTION
Metal does not cause infection, but if a wound is contaminated the presence of any foreign body limits the access of normal defence mechanisms.   Consequently infection may flourish and may persist until the metal is removed.   The remedy is not antibiotics but rigid asepsis and the avoidance of haematoma.

WEAKNESS
Metal plates and screws may not be strong enough to resist angulation at a fracture. Moreover, the bone may have been weakened by drill holes and some of its cells damaged by heat if a motor drill was used.   Consequently with a recently plated fracture plaster is often needed; it is in this situation that 'delayed splintage' (page 321) is especially valuable.

CORROSION
The main causes of corrosion are damage to the surface of the metal and electrolysis between dissimilar metals.   Its effects include loosening, pain and metal fracture. Corrosion is rarely a problem except with plates and screws: here it can be initiated if the screws are of different composition from the plate, if pieces of drill have been trapped between the two, or if the smooth surface of either has been scratched. Consequently it is important to insist upon immaculate standards of manufacture and supply, and to handle metals with almost loving care.

ABSORPTION

Minute particles of metal may be abraded by friction. Some of these contribute to the sludge which can be seen locally, others are absorbed and can be detected in hair, nails and other tissues. Neither effect is known to be harmful, but some heavy metals (e.g. cobalt) could possibly be concentrated in certain tissues and might after many years prove deleterious. The problem only arises where both surfaces of an implanted joint are metallic; little or no metal abrasion occurs where the friction is between metal and plastic, or between metal and bone.

OTHER IMPLANTS

PLASTICS

These are being used increasingly as one component of a total joint replacement. 'Teflon' proved too soft, and ultra-high molecular weight polyethylene is now almost universally used. It has considerable resistance to wear and the few abraded particles have no known harmful effect.

Bone cement (methyl methacrylate) is a special variety of plastic, used extensively for bonding implants to bone. We owe a great debt to John Charnley for its development. The polymer (a powder) is supplied in a pre-sterilized package, the liquid monomer in an ampoule. When mixed they form a doughy mass which sets hard in 5–7 minutes, becoming too hot to handle in the process. The doughy mass must not be placed in the bone until it forms a surface skin; otherwise the toxic monomer may be absorbed causing considerable and possibly dangerous hypotension. Cement can be impregnated with an antibiotic (usually gentamicin).

SILICONES

An entire chemistry, analogous to the organic chemistry of carbon, can be built up around silicon compounds. A multiplicity of physical properties can be achieved, from liquids to hard (Silastic) rubbery materials; all are inert in the body, so the possibilities are endless. Orthopaedic uses already include: silicone oils and grease for joint lubrication; hard Silastic replacements after excision of the carpal scaphoid, lunate or trapezium (and similar replacements at other sites); firm but flexible one-piece finger-joint prostheses; soft sponges for insertion between a prominent meta-tarsal head and an excised diabetic ulcer; and malleable rods for flexor tendon grafting—the rods are first sutured at the proposed site of the definitive tendon graft, then removed leaving an endothelial-lined channel within which the graft can slide smoothly.

NOTE — Prostheses incorporating ceramic components are being tried; they seem likely to have little tissue reaction and to wear well.

LEG EQUALIZATION

Inequality of leg length amounting to more than one inch needs treatment. The possibilities are:

(1) *Lengthening the shorter leg* — The simplest and safest method is a raised shoe. The alternative is operation, after which 5 or 8 cm of length can be gained in the tibia or femur. The bone is osteotomized, with minimum disturbance of perio-steum, and distracted by four skeletal pins (Fig. 11.10). Note that a piece of fibula has been excised and the lower end fixed to the tibia; otherwise the ankle becomes deformed. Distraction must be gradual to avoid damaging nerves or vessels.

(2) *Shortening the longer leg* — In children epiphyseal arrest is an effective method; it can be temporary, using staples; or permanent, using bone grafts. In deciding at what age to operate Menelaus' formula, though approximate, is useful: he assumes

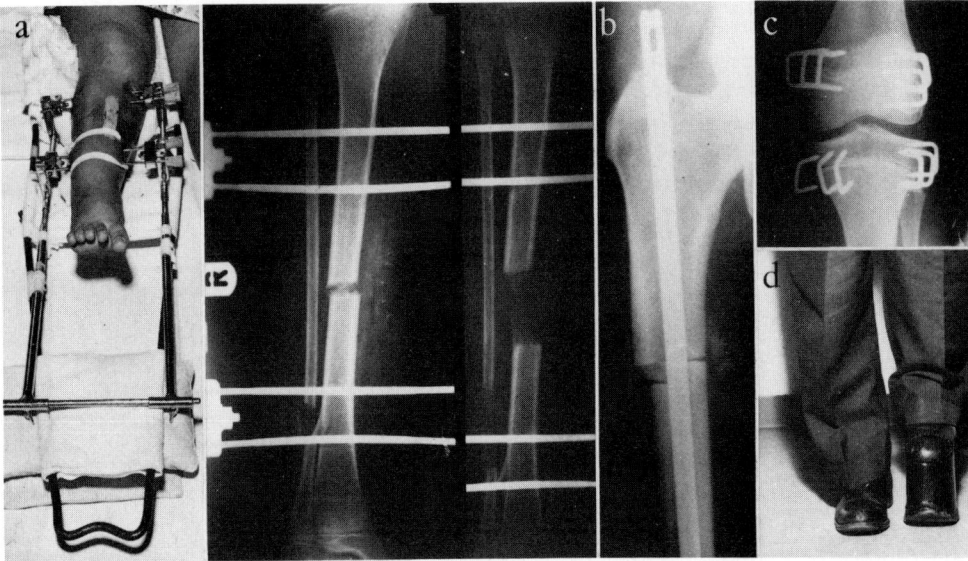

11.10 Leg equalization
The short leg may be lengthened by osteotomy and traction (a). The longer leg may be shortened by excising a length of bone (b), or by arresting epiphyseal growth (c). But the simplest way to equalize length is with a raised shoe (d).

that each year the lower femoral and upper tibial epiphyses contribute $\frac{3}{8}$ inch and $\frac{1}{4}$ inch respectively to length; and that these epiphyses fuse at 14 in boys and 16 in girls. In adults a piece of bone can be excised, preferably using a step osteotomy, and the approximated ends held by internal fixation.

The danger with either method stems from the fact that the longer leg is usually the normal one; should serious complications ensue, the patient may not 'have a leg to stand on'.

(3) *Combined methods* — Merle d'Aubigné (1971) advocates removing bone from the longer femur and inserting it into the shorter one. When this combination is augmented by subsequent tibial lengthening remarkable gains can be achieved.

MICROSURGERY AND LIMB REPLANTATION

Microsurgical techniques, originally used for aural and ophthalmic surgery, have been adapted for orthopaedics. In addition to the operating microscope important pre-requisites are special instruments, microsutures, a chair with arm supports and — not least — a surgeon with a steady hand. While interfascicular nerve suture is of value, the main use of microtechniques is in repairing blood vessels and — occasionally — in reattaching a severed limb or digit. An artery of 1 mm diameter needs 7 or 8 circumferential sutures. Only healthy ends of approximately equal diameter should be sutured; tension, kinking and torsion must be avoided.

Replantation of a severed limb or digit is time-consuming for patient and doctor, seldom successful, and at best achieves only modest function — but it is not impossible. The operation is a virtuoso performance. The surgeon should have practised his technique with the dedication of a concert pianist and his team should be as well drilled as a chamber orchestra. The severed digit or limb should be kept cool during transport. Shortly before operation it is soaked in aqueous chlorhexidine solution. Two teams now dissect, identify and mark each artery, nerve and vein of the stump and the limb. Following careful débridement the bones are shortened to reduce tension and fixed together by K-wires, nails or plates. Next the vessels are sutured — veins first and (if possible) two veins for each artery. Nerves and tendons next need suturing; the excision of less important muscles is another way of reducing tension. Macrodex at the end of the operation and heparin for a few days afterwards are useful. Decompression of skin and fascia, as well as thrombectomy may be needed in the post-operative period.

AMPUTATIONS

INDICATIONS

Colloquially the indications are 3 D's — Dead, Dangerous and Damn nuisance.

(*a*) DEAD LIMB — A limb may be dead because of *severe trauma*, especially to blood vessels, or *gangrene*, due to arteriosclerosis, embolism, thrombosis, or diabetes.

(*b*) LETHAL LIMB — A limb which may kill the patient because of a *malignant tumour*, or *severe sepsis*, especially gas gangrene, or a *crush injury*, in which releasing the compression force may result in renal failure (crush syndrome).

(*c*) NUISANCE — A limb may be inferior to an artificial limb or worse than no limb at all. This may be because the limb is *painful*, *useless*, that is, too flail or too stiff, or *septic*; a leg with recurrent flares from osteomyelitis may be more nuisance than it is worth.

VARIETIES

A *provisional amputation* is performed where re-amputation may be necessary because primary healing is unlikely. The limb is amputated as distal as the causal condition will allow. Skin flaps sufficient to cover the deep tissues are cut and sutured loosely over a pack.

Definitive end-bearing amputation is performed when weight is to be taken through the end of a stump. Therefore the scar must not be terminal, and the bone end must be solid, not hollow, which means it must be cut through or near a joint. Examples are through-knee and Syme's amputations.

Definitive non-end-bearing amputations are the commonest variety. All upper limb and most lower limb amputations come into this category. Because weight is not to be taken at the end of the stump, the scar should be terminal.

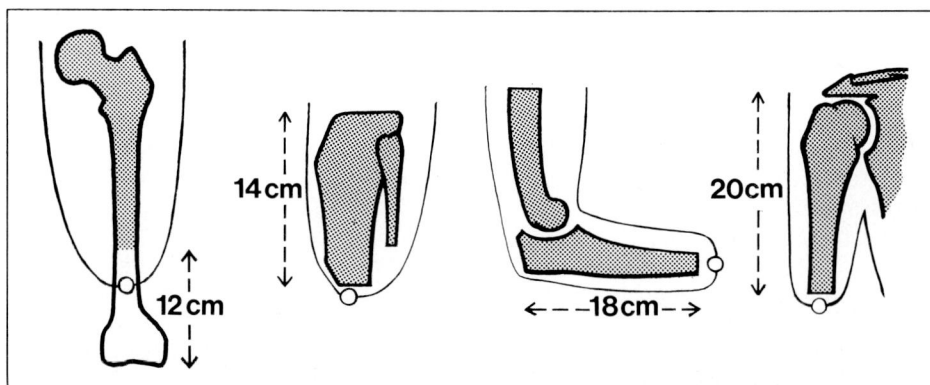

11.11 AMPUTATIONS (1)
The traditional sites of election; the scar is made terminal because these are not end-bearing stumps.

AMPUTATIONS AT THE SITES OF ELECTION

Most lower limb amputations (80 per cent) are for ischaemic disease and are performed through the site of election below the most distal palpable pulse. When deciding the optimum for an individual patient the limb-fitting surgeon should be consulted. The problem with too short a stump is that it slips out of the prosthesis. The dangers of too long a stump are that the disease process may not have been eradicated or the circulation may be precarious.

PRINCIPLES OF TECHNIQUE

A tourniquet is used unless there is arterial insufficiency. Skin flaps are cut — too long at first and subsequently tailored. As a rule anterior and posterior flaps of equal length are used for the upper limb and for above-knee amputations; below the knee a long posterior flap is usual.

Muscles are divided distal to the proposed site of bone section; subsequently opposing groups are sutured over the bone end to each other and to the periosteum, thus providing better muscle control as well as better circulation. Nerves are divided proximal to the bone cut.

The bone is sawn across at the proposed level. In below-knee amputations the front of the tibia is bevelled and the fibula cut 3 cm shorter.

The main vessels are tied, the tourniquet removed and every bleeding point meticulously ligated. The skin is sutured carefully without tension. Suction drainage is advised and the stump firmly bandaged.

AFTER-CARE

If a haematoma forms, it is evacuated at 5–6 days from operation. Repeated firm bandaging or a temporary pylon help to make the stump conical. The muscles must be exercised, the joints kept mobile and the patient taught to use his prosthesis.

AMPUTATIONS OTHER THAN AT THE SITES OF ELECTION

UPPER LIMB

FOREQUARTER AMPUTATION — This mutilating operation should be done only when there is hope of eradicating malignant disease or palliating otherwise intractable pain.

DISARTICULATION AT THE SHOULDER — This operation is rarely indicated, and if the head of the humerus can be left, the appearance is much better. If an inch of humerus can be left below the anterior axillary fold, it is possible to hold the stump in a prosthesis.

BELOW THE ELBOW — The shortest stump which will stay in a prosthesis is an inch measured from the front of the flexed elbow. However, an even shorter stump may be useful as a hook to hang things from. Long below-elbow amputations are no better than those of standard length, for pronation and supination cannot be usefully employed with a prosthesis.

AMPUTATIONS IN THE HAND — These operations are discussed on page 187.

LOWER LIMB

HINDQUARTER AMPUTATION — This operation is only performed for malignant disease. Sir Gordon Gordon-Taylor's technique should be followed in detail.

DISARTICULATION THROUGH THE HIP — This is rarely indicated and very difficult to fit with a prosthesis. If the femoral head, neck and trochanters can be left it is possible to fit a tilting-table prosthesis in which the upper femur sits flexed.

THIGH AMPUTATIONS — A longer stump offers the patient better control of the prosthesis, but at least 12 cm must be left below the stump for the knee mechanism. With less than 18 cm from the top of the greater trochanter it is difficult to keep the stump in the socket.

AROUND THE KNEE — The Stokes-Gritti operation (in which the trimmed patella is apposed to the trimmed femoral condyle) is rarely performed because the bone may not unite securely, the end-bearing stump is rarely satisfactory, and there is no room for a sophisticated knee mechanism.

Amputation through the knee is becoming increasingly popular especially for vascular insufficiency. A long anterior or equal medial and lateral flaps are used. The patella is left in situ and the patellar ligament sutured to the cruciate ligaments. A temporary pylon can be fitted within a few days. Through-knee amputations are also of value in children, because the lower femoral growth disc is preserved.

A very short below-knee amputation with only 3 cm of tibia is occasionally used; the patient takes weight by kneeling on a peg leg.

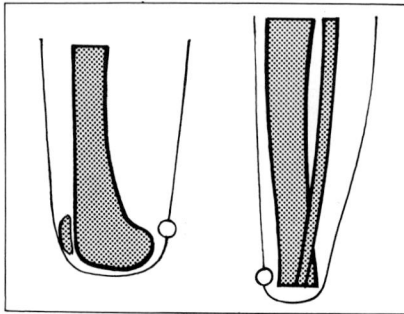

11.12 AMPUTATIONS (2)
Through-knee and Syme's amputations are end-bearing; consequently the scars are not terminal.

BELOW-KNEE AMPUTATIONS — Healthy below-knee stumps can be fitted with excellent prostheses allowing good function and nearly normal gait. Even a 5 or 6 cm stump may be fittable in a thin patient; more makes fitting easier, but there is no advantage in prolonging the stump beyond the conventional 14 cm. With a long posterior flap and suction drainage, healing can often be achieved even when the blood supply is impaired.

ABOVE THE ANKLE — Syme's amputation is sometimes very satisfactory, providing the circulation of the limb is good. The indications are few, and the operation is difficult to do well. Because the stump is designed to be end-bearing, the scar is brought away from the end by cutting a long posterior flap. This flap must contain not only the skin of the heel, but also all the fibro-fatty tissue, to provide a good pad for weight bearing, and therefore in cutting the flap the bone must be picked clean. The bones are divided just above the malleoli to provide a broad area of cancellous bone, to which the flap should stick firmly, otherwise the soft tissues tend to wobble about. Pirogoff's amputation is similar in principle to Syme's, but is rarely performed. The back of the os calcis is stuck on to the cut end of the tibia and fibula.

PARTIAL FOOT AMPUTATIONS — The problem is that the tendo achillis tends to pull the foot into equinus; this can be avoided by splintage, tenotomy, or tendon transplants. The foot may be amputated at any convenient level, e.g. through the mid-tarsal joints (Chopart), through the tarso-metatarsal joints (Lisfranc), through the metatarsal bones or through the metatarso-phalangeal joints. It is best to disregard the classical descriptions and to leave as long a foot as possible providing it is plantigrade and that an adequate flap of plantar skin can be provided. The only prosthesis needed is a specially moulded slipper worn inside a normal shoe.

IN THE FOOT — Where feasible, it is better to amputate through the base of the proximal phalanx rather than through the metatarso-phalangeal joint. With diabetic gangrene, septic arthritis of the joint is not uncommon; the entire ray (toe plus metatarsal bone) should be amputated.

PROSTHESES

All prostheses must fit comfortably; they should also function well and look presentable. The patient accepts and uses a prosthesis much better if it is fitted soon after operation; delay is unjustifiable now that modular components are available and only the socket need be made individually. Powered prostheses are being developed.

In the upper limb, the distal portion of the prosthesis is detachable and can be replaced by a 'dress hand' or by a variety of useful gadgets.

In the lower limb weight can be transmitted through the ischial tuberosity, the patellar tendon, the upper tibia or the soft tissues; combinations are permissible and near-total-contact sockets are available for below-knee stumps. The prosthesis is held on by braces, or belt, or a tight thigh corset; for above-knee stumps a suction socket is often preferred.

COMPLICATIONS OF AMPUTATION STUMPS

EARLY COMPLICATIONS

In addition to the complications of any operation (especially secondary haemorrhage from infection), there are two special hazards.

(1) *Breakdown of skin flaps*: this may be due to ischaemia, to suturing under excessive tension, or (in below-knee amputations) to an unduly long tibia pressing against the flap.

(2) *Gas gangrene:* Clostridia and spores from the perineum may infect a high above-knee amputation (or re-amputation) especially if performed through ischaemic tissue.

LATE COMPLICATIONS

SKIN — Eczema is common, and tender purulent lumps may develop in the groin. A rest from the prosthesis is indicated.

Ulceration is usually due to poor circulation and re-amputation at a higher level is then necessary. If, however, the circulation is satisfactory and the skin around an ulcer is healthy, it may be sufficient merely to excise an inch of bone and resuture.

MUSCLE — If too much muscle is left at the end of the stump, the resulting unstable 'cushion' induces a feeling of insecurity which may prevent proper use of a prosthesis; if so, the excess soft tissue must be excised.

ARTERY — Poor circulation gives a cold, blue stump which is liable to ulcerate. This problem chiefly arises with below-knee amputations and often re-amputation is necessary.

NERVE — A cut nerve always forms a bulb and occasionally this so-called neuroma is painful and tender. The treatment is to excise 3 cm of the nerve well above the neuroma.

'Phantom limb' is the term used to describe the feeling that the amputated limb is still present. The patient should be warned of the possibility; eventually the feeling recedes or disappears.

A painful phantom limb is very difficult to treat; intermittent percussion to the end of the stump has been recommended both for phantom limb and for painful neuroma; it sounds brutal but success is claimed.

JOINT — The joint above an amputation may be stiff or deformed. A common deformity is fixed flexion and fixed abduction at the hip in above-knee stumps (because the adductors and hamstring muscles have been divided). It should be avoided by exercises. If it becomes established, subtrochanteric osteotomy may be necessary. Fixed flexion at the knee makes it difficult to walk properly and should also be avoided.

BONE — A spur often forms at the end of the bone, but is usually painless. If there has been infection, however, the spur may be large and painful and it may be necessary to excise the end of the bone with the spur.

If the bone is transmitting little weight it becomes osteoporotic and liable to fracture. Such fractures are best treated by internal fixation.

Suggestions for further reading

Burwell, R. G. (1969). 'The Fate of Bone Grafts.' In *Recent Advances in Orthopaedics*, Ed. by A. Graham Apley. London; Churchill

Campbell, W. C. (1971). *Operative Orthopaedics*, 5th. Edn. London; Kimpton

Charnley, J. (1970). *Acrylic Cement in Orthopaedic Surgery*. London; Churchill-Livingstone

Gordon-Taylor, G., Wiles, P., Patey, D. H., Turner-Warwick, W. and Monro, R. S. (1952). 'The Interinnomino-abdominal Operation.' *J. Bone Jt Surg*. **34B**, 14

Helal, B. (1969). 'Silicones in Orthopaedic Surgery.' In *Recent Advances in Orthopaedics*, Ed. by A. Graham Apley. London; Churchill

Imamaliev, A. S. (1969). 'The Preparation, Preservation and Transplantation of Articular Bone Ends.' In *Recent Advances in Orthopaedics*, Ed. by A. Graham Apley. London; Churchill

McKee, G. K., Charnley, J., Hicks, J. H. and Zarek, J. M. (1957). Symposium: 'The Use of Metal in Bone Surgery.' *Proc. R. Soc. Med.* **50,** 837

Menelaus, M. B. (1966). 'Correction of Leg Length Discrepancy by Epiphyseal Arrest.' *J. Bone Jt Surg.* **48B,** 336

Merle d'Aubigné, R. and Debousset, J. (1971). ' Surgical Correction of Large length discrepancies in the lower extremities of children and adults.' *J. Bone Jt Surg.* **53A,** 411

O'Brien, B. McC. (1977). *Microvascular Reconstructive Surgery*. Edinburgh; Churchill Livingstone

Perkins, G. (1961). *Orthopaedics* London; Athlone Press

Robinson, K. P. (1976). ' Amputations of the Lower Limb.' *Br. J. Hosp. Med.* **16,** No. 6

'Symposium on Limb Ablation and Limb Replacement' (1967). *Ann. R. Coll. Surg. Eng.* **40, 4**

CHAPTER 12

THE SHOULDER JOINT

EXAMINATION OF THE SHOULDER

SYMPTOMS

Pain may be felt at the point of the shoulder or anteriorly. More often it is felt at the insertion of the deltoid muscle and radiates to the outer side of the elbow and to the dorsum of the forearm and wrist. Stiffness may cause difficulty in dressing, brushing the hair, or similar activities in which the arm is raised. Weakness is only occasionally a symptom.

SIGNS

LOOK

Skin — Scars or sinuses are noted.

Shape — There may be wasting of the deltoid muscle. When the acromio-clavicular joint is dislocated, the outer end of the clavicle forms an obvious lump.

Position — The position in which the arm is held may be of diagnostic value.

FEEL

Skin — Because the joint is well covered inflammation rarely influences the skin temperature.

Soft tissues — Fluid and synovial thickening are not detectable. Muscle bulk and tautness, especially of the deltoid muscle, are tested.

Bony points — The clavicle, acromion process and humeral head are systematically palpated. Tenderness is sometimes difficult to localize.

MOVE — Movements occur not only at the gleno-humeral joint but also between the scapula and the chest wall. The combined movements are tested first, then gleno-humeral movement is assessed separately.

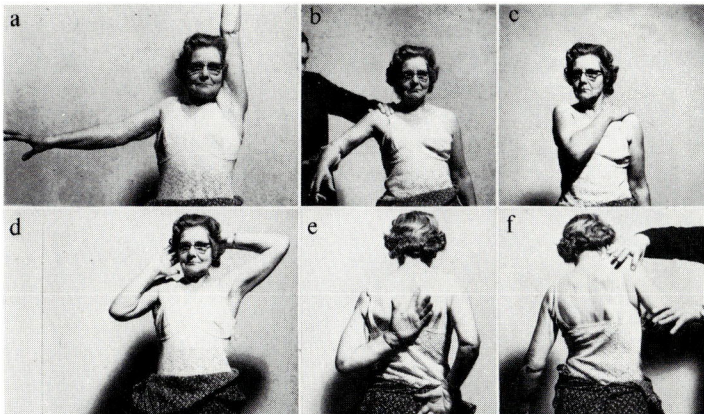

12.1 EXAMINATION OF THE SHOULDER Exemplified in a patient with a frozen right shoulder: all movements are limited. (a) active abduction, (b) anchoring the acromion to isolate gleno-humeral abduction, (c) adduction, (d) external rotation, (e) internal rotation, (f) testing power in the deltoid muscle.

Active movements — The patient is asked to raise his arms sideways until they point to the ceiling. Abduction may be (*a*) diminished in range; (*b*) painful; (*c*) altered in rhythm, that is, the scapula begins to move too early, producing a shrugging effect.

To test adduction the patient is asked to touch the opposite shoulder blade by moving his arm in front of the body; and then behind the body to test internal rotation. External rotation may be examined in two ways: by trying to touch the back of the neck while keeping the elbows well back; or by tucking the elbows into the side, bending them to 90 degrees, and then separating the hands. Flexion and extension can be examined by raising the arms forwards and then backwards.

Passive movements — If the patient is unable to abduct his arm fully, passive abduction is tried. With a complete tear of the supraspinatus tendon, active abduction is grossly limited, but passive abduction is full. Internal and external rotation may also be examined passively, and, if the shoulder can be abducted to a right-angle, about 90 degrees of rotation in each direction is normally possible.

If movement at the shoulder is limited, gleno-humeral movement is tested separately, for, even when the gleno-humeral joint has been arthrodesed, the arm can be raised to nearly 90 degrees; the scapula is therefore anchored by placing one hand on the acromion process while the other hand moves the patient's arm.

Power — The patient is asked to abduct the arm actively. With one hand the surgeon resists the movement, with the other he feels the deltoid muscle.

X-RAY — The antero-posterior view is the most useful. The film is examined in an orderly sequence, noting the density as a whole, the joint position and line, and the detail of the individual bones. A calcified area may be seen just above the great tuberosity.

SCAPULAR DISORDERS

SPRENGEL'S SHOULDER (CONGENITAL UNDESCENDED SCAPULA)

The scapulae normally complete their descent from the neck by the third month of foetal life. Rarely one remains unduly high.

CLINICAL FEATURES

Deformity is the only symptom, even though movement is limited. The signs are:

LOOK — The shoulder on the affected side is higher and a 'web' of skin may run from it to the side of the head.

FEEL — The scapula feels abnormally high and is small.

MOVE — Movements are painless, but abduction may be considerably limited by fixation of the scapula.

X-RAY — This often shows abnormalities of ribs and vertebrae, and sometimes an extra bone (omo-vertebral) between the upper scapula and the cervical spine.

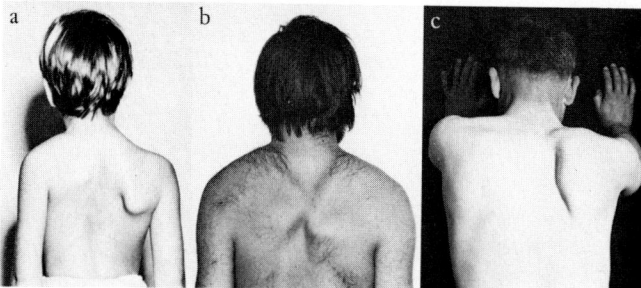

12.2 SCAPULAR DISORDERS
(a) Sprengel shoulder;
(b) Klippel–Feil syndrome;
(c) winged scapula.

TREATMENT

Mild cases are best left untreated.   When abduction is restricted by an omo-vertebral bone its excision considerably improves function.   If the supero-medial portion of the scapula also is excised, the shoulder may look less deformed.   An alternative is vertical osteotomy of the scapula near its vertebral border; the main mass of the bone is pulled distally and fixed back to the undisturbed medial portion.

> NOTE — In the Klippel-Feil syndrome there is bilateral failure of scapular descent.   The patient looks as if he has no neck; there is a low hair line, bilateral neck webbing, and gross limitation of movement.   Other congenital abnormalities are present.
>
> Bilateral shortness of the sternomastoid muscle is another rare condition in which the patient looks as if he has scarcely any neck, but his head is poked forwards and his chin sticks up; in contrast with Klippel-Feil syndrome, there are no associated congenital deformities.

WINGED SCAPULA

The serratus anterior muscle is paralysed, usually by trauma from carrying a heavy weight on the shoulder or from damage to the long thoracic nerve during radical mastectomy.   Some cases appear to be infective in origin.   Traumatic rupture of the muscle has also been described.

The patient is asked to raise his arms 90 degrees and to push with his hands against a wall.   Winging (backward projection of the vertebral border) then becomes obvious.   Movements are usually full and power only slightly reduced.   The disability is slight and is best accepted.

GRATING SCAPULA

The patient complains of noisy grating or clicking on moving the arm.   It is painless, and the cause is unknown, though bony, muscular, or bursal abnormalities have been blamed.   No treatment is advised.

TUBERCULOSIS OF THE SHOULDER

(See also page 34)

Although the disease process starts as a synovitis or osteomyelitis, it is rarely seen until arthritis has supervened.   Abscess and sinus formation are quite common (florid type).   If there is no discharge at any stage the term 'caries sicca' is used; one suspects, however, that many cases of reputed caries sicca were examples of frozen shoulder.

SYMPTOMS AND SIGNS

A constant grumbling ache may last many months or years, and the patient may complain of stiffness.

Adults are mainly affected.   The general signs of tuberculosis are often slight, though pulmonary tuberculosis may coexist.

> LOOK — A sinus may be present, but the striking feature is marked wasting of the deltoid muscle and, to some extent, of the scapular muscles.
>
> FEEL — Diffuse tenderness is common and slight warmth may be detectable.
>
> MOVE — All movements are considerably limited and may cause pain.
>
> X-RAY — Generalized rarefaction is present, usually with some erosion of both joint surfaces; there may be a ragged abscess cavity in the humeral head.

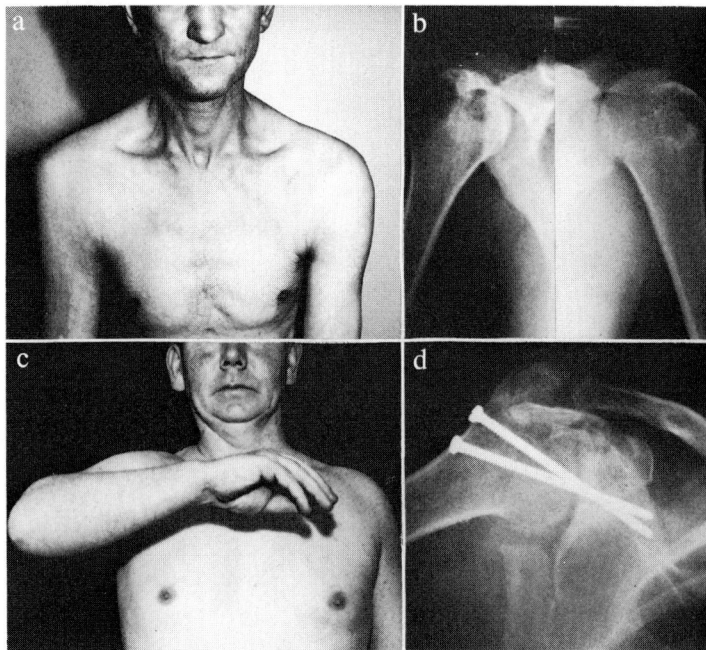

12.3 TUBERCULOSIS
OF THE SHOULDER

(a) marked wasting
of right deltoid;

(b) bone rarefaction
and joint damage in
arthritis, compared
with the normal;

(c, d) after arthro-
desis of the gleno-
humeral joint
scapulo-thoracic
movement remains,
permitting useful
abduction.

TREATMENT

In addition to general treatment (page 35) the shoulder may be rested on an abduction splint. Healing occurs by fibrosis and, because of the prolonged action of gravity, the fibrous joint gradually elongates, so that some surgeons are content merely to rest the arm in a sling from the start. Unless the disease is obviously settling within two months a clearance operation is advisable (page 39).

If flares subsequently occur, or if the shoulder continues to be painful, the joint is arthrodesed by turning down the outer end of the acromion process and clavicle and embedding them into the humeral head.

MUSCULOTENDINOUS CUFF LESIONS

The supraspinatus, infraspinatus, subscapularis and teres minor muscles become tendinous at their outer ends, and the tendons blend with the capsule to form a cuff. This tendinous area, and especially the supraspinatus tendon, is liable to a variety of lesions. The differing clinical pictures stem directly from the underlying pathology; in all there is a mixture of three factors—degeneration, trauma and reaction.

Degeneration — It has been shown that, in the resting position, blood is squeezed out of the supraspinatus tendon. This may explain the frequent autopsy finding (even with symptomless shoulders) of areas of avascular degeneration—increasing with advancing age. As in other avascular areas, calcification may occur.

Trauma — The supraspinatus tendon is liable to injury if its contraction is resisted. This may occur when lifting a weight, or when the patient uses his arm to save himself from falling. It is very difficult to injure the cuff unless it is already degenerate; and the more degenerate it is the more easily it tears.

Reaction — In an attempt to repair a torn tendon or to revascularize a degenerate area, new blood vessels grow in; probably it is this 'inflammatory reaction' which results in pain.

WEAR, TEAR AND REPAIR — The three pathological processes may be summed up as 'wear', 'tear', and 'repair'. In the young patient the 'repair' process is vigorous; consequently, healing is relatively rapid but (because the repair process itself causes pain) it is accompanied by considerable distress. The older patient has more 'wear', but less vigorous 'repair'; healing will be slower but pain less severe. Thus acute tendinitis (the youngest lesion) is intensely painful but rapidly better; chronic tendinitis and frozen shoulder (a middle group) are only moderately painful but take many months to recover; and a complete tear (usually elderly) becomes painless soon after injury, but never mends.

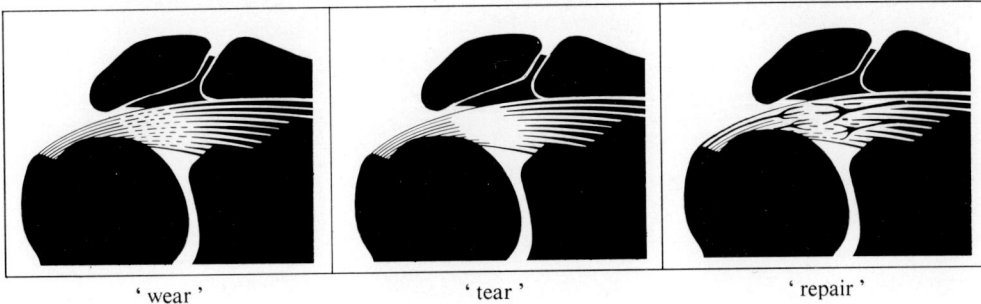

' wear '   ' tear '   ' repair '

12.4   THE PATHOLOGY OF SUPRASPINATUS LESIONS

Age	Lesion	Wear	Tear	Repair	Pain	Recovery
Young	Acute tendinitis	?	?	+ + + +	+ + + +	Rapid
Old	Complete tear	+ + + + +	+	O	O	O
Middle	Partial tear Painful arc Frozen shoulder	+ + +	+ or −	+ +	+ +	Slow

ACUTE TENDINITIS (ACUTE CALCIFICATION)

Degeneration in a small localized area of the supraspinatus tendon probably accounts for the deposition of calcium. Trauma is insignificant; no more, as a rule, than a little over-use.

The reaction is tremendous. There is rapid swelling, and tension within the tendon rises, like a boil before it bursts. Once the calcified substance has erupted into the bursa, tension and pain quickly subside and the calcium is absorbed.

SYMPTOMS

A young adult, usually aged 25–45, though occasionally older, complains of dull aching sometimes following slight over-use. Hourly the pain increases in severity, rising in a crescendo to an agonizing climax. After a few days, pain subsides and the shoulder then gradually returns to normal. In some patients the process is less dramatic; pain is less severe and recovery slower.

SIGNS

LOOK — The patient holds the arm almost immobile.

FEEL — The joint is too tender to permit precise palpation.

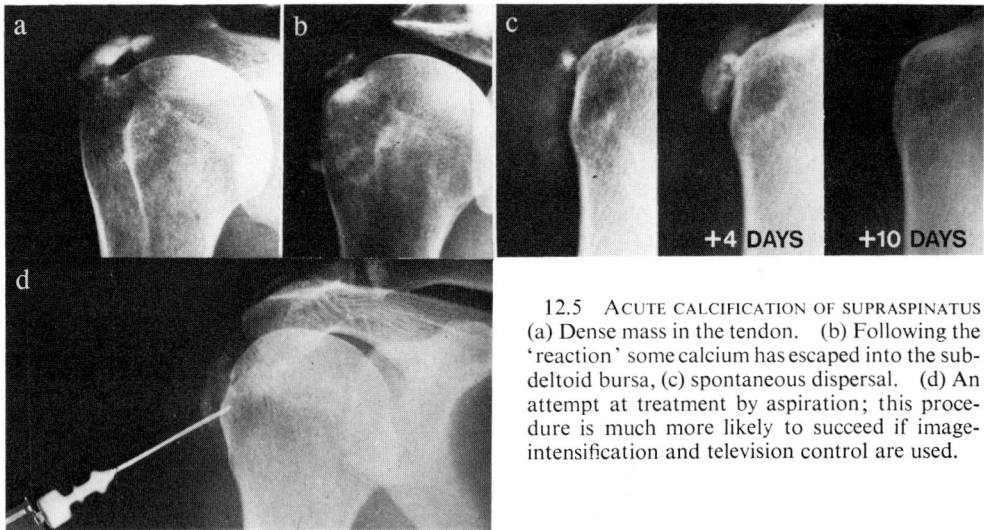

12.5 ACUTE CALCIFICATION OF SUPRASPINATUS
(a) Dense mass in the tendon.   (b) Following the
'reaction' some calcium has escaped into the subdeltoid bursa, (c) spontaneous dispersal.   (d) An
attempt at treatment by aspiration; this procedure is much more likely to succeed if image-
intensification and television control are used.

MOVE — Active abduction is very painful and, if the condition is severe, movement is impossible.

X-RAY — Calcification is always present and shows as a dense area just above the great tuberosity.   As pain subsides the calcium appears to have spilt into the subdeltoid bursa; eventually it disappears.

TREATMENT

The patient is given morphine and a sling; spontaneous recovery usually occurs within a very few days and full shoulder movements return.   Relief of pain can often be hastened by injecting local anaesthetic into the affected area and then attempting to aspirate the toothpaste-like calcified material.   Usually nothing can be withdrawn, even when the area is pin-pointed by using an image intensifier; nevertheless the needle puncture relieves tension by facilitating eruption into the bursa.

If symptoms are severe, rapid relief can be obtained by operation.   Through a small vertical incision just below the acromion process the deltoid fibres are separated and, on rotating the humerus, the affected area of tendon is seen.   The calcified material is scooped out.

CHRONIC TENDINITIS (PAINFUL ARC)

Degeneration of moderate degree affects a small area of the supraspinatus tendon near its insertion.   The vascular response may be triggered off by an injury (such as a small tear) or merely by over-use.   The resulting swelling is often slight, but is so situated that, on abduction, it impinges upon the under surface of the acromion.

SYMPTOMS

The patient, usually aged 45–60 years, complains that certain movements and certain positions of the shoulder are painful.   These symptoms come on gradually or may follow a few weeks after an injury.

SIGNS

LOOK — The shoulder looks normal.

FEEL — There may be tenderness below the acromion process or further forward.

MOVE — In mid-abduction there is a painful arc of movement, often with a characteristic jerk as the affected area of tendon comes into contact with the under surface of the acromion process. Once this point is passed abduction is painless, because the swollen area is no longer pressing against bone.

If the tendinitis has followed a partial tear, there may also be some loss of power and faulty rhythm.

X-RAY — Usually the appearance is normal, but occasionally calcification just above the greater tuberosity is seen.

DIFFERENTIAL DIAGNOSIS

Acromio-clavicular osteoarthritis also may cause pain on abduction; the pain is not limited to a small arc of movement but is usually felt through the entire range of abduction above a right-angle. Adduction also is painful, and the joint feels thick and tender. X-ray shows sclerosis and lipping. The condition may be treated by heat, injections, or very rarely by excising the outer end of the clavicle.

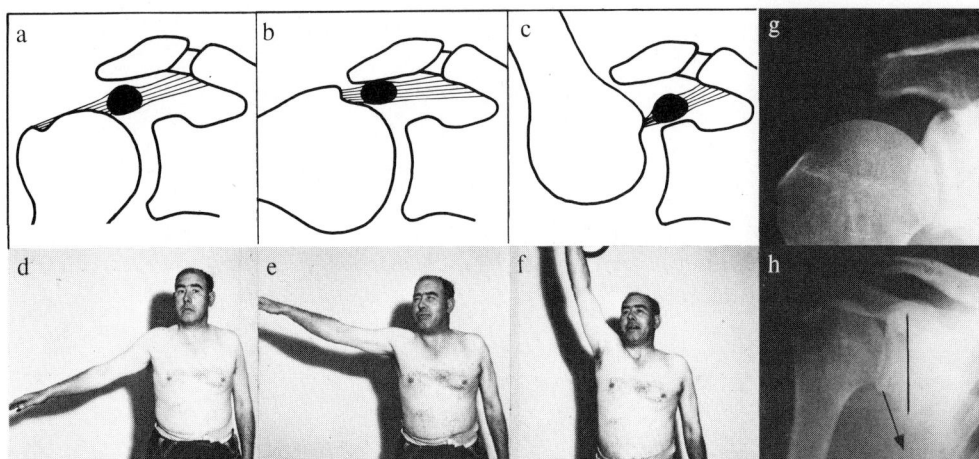

12.6 PAINFUL ARC
(a-f) The patient registers pain over only a limited arc of abduction, and the diagrams show why. Operation is rarely needed: the possibilities are (g) acromionectomy, and (h) glenoid osteotomy.

TREATMENT

Chronic tendinitis usually responds to conservative treatment, which consists of heat, exercises and injections. Heat (infra-red or short-wave diathermy) is soothing. For exercises the patient is told to use his arm but to try and avoid the actual arc of pain. Injection of local anaesthetic and hydrocortisone into the tender area is often helpful and if so can be usefully repeated after 3 or 4 weeks.

Rarely, if conservative treatment fails and pain is considerable, operation is indicated. Anterior acromionectomy may be performed; or Stamm's operation, in which an oblique osteotomy through the neck of the glenoid enables the shoulder joint to be displaced downwards and medially.

FROZEN SHOULDER (ADHESIVE CAPSULITIS, PERI-ARTHRITIS)

Probably the process is initiated by injury or over-use in the usual part of the supraspinatus tendon; but it spreads to involve the entire tendinous cuff. This becomes thick, vascular and infiltrated with lymphocytes and plasma cells; it sticks to the humeral head, and the infra-articular 'gusset' of capsule may be obliterated by adhesions. It seems likely that the cause is an auto-immune response to the breakdown of collagen fascicles or their mucopolysaccharide sheaths.

SYMPTOMS

The patient, aged 45–60, may give a history of trauma, often trivial, followed by pain and stiffness. The pain is felt at the deltoid insertion and radiates along the outer side of the arm to the back of the forearm and hand. Gradually it increases in severity and often prevents the patient from sleeping on the affected side. After several months it slowly subsides. Stiffness also increases in severity for some months, and becomes more and more of a handicap. It outlasts the pain by a few months, then gradually movement returns, almost to normal.

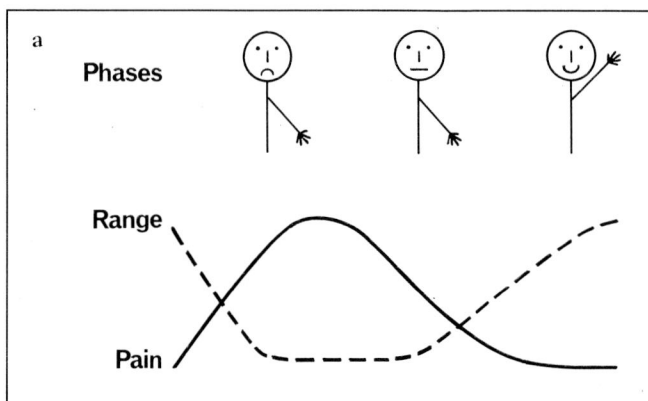

12.7   FROZEN SHOULDER (*see also* Fig. 12.1, page 147) (a) Natural history of frozen shoulder. The face tells the story.

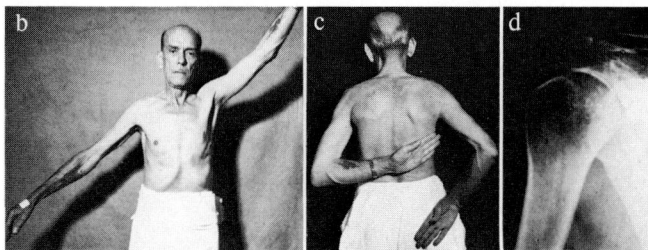

(b, c, d) Patient in phase 2: limited abduction (b); limited internal rotation (c); localized rarefaction (d).

There are thus three phases: (1) increasing pain and increasing stiffness; (2) decreasing pain with persistent stiffness; (3) painless return of almost full movement. Each phase lasts 4–8 months.

SIGNS

LOOK — Occasionally there is slight wasting.

FEEL — Tenderness may be felt below the acromion process or in front.

MOVE — In a severe case movements, both active and passive, are grossly restricted in all directions from the sling position. With recovery the range slowly increases. (There is great variation in the severity of frozen shoulder. In the mildest type there may be only slight restriction of the extremes of range, with gradual recovery after a few months.)

X-RAY — The x-ray appearance of a frozen shoulder is widely accepted as normal; but usually there is a little rarefaction beneath the greater tuberosity.

DIFFERENTIAL DIAGNOSIS

The following conditions must be distinguished from frozen shoulder.

POST-TRAUMATIC STIFFNESS — After a fractured neck of humerus stiffness may persist for some months. There is, however, a history of injury followed by a bruise; the stiffness is maximal at the start and gradually lessens (unlike the pattern of a frozen shoulder), and x-rays show the fracture.

TUBERCULOSIS — Tuberculosis, like frozen shoulder, has a long history of ache and stiffness, but wasting is much more marked and x-rays show bone destruction. Caries sicca ('dry tuberculosis') is said to enjoy a good prognosis; this is readily explicable if the term is erroneously applied to cases of frozen shoulder.

OSTEOARTHRITIS — Contrary to popular belief, osteoarthritis of the shoulder is rare. It should not be diagnosed unless the phasic story of a frozen shoulder is lacking and x-rays show osteophytes. If there is subsequent recovery of painless movement it indicates that the true diagnosis of frozen shoulder had been missed.

TREATMENT

Conservative treatment aims at alleviating pain while recovery is awaited; it is important not only to administer analgesics but also to reassure the patient that recovery is certain. Heat sometimes helps, though often ice-packs are more soothing. Exercises are encouraged, but the patient is warned that moderation and regularity will achieve more than sporadic masochism. Serial injections of hydrocortisone with local anaesthetic sometimes help.

Manipulation under anaesthesia often hastens recovery; hydrocortisone and local anaesthetic are injected, then external rotation is restored, and finally abduction is gently but firmly regained. Alternatively range can be increased by distending the joint with a large quantity (up to 200 cc) of fluid. Arthrographic studies demonstrate that distension or manipulation achieve their effect by rupturing the capsule.

SUPRASPINATUS TEARS

PATHOLOGY

Degeneration is an essential prerequisite for a supraspinatus tear. The injury need not be severe; with gross degeneration relatively slight trauma may cause a complete tear.

The reaction to a partial tear consists of the ingrowth of blood vessels to the damaged area; the intact tendon fibres provide sufficient splintage to enable the torn fibres to be repaired. With a complete tear there is little or no reaction; no repair occurs and the lateral stub of tendon (about half an inch) is rubbed away.

SYMPTOMS

The patient is usually aged 45–65; the younger he is the more likely is the tear to be a partial one. While lifting a weight or protecting himself from falling he 'sprains' the shoulder. Pain is felt immediately, radiating from the deltoid insertion, and he is unable to lift the arm sideways.

Often the patient seeks no advice, or is given no effective treatment. If the tear is partial he may (a) gradually recover fully; (b) partly recover, but with a persistent painful arc of abduction; or (c) gradually develop a frozen shoulder. If the tear is complete the pain soon subsides, but gross weakness of abduction persists; other movements return and frozen shoulder is never the sequel to a complete tear. Several years after a complete tear the power of abduction may apparently recover; possibly the teres minor hypertrophies and holds down the humeral head.

SIGNS

LOOK — The appearance is normal.

FEEL — Tenderness may be diffuse or may be localized to just below the tip of the acromion process, and in this situation a gap can occasionally be felt.

MOVE — With a recent injury active abduction is grossly limited, its rhythm is faulty and the attempt is painful. Passive abduction also is limited or prevented by pain. These signs apply to both partial and complete tears, but if, as commonly happens, some weeks have elapsed since injury, the two types are easily differentiated. With a complete tear pain has by then subsided and the clinical picture is unmistakable: active abduction is impossible and attempting it produces a characteristic shrug; but passive abduction is

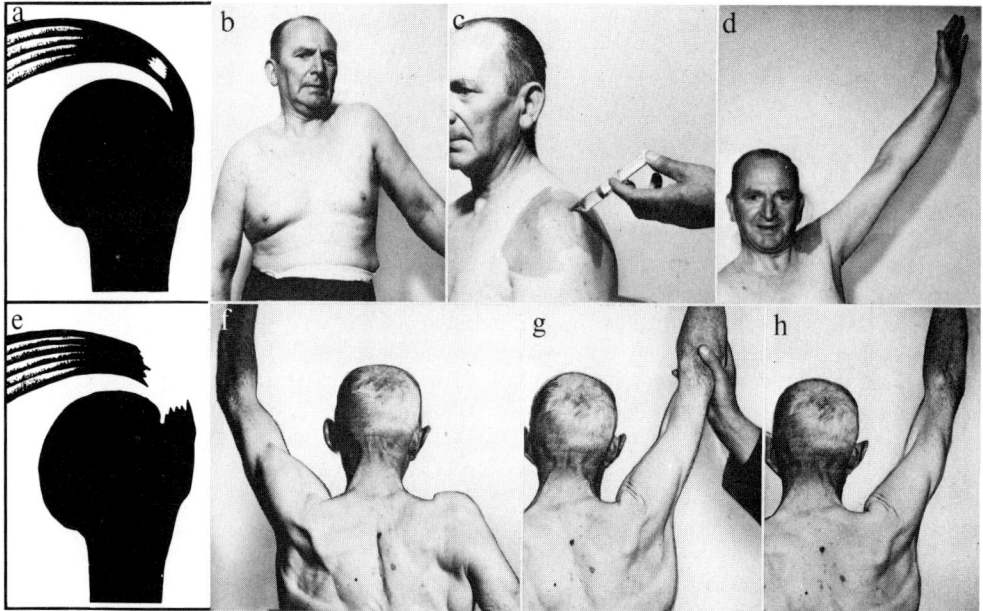

12.8 TORN SUPRASPINATUS

(a, b, c, d) Partial tear of left supraspinatus: the patient can abduct actively once pain has been abolished with local anaesthetic.

(e, f, g, h) Complete tear of right supraspinatus: active abduction is impossible even when pain subsides (f), or has been abolished by injection; but once the arm is passively abducted (g), the patient can hold it up with his deltoid muscle (h).

full, and once the arm has been passively lifted above a right angle the patient can keep it up by using his deltoid (the abduction paradox); when he lowers it sideways it suddenly drops (the drop arm sign).

X-RAY — The presence and extent of the tear can be demonstrated by arthrography. With old tears the gap between the humeral head and the acromion process becomes narrowed.

PARTIAL OR COMPLETE? — Soon after injury it may be difficult to distinguish a partial from a complete tear because, in both, pain prevents even passive abduction. Local anaesthetic is therefore injected until passive abduction is painless. If the patient can then abduct his arm actively and without shrugging, the tear must be only partial. This test is simpler than arthrography.

TREATMENT

PARTIAL TEAR — Treatment is always conservative and consists of (*a*) heat, which is soothing; (*b*) exercises, the most valuable in the early stages being 'pendulum' exercises, in which the patient leans forward at the hips and moves his arm as if stirring a giant pudding; and (*c*) one or two injections of local anaesthetic into the tender area.

COMPLETE TEAR — In early cases repair is desirable.   The best approach is postero-superior, with the patient prone; should the tear be difficult to close the muscle can be advanced laterally.   The sutures are liable to cut out because the tendon is degenerate and the operation is unwise unless the patient is younger than usual; an untreated tear becomes painless and useful function is achieved by trick movements.

LESIONS OF THE BICEPS TENDON

TENDINITIS

A primary biceps tendinitis may follow unaccustomed use, such as home decorating or vigorous tennis, in patients aged 30–40 years.   The shoulder is normal except for pain on external rotation and tenderness in the bicipital groove.   Rest and local heat are usually sufficient treatment, but if recovery is delayed local anaesthetic injections or deep transverse frictions to the tender area are useful.

Secondary tendinitis occurs in cuff lesions when the reaction to degeneration spreads to the biceps.   Signs of biceps tendinitis are added to those of the underlying lesion, and both conditions may require treatment.

RUPTURED BICEPS TENDON

It used to be thought that the tendon of the long head of the biceps ruptured because it rubbed against osteophytes in an osteoarthritic shoulder.   Most orthopaedic surgeons now agree that it is simply a tear through an area of avascular degeneration, comparable to that occurring in the supraspinatus tendon.

The patient is always aged over 50.   While lifting he feels something snap and the shoulder, which previously felt normal, aches for a time.   Soon his ache disappears and good function returns.   The clinical picture is unmistakable.   The

12.9   THE BICEPS TENDON
Tendinitis: localized tenderness (a), and pain on flexion against resistance (b).

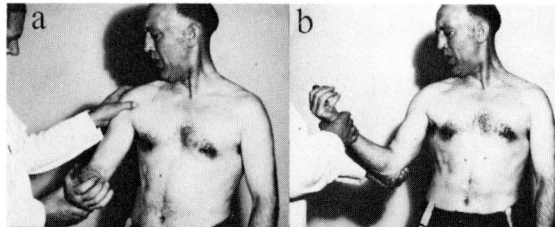

(c) Ruptured long head of right biceps: compared with the normal side, the belly of biceps is lower and rounder.

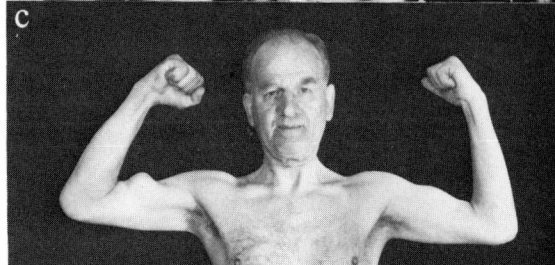

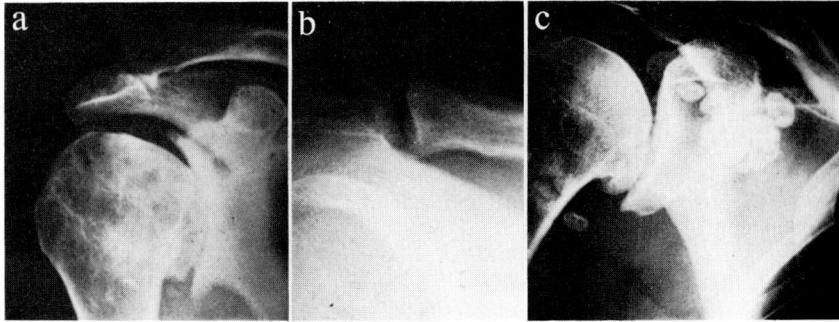

12.10
(a) Osteoarthritis of the gleno-humeral joint, which is less common than (b) osteo-arthritis of the acromio-clavicular joint.   (c) Synovial osteochondromatosis.

belly of the muscle is too low; and when in action it does not tauten properly and looks semi-circular instead of semi-oval.   Shoulder movements are normal and no treatment is required.   Occasionally the biceps insertion is avulsed; the muscle belly then retracts to a more proximal position.

BRACHIAL NEURALGIA

The term 'brachial neuralgia' is usually applied to pain extending over a large part of the upper limb.   The common causes may conveniently be classified on an anatomical basis.

DISORDERS AROUND THE SHOULDER

In all these, movement at the shoulder joint itself is painful or limited.

MUSCULOTENDINOUS CUFF — The onset of cuff lesions may be gradual or follow trauma, often trivial.   X-rays show calcification or no abnormality.

BONES — A fracture may have been missed.   The history is one of injury followed by a bruise, and x-rays show the fracture.

JOINT — (a) In tuberculosis the onset is gradual, muscle wasting marked and x-rays show bone destruction; (b) in rheumatoid arthritis, other joints are also affected; (c) pyogenic arthritis rarely occurs and is liable to give a totally stiff but painless shoulder; (d) osteo-arthritis is also a rarity.

SHOULDER–HAND SYNDROME — Not only is the shoulder painful and stiffish, but the same hand is similarly affected.   Moreover the hand may be swollen and the skin looks shiny and trophic; contractures may develop.   The cause is unknown but there is often associated cardio-pulmonary disease and 25 per cent of cases are bilateral.   A short course of steroids in fairly high doses is said to be the most effective treatment.

DISORDERS PROXIMAL TO THE SHOULDER

In all of these, the shoulder itself has normal movement and a normal x-ray appearance.

TRUNK — Disorders of the diaphragm, heart, pericardium or pleura may cause pain in the arm.

NECK — (a) Disc disorders (prolapse or spondylosis) may cause pain and weakness or numbness in the appropriate root distribution, usually C.6 or C.7; neck movements are limited and the disc spaces narrowed on x-ray; (b) vertebral disease, such as tuberculosis,

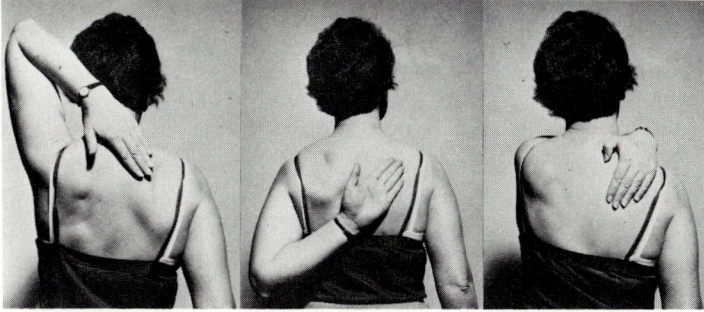

12.11 THE 'SCRATCH TEST'
If a patient with brachial neuralgia can, without pain, scratch the opposite scapula
in these three ways, the shoulder joint and its tendons are unlikely to be at fault.

may cause limited neck movement, there is sometimes an abscess, and x-rays show bone
destruction affecting two adjacent vertebrae: (c) vertebral-body tumours may cause
limitation of neck movements and root symptoms, and x-rays show that one body only
is affected; (d) cord or root tumours have a gradual onset and a characteristic distribution
of neurological signs.

NECK-ARM JUNCTION — (a) With a cervical rib, pain is usually ulnar in distribution and
any wasting is in the small muscles of the hand (first thoracic nerve)—the rib or a large
transverse process may show on x-ray; (b) in Pancoast's syndrome there is a hard lump
at the root of the neck, a Horner's syndrome, and x-rays show a bronchial carcinoma.

DISORDERS DISTAL TO THE SHOULDER

In these, the shoulder and neck move normally and the x-ray appearance is normal.

ELBOW — Pain from a tennis elbow may radiate to the entire limb, but tenderness is
localized to the lateral epicondyle and there is pain on dorsiflexing the wrist against
resistance.

WRIST — The pain in carpal tunnel syndrome is mainly in the median area of the hand
and is worse at night. Any wasting is of the opponens pollicis muscle.

INVESTIGATION

To investigate the cause of brachial neuralgia the following points must be considered.

HISTORY — Was there an injury? What is the nature and distribution of pain?

GENERAL FEATURES — What is the patient's age? Is there any evidence of general disease?

LOCAL FEATURES — Is there limitation of neck movement? Is there limitation of shoulder
movement? Can the distribution of any neurological signs be related to a single peripheral nerve or root? Are there abnormal x-ray findings in the neck or shoulder?

Suggestions for further reading

Debeyre, J., *et al.* (1965). 'Repair of Ruptures of the Rotator Cuff of the
  Shoulder.' *J. Bone Jt Surg.* **47B**, 1, 36
Hammond, G. (1971). 'Complete Acromionectomy in the Treatment of
  Chronic Tendinitis of the Shoulder.' *J. Bone Jt Surg.* **53A**, 173

Hensinger, R. N., *et al.* (1974). 'Klippel-Feil Syndrome.' *J. Bone Jt Surg.*
    56A, 1246
MacNab, I. (1973). 'Rotator Cuff Tendinitis.' *Ann R. Coll. Surg. Eng.* **53,**
    271
McLaughlin, H. L. (1962). 'Rupture of the Rotator Cuff.' *J. Bone Jt Surg.*
    44A, 979
Moseley, H. F. (1969). *Shoulder Lesions*, 3rd Edn. Edinburgh; Livingstone
Richardson, A. T. (1975). 'The Painful Shoulder.' *Proc. Roy. Soc. Med.*
    68, 11, 731
Wolfgang, G. L. (1974). 'Surgical Repair of Tears of the Rotator Cuff of the
    Shoulder.' *J. Bone Jt Surg.* **56A,** 14

CHAPTER 13

THE ELBOW JOINT

EXAMINATION OF THE ELBOW

SYMPTOMS

The common symptoms of elbow disorders are pain, stiffness, deformity and occasionally locking. Pain at the elbow may be referred from neck or shoulder disorders; numbness or weakness of the hand may be the result of elbow disorders.

SIGNS

LOOK — The patient holds his arms alongside his body with palms forwards. Varus or valgus deformity is then obvious, but it cannot be accurately assessed unless the elbow is straight. He then holds his arms out sideways at right angles to the body with palms upwards and elbows straight. In this position, wasting or lumps are easily seen.

FEEL — The back and sides of the joint are palpated for warmth, tenderness (which must be accurately localized) and fluid, and to determine whether the bony points are correctly related.

MOVE — Flexion and extension are compared on the two sides. Then, with the elbows tucked into the sides and flexed to a right angle, the radio-ulnar joints are tested for pronation and supination.

X-RAY — The position of each bone is noted, then the joint line and space. Next, the individual bones are inspected for evidence of old injury or bone destruction. Finally, loose bodies are sought.

NOTE — Where appropriate, other parts are examined: the neck (for cervical disc lesions), the shoulder (for cuff lesions) and the hand (for nerve lesions).

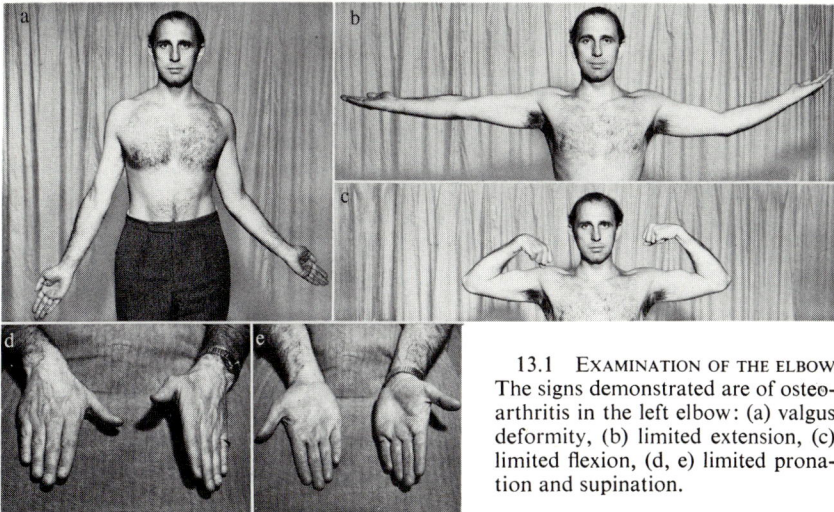

13.1 EXAMINATION OF THE ELBOW The signs demonstrated are of osteo-arthritis in the left elbow: (a) valgus deformity, (b) limited extension, (c) limited flexion, (d, e) limited pronation and supination.

ELBOW DEFORMITIES

CUBITUS VARUS ('Gun-stock' deformity)

The commonest cause is mal-union of a supracondylar fracture. The deformity is obvious only when the elbow is extended, but it looks rather ugly and the hand brushes against the body in walking. The deformity can be corrected by a wedge osteotomy of the lower humerus, after which the arm is held in plaster in full extension and slight valgus.

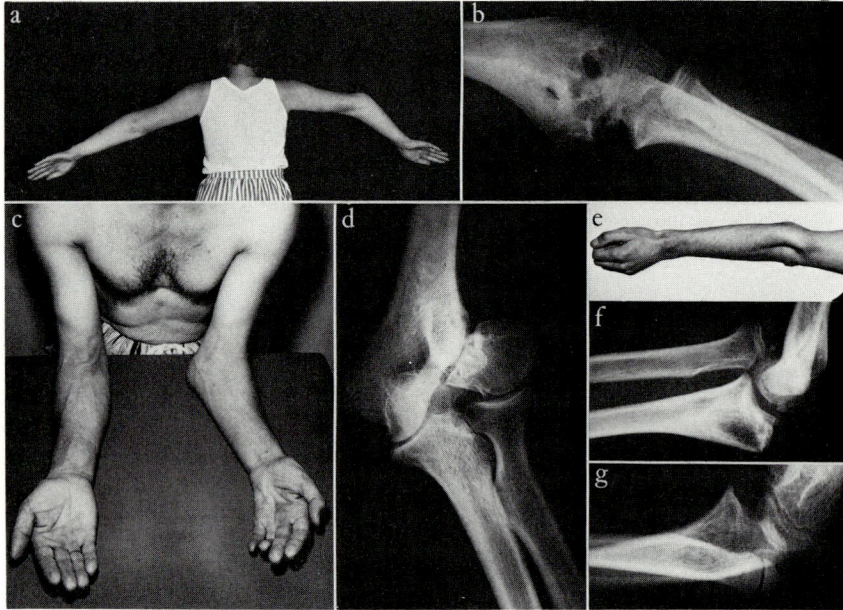

13.2 ELBOW DEFORMITIES
(a, b) Varus deformity following old supracondylar fracture; (c, d) valgus deformity following non-union of the lateral condyle; (e, f) old traumatic anterior dislocation of the radial head; (g) congenital posterior dislocation of the radial head — in contrast with acquired dislocations the head is dome-shaped.

CUBITUS VALGUS

The commonest cause is non-union of a fractured lateral condyle; this may give gross deformity and a bony knob on the outer side of the joint. The importance of valgus deformity is the liability for delayed ulnar palsy to develop; years after the causal injury the patient notices weakness of the hand with numbness and tingling of the ulnar fingers. The deformity itself needs no treatment but for delayed ulnar palsy the nerve should be transposed to the front of the elbow.

DISLOCATED HEAD OF RADIUS

This may be congenital or follow the failure to reduce a pronation type of elbow injury (page 383). The patient may notice the lump which is easily palpable and can be felt to move when the forearm is rotated. X-rays reveal the dislocation; if congenital, the radial head may be anterior or posterior, and is characteristically dome-shaped; if part of a Monteggia fracture-dislocation the forward curve of the mal-united ulna can be seen. If the lump limits elbow flexion it can be excised.

Congenital subluxation of the radial head, usually lateral, is commonly associated with a wide variety of bone dysplasias.

STIFFNESS OF THE ELBOW

BOTH ELBOWS

The commonest cause of bilateral stiffness is rheumatoid arthritis; other causes include arthrogryposis multiplex congenita and ankylosing spondylitis. If both elbows are completely stiff at impractical angles, disability is severe; arthroplasty or joint replacement, to enable at least one hand to reach the mouth, is needed.

ONE ELBOW

Congenital synostosis of the superior radio-ulnar joint (with loss of rotation) is only moderately inconvenient, but if the humerus shares in the synostosis the disability is considerable; a more useful angle can be achieved by osteotomy, although the stiffness is, of course, unaffected.

Acquired causes of limited elbow movement are much less rare. Three are described below; a fourth (pulled elbow) is described on page 383.

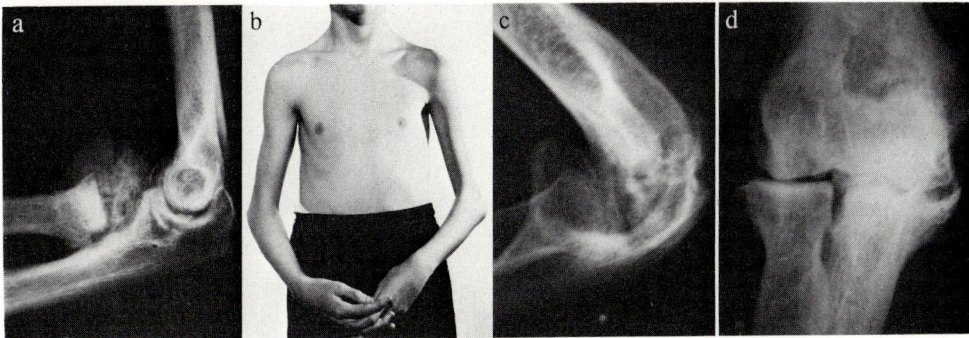

13.3 STIFFNESS OF THE ELBOW
(a) Myositis ossificans following excision of a fractured head of radius; (b, c) wasting and joint destruction in tuberculosis; (d) osteoarthritis.

POST-TRAUMATIC STIFFNESS

Temporary stiffness may follow any elbow injury. Permanent limitation of movement is likely after severe fractures into the joint in adults, or when injury has been complicated by myositis ossificans. Unless the fracture was recent there is neither warmth nor tenderness. X-rays reveal the old fracture or the tell-tale calcification of myositis ossificans.

To minimize post-traumatic stiffness, an injured elbow should be rested and passive movements absolutely prohibited. At the first suggestion of myositis ossificans, complete rest in a plaster gutter is imperative; later, when the calcified area has become well-defined, it may be removed, though the gain in movement is not often great.

TUBERCULOSIS (see also page 34)

Although the disease begins as synovitis or osteomyelitis, tuberculosis of the elbow is rarely seen until arthritis supervenes, by which time complete resolution cannot occur. Because the elbow is a superficial joint, sinus formation is common.

The onset of symptoms is insidious and the patient gives a long history of aching and stiffness. The most striking physical sign is the marked wasting. While the disease is active the joint is held flexed, looks swollen, feels warm and diffusely tender; movement is considerably limited and accompanied by pain and spasm. X-rays show generalized rarefaction, and often an apparent increase of joint space because of bone erosion. With healing a little movement returns, but the arm remains thin.

In addition to general treatment (page 35), the elbow is rested. At first, it may be held in a plaster gutter flexed more acutely than a right angle and in mid-rotation. Later a removable polythene splint, or collar and cuff, is sufficient and even these are sometimes discarded. Healing is by fibrosis. The fibrous tissue gradually elongates because of the weight of the arm; hence the need to splint the elbow well above the right angle during the acute stage.

OSTEOARTHRITIS

Osteoarthritis may result from articular damage when the joint contains a loose body (especially with osteochondritis dissecans), or multiple loose bodies (synovial chondromatosis), or it may follow severe fractures.

The symptoms are few. Until stiffness is considerable it often passes unnoticed. There is rarely much pain; occasionally the joint may lock. Symptoms of ulnar palsy may be the presenting feature. Apart from limited movement the signs are few: the joint may look and feel somewhat enlarged, but there is no wasting or tenderness. X-rays show diminution of the joint space with bone sclerosis and osteophytes; one or more loose bodies may be seen.

The osteoarthritis itself rarely requires treatment. Loose bodies, however, if they cause locking, should be removed; and if there are signs of ulnar neuritis, the nerve should be transposed.

FLAILNESS OF THE ELBOW

A flail elbow often causes surprisingly little disability, though a removable leather or polythene splint is usually helpful. There are three causes.

GUNSHOT WOUND — There is a scar, the elbow is flail, and often there is ulnar nerve palsy. X-rays show that the bones have been shot away.

CHARCOT'S DISEASE — There is flailness, but no scar and no ulnar palsy. The joint is enlarged and can be moved painlessly in any direction. X-rays show dislocation, bone destruction and calcification in the capsule.

POLIOMYELITIS — With a balanced paralysis the elbow may be flail, but flailness is not a presenting symptom.

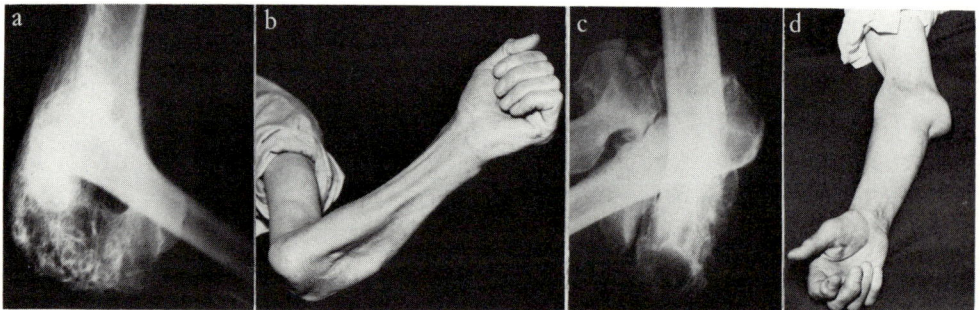

13.4   FLAIL ELBOW
(a, b) Following gun-shot wound; (c, d) Charcot's disease.

OTHER DISORDERS OF THE ELBOW

TENNIS ELBOW

This, the commonest elbow disorder, is only occasionally due to tennis. Most cases follow minor and often unrecognized trauma; the common extensor origin is damaged and subsequent adhesions bind torn to untorn fibres and to the joint capsule.

Other possible explanations include tendinitis, fibrillation of the radial head, and entrapment of a branch of the radial nerve.

CLINICAL FEATURES

The onset is commonly gradual, rarely sudden, and hardly ever at tennis. The patient complains of pain on certain movements such as pouring out tea, turning a stiff door-handle or lifting with the forearm pronated. The pain in severe cases may radiate widely.

The elbow looks normal and flexion and extension are full and painless (though extension is sometimes temporarily painful). The x-ray appearance is normal.

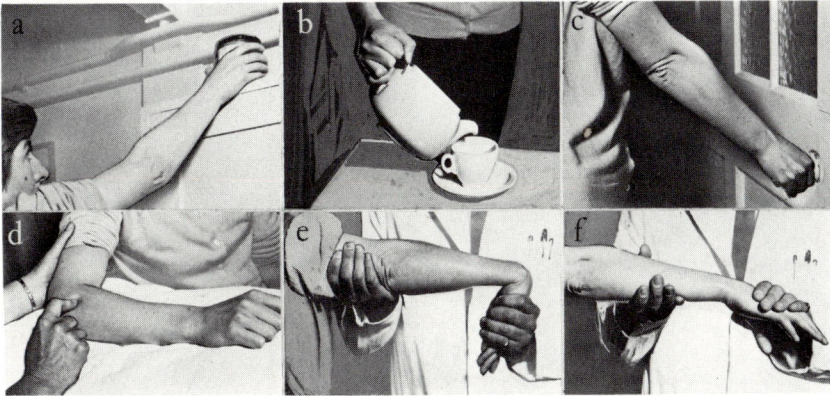

13.5 TENNIS ELBOW
(a, b, c) Movements which cause pain — in all three extensor carpi radialis brevis is in action. (d) Localized tenderness. (e) Pain on passive stretching. (f) Pain on resisted dorsiflexion.

There are three positive physical signs: (a) localized tenderness (over the lateral epicondyle); (b) pain on passive stretching (the wrist extensors are stretched by holding the elbow straight, the forearm prone and the wrist palmarflexed); and (c) pain on active contraction against resistance (the elbow is held straight and the forearm prone and the patient is prevented from dorsiflexing his wrist).

TREATMENT

Of the many methods of treatment, it is impossible to predict which is likely to be successful in any given case, and a useful sequence in which they may be tried is as follows.

(1) INJECTION — The tender area is injected with a mixture of 3 ml of 1 per cent Xylocaine and 1 ml of hydrocortisone acetate containing 25 mg. If the condition is improved, but not cured, the injection is repeated 3 weeks later.

(2) PHYSIOTHERAPY — Deep transverse frictions, though sometimes effective, are painful; a more comfortable alternative is ultra-sound.

(3) MANIPULATIONS — The elbow is forcibly extended with the forearm prone and the wrist fully palmar flexed.

(4) REST — If the patient will submit to resting the arm in a sling or, better still, in plaster, for several weeks recovery is usual.

(5) OPERATION — A few cases are sufficiently persistent or recurrent for operation to be necessary. The origin of the common extensor muscle is detached from the lateral epicondyle, the orbicular ligament divided and any nerve entrapment released.

SPORTS ELBOWS

Golfer's elbow is comparable to tennis elbow except that the flexor origin (not the extensor) is affected. Treatment is similar.

Javelin throwers using the over-arm action may avulse the tip of the olecranon; with the round-arm action the medial ligament may be avulsed.

Baseball pitchers may suffer extensive elbow damage with hypertrophy of the lower humerus which no longer fits into the olecranon, and loose-body formation. The junior equivalent (little leaguer's elbow) is partial avulsion of the medial epicondyle.

LOOSE BODIES

Possible causes include:

INJURY — A fracture, dislocation or repeated minor injury may break off a piece of bone into the joint. Osteochondritis dissecans, in which a piece of bone becomes detached from the capitulum, is possibly traumatic in origin.

DEGENERATION — In osteoarthritis small osteophytes may break off, and in Charcot's disease large pieces of bone are found in the joint.

INFLAMMATION — Small fibrinous loose bodies may occur in inflammatory disease, but the inflammatory process overshadows the loose bodies.

IDIOPATHIC — Synovial osteochondromatosis occasionally occurs, producing many loose bodies.

The patient may complain of sudden locking and unlocking of the joint. Symptoms of osteoarthritis may co-exist.

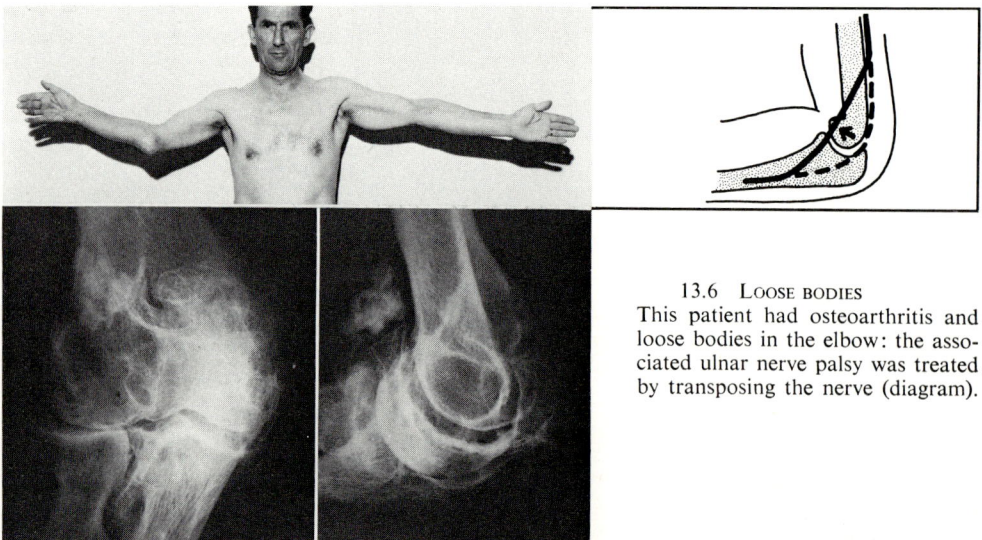

13.6 LOOSE BODIES
This patient had osteoarthritis and loose bodies in the elbow: the associated ulnar nerve palsy was treated by transposing the nerve (diagram).

A loose body is rarely palpable. When degenerative changes have occurred, extremes of movement are limited. X-rays nearly always reveal the loose body or bodies; and in the special case of osteochondritis dissecans there is a rarefied cystic area in the capitulum and enlargement of the radial head.

If loose bodies are troublesome they can be removed.

NERVE LESIONS

ULNAR PALSY is often the sequel to elbow disorders such as osteoarthritis, valgus deformity or constriction of the nerve by a fibrous band at the proximal end of the flexor carpi ulnaris muscle (ulnar tunnel). Occasionally the nerve repeatedly dislocates forwards.

There may be no pain. The usual presenting symptom is numbness or weakness in the hand. The hand becomes clawed and the interossei (especially the first) are wasted. The nerve may be tender in the region of the elbow.

The nerve should be freed by dividing the roof of the ulnar tunnel if this is the cause; otherwise it is best transposed to the front of the elbow.

ULNAR NERVE TRANSPOSITION — The nerve is exposed by a long incision centred over the medial epicondyle. It is freed upwards to the point where it runs through the medial intermuscular septum, and the septum in this area must be divided. Mobilization of the distal portion is facilitated by careful stripping of the branches. A bed is prepared in the flexor muscles and, when the nerve can lie easily in it without tension, one or two catgut sutures are placed to hold the nerve in its new bed.

POSTERIOR INTEROSSEOUS NERVE lesions just below the elbow can give rise to palsy. Tumour (for example lipoma), ganglion, fibrosis and traumatic neuritis have all been described. The treatment is operative decompression.

BURSAE

The olecranon bursa sometimes becomes enlarged as a result of pressure or friction, and if the enlargement is a nuisance the fluid may be aspirated. Occasionally, the bursa is affected by gout, syphilis or tuberculosis. A chronically enlarged bursa may need excision. In rheumatoid arthritis, also, the bursa may become enlarged, but more often a fibrous lump develops just distal to the olecranon process.

Suggestions for further reading

Capener, N. (1966). 'The vulnerability of the posterior interosseous nerve of the forearm.' *J. Bone Jt Surg.* **48B**, 1, 770 (see also 3 following articles)

Godshall, R. W. and Hansen, C. A. (1971). 'Traumatic Ulnar Neuropathy in Adolescent Baseball Pitchers.' *J. Bone Jt Surg.* **53A**, 359

Roles, N. C. and Maudsley, R. H. (1972). 'Radial Tunnel Syndrome.' *J. Bone Jt Surg.* **54B**, 499

Smith, F. D. (1954). *Surgery of the Elbow.* Springfield; Thomas

CHAPTER 14

THE WRIST JOINT

EXAMINATION OF THE WRIST

SYMPTOMS

The common symptoms are pain, deformity, swelling or a lump.

SIGNS

Examination of the wrist is not complete without also examining the elbow, forearm and hand.

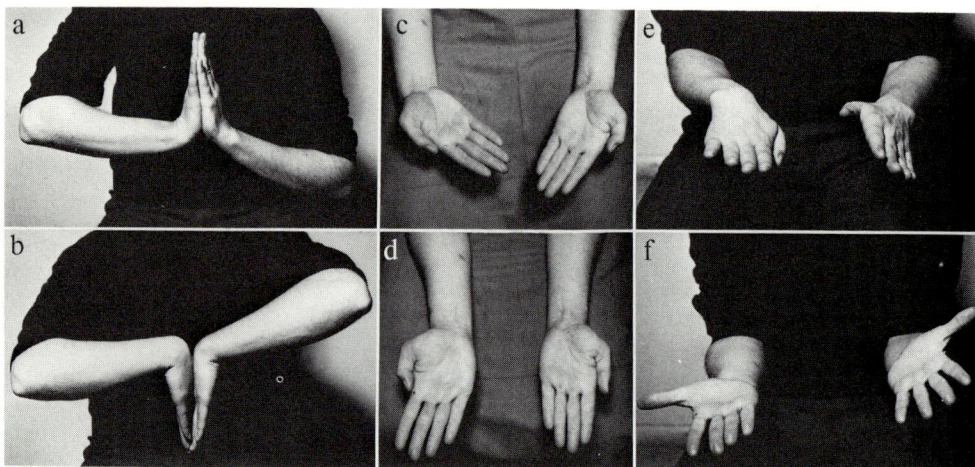

14.1   EXAMINATION OF THE WRIST
All movements of the left wrist are limited.   (a) dorsiflexion, (b) palmarflexion, (c) ulnar deviation, (d) radial deviation, (e) pronation, (f) supination.

LOOK — The skin is inspected for scars.   Both wrists and forearms are compared to see if there is deformity.   Swelling, lumps and wasting of the forearm are noted.

FEEL — Undue warmth is noted.   Tender areas must be accurately localized, and the bony landmarks compared with those of the normal wrist.   Lumps are palpated separately.

MOVE — To compare dorsiflexion of the wrists the patient places his palms together in a position of prayer, then elevates his elbows.   Palmarflexion is examined in a similar way.   With the elbows at right angles and tucked in to the sides, radial and ulnar deviation are next examined, then pronation and supination.

X-RAY — Antero-posterior and lateral views are necessary, and often both wrists must be x-rayed for comparison.   General rarefaction, alteration of joint spaces (in the radio-carpal or intercarpal joints) and abnormalities in shape or density of the individual bones are noted.

168

WRIST DEFORMITIES

RADIAL CLUB HAND — The whole or part of the radius is missing. The wrist is palmar-flexed and radially deviated, the hand lacks a thumb, and other anomalies of the fingers and of the elbow usually co-exist. Operations to stabilize and centralize the carpus may be cosmetically attractive, but they seldom improve function; the untreated deformity may already be in the hand-to-mouth position.

MADELUNG'S DEFORMITY — This may be congenital in origin, but is probably due to injury affecting the lower radial epiphysis or rupturing the triangular fibrocartilage. The deformity (sometimes bilateral) is rarely seen before the age of 10 years and increases until growth is complete. The lower radius curves forwards, carrying with it the carpus and hand, but leaving the lower ulna sticking out as a lump on the back of the wrist.

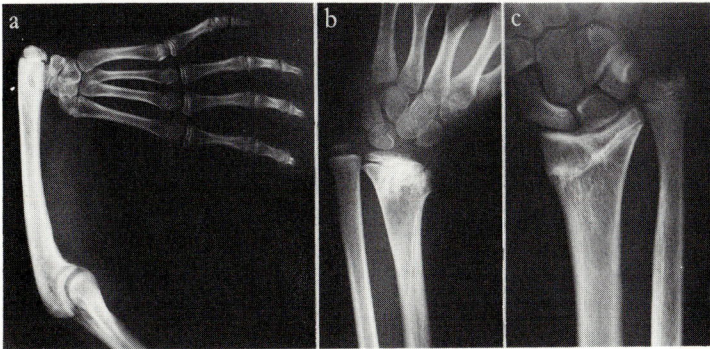

14.2 WRIST DEFORMITIES
(a) Absent radius and first ray, (b) damage to radial growth disc; this type of injury might cause (c) Madelung's deformity.

If deformity is severe the lower ulna may be excised, or osteotomy of the lower radius may be combined with shortening of the ulna.

POST-TRAUMATIC — After a Colles' fracture radial deviation and posterior angulation are common. These deformities cause little disability but may look ugly.

POST-INFLAMMATORY — After long-standing tuberculous or rheumatoid arthritis of the wrist forward subluxation at the radiocarpal joint commonly develops.

STIFFNESS OF THE WRIST

TUBERCULOSIS (see also page 34)

At the wrist, tuberculosis is rarely seen until it has progressed to a true arthritis. Pain and stiffness come on gradually and the hand feels weak.

The forearm looks wasted, the wrist is swollen, the carpus subluxed forwards, and there may be a sinus. Movements are restricted and painful. The x-ray looks hazy, with narrowing and irregularity of the radio-carpal and intercarpal joints, and sometimes bone erosion.

The condition must be differentiated from rheumatoid arthritis. Bilateral arthritis of the wrist is nearly always rheumatoid in origin, but when only one wrist is affected the signs strongly resemble those of tuberculosis; serological tests may establish the diagnosis, but often a biopsy is necessary.

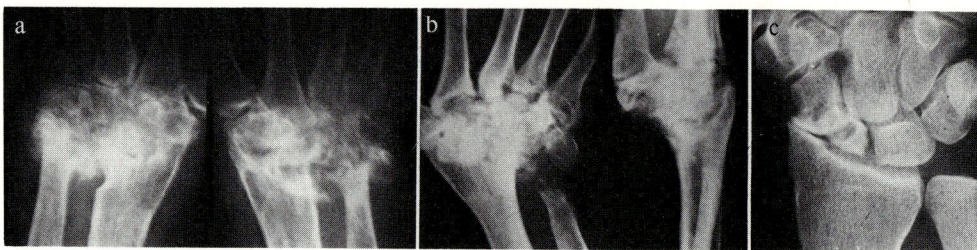

14.3 STIFFNESS OF THE WRIST
(a) Bilateral in rheumatoid arthritis; (b) unilateral in tuberculous arthritis; (c) localized osteoarthritis following fractured scaphoid.

Anti-tuberculous drugs are given and the wrist is rested in plaster which extends from the upper forearm to the proximal palm crease (permitting finger flexion) and holds the wrist 20 degrees dorsiflexed. Later a removable splint is used. Only rarely is arthrodesis necessary.

KIENBÖCK'S DISEASE

The name refers to avascular necrosis of the carpal lunate. Trauma (a single definite injury or repeated minor ones) may be the precipitating cause; but in a significantly high proportion of cases the ulna is too short (relative to the radius).

The patient, often a young adult, complains of ache and stiffness. Localized tenderness and limited dorsiflexion are usual. X-rays at first show increased density of the lunate; later the bone looks squashed and irregular; still later the wrist may become osteoarthritic.

In early cases, shortening the radius or lengthening the ulna may lead to improvement. Later, replacing the lunate with a prosthesis (made of plastic or Silastic) has been advocated. Once osteoarthritis has supervened the alternatives are splintage or arthrodesis.

OSTEOARTHRITIS

Osteoarthritis of the wrist is uncommon except as the sequel to injury. Any fracture into the joint may predispose to degeneration, but the commonest is a fractured scaphoid, especially with non-union or avascular necrosis. Kienböck's disease is a less frequent cause.

The patient may have forgotten the original injury. Years later he complains of pain and stiffness. At first these occur intermittently after use; later they become more constant, and recurrent 'wrist sprains' are common.

The appearance is usually normal and there is no wasting. Movements at the wrist and radio-ulnar joints are limited and painful. X-rays show irregular narrowing at the radio-carpal joint, with bone sclerosis; the proximal portion of the scaphoid or the lunate may be irregular and dense.

Rest, in a polythene splint, is often sufficient treatment. Excision of the radial styloid process is helpful when osteoarthritis has followed scaphoid injury. Arthrodesis of the wrist is rarely necessary.

Note — At the carpo-metacarpal joint of the thumb osteoarthritis is much commoner than at the wrist, because the thumb is an ' extreme-range joint ' (page 47), and the patient soon complains of pain on using the hand. Often there is no history of injury. The joint is tender, and full extension and adduction are painful. X-rays show narrowing of the space between the trapezium and first metacarpal, often with sclerosis. If short-wave diathermy and restriction of activity do not give relief, operation may be advisable. Excision of the trapezium (possibly with a Silastic replacement) gives relief of pain and often rapid return of full function; arthrodesis always gives a good result, but involves 3 months in plaster.

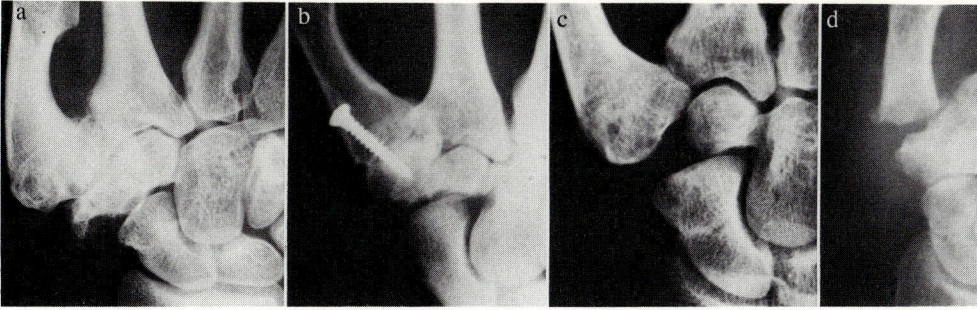

14.4 OSTEOARTHRITIS OF THE CARPO-METACARPAL THUMB JOINT
(a) Narrowed joint space and osteophytes. If operation is needed the possibilities
are arthrodesis (b), or arthroplasty (c, d); in (c) the trapezium has been excised, in
(d) the metacarpal base.

SWELLINGS AROUND THE WRIST

GANGLION

It seems that ganglia arise not by synovial herniation from a joint or tendon sheath,
but from small bursae within the substance of the joint capsule or the fibrous tendon
sheath. These bursae become distended, possibly following trauma, giving rise to a
main 'cyst' containing viscous fluid and smaller pseudopodia.

The patient, often a young adult, presents with a painless lump, though occasionally
there is slight ache and weakness. The lump is well-defined, cystic and not tender;
it can sometimes be transilluminated and may feel more tense when the tendons are
put into action. The back of the wrist is the commonest site, but ganglia in front
may compress a nerve or penetrate between the fibres, causing numbness or weakness.

Squashing the lump may disperse it, but recurrence is common. If it recurs and
is troublesome the best treatment is operative excision. A tourniquet is used; the
ganglion is removed together with all the pseudopodia and the fibrous layer from
which they arise.

> *Note* — Ganglia occasionally occur in the palm or fingers. They are then small, hard and
> tender, so that diagnosis is not easy until the lump is exposed.

COMPOUND PALMAR GANGLION

Chronic inflammation distends the common sheath of the flexor tendons both
above and below the flexor retinaculum. Rheumatoid arthritis and tuberculosis are
the commonest causes. The synovial membrane becomes thick and villous. The
amount of fluid is increased and it may contain fibrin particles moulded by repeated
movement to the shape of melon seeds. The tendons may eventually fray and
rupture.

Pain is unusual, but paraesthesia due to median nerve compression may occur.
The swelling is hour-glass in shape, bulging above and below the flexor retinaculum;
it is not warm or tender; fluid can be pushed from one part to the other (cross-
fluctuation).

If the condition is tuberculous, general treatment is begun (page 35). The contents of the ganglion are evacuated, streptomycin instilled, and the wrist is rested in
a splint. If these measures fail the entire flexor sheath is dissected out. Complete
excision is also the best treatment when the cause is rheumatoid disease.

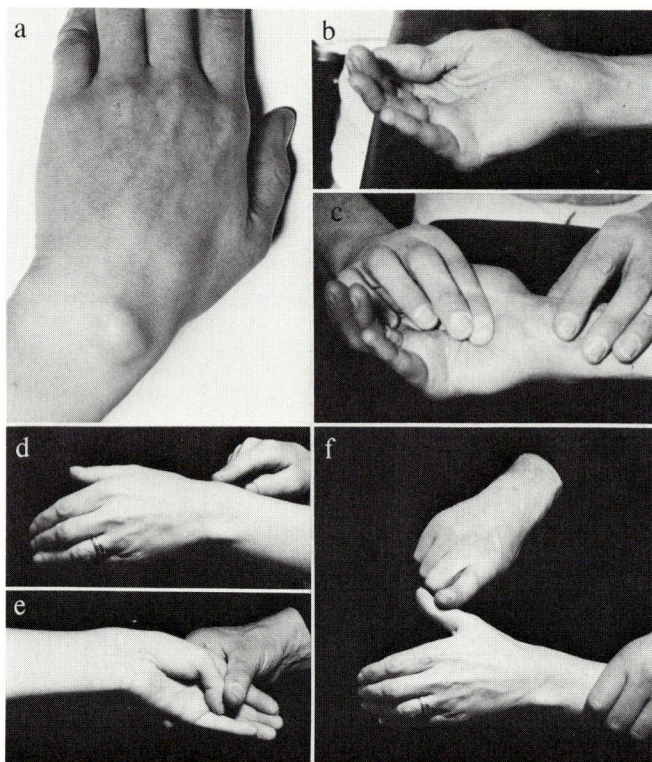

14.5 WRIST SWELLINGS
(a) Simple ganglion; (b, c) compound palmar ganglion with cross-fluctuation.

de Quervain's disease; (d) the patient can point to the painful area; (e) forced adduction is painful; (f) pain on active extension against resistance.

STENOSING TENOVAGINITIS (de Quervain's disease)

In this common variety of tunnel syndrome the fibrous sheath containing the extensor pollicis brevis and abductor pollicis longus tendons becomes thickened, possibly as a result of degenerative changes or over-use. There may be an underlying abnormality in the number of tendons.

The condition is commonest in women aged 40–50 years who complain of pain on the radial side of the wrist, worse after such actions as wringing clothes. A small lump is visible on the radial side three-quarters of an inch above the wrist. The lump feels almost bony hard, so that it is frequently mistaken for an exostosis (but the x-ray appearance is always normal); tenderness is precisely localized to the lump. Pain is felt if the patient extends the thumb against resistance, or if it is passively adducted across the palm.

Rest, transverse frictions or injections of hydrocortisone sometimes give relief. Operation, which consists of slitting the sheath, is uniformly successful and the patient wakes up cured.

Suggestions for further reading

Andren, L. and Elken, O. (1971). 'Arthrographic Studies of Wrist Ganglions.' *J. Bone Jt Surg.* **53A**, 299

Lamb, D. W. (1972). 'The Treatment of Radial Club Hand.' *The Hand*, **4**, 22

Ranawat, M. D., *et al.* (1975). 'Madelung's Deformity.' *J. Bone Jt Surg.* **57A**, 772

Roca, J., *et al.* (1976). 'Treatment of Kienböck's Disease Using a Silicone Rubber Implant.' *J. Bone Jt Surg.* **58A**, 373

CHAPTER 15

THE HAND

EXAMINATION OF THE HAND

SYMPTOMS

The common symptoms in the hand are pain, paraesthesia, deformity, stiffness and weakness.   Pain may be local or referred from a lesion in the neck, thoraco-brachial junction, shoulder, elbow or wrist.

SIGNS

Both upper limbs should be bared for comparison.

LOOK — The skin may be scarred, altered in colour, dry or moist, and hairy or smooth. Wasting and deformity, and the presence of any lumps should be noted.   The position in which the fingers are naturally held is often important.

FEEL — The skin temperature is noted and sensation tested, especially two-point discrimination.

MOVE — Active movements are tested by examining the motor functions of the hand as pincers (as in writing); as a vice (as in holding a hammer); and for tapping (as in typewriting).

15.1   EXAMINATION OF THE HAND Positions: (a) resting posture, (b) full flexion, (c) full extension.

Strength: (d) power grip, (e) finger abduction, (f) pinch grip.

Sensation: (g) pin prick, (h) light touch, (i) stereognosis.

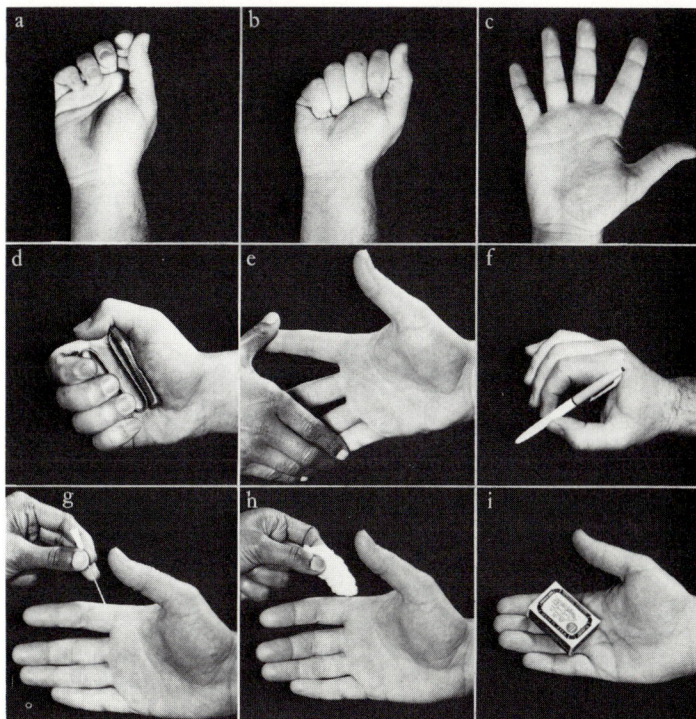

173

Individual finger and thumb movements must be examined when a nerve or tendon is suspect.   Passive movements must be examined, especially if there is deformity.

X-RAYS — X-rays are necessary to exclude bony damage.

DEFORMITIES OF THE HAND

CONGENITAL DEFORMITIES

SYNDACTYLY (congenital webbing) — This condition may be corrected by separating the fingers and repairing the defects with skin grafts.

LOBSTER HAND — This is usually familial.   There is congenital absence of the middle three fingers.   Function is usually good.

FLEXION OF THE LITTLE FINGER (CAMPTODACTYLY) — This is often bilateral.   The proximal finger joint is fixed flexed.   Although it is congenital, the deformity is rarely seen until the child is aged 10 years.   Function is good and the condition is best left untreated.

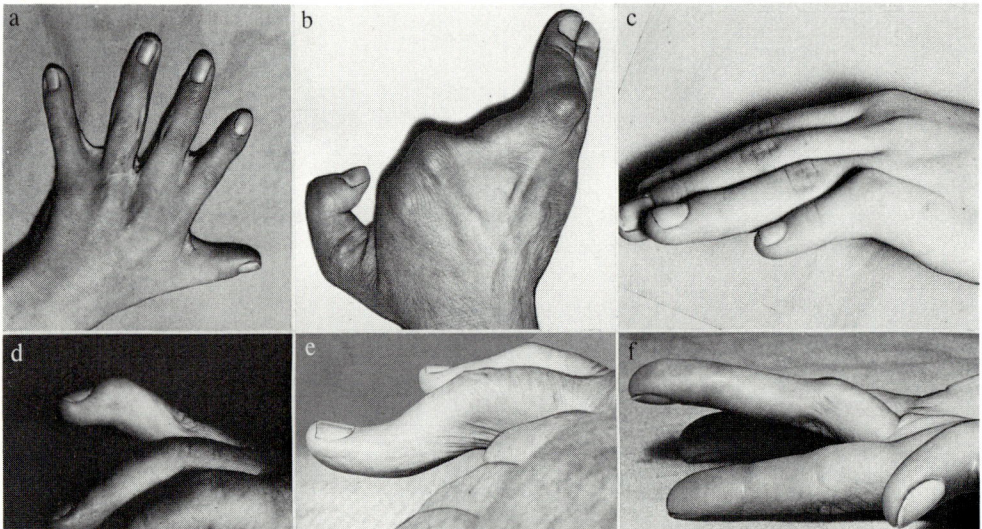

15.2   HAND DEFORMITIES
Upper row — congenital. (a) Webbing (syndactyly); (b) lobster hand (not a typical case); (c) congenital contracture of little finger.
Lower row—following tendon injury. (d) Terminal slip of extensor (mallet finger); (e) middle slip of extensor (boutonnière); (f) sublimis tendon (swan-neck deformity);

DEFORMITIES FOLLOWING TRAUMA

SKIN

CUTS — Cuts on the palm are liable to heal with contracture; accordingly, incisions should never cross the skin creases; ideally they should be parallel with and immediately adjacent to the creases.   In the fingers, either a mid-axial incision or Bruner's zig-zag incision is best.

BURNS — Burns may heal with contracture and may then require excision and grafting.

NERVES (*see also* pages 120–124)

ULNAR PALSY — The ulnar two fingers are ' clawed ', each is hyperextended at the meta-carpophalangeal joint and flexed at the proximal finger joint.   The distal joint is straight

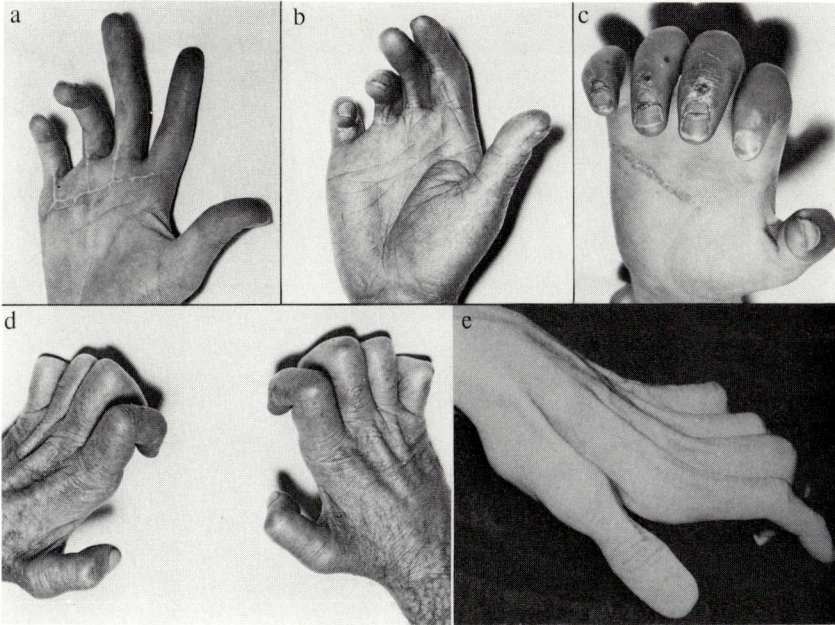

15.3 EXAMPLES OF CLAW HAND
(a) Following badly placed incisions; (b) ulnar nerve palsy. (c) Volkmann's contracture. (d) Bilateral clawing in peroneal muscular atrophy; (e) associated with the nerve lesions of leprosy.

if the lesion is high (because half the flexor profundus digitorum muscle is paralysed), but flexed if the lesion is low. The interosseus muscles are wasted, most noticeably in the first cleft. Ulnar sensation is lost.

OTHER NERVE LESIONS — Other nerve lesions may not produce obvious deformity, but the hand is held in an unnatural resting position.

Median nerve — Paralysis of the thenar muscles allows the thumb to fall into the simian position and the thenar eminence becomes flat; the index finger is held out straight because its profundus muscle is paralysed; sensation is lost over the median nerve area.

Musculospiral nerve — With musculospiral nerve lesions there is drop wrist; the fingers cannot be actively straightened at the metacarpo-phalangeal joints, but the interphalangeal joints can be extended with the lumbrical muscles.

Brachial plexus — Lesions of the plexus or roots may cause deformity, but neither the muscle weakness nor the sensory loss follows the pattern of a peripheral nerve lesion.

ARTERIES

ISCHAEMIC CONTRACTURE OF THE FOREARM (Volkmann, page 333)—This follows damage to the brachial artery in elbow injuries. The forearm flexor muscles may subsequently fibrose and shrink.   The forearm is thin and the finger joints flexed; they can be straightened only when the wrist is flexed.

ISCHAEMIC CONTRACTURE OF THE HAND (Bunnell; page 334)—This follows forearm injuries, especially when swelling of the hand is associated with a tight plaster or bandage The intrinsic hand muscles fibrose and shrink. The metacarpophalangeal joints are therefore flexed, the finger joints straight, and the thumb adducted across the palm.

TENDONS

MALLET FINGER — Mallet finger results from injury to the extensor tendon of the terminal phalanx. It occurs if the finger tip is forcibly bent during active extension, as in making a bed or catching a ball. The terminal joint is held flexed and the patient cannot straighten it, though the surgeon can. The tendon insertion may have been avulsed or may have pulled off a fragment of bone. The finger should be held for six weeks in a splint with the distal joint hyperextended; an Oatley splint, which leaves the proximal joint free and is removable, is ideal for this purpose (see also page 396).

MALLET THUMB — Mallet thumb resembles mallet finger in that the terminal joint is held flexed and can only be straightened passively. The long thumb extensor may be cut anywhere, or it may rupture at the wrist in rheumatoid arthritis, or following a fractured lower radius. Except after an open cut, direct repair is not advisable, for the ends are frayed. It is better to attach the cut distal end to another tendon (extensor indicis proprius, extensor pollicis brevis or extensor carpi radialis longus).

BOUTONNIÈRE — This deformity (which the French call le buttonhole) follows division or avulsion of the central slip of the extensor tendon proximal to its insertion into the middle phalanx. The lateral slips separate and the joint buttonholes backwards, resulting in fixed flexion of the proximal joint and hyperextension of the distal joint. (If caused by a small cut on the dorsum the injury is often missed.) Holding the finger straight in plaster probably leads to union, but the finger should not be splinted straight for longer than 3 weeks. The alternative is direct suture. In the established case one lateral slip can be transposed to the base of the middle phalanx.

SWAN-NECK DEFORMITY — This follows division, avulsion, or faulty function of the flexor sublimis tendon. The deformity is exactly the reverse of the familiar 'buttonhole' deformity, in that the proximal joint is hyperextended and the distal joint slightly flexed. Attempted repair of an avulsed sublimis tendon produces adhesions which limit the action of the profundus; if there is disability or the retracted proximal end is tender, the sublimis tendon should be excised through a small palmar incision.

DIVISION OF PROFUNDUS TENDON — Division of the profundus tendon alone produces no obvious deformity, but the resting posture of the finger is straighter than normal; the terminal joint cannot be actively flexed. For treatment of a cut profundus tendon see page 184: an avulsed profundus tendon should be reattached to the terminal phalanx.

DIVISION OF BOTH SUBLIMIS AND PROFUNDUS TENDONS — Division of both these tendons only follows open injuries (see page 185). There is no deformity but the finger is held straighter than normal and neither joint can be actively flexed; the patient may develop the trick of flexing the finger with its neighbour. Sometimes the retracted proximal ends of the tendons can be felt in the palm.

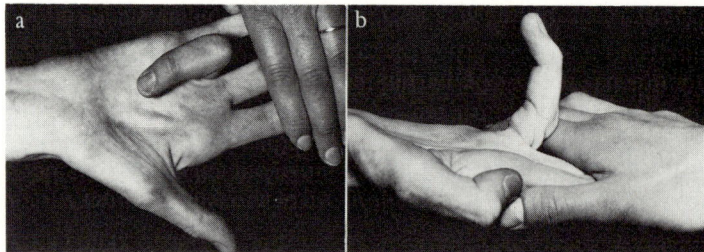

15.4 TESTING SUBLIMIS
To detect sublimis competence, first anchor the profundus, which is a 'mass action' muscle. In (a) the sublimis is normal; it alone is flexing the annularis — the tip is flail. In (b) sublimis is not working; only by using profundus (with difficulty) can the annularis be flexed, consequently the tip is not flail. (Apley, 1956.)

BONES AND JOINTS (*see also* page 393)

FINGER STIFFNESS — Some finger injuries, notably comminuted intra-articular fractures, inevitably cause stiffness. In most other cases stiffness is avoidable and results from inadequate management. Swelling and faulty splintage are the culprits. An injured hand must not be allowed to dangle idly in a sling; elevation and exercises are essential. When splintage is needed the metacarpo-phalangeal joints must never be straight, they should be as near a right angle as possible; interphalangeal joints, however, should, if splinted, be straight or nearly straight (*see* Fig. 15.10, page 185).

DEFORMITIES FOLLOWING INFLAMMATIONS

TENDON SHEATHS

ACUTE INFECTION — This is liable to leave a permanently stiff, bent finger. If this is a nuisance, it should be amputated.

CHRONIC INFECTION — Chronic synovitis occasionally follows implantation of a low-grade pyogenic infection or, rarely, of tuberculosis. From the thumb or little finger infection may spread to the common flexor sheath producing a compound palmar ganglion (page 171). In the middle three fingers infection remains confined to the sheath; the finger is bent and swollen. If antibiotics combined with aspiration, drainage and irrigation prove ineffective, a finger may need to be amputated.

BONES

TUBERCULOUS OSTEOMYELITIS (DACTYLITIS) — This condition is rare but may occur in a metacarpal or phalanx. There is slight swelling and tenderness and often a sinus. X-rays show rarefaction, and ballooning of the affected bone. If general treatment and splintage fail, amputation of the affected finger or ray may be advisable.

JOINTS

RHEUMATOID ARTHRITIS (*see* Chapter 3) — Rheumatoid arthritis causes multiple deformities in both hands. The joints are knobbly and the muscles wasted. The metacarpo-phalangeal joints are fixed flexed and the fingers deviated to the ulnar side.

GOUT — Gout may involve the hands and, if there have been a number of attacks, joint deformities may follow. Usually the characteristic tophi can be seen.

OTHER DEFORMITIES

DUPUYTREN'S CONTRACTURE

CAUSE — This curious disorder is of autosomal dominant inheritance; it is almost confined to individuals of European descent, in whom it becomes increasingly common with advancing age. It occurs commonly in association with epilepsy; associations with alcoholic cirrhosis, pulmonary tuberculosis, and with post-fracture splintage are less convincingly documented.

PATHOLOGY — A fibrous plaque develops in the palmar fascia, usually opposite the ring finger. Histologically it contains torn collagen fibres and altered blood pigment. As the fascia thickens and shrinks, its distal prolongations pull the fingers into flexion and its superficial attachments pucker the palmar skin.

SYMPTOMS — In the early stage the patient may complain of pain on grasping; later the condition is painless but, as deformity increases, the grip is impaired, there is difficulty in releasing objects and the bent fingers get in the way.

SIGNS — Ninety per cent of patients are men. Nearly always, both hands are involved, one more than the other. The ulnar palm is puckered, nodular and thick, with obvious fibrous bands. The affected fingers (chiefly the ring and little fingers) are flexed at

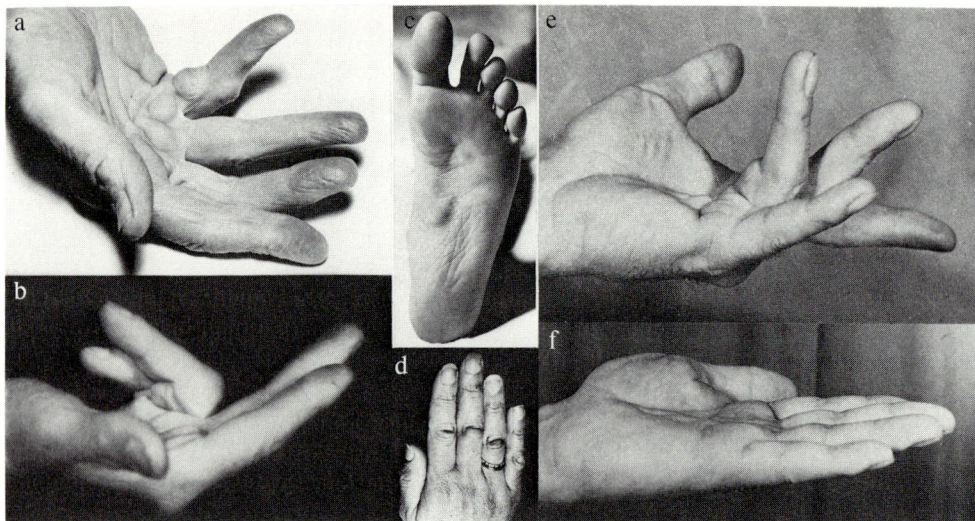

15.5 Dupuytren's contracture
(a) Moderately severe, with diagnostic nodules and pits; (b) severe contracture.
(c) Dupuytren's nodule in the sole; (d) Garrod's pads. (e, f) Before and after subcutaneous fasciotomy.

the metacarpo-phalangeal and proximal finger joints; the distal joint is never flexed but may be hyperextended in severe deformities when the finger tips dig into the palm. Garrod's pads (thickening of the dorsum of the proximal finger joints) are sometimes seen, and nodular thickening comparable to that in the palm may occur in the foot. An occasional association with fibrosis of the corpus cavernosum is called Peyronie's disease.

TREATMENT — Operation is indicated if the deformity is a nuisance or rapidly progressing. The aim is reasonable, not complete, correction. After operation, a removable splint is used to maintain correction and is removed daily for wax baths and exercises. After 6 weeks it is used only as a night splint for a further 6 months. The following operations may be used.

Fasciotomy — A tenotome is inserted horizontally, the skin is carefully separated from the fascia and then deforming bands are divided. This manœuvre is repeated from other points of entry until reasonable correction has been obtained. In experienced hands this is a good operation.

Fasciectomy — Through an incision in the distal palmar crease the palmar fascia is carefully dissected free and excised. Where necessary, a Z-shaped incision over the proximal phalanx may be used in addition. The long term results are better than with fasciotomy, but the period of disability is longer and the complication rate higher.

Amputation — Amputation of a severely affected fifth finger is sometimes advisable, especially if the joint capsules have secondarily contracted.

MISCELLANEOUS CAUSES OF DEFORMITY

NEUROLOGICAL DISORDERS — Disorders such as syringomyelia, poliomyelitis, or tumours of the spinal cord or roots may cause a variety of hand deformities. Upper motor neurone disorders (hemiplegia or cerebral palsy) cause fixed flexion of the wrist and fingers with adduction of the thumb.

MYOPATHIES — Myopathies which affect peripheral muscles first and most severely (for example, peroneal muscle atrophy) may cause marked clawing of hands and feet. The forearm is thin, the metacarpo-phalangeal joints are hyperextended and the finger joints flexed; the thumb is abducted and flexed (the 'intrinsic minus' hand).

MULTIPLE CHONDROMATA — These lesions may deform the hand considerably in Ollier's disease (see page 65). A single chondroma rarely presents as a deformity.

HYSTERICAL DEFORMITY — Hysteria should not be diagnosed until everything else has been excluded. The commonest hysterical deformity in the hand is flexion at the metacarpo-phalangeal joints, extended fingers and an adducted thumb.

TUNNEL SYNDROMES

CARPAL TUNNEL SYNDROME

There is insufficient space for the median nerve beneath the anterior carpal ligament. In the normal carpal tunnel there is barely room for all the tendons and the median nerve; consequently any swelling is likely to result in compression. Usually the cause eludes detection; the syndrome is, however, common in menopausal women, in rheumatoid arthritis, and in pregnancy.

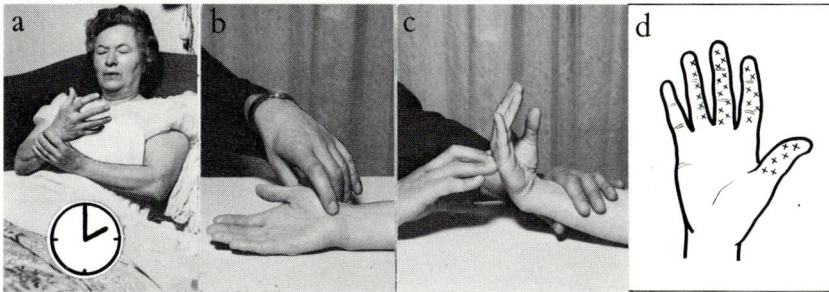

15.6 CARPAL TUNNEL SYNDROME
(a) The patient is woken in the early hours. (b, c) Pressure on the tunnel, or forced palmarflexion, may reproduce pain or tingling; (d) a positive 'map test'.

SYMPTOMS

Pain and paraesthesia occur in the distribution of the median nerve in the hand. Night after night the patient is woken in the early hours with burning pain, tingling and numbness; the fingers may feel swollen and the whole arm heavy. Hanging the arm over the side of the bed, or getting up and walking about may, after an hour or so, relieve the pain. During the day little pain is felt except with such activities as knitting. The pain may radiate up the arm. There is often clumsiness and difficulty in fine movements such as sewing.

SIGNS

The condition is eight times more common in women than men. The usual age group is 40–50 years; in younger patients it is not uncommon to find related factors such as pregnancy, rheumatoid disease or tenosynovitis.

Both hands, or only the master hand, may be involved. Abnormal physical signs are usually absent and indeed the condition should be diagnosed before signs are obvious. The pattern of sensory changes can sometimes be reproduced by holding the wrist fully palmarflexed for one minute, or by tapping the front of the wrist. The patient is often unsure of the precise distribution of paraesthesia, and it is helpful to ask her to return after a few days when she has mapped it out. The diagnosis can be confirmed by electromyography.

In late cases there is wasting of the thenar muscles with altered sensation in the median area.

TREATMENT

Conservative treatment consists of injecting hydrocortisone into the flexor sheath or wearing a cock-up splint. If these fail, or if there is already clinically detectable neurological deficit, operation is advised. The anterior carpal ligament is divided. The patient wakes up relieved of pain and from then on is not disturbed at night; but neurological deficit may not recover fully.

STENOSING TENOVAGINITIS OF FLEXOR TENDONS

There is insufficient space for normal tendon action. This may be due to rheumatoid tenosynovitis, to thickening of the fibrous sheath (stenosing tenovaginitis) or to nodular thickening of the tendon.

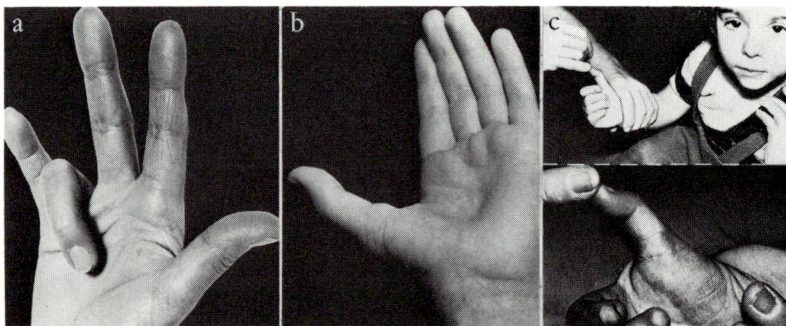

15.7 STENOSING TENOVAGINITIS
(a) Trigger finger; (b) trigger thumb — the only variety which also occurs in children, in whom (c) the thumb may be stuck bent.

CLINICAL FEATURES

In adults any finger or the thumb may be affected, but the ring and middle fingers most commonly. The patient first notices that the finger clicks, often painfully, when he bends it. Later, he complains that when the hand is unclenched the affected finger remains bent; it may suddenly straighten with a snap (trigger finger) or may remain flexed until forced straight with the other hand. A tender nodule can be felt in front of the affected metacarpo-phalangeal joint, and the finger or thumb clicks when actively moved.

In babies only the thumb is affected and the mother notices that the thumb remains bent. A hard nodule is palpable, and often dislocation is wrongly diagnosed.

TREATMENT

Through a transverse incision in the distal palmar crease, or in the metacarpo-phalangeal crease of the thumb, the fibrous sheath is incised until the tendon moves freely. In babies it is worth waiting a few months, as spontaneous recovery may occur.

ACUTE INFECTIONS OF THE HAND

Almost invariably, staphylococci have been implanted by trivial or unobserved injury. Streptococcal infections occasionally occur and cause widespread disturbance.

CLINICAL FEATURES

Usually there is a history of trauma, but it may have been so trivial as to pass unnoticed. A few hours or days later the finger becomes painful and swollen. The patient may be ill and pyrexial. The local signs are as follows:

LOOK — The finger may be red and swollen. Oedema of the dorsum of the hand is common in any infection. Red streaks on the forearm indicate lymphangitis.

FEEL — Palpation must be gentle, but the site of maximal tenderness is important for diagnosis and treatment, and must be carefully pinpointed. Sometimes fluctuation can be elicited. Enlarged axillary lymph nodes may be palpable.

MOVE — With superficial infections the patient can move his finger, though he may be unwilling to do so. With deep infections the finger is immobile.

X-RAY — Severe pulp infections may lead to bone necrosis which is shown by x-ray.

TREATMENT

Superficial hand infections are common; if their treatment is delayed or inadequate, infection may rapidly extend, with serious consequences.

The essentials of treatment are as follows.

PENICILLIN — Penicillin must be given in large doses immediately a hand infection is seen, and suitable antibiotic therapy continued until there is healing.

DRAINAGE — Drainage is essential as soon as pus forms or its presence is suspected. A tourniquet and adequate anaesthesia are necessary. There are no standard incisions, but no incision should cross a skin crease. Nearly always the incision should be small and at the site of maximal tenderness. (With the use of antibiotics, the old-fashioned long incisions are hardly ever necessary.) When pus is encountered it must be carefully mopped away and a search made for deeper pockets of infection. It may be necessary to snip away necrotic skin. A drain is unnecessary, and only dry dressings are used. The pus obtained is sent for culture.

REST AND ELEVATION — Rest and elevation are important in all hand infections. Once the acute inflammation has subsided, gentle active movements are begun.

INFECTIONS AT SPECIAL SITES

SUBCUTANEOUS TISSUES

NAIL BED (PARONYCHIA) — Infection beneath the horny layer of skin at the nail base or edge is common. The infected area is slightly swollen, red or purulent, and locally tender. Finger movements are full.

Unless discharge is already free, a portion of the nail may need to be excised.

PULP (WHITLOW) — Pulp infection is common. Swelling is resisted by the fibrous bands connecting bone to skin, so that pain is severe and bone necrosis may occur. The finger tip is swollen, red and locally very tender. The patient guards the finger against contact; he is unwilling but able to move the finger.

Early drainage is essential. Under antibiotic cover a small incision over the site of maximal tenderness is usually sufficient, but the incision may need to be enlarged in late cases when the pus has extended. If healing is delayed x-rays may show a sequestrum which should be removed.

ELSEWHERE IN THE HAND — Anywhere in the hand a blister or superficial cut may become infected, causing local redness, swelling and tenderness. A local collection of pus should be drained through a small incision over the site of maximal tenderness. It is important to exclude a deeper pocket of pus.

Subcutaneous infection over the front of the middle phalanx carries the risk of involving a tendon sheath. Infection in a web space may also extend, usually along the lumbrical canal and thence either forwards through the palmar fascia or backwards between the metacarpal bones. In all these instances the importance of seeking a deeper pocket of pus is obvious.

Erysipeloid — Erysipeloid is a specific infection of one finger in meat or fish porters. It is rapidly cured by penicillin.

TENDON SHEATHS (SUPPURATIVE TENOSYNOVITIS)

Pus in a tendon sheath is uncommon but dangerous and painful. It is liable to leave a stiff finger because of synovial adhesions.

MIDDLE THREE FINGERS — The affected finger is swollen and looks like a sausage. It is held bent, is very tender and the patient will not move it or permit it to be moved.

Usually two transverse incisions are necessary, one near the distal end of the sheath and one near the proximal end; using a ureteric catheter the sheath is then irrigated with penicillin; with localized infections one incision is sometimes sufficient. Delayed healing may be caused by necrosis of tendon, and if so the tendon should be removed or the finger amputated.

THUMB AND LITTLE FINGER — Tendon sheath infection in the thumb may spread to the radial bursa, and in the little finger to the ulnar bursa. The affected digit is swollen, bent, tender and held still, and swelling and tenderness extend proximally.

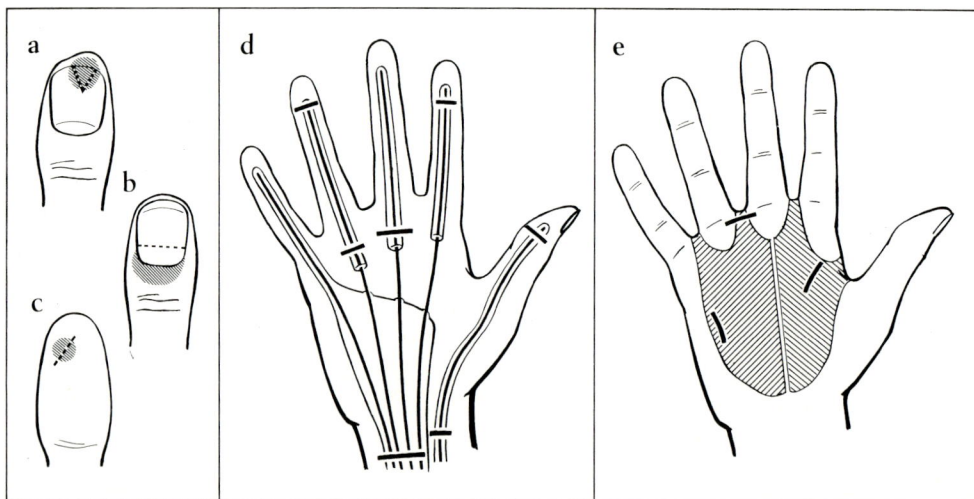

15.8 THE TREATMENT OF HAND INFECTIONS
(a) To drain an apical abscess it is often best to excise a triangle of nail. (b) Acute paronychia is most efficiently drained by excising the proximal part of the nail. (c) A pulp abscess should be drained over the point of maximal tenderness. (d) Synovial sheath infections can be drained by incisions near their proximal or distal ends, or both. (e) Incisions for web abscess and for the rare infections of the mid-palmar and thenar spaces (partly re-drawn from *Infections of the Hand* by D. N. Bailey, published by H. K. Lewis, London).

In addition to draining the digital portion of the sheath the ulnar or radial bursa may need to be drained through transverse incisions just above the wrist; the sheath is then irrigated with penicillin.

FASCIAL SPACES

Infection from a web space or from an infected tendon sheath may spread to either of the deep fascial spaces of the palm.

MEDIAL SPACE (MIDPALMAR) — The palm is ballooned so that its normal concavity is lost.   There is extensive tenderness and the whole hand is held still.   For drainage an incision is made directly over the abscess, and sinus forceps inserted; if the web space also is infected it too should be incised.

LATERAL SPACE (THENAR) — The palm is flat, there is deep tenderness, and the thumb and index finger are held still.   For drainage the skin is incised in the first web and the abscess opened with sinus forceps.

PROXIMAL EXTENSIONS — From medial or lateral space infections, pus may track up the forearm where it can be drained by antero-medial or antero-lateral incisions.

MANAGEMENT OF OPEN INJURIES OF THE HAND

In the U.S.A. 2 million disabling work injuries occur annually; 75 per cent affect the hand.   In Britain the problem is equally serious.   Early and expert surgery is essential to minimize disability; the care of the injured hand is no job for the junior casualty officer.   He should, however, be cautioned, to avoid irritants such as iodine or spirit; only bland substances (e.g. cetrimide) should be applied.

SIGNS

Detailed examination may have to await exploration, but careful pre-operative assessment is important if needless groping is to be avoided.   The spectrum of open injuries embraces tidy or ' clean ' cuts, lacerations, crushing and injection injuries, burns and pulp defects.   The patient's occupation and social status are important.

LOOK — Skin damage is the dominant factor.   ' Untidy' wounds, degloving and crushed skin are all serious, but even a tiny clean cut may conceal nerve or tendon damage. Localized swelling may suggest an injection injury or a traumatic aneurysm.

FEEL — Sensation is tested and re-tested several times.

MOVE — Active movements are tested to assess tendon damage, but if this is too painful the resting attitude of the fingers is a useful guide.

X-RAY — Fractures, dislocations, or foreign bodies may be seen by x-ray.

PRIMARY TREATMENT

PRE-OPERATIVE PROCEDURES

(1) PROPHYLAXIS — Antibiotics, if indicated are given as soon as possible, and suitable prophylactics against tetanus and gas-gangrene.

(2) ANAESTHETIC — General anaesthesia is preferable, though brachial block can be used, or even digital block for finger-tip injuries.

(3) TOURNIQUET — A high pneumatic tourniquet, applied after elevating the limb, is helpful but not essential.   It should certainly not be used with crush injuries, where muscle viability is in doubt.

(4) CLEANING — The wound is covered with a sterile pack while the neighbouring skin is cleaned with cetrimide.

(5) POSITION — The hand must be placed on an arm table in a good light.   The sterile pack is removed, the wound itself gently cleaned with cetrimide, and towelled off.

WOUND EXCISION AND DEEP REPAIR

SKIN — Do not excise a strip of skin around the wound — skin is too precious to waste. Only obviously dead skin should be removed.   For adequate exposure the wound may need enlarging, but incisions must not cross a skin crease, nor an interdigital web. Through the enlarged wound, loose débris is picked out.

Burns with only partial skin loss are cleaned, covered with non-stick dressings backed by wool and elevated.   The dressing is left undisturbed for 10–14 days, but finger movements are encouraged.   (Treatment by exposure, practised in some burns units, demands a specially clean environment.)   With whole thickness skin loss, devitalized tissue is excised, the wound cleaned and dressed, and five days later skin grafted.   Electric burns may cause extensive damage and thrombosis which become apparent only after several days.

SUBCUTANEOUS TISSUES — *Injection injuries* of oil or paint under pressure are damaging because of tension, toxicity or both.   Immediate decompression and removal of the foreign substance offers the best hope, but most reported series feature a high incidence of finger or partial hand amputation.

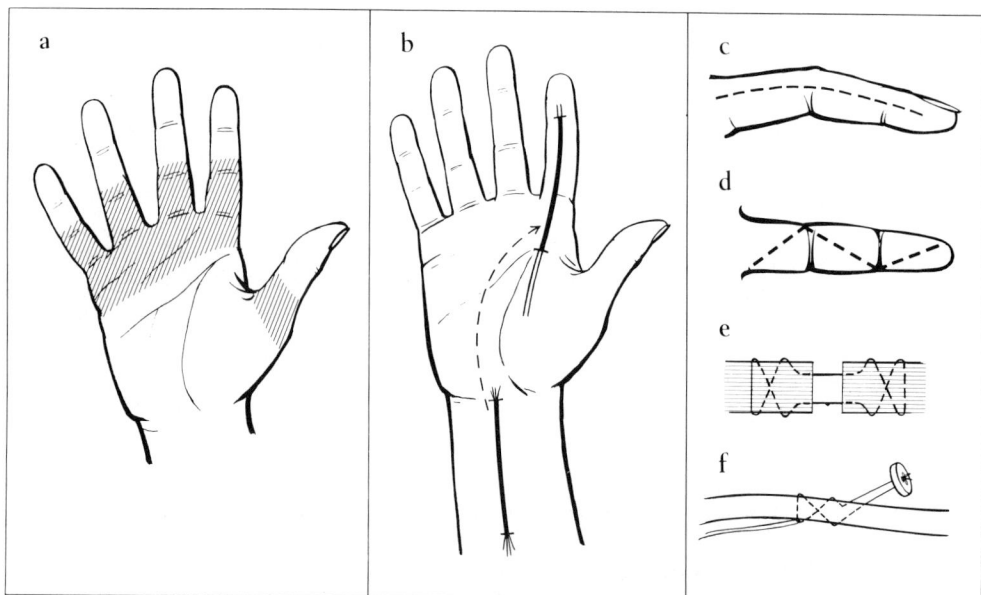

15.9   TENDON INJURIES (BUNNELL'S TECHNIQUE)
(a) Zones of the hand (re-drawn from *Injuries of the Hand* by R. J. Furlong, published by Churchill, London).   The intermediate zone (shaded) contains two tendons and two sheaths; primary suture usually fails. (b) The principle of tendon grafting to replace a cut profundus. (c) Mid-axial incision. (d) Bruner's zig-zag incision. (e) One method of tendon suture. (f) Bunnell's pull-out technique.

TENDONS — Repair must not be attempted if the wound is grossly contaminated, or if the ends of the tendon can be found only by extensive dissection.

Extensor tendons are relatively easy and safe to repair, but with flexors the situation is complex.   Successful primary repair of one or both tendons at all levels is feasible but only with a clean cut and early operation by an expert hand surgeon.   Where these conditions are lacking the wisest policy (advocated by Bunnell) is as follows:

Proximal zone (*from carpus to distal palmar crease*) — Tendon suture is permissible and relatively easy because the cut ends do not retract far; the lumbrical muscle should be lightly stitched round the suture line.

Intermediate zone (*distal palmar crease to proximal finger joint*) — There are two tendons inside two sheaths (fibrous and synovial); tendon suture leads to adhesions but is occasionally done to prevent the sheath from narrowing.

Distal zone — If the profundus tendon has been divided, primary suture is advisable unless the proximal end has retracted or the wound is dirty. If possible, the fibrous sheath is excised except for one band opposite the middle phalanx which is left as a pulley.

MUSCLE — Muscle damage occurs only in the palm and mainly in the thenar and hypo-thenar eminences. Dead or doubtfully viable muscle is excised with meticulous care to avoid nerves.

NERVE — Digital nerves are best repaired at the primary operation, providing the wound is not too dirty and no extensive dissection is needed.

JOINTS — Suture of torn capsule and ligaments helps to restore stability and permit early movement.

BONES — Fractures are reduced and subsequently treated as described in Chapter 23. If the fracture is unstable internal fixation is sometimes employed. The risk is worth taking because stiffness in the hand from prolonged external splintage is so disabling; percutaneous pinning techniques are used.

Amputation — Amputation of a finger as a primary procedure should be avoided unless the damage involves many tissues and is clearly irreparable. Even when a finger has been amputated by the injury, the possibility of re-attachment should be considered.

WOUND CLOSURE

HAEMOSTASIS — The tourniquet is removed and meticulous haemostasis obtained. The success of the operation depends largely upon this and skin healing.

SKIN CLOSURE — Only if the wound is grossly contaminated is closure delayed for a few days. Nearly always immediate closure is carried out by one of three methods.

Direct suture — This method is preferred if it can be achieved without tension and with only slight undercutting of skin edges.

Free skin grafts — These are often useful as temporary cover. They are usually taken from the front of the forearm and stitched into place. Partial thickness grafts take better, though it may be necessary later to replace them with full thickness grafts.

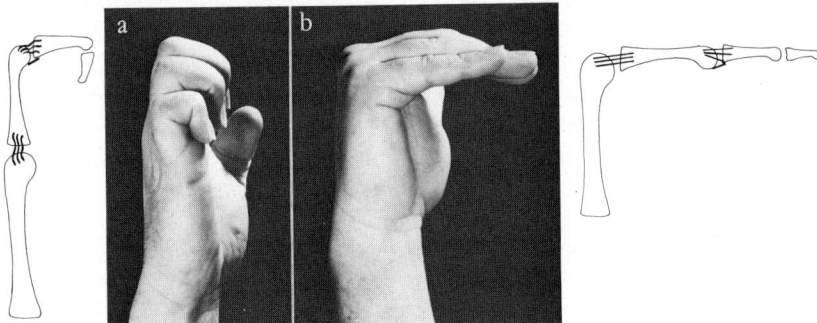

15.10 POSITION FOR FINGER SPLINTAGE
Fingers must not be splinted in position (a). The ligaments must be kept taut, otherwise they contract, causing stiffness. At the metacarpo-phalangeal joints the collateral ligaments are taut at 90 degrees; at the interphalangeal joints the important ligaments linking the volar plate to the collaterals are taut when the joint is fully straight. This is why James (1970) rightly insists on position (b) as the only safe one for splintage.

Flap grafts — Flap grafts are necessary if tendon or bare bone is exposed, for thin grafts do not take on these tissues. Flap grafts may be taken from local or distant sites. Sometimes a severely mutilated finger is sacrificed and its skin used as a rotation flap. A skin graft must be fixed securely and without dead space.

Pulp and finger-tip injuries — Split skin or full thickness grafts are conventional, but in most children and selected adults spontaneous healing (carefully supervised) offers an equally good appearance, with better sensation.

DRESSING — The wound is covered with several thicknesses of dry gauze, and ample wool soaked in flavine-paraffin emulsion. A firm crepe bandage ensures even pressure and a light plaster slab holds the wrist and hand with the metacarpo-phalangeal joints in flexion. If possible, the finger tips are left visible.

POST-OPERATIVE PLAN

IMMEDIATE AFTER-CARE — The hand is kept elevated and at rest. Antibiotics are continued as necessary. For the first 3 weeks the dressing is not disturbed unless the fingers become unduly swollen or blue or numb.

ASSESSMENT — At 3 weeks the dressings are taken off. It is now possible to estimate, from the state of healing and a knowledge of the operative findings, what the future function of the hand is likely to be.

The sensory and the various motor functions (*see* page 173) are separately assessed. With this information, and a knowledge of the patient's work and hobbies, the nature of further treatment can be decided; it may be conservative (rehabilitation) or operative.

REHABILITATION — When the wound has healed, active exercises and wax baths are started. The hand is increasingly used for more and more arduous and complex tasks, especially those which resemble the patient's normal job, until he is fit to start work; if necessary, his work is modified temporarily. Even if further surgery is required, tendon or nerve repair is postponed until the skin is healthy, there is no oedema, and the joints have regained a normal range of passive movement.

SECONDARY OPERATIONS

One of three procedures may be necessary: secondary repair or replacement of damaged structures, amputation of fingers, or reconstruction of a mutilated hand.

SECONDARY REPAIR

SKIN — If the skin cover has broken down or is unsuitable for surgery it is replaced by a graft. As always, the skin creases must be respected. Contractures are dealt with by Z-plasty or skin replacement. When important volar surfaces are insensitive, a flap of skin complete with its nerve supply may be transposed (sensory flap).

TENDONS

Proximal zone — If the tendons were not sutured at the primary operation, it is safe to carry out direct suture as a secondary procedure. The suture line of the profundus tendon is protected by wrapping the lumbrical muscle round it. The sublimis tendon may either be repaired or sacrificed.

Intermediate zone — If the sublimis tendon alone is cut and the proximal end forms an uncomfortable lump, it should be excised. A cut profundus tendon may be left if the patient is willing to accept the disability; otherwise a tendon graft is necessary.

Technique of tendon graft — Three donor sites can be used: (*a*) sublimis tendon from the injured finger (but this has no paratenon); (*b*) the fourth toe extensor (but this is rather thin, and the foot operation keeps the patient in bed); (c) palmaris longus tendon (the best) which must be excised with a wide margin of paratenon. It is absent in some people and its presence must be confirmed before operation.

The cut tendon is exposed by a longitudinal incision just behind the flexor finger creases (mid-axial), or by a zig-zag incision (Fig. 15.9, page 184).

The fibrous sheath is next excised, leaving a pulley opposite the proximal phalanx and one opposite the middle phalanx. Through a separate incision in the proximal palmar crease the sublimis tendon is excised and the profundus tendon trimmed. The graft is then sutured to the proximal profundus stump, threaded through the pulleys and sutured to the distal profundus stump with the finger flexed. (In difficult situations a Silastic tendon is used as a spacer at this stage; 10 weeks later it is replaced by the tendon graft.)

Distal zone — Only the profundus tendon can have been cut. The disability of a flail terminal phalanx may require surgery. Possible procedures are (a) a tenodesis to stabilize the joint in 30 degrees of flexion; (b) an arthrodesis in the same position; (c) a tendon graft as described above, which is capable of restoring normal function but necessitates excision of an undamaged sublimis tendon, thus entailing a risk of leaving the finger worse than before operation; or (d) advancing the profundus tendon and re-attaching it to the terminal phalanx.

NERVES — Cut median or ulnar nerves are repaired in the usual way. Digital nerves also are sutured if the finger has satisfactory motor function, but suture distal to the knuckle often fails. Useful sensation can sometimes be restored by using a sensory cross-finger pedicle graft.

JOINTS — Joint stiffness is best treated by active exercises. Stiff knuckle joints are sometimes helped by capsulotomy. Flail joints are stabilized by tenodesis or arthrodesis.

BONES — Mal-union hardly ever requires treatment. Non-union is exceedingly rare, but grafting may be required.

AMPUTATION

INDICATIONS — A finger is amputated only if it remains painful or unhealed, or a nuisance (that is if the patient cannot flex it, or cannot straighten it or cannot feel with it) and then only if repair is impossible or uneconomic.

TECHNIQUE — The aim is a mobile digit covered by healthy skin with normal sensation. A palmar flap is best and must always be ample in size; a tight flap usually gives pain. (Unless the flap seems too loose it is too tight.)

In the thumb every millimetre is worth preserving; even a stiff or deformed thumb is worth keeping. The index and little fingers are amputated as distally as possible, provided there is voluntary control of the proximal phalanx; if not, oblique amputation through the metacarpal shaft gives a good cosmetic result.

The middle and ring fingers should not be amputated through the knuckle joint, or the hand will be ugly and coins fall through it. If the proximal phalanx can be left, the hand is still ugly but stronger. Alternatively the entire finger with most of its metacarpal may be amputated; the hand is weakened but the amputation is less noticeable.

LATE RECONSTRUCTION

A severely mutilated hand should be dealt with by a hand expert. Three possibilities may be considered in exceptional cases.

(a) If all the fingers have been lost but the thumb is present, a new finger can sometimes be constructed with cancellous bone, covered by a tube flap of skin.

(b) If the thumb has been lost the three possibilities are: pollicization (rotating a finger to oppose the other fingers); osteoplastic reconstruction (which requires several operations but may provide a good grip); and toe transplant (usually from the hallux).

(*c*) If the thumb and all the fingers have been lost, making a cleft between two metacarpal bones may permit pincer action.

Suggestions for further reading

Apley, A. Graham (1956).   'Test for the Power of Flexor Digitorum Sublimis.'
   Br. med. J. **1**, 25
Bailey, David N. (1964).   *The Infected Hand.*   London; Lewis
Bunnell, S. (1971).   *Surgery of the Hand*, 5th ed. revised by J. H. Boyes.   Phila-
   delphia; Lippincott
Horn, J. S. (1969).   'The Reattachment of Severed Extremities.'   In *Recent
   Advances in Orthopaedics*, Ed. by A. Graham Apley.   London; Churchill
Hunter, J. M. *et al.* (1971).   'Flexor-tendon Reconstruction in Severely Damaged
   Hands.'   *J. Bone Jt Surg.* **53A**, 829
James, J. I. P. (1970).   ' The Assessment and Management of the Injured Hand.'
   The Hand, **2**, 2
Lamb, D. W. (1977).   ' Radial Club Hand.' *J. Bone Jt Surg.* **59A**, 1
Pulvertaft, R. G. (1973).   ' Twenty-five Years of Hand Surgery.'   *J. Bone Jt
   Surg.* **55B**, 32
Pulvertaft, R. G. (Ed.) (1977).   *Operative Surgery*, 3rd ed., Vol. 11, *The Hand.*
   London; Butterworths
Rank, B. K. and Wakefield, A. R. (1973).   *Surgery of Repair as Applied to
   Hand Injuries.*   4th ed.   Edinburgh; Churchill Livingstone
Stack, H. G. (1973).   *The Palmar Fascia.*   Edinburgh; Churchill Livingstone
Takayuki Mura *et al.* (1976).   ' Reconstruction of the Mutilated Hand.'   *The
   Hand.* **8**, 1, 78
Wynn Parry, C. B. (1973).   *Rehabilitation of the Hand.*   3rd ed.   London;
   Butterworths

CHAPTER 16

THE NECK

SYMPTOMS

The common symptoms of neck disorder are pain in the neck, scapular region or upper limbs; stiffness, either intermittent or constant; deformity, especially wry neck; and tingling, numbness or weakness in the upper limb. (Symptoms in both upper limbs usually indicate a neck disorder.)

SIGNS

No examination of the neck is complete without examination of both upper limbs.

LOOK — Any deformity is noted; the neck may be flexed forward, tilted sideways or twisted. From the back, skin blemishes or scapular abnormalities can be seen. One shoulder may be higher and there may be muscle wasting in the upper limb.

16.1 EXAMINATION
OF THE NECK
(a) Flexion, (b) extension, (c) rotation, (d, e) sideways tilt; (f, g) testing power in the elbow and wrist extensors. In this patient with signs of a prolapsed disc, flexion and tilting to the left are limited.

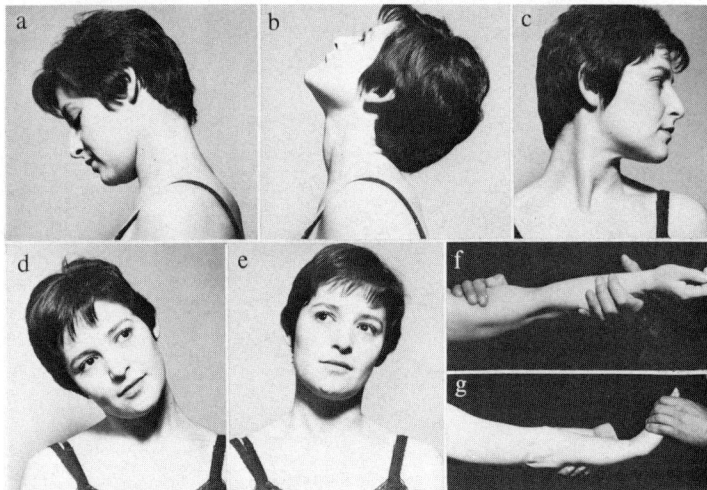

FEEL — The neck is palpated for tender areas or lumps. The radial pulses are examined and the skin tested for sensation.

MOVE — Forward flexion, extension, lateral flexion and rotation are tested, then shoulder movements. If necessary, muscle power and tone in the limbs are assessed.

X-RAY — In the lateral view, the cervical curve is inspected, then the individual vertebrae, the disc spaces and finally the intervertebral articulations. An antero-posterior view of the lower cervical spine is rarely of value except to demonstrate a cervical rib; for the upper cervical spine, a projection through the mouth may be required. Occasionally, lateral films taken with the head alternately flexed and extended are required to demonstrate instability.

INFANTILE TORTICOLLIS (Congenital Muscular Torticollis)

The sternomastoid muscle on one side is fibrous and fails to elongate as the child grows; consequently progressive deformity develops. The cause is unknown; the muscle may have suffered ischaemia from a distorted position *in utero* (the association with hip dysplasia is supporting evidence), or it may have been injured at birth.

CLINICAL FEATURES

A history of difficult labour or breech delivery is common. In 20 per cent of patients a lump is noticed in the first few weeks of life; it is well-defined and involves one or both heads of the sternomastoid. At this stage there is neither deformity nor obvious limitation of movement and within a few months the lump has disappeared.

Deformity does not become apparent until the child is 3 or 4 years old. During growth, as the normal sternomastoid gradually elongates, discrepancy becomes more obvious. It is as though, on the affected side, the mastoid process were growing closer to the sternal notch; consequently, the ear becomes lower and further forward. In fact, on the affected side the entire face is tilted downwards, twisted forwards and is shorter than on the normal side. The sternomastoid tendon feels tight and cord-like, restricting movements away from the deformity. X-rays are normal.

TREATMENT

PROPHYLAXIS — If a child has had a sternomastoid 'tumour' every effort should be made to prevent torticollis from developing. Each day a physiotherapist or the mother manipulates the neck into a position which elongates the affected sternomastoid to the full. The baby is laid to sleep on alternate sides.

STRETCHING AND SPLINTAGE — If, when the child is first seen, the head cannot be tilted fully in the direction opposite to that of the deformity, daily stretching is followed by

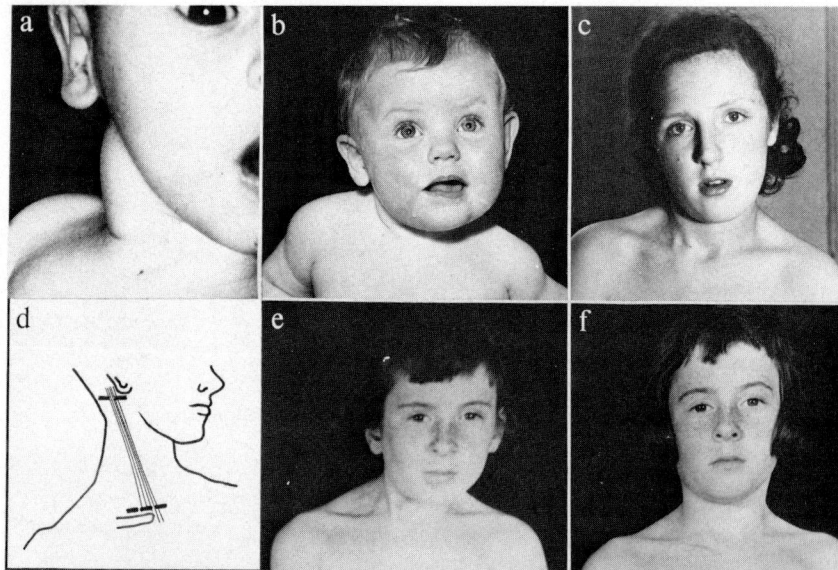

16.2 TORTICOLLIS
Upper row — natural history: (a) sternomastoid tumour in a young baby, (b) early wry neck, (c) deformity with facial hemi-atrophy in the adolescent.
Lower row — surgical treatment: (d) two sites at which the sternomastoid may be divided; (e, f) before and a few months after operation.

the application of a splint or a linen skull-cap attached by tapes tied under the axilla. This treatment is continued until the child naturally comes to hold its head correctly and the cap is worn at night for a further 6 months at least. A careful watch is kept for recurrence of the deformity.

OPERATIONS — One of three procedures designed to elongate the sternomastoid is indicated if stretching fails or the deformity is not seen until the age of 3–4 years.

Subcutaneous tenotomy at the lower end — This must be carefully performed if the vessels are to be avoided, but leaves no visible scar—an important consideration in an operation which is performed only for cosmetic reasons.

Open division of the lower end — A transverse incision is used, and the tendon divided. The anaesthetist then twists the child's head so as to obtain further correction of the deformity, and tight fascial bands are divided; this must be repeated until complete overcorrection is achieved. The operation is completely safe and the scar hardly visible.

Division of the upper end — This procedure may be performed alone, or may be combined with either of the above methods, the advantage being that the scar is hidden by the hair.

After operation correction must be maintained, at first by a skull cap tied under the axilla, then by a polythene collar which holds the head over and is worn for several months until the child has learnt to hold his head correctly.

SECONDARY TORTICOLLIS

A tilt or twist of the neck may develop secondarily as a result of acute disc prolapse (the commonest cause in adults), so-called fibrositis (usually a prolapsed cervical disc), skin scarring (especially after burns), inflamed neck glands, vertebral tuberculosis, ocular disorders or injuries of the cervical spine. In all these the diagnosis is usually obvious; the condition does not necessarily date from infancy and there is no facial asymmetry.

'Spasmodic' torticollis is also a secondary deformity, and is associated with neurological or psychological disorder. The sternomastoid muscle is in marked spasm, and the head grossly twisted. Sometimes violent jerking movements occur or are provoked by attempted correction.

The treatment of secondary torticollis is that of the primary cause.

PROLAPSED CERVICAL DISC

CAUSE AND PATHOLOGY

The factors responsible for a prolapsed cervical disc are the same as those of lumbar disc prolapse, namely injury (especially sudden unguarded movements), absorption of fluid causing nuclear tension to increase, and degenerative changes in the annulus (*see* page 216).

Prolapsed material may press on (*a*) the dura mater, causing neck pain and stiffness; or (*b*) the nerve roots, causing pain and paraesthesia in one or both arms. Prolapse occurs immediately above or below the sixth cervical vertebra, so that the nerve roots affected are C.6 or C.7.

CLINICAL FEATURES

The original attack, unlike that of lumbar disc prolapse, can seldom be related to definite and severe strain. It often occurs when a patient stretches himself on waking.

Subsequent attacks may be sudden or gradual in onset, and with trivial cause. The patient may complain of:

(*a*) Pain and stiffness of the neck; the pain often radiates to the scapular region and sometimes to the occiput.

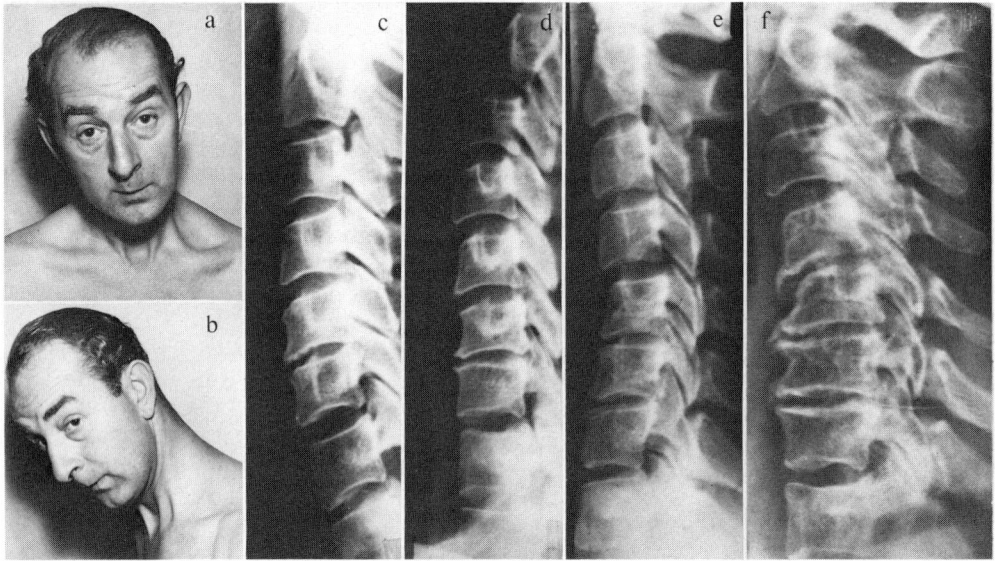

16.3   CERVICAL DISC LESIONS
(a, b) Acute wry neck due to prolapsed disc.   (c) A reduced disc space at C.5/6 is
not necessarily significant when the cervical lordosis is normal: in (d) the lordosis is
obliterated, and in (e) it is reversed — both strongly suggest a prolapsed disc.   (f)
Spondylosis, with multiple disc degeneration.

(*b*) Pain and paraesthesia in one upper limb (rarely both), often radiating to the
outer elbow, back of the wrist and to the index and middle fingers.   Weakness is rare.

Between attacks the patient feels well.   There are no general signs and the patient
is a fit adult.

NECK SIGNS (DURING AN ATTACK)

LOOK — The neck may be tilted forwards and may also be tilted sideways.

FEEL — Tender areas are felt in the posterior neck muscles, the trapezius and the scapular
region.

MOVE — Some movements are restricted and painful, but at least one movement is full
and painless unless the attack is very severe.   Shoulder movements are full.

X-RAY — At the affected level the normal lordosis is interrupted and the disc space is
often narrowed.

ARM SIGNS

The joints are normal but the arms should be examined for neurological deficit.
The C.6 root innervates the biceps jerk, the biceps muscle and wrist dorsiflexors,
and sensation of the lateral forearm, thumb and index finger; C.7 innervates the
triceps and radial jerks, the triceps muscle, wrist palmarflexors and finger extensors,
and sensation in the middle finger.

DIFFERENTIAL DIAGNOSIS

CERVICAL RIB SYNDROME — Pain is felt usually in the ulnar forearm and hand, a lump
may be palpable in the neck and the rib may show on x-ray.

CARPAL TUNNEL SYNDROME — Although pain may be referred up to the neck, neck movements are painless, and the pain in the hand is felt on the palmar surface in the distribution of the median nerve.

SUPRASPINATUS TENDON LESIONS — Although the distribution of pain may resemble that of a prolapsed cervical disc, movements at the shoulder joint are abnormal.

CERVICAL TUMOURS — With tumours of the spinal cord, nerve roots or cervical lymph nodes, the symptoms are not intermittent and the x-ray picture may be abnormal. Tumours of the cervical vertebrae are seen on x-ray.

CERVICAL SPINE INFECTIONS — The symptoms do not occur in attacks, there may be an abscess, and x-rays show narrowing of a disc space, and bone destruction.

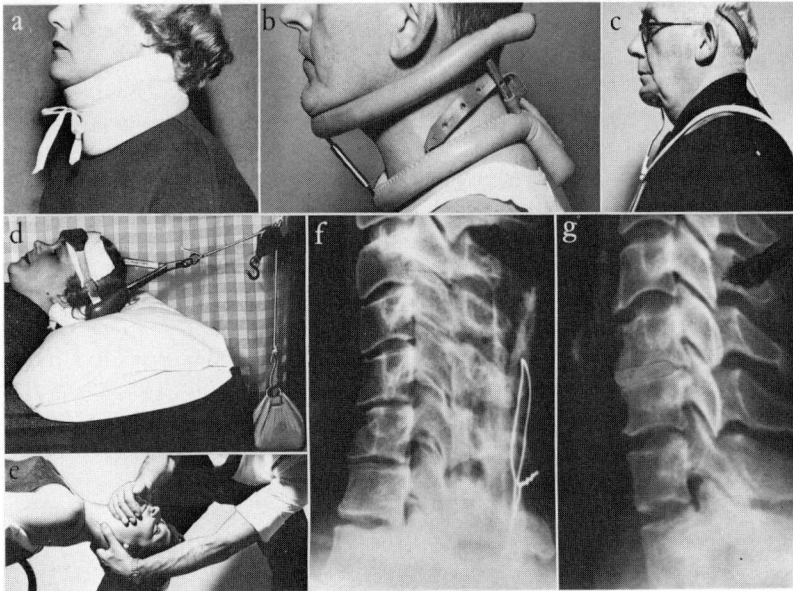

16.4 CERVICAL DISC TREATMENT
(a, b, c) Varieties of collar; (d) out-patient traction; (e) manipulation. Operation is rarely needed; grafting from the back (f) is being superseded by anterior fusion (g), which necessarily includes disc removal.

TREATMENT

Heat and analgesics are soothing but, as with lumbar disc prolapse, there are only three satisfactory ways of treating the prolapse itself.

REST — A collar is comforting and prevents unguarded movement; it may be made of cardboard and felt, stiff sponge-rubber, or polythene and metal.

REDUCE — Traction may enlarge the disc space, thus permitting the disc to slip back into place. The head of the couch is raised and weights tied to a harness fitting under the chin and occiput. Up to 40 lb. may be used for 20 minutes daily. Continuous traction using up to 10 lb. for 48 hours is more effective but the patient must be in hospital and sedated. Rapid reduction by manipulation (without anaesthetic) can be effective, and is probably safe providing the neck is first pulled in the extended position.

REMOVE — If symptoms are severe enough for operation the disc is removed through an anterior approach; bone grafts are inserted to fuse the affected area and to restore the normal intervertebral height.

CERVICAL SPONDYLOSIS

Spondylosis is the commonest disorder of the cervical spine. The lower cervical discs degenerate and disc material extrudes; surrounding fibrosis may spread to the root sleeves. The edges of the vertebral bodies hypertrophy (lipping) and later the intervertebral joints degenerate.

SYMPTOMS

The patient, aged over 40, complains of neck pain which comes on gradually and is often worse on first getting up. The pain may radiate widely: to the occiput and frontal region; to the scapular muscles; and down one or both arms. Paraesthesia, weakness and clumsiness are occasionally symptoms.

SIGNS

LOOK — The appearance is normal.

FEEL — Tenderness in the posterior neck muscles and scapular region is common.

MOVE — All movements are slightly limited by pain at their extremes.

X-RAY — Several disc spaces are diminished, and the corners of the vertebrae show lipping. (Identical x-ray changes may be present in a patient with no symptoms.)

NOTE — When a normal neck is moved the vertebral and basilar arteries have a considerable excursion. If the fibrosis associated with spondylosis sufficiently restricts this excursion the patient, on twisting his neck, may feel dizzy or even black out and fall. Angiography demonstrates the lesion.

LIMB SIGNS — In one or both upper limbs numbness or weakness may occasionally be found. Very rarely the lower limbs may have increased tone and brisk reflexes from upper motor neurone pressure.

TREATMENT

Heat and massage are often soothing, but restricting neck movements in a collar is the most effective treatment.

Operation is very rarely indicated. If severe symptoms are relieved only by a rigid and irksome support, spinal fusion is valuable. Very rarely, when abnormal signs in upper and lower limbs are not abolished by splintage or traction, decompression by laminectomy is performed.

CERVICAL RIB SYNDROME

The subclavian artery and first thoracic nerve pass through a triangle based on the first rib and bordered by scalenus anticus and medius. Even under normal circumstances these structures bend acutely when the arm rests by the side; an extra rib (or its fibrous equivalent extending from a large costal process), or an anomalous scalene muscle, sharpens the angle by forcing the vessel and nerve still higher. Even with normal ribs and muscles a post-fixed brachial plexus is excessively angulated.

These anomalies are all congenital; yet symptoms are rare before the age of 30. This is probably because, with declining youth the shoulders sag, increasing the angulation; indeed drooping shoulders alone may cause the rib syndrome.

As a result of increased angulation the first thoracic nerve may be stretched or compressed, causing sensory changes along the post-axial forearm and hand, with weakness of the intrinsic hand muscles. The subclavian artery is rarely compressed but may be narrowed by irritation of its sympathetic supply, or its wall damaged leading to the formation of small emboli.

CLINICAL FEATURES

There are no general symptoms or neck symptoms. In the arm the patient, usually a female in her thirties, may complain of: (*a*) pain in the ulnar forearm and hand, worse after household chores; (*b*) weakness or clumsiness; and (*c*) excessive sweating, or blueness and coldness of the fingers.

NECK SIGNS

LOOK — The shoulder on the affected side may be lower; or both may sag.

FEEL — A lump (the abnormally elevated subclavian artery) may be palpable above the clavicle. It pulsates, is tender, and pressure on it may increase symptoms.

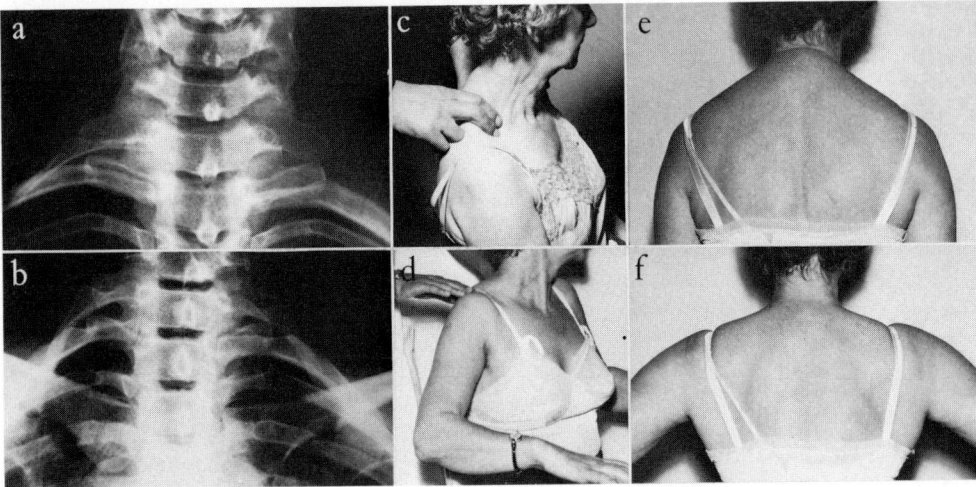

16.5 CERVICAL RIBS
(a) Unilateral; (b) bilateral. (c) A pulsating lump (the elevated subclavian artery) is usually palpable. (d) Teaching the patient shrugging exercises; before exercises the shoulders sag (e) — the aim is to restore the posture shown in (f),

MOVE — Neck and shoulder movements are normal, but pulling the arm downwards while pushing the neck away may obliterate the pulse too readily.

X-RAY — Occasionally a well-formed rib is seen, but more often there is merely enlargement of the transverse process of the seventh cervical vertebra.

ARM SIGNS

LOOK — The small muscles of the hand may be wasted: thenar, hypothenar and interosseus muscles are affected because all are supplied by the first thoracic nerve. Occasionally increased sweating or cyanosis is seen.

FEEL — If there are sensory changes they occur in the distribution of the first thoracic nerve root and are not confined to the distribution of a single peripheral nerve.

MOVE — If there is wasting, muscle power is reduced.

DIFFERENTIAL DIAGNOSIS

Many disorders resemble cervical rib syndrome.

CARPAL TUNNEL SYNDROME —Until this common disorder was widely recognized many cases were wrongly called cervical rib syndrome. Even when x-rays show a rib the symptoms may still be due to median nerve compression in the carpal tunnel. The nocturnal pain and its distribution are characteristic.

ULNAR TUNNEL SYNDROME — The symptoms and signs are sharply confined to the distribution of the ulnar nerve, and the neck is unaffected.

ACROPARAESTHESIA — There is sensory disturbance in both hands and sometimes the feet. When only the hands are affected the diagnosis is usually wrong, and the patient is probably suffering from a carpal tunnel syndrome.

PANCOAST SYNDROME — Apical carcinoma of the bronchus may infiltrate the structures at the root of the neck, causing pain, numbness and weakness of the hand. A hard mass may be palpable in the neck and x-ray of the chest shows a characteristic opacity.

CERVICAL SPINE LESIONS — In disc prolapse or spondylosis, pain is not post-axial in distribution and neck movements are limited. In tuberculosis and secondary deposits the x-ray appearance is characteristic.

SPINAL CORD LESIONS — Syringomyelia or other spinal cord lesions may cause wasting of the hand, but other neurological features establish the diagnosis (*see* page 207).

CUFF LESIONS — With supraspinatus tendon lesions pain sometimes radiates to the arm and hand but shoulder movement is limited and painful.

TREATMENT

CONSERVATIVE — The patient is taught exercises to strengthen the shrugging muscles. She is given analgesics, and advised to reduce her own weight and that of her shopping basket. These measures are usually adequate.

OPERATIVE — Operation is indicated if pain is severe, if muscle wasting is obvious, or if there are vascular disturbances.

Technique — The neurovascular bundle is exposed through a transverse incision half an inch above the clavicle. The scalenus anticus muscle is identified, the phrenic nerve retracted and the muscle is cut across. The rib (or its fibrous counterpart) also is divided; if none is present an inch of the first rib is excised.

TUBERCULOSIS OF THE CERVICAL SPINE
(*See also* Chapter 4)

Cervical spine tuberculosis is very rare. The presenting symptoms may vary from trivial neck pain to tetraplegia. Deformity is usually slight, though the normal cervical lordosis may be lost and there may be torticollis. Movements are limited, provoking pain and spasm when attempted. X-rays usually show bone destruction with a narrowed disc space and forward angulation. If there is an abscess it may be retropharyngeal, or present behind the sternomastoid muscle.

Anti-tuberculous drugs are given (page 35). The neck must be held still, but this is so irksome that, when the general condition permits, operation is advised. Through an anterior approach caseous material is evacuated and bone grafts used to fix the diseased vertebrae together.

Suggestions for further reading

Brain, R. (1954). 'Spondylosis.' *Lancet*, **1,** 687
Editorial (1972). 'Signs and Symptoms in Cervical Spondylosis.' *Lancet* **2**, 70
Frykholm, R. (1952). 'Cervical Nerve Root Compression resulting from Disc Degeneration and Root Sleeve Fibrosis.' *Acta chir. scand.* Suppl. 160
Hulbert, K. F. (1950). 'Congenital Torticollis.' *J. Bone Jt Surg.* **32B,** 50

Hummer, C. D. and Macewen, G. D. (1972). 'The Coexistence of Torticollis and Congenital Dysplasia of the Hip.' *J. Bone Jt Surg.* **54A**, 1255

Macdonald, D. (1969). 'Sternomastoid Tumour and Muscular Torticollis.' *J. Bone Jt Surg.* **51B**, 432

Osmond-Clarke, H. (1959). 'Pain in the Neck and Arm.' In *Text-Book of British Surgery*. Ed. by Souttar, H. and Goligher, J. C. London; Heinemann

Telford, E. D. and Mottershead, S. (1948). 'Pressure at the Cervicobrachial Junction.' *J. Bone Jt Surg.* **30B**, 249

CHAPTER 17

THE THORACO-LUMBAR SPINE

EXAMINATION

SYMPTOMS

The most common presenting symptoms of thoraco-lumbar spine disorders are pain, stiffness, deformity or a lump in the back; and pain, paraesthesia or weakness of the legs (the effects of nerve root pressure).

SIGNS WITH THE PATIENT STANDING

LOOK

Skin — Scars, abnormal hair, skin creases or pigmentation may be seen.
Shape and position — From behind, any asymmetry of the chest, trunk, pelvis or hips is noted and any lumps are observed. If the spine is deviated from the midline or rotated, there is scoliosis.

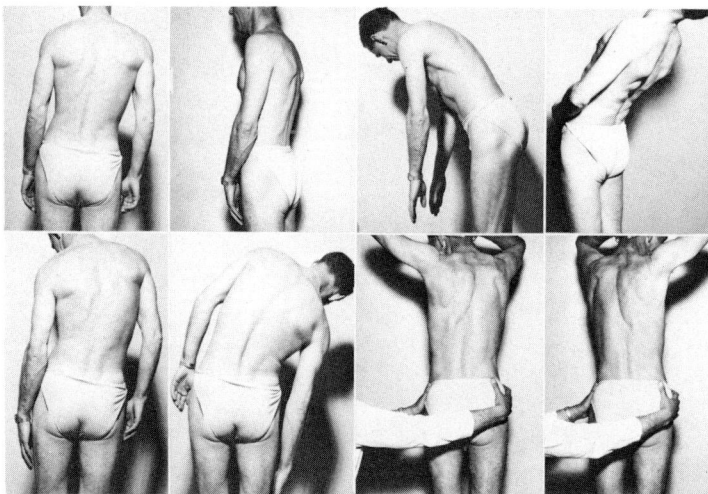

17.1 EXAMINATION OF THE SPINE (1) STANDING This patient has a prolapsed lumbar disc. He stands with a tilt. Forward flexion and tilting to the left are limited—other movements full.

From the side, any abnormalities of the antero-posterior curves are seen. The thoracic spine may be unduly bent (kyphosis) or angulated forwards (kyphos, which shows clearly as a knuckle when the patient bends). The lumbar spine may be unduly flat or excessively lordosed.

FEEL

Warmth is not detectable and tenderness is only occasionally useful. The spinous processes should be palpated, noting any kyphos or a 'step'.

MOVE

Forward flexion of the lumbar spine is tested by watching the patient try to touch his toes. Even with a stiff back he may be able to do this by flexing the hips;

198

17.2 EXAMINATION OF THE SPINE (2) In both diagrams the hands nearly reach the toes. To distinguish hip flexion (top diagram) from spine flexion, watch the lumbar lordosis, or note the separation of fingers placed on the spinous processes.

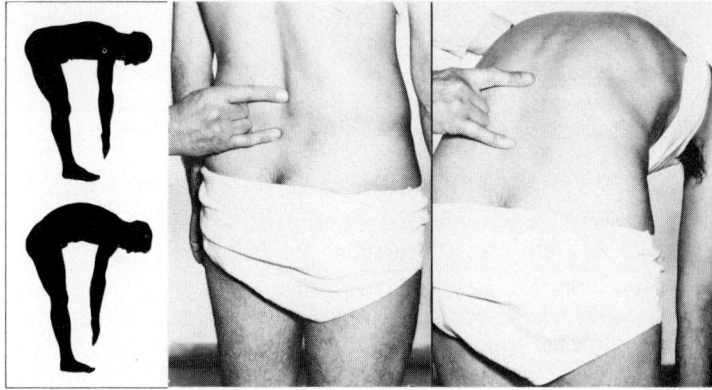

so watch the back to see if the normal lordosis straightens and reverses. Extension is tested by asking him to lean backwards; again the lumbar spine is watched. Lateral flexion is tested by asking the patient to bend sideways, sliding his hand down the outer side of his leg. Rotation is examined by asking him to twist the trunk to each side in turn; the pelvis is anchored by the surgeon's hands, or by the patient sitting on a couch.

Thoracic spine movements are difficult to detect — except breathing; the respiratory excursion must be noted.

SIGNS WITH THE PATIENT LYING ON HIS BACK

It is important to test for cord or root involvement and to examine the hips; where infection is suspected an abscess should be sought. Muscle tone and power are

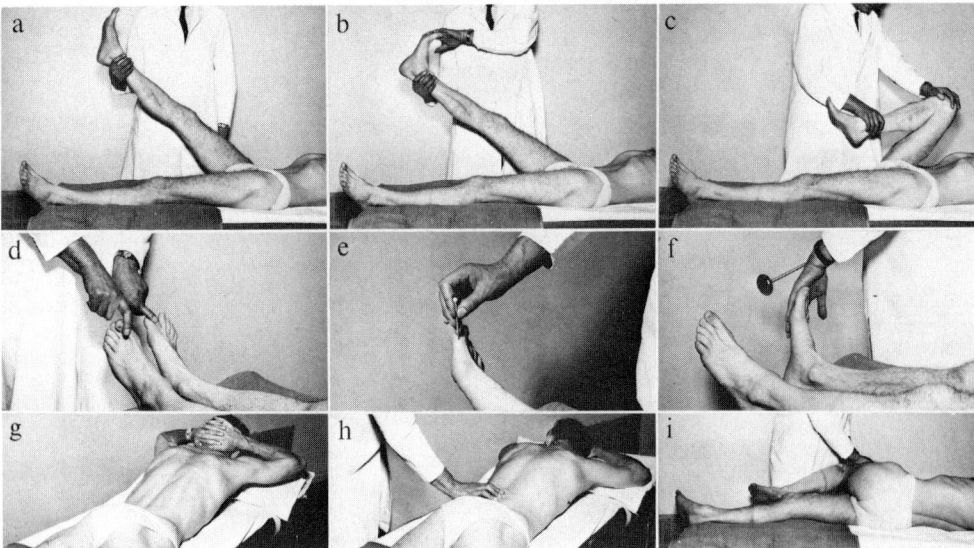

17.3 EXAMINATION OF THE SPINE (3) WITH THE PATIENT LYING
The legs are examined for nerve root involvement. (a) Straight leg raising is limited, and (b) the sciatic stretch is positive; but (c) flexion of the hip with the knee bent is painless, demonstrating that the hip is not at fault. (d) Muscle power, (e) skin sensation, and (f) the tendon reflexes are tested. With the patient prone he is examined for (g) muscle power, and (h) tenderness; (i) the sacro-iliac joints also may be examined.

examined, sensory changes noted and the reflexes tested. In examining for lumbar root involvement the straight legs are lifted alternately. If straight-leg raising is limited by pain, the leg is lowered 2 degrees from the painful angle; if dorsiflexing the foot causes pain to return, the limitation of straight-leg raising was due to abnormal stretching of the sciatic nerve or its roots and other causes are excluded.

SIGNS WITH THE PATIENT LYING ON HIS FACE

The presence of tenderness, deformity or abscess is confirmed. The tone and bulk of the back and buttock muscles are examined and the hips tested for full extension.

SACRO-ILIAC JOINTS — The sacro-iliac joints are difficult to examine because they are too deep to feel and because it is almost impossible to be sure that movement is not occurring at the lumbar spine or hips. The iliac crests may be squeezed together, pushed apart or, with the patient lying on either side, rotation may be attempted. If any of these movements is painful, the sacro-iliac joint may be at fault.

X-RAY APPEARANCES

First look at the spine as a whole. In the antero-posterior view it should be perfectly straight; in the lateral view the normal thoracic kyphosis and lumbar lordosis should be smooth and uninterrupted.

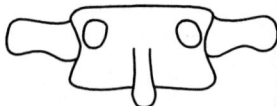

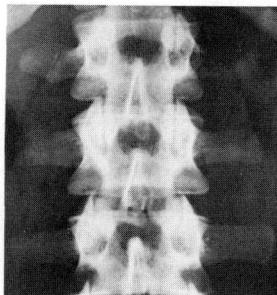

17.4   SPINE X-RAY
The AP resembles a face; the ears are transverse processes, the eyes pedicles and the nose is the spinous process (after Hoppenfeld).

Next look at the individual vertebrae and count them. In the antero-posterior view each should look like a face (Hoppenfeld, 1967), with ears (the transverse processes), eyes (the pedicles seen end-on) and a nose (the spinous process). In the lateral view the body should look like a rectangular box with straight or only slightly indented sides, the neural arch should be unbroken and the intervertebral joint surfaces smooth and parallel. Oblique films may be needed to display laminar defects.

TUBERCULOSIS OF THE SPINE

The spine is the commonest site of skeletal tuberculosis, and also the most dangerous.

PATHOLOGY

OSTEOMYELITIS — Blood-borne infection settles in a single vertebra which squashes down into the one below and infects it; or two neighbouring vertebrae are infected simultaneously. The neural arches are usually unaffected so that, as the bodies collapse, forward angulation (kyphos) develops.

SPREAD — The collapse squeezes out caseous material which may infect neighbouring vertebrae, or press on the cord, or escape into the soft tissues as a cold abscess. As the disease progresses, destruction, wedging and forward angulation increase and may, in the thoracic spine, become severe.

HEALING — With healing, the vertebrae recalcify and bony fusion may occur between them. Nevertheless, if there has been much forward angulation, the spine is usually 'unsound', and flares are common, with further illness and further collapse.

CLINICAL FEATURES

There is a long history with insidious onset and vague ill health. Pain is usually slight, often only a dull ache, worse after standing or jolting. Sometimes a lump (the kyphos or an abscess) is the presenting symptom; occasionally paraesthesia or weakness of the legs due to paraplegia.

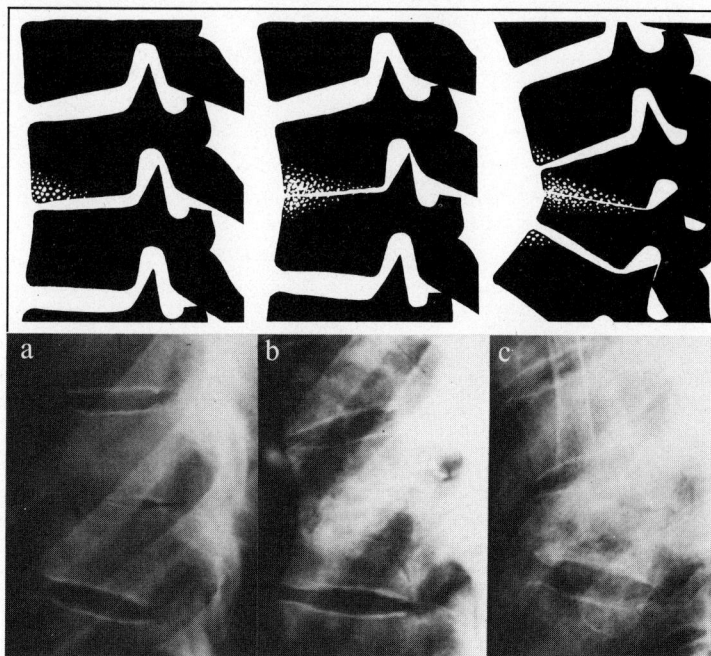

17.5 SPINE TUBERCULOSIS (1) PATHOLOGY
(a, b, c) Progressively increasing destruction of the front of the vertebral bodies leads to forward collapse.

In the active stage the local signs are as follows:

LOOK — A characteristic feature in the thoracic spine is an angular kyphos, best seen from the side. In advanced cases the patient is a hunchback. In the lumbar spine the kyphos is scarcely visible, but an abscess in the loin or groin may be obvious.

FEEL — The fingers can detect a kyphos, however slight; one need only run the hand down the spinous processes. Abscesses are fluctuant and the skin over them slightly warm (the term 'cold abscess' is merely a reminder that they lack the heat of a pyogenic abscess).

MOVE — Diminished movement is undetectable in the thoracic region, but easy to observe in the lumbar spine; the back should be carefully watched while movements are attempted. Usually all are limited and the attempt provokes muscle spasm. Formerly the coin test was used; a child with lumbar spasm prefers bending at the hips and knees rather than at the spine.

The legs also must be examined for neurological deficit.

X-RAY — In lateral films two adjacent bodies show destruction and the intervening disc space is narrowed; a characteristic feature in the antero-posterior view of thoracic disease is a paravertebral abscess.

In the healing stage pain vanishes and the patient is fit again. The bones recalcify

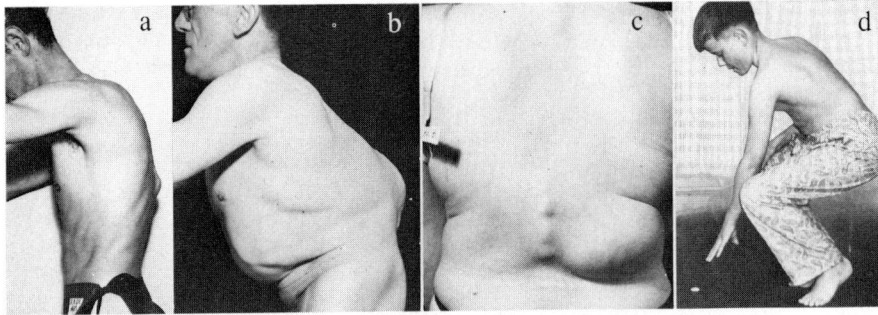

17.6 SPINE TUBERCULOSIS (2) CLINICAL FEATURES
(a) This kyphos is slight but diagnostic. If collapse continues (b) kyphos becomes severe. (c) Large lumbar abscess. (d) The coin test.

and look 'harder' on x-ray; even the abscesses may become calcified. Deformity is permanent and with an exaggerated thoracic kyphos the spine remains 'unsound' and liable to flare.

IMPORTANT NOTE — The description given refers specifically to British Nationals, in whom the general illness is usually mild, only one area of the thoraco-lumbar spine is affected and two neighbouring vertebrae together with the intervening disc space are involved. By contrast in immigrants from the West Indies, Africa or India the general illness is often more severe and the disease more likely to affect multiple sites (including the cervical spine); but the affected vertebral bodies are not always contiguous, the disc spaces not necessarily narrowed and neural arches or processes are not uncommonly affected.

DIFFERENTIAL DIAGNOSIS

Thoracic tuberculosis must be differentiated from other causes of kyphosis (page 210): the diagnostic x-ray features are the narrowed disc space between two affected vertebrae, and the tell-tale shadow of a paravertebral abscess.

Lumbar tuberculosis must be differentiated from other causes of backache (page 219) in a slightly unfit patient. Confusion sometimes arises with osteochondritis which, in the lumbar spine, usually presents in adolescence: x-ray shows the anterior corner of one (or two) vertebrae eroded and slight narrowing of the disc space; but the erosion has a sclerosed margin, the vertebra below the narrow disc looks bigger from the side and, of course, the patient is not ill. A brief period of rest settles the problem.

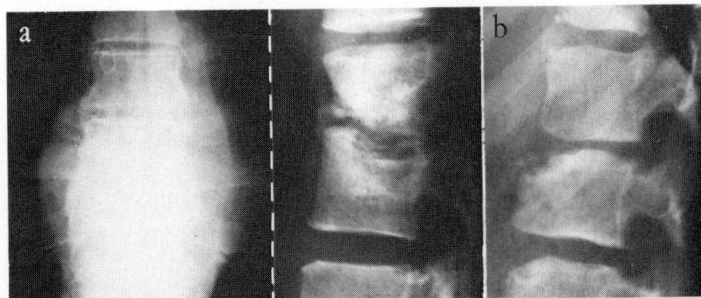

17.7 SPINE TUBERCULOSIS (3) X-RAYS
(a) Paravertebral abscess and erosion of two adjacent vertebrae is characteristic; by contrast in (b) lumbar osteochondritis, one body is normal and the 'eroded' vertebra is bigger.

TREATMENT

Anti-tuberculous drugs are essential in every case. In other respects methods vary widely and three régimes are used:

(1) No treatment other than drugs, except out-patient observation; sometimes a plaster back support or a brace is added.

(2) In-patient conservative treatment; simple bed rest, or a plaster bed or even (for thoracic disease in children) a hyperextension frame: no operation, except perhaps minimal débridement.

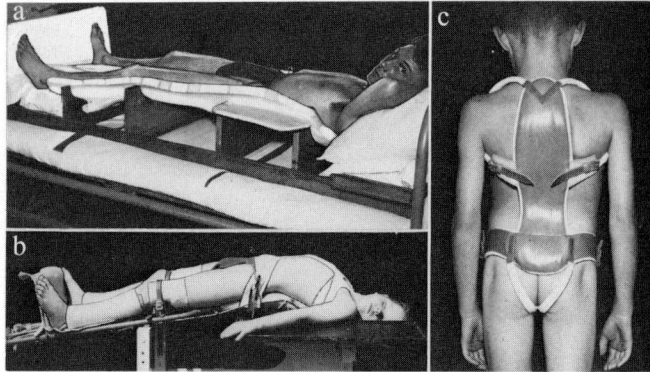

17.8 SPINE TUBERCULOSIS (4) ASPECTS OF CONSERVATIVE TREATMENT Splintage is sometimes used. (a) Adult on plaster bed; (b) child on hyperextension frame; (c) Jones' back brace.

(3) Operative excision of the disease as soon as the general condition permits. Anterior approaches as practised in Hong Kong are popular (trans-thoracic or retroperitoneal). The abscess is evacuated, caseous bone and disc material gently removed and the cavity plugged with strong iliac bone grafts. Sometimes streptomycin powder also is inserted.

Extensive trials on non-paraplegic patients have been conducted by the Medical Research Council (Seddon, 1976). Treatment by drugs alone gave good results (more than 80 per cent of patients well, with sinuses dry, no paraplegia and x-ray healing); but the kyphos usually increased slightly (average 15 degrees). Treatment by extensive surgery gave a slightly higher percentage of good results with no increase of kyphos. Clearly operative treatment is preferable, but it is not without hazard and should be restricted to those centres where a high standard of operative expertise is available.

Whatever method is used, drug treatment is continued until the patient has fully recovered and for a minimum of 18 months. Even then periodic observation is esential, the two important complications being:

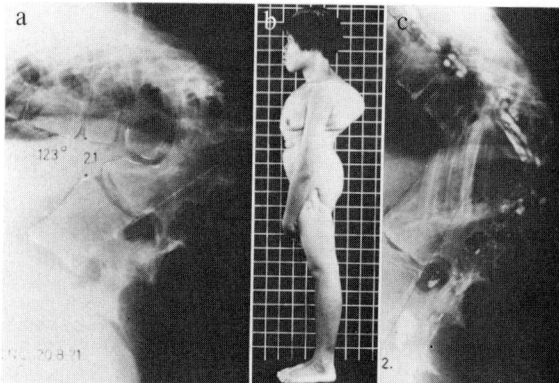

17.9 SPINE TUBERCULOSIS (5) OPERATIVE TREATMENT A very severe kyphos (a, b,) has been partially corrected and (c) held with anterior grafts (by courtesy of Professor Arthur Yau, Hong Kong).

(1) Flare of the disease (malaise, pain, an abscess or sinus or x-ray changes); and (2) Paraplegia.

POTT'S PARAPLEGIA

The spinal cord may be compressed by soft inflammatory material (an abscess, a caseous mass, or granulation tissue); or by hard solid material (a bony sequestrum, a sequestrated disc, or the ridge of bone at the kyphos). Occasionally fibrous tissue is the compressing agent.

Clinically the patient presents with signs of paraplegia added to those of spine tuberculosis. Clumsiness, incoordination and weakness are early symptoms; later, voluntary power is reduced, muscle tone increased and the tendon reflexes brisk; clonus and extensor plantar responses may occur. Paraesthesia or numbness, and disturbance of bladder control are common.

The patient is rested on a plaster bed and given anti-tuberculous drugs. Unless the paraplegia soon begins to subside operation is advised. The antero-lateral approach is traditional, but a trans-thoracic approach easier. The cord is extensively decompressed, necrotic material removed and the spine grafted. If recovery does not follow, the management is similar to that for traumatic paraplegia (page 411).

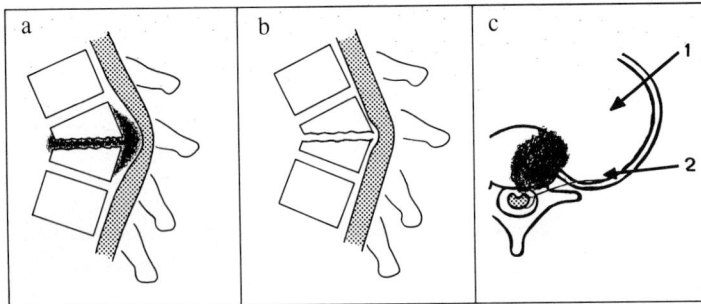

17.10 SPINE TUBERCULOSIS (6) PARAPLEGIA
Pott's paraplegia may follow pressure of (a) soft material (an abscess), or (b) hard material (the bony kyphos); (c) routes for decompression—
1. transthoracic,
2. antero-lateral.

REGIONAL SUMMARY OF SPINAL TUBERCULOSIS

The following Table, based on that of Perkins, draws attention to the leading features at various levels of the spine.

Level	Deformity	Abscess	Spasm	X-ray	Comments
C.1–C.2	None	Retropharyngeal	Present	Difficult to interpret	Very rare
C.3–Th.2	Sometimes torticollis or loss of lordosis	Behind sternomastoid muscle	Present	Wedging obvious	Rare: may give rise to tetraplegia
Th.3–Th.11	Kyphos and kyphosis	Often only seen by x-ray	Absent	Collapse, wedging, abscess	Common: may give rise to paraplegia
Th.12–L.4	Often none	Common, especially psoas abscess	Present	Narrow disc, sometimes wedging	Common: diagnosed late
L.5–S.1	None	Usually in buttock	Absent	Often only narrow disc	Often diag-nosed as disc prolapse

SCOLIOSIS

Seen from behind the normal spine is straight; deviation to one side constitutes scoliosis. The slight deviation which may follow fracture or tuberculosis (osteogenic scoliosis) is not considered in this section; nor is the curvature (thoracogenic) which may follow extensive chest surgery. The two main groups discussed are mobile and fixed scoliosis.

MOBILE SCOLIOSIS (Transient)

The vertebrae are not rotated. The curve is essentially transient and never develops into fixed scoliosis. There are three varieties:

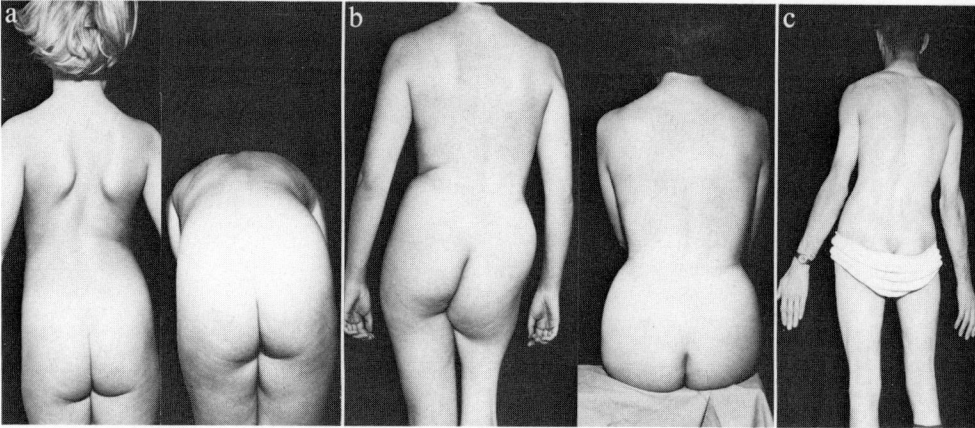

17.11 MOBILE SCOLIOSIS
(a) Postural scoliosis disappears on flexion. (b) Short leg scoliosis disappears when the patient sits. (c) Sciatic scoliosis disappears when the underlying cause (a prolapsed disc) has been treated.

POSTURAL — This is common, especially in adolescent girls. The curve is mild and usually convex to the left. The diagnostic feature is that when the child bends forward the spine straightens completely (in marked contrast to fixed curves which become more obvious on bending). Spontaneous recovery is invariable and exercises serve only to placate the parents.

COMPENSATORY — The most important cause is a short leg; the diagnostic feature is that when the patient sits (thereby cancelling leg inequality) the curve disappears. Other causes of compensatory scoliosis, such as a short sterno-mastoid, ocular disorders and empyema are usually self-evident.

SCIATIC — This term is applied to the lateral tilt which may accompany a prolapsed lumbar disc. The clinical features of the underlying cause are manifest, and the tilt disappears when the cause is remedied.

FIXED SCOLIOSIS (Structural)

With fixed scoliosis deviation from the midline is always accompanied by rotation of the vertebrae; the bodies rotate towards the convexity of the curve, the neural arches and spinous processes towards the concavity.

Once the deformity has developed it is liable to increase, probably because the greater pressure through epiphyses on the concave side slows their growth. The curve stops increasing when the spine stops growing; a reliable guide to spinal maturity is the complete appearance of the iliac apophyses on x-ray (Risser's sign).

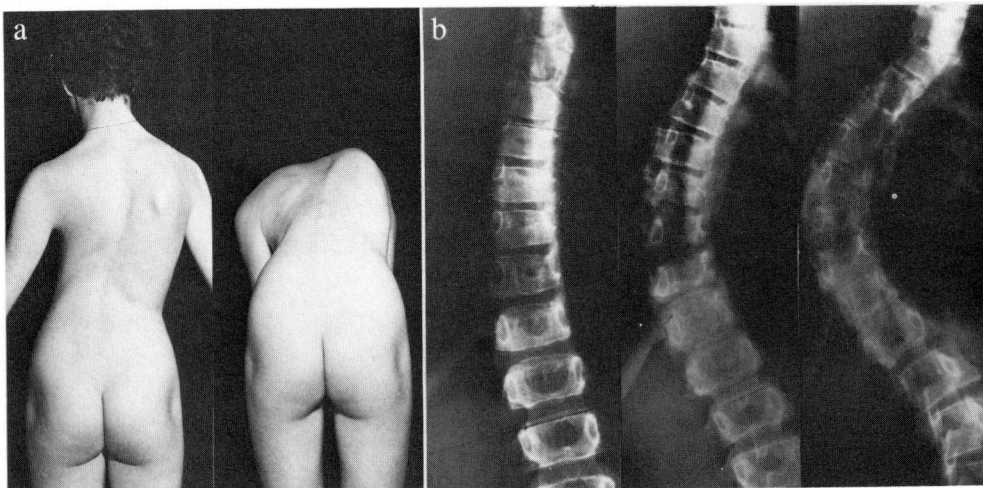

17.12 FIXED SCOLIOSIS (1)
(a) A fixed (structural) curve is more obvious on flexion. (b) Over a period of 4 years this curve has steadily increased.

There are usually three curves; the middle one is primary and fixed from the start; the compensatory curves above and below may later become fixed.

VARIETIES

IDIOPATHIC — This is the commonest variety. As its name implies the cause is unknown, but genetic factors certainly play a part. It is not the sequel to postural scoliosis, nor is it due to unrecognized poliomyelitis. Mental defect is distinctly commoner than in the rest of the population. The diagnosis is reached by excluding identifiable causes. Fig. 17.13 illustrates the five main curve patterns.

Infantile scoliosis is rare in North America, probably because most babies there sleep prone (Wynne-Davies, 1975). If mild, this variety may resolve; the distinction from progressive scoliosis can be made by serial observation, or better by comparing the rib-vertebra angle on the two sides (Mehta, 1972).

CONGENITAL — In order to label scoliosis as congenital there should be radiologically demonstrable anomalies such as hemivertebrae, absent discs, fused vertebrae, absent ribs or fused ribs. The overlying tissues often show tell-tale abnormalities such as angiomas, naevi, excess hair, dimples or a pad of fat. Although congenital scoliosis often remains mild sometimes it becomes extremely severe. When there is also spina bifida, neurological changes may be present in one or both legs.

PARALYTIC — Paralytic disorders associated with scoliosis include poliomyelitis, muscular dystrophies and cerebral palsy. With poliomyelitis the curve may not appear for some years after the original disease; unbalanced paralysis, especially of the intercostal or lateral abdominal muscles, causes a curve which then increases progressively. Patients with muscle dystrophy may have no supporting trunk muscles at all; they develop a floppy unstable spine. With paralytic scoliosis extensive fusion may be needed.

NEUROFIBROMATOSIS (page 101) — Thirty per cent of patients with multiple neurofibromatosis develop scoliosis, often a short sharp thoracic curve which is liable to become severe. Characteristic café-au-lait spots are nearly always obvious.

Infantile Thoracic

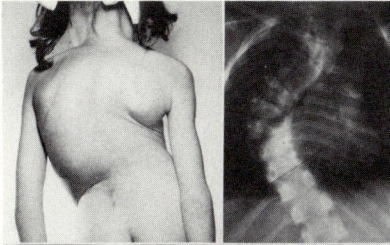

60% male.
90% convex to left.
Associated with ipsilateral plagiocephaly.
  May be resolving or progressive.
Progressive variety becomes severe.

Adolescent Thoracic

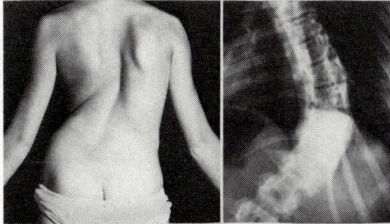

90% female.
90% convex to right.
Rib rotation exaggerates the deformity.
50% develop curves of greater than 70
  degrees.

Thoraco-lumbar

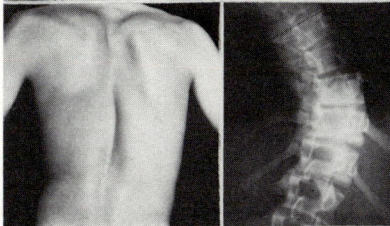

Slightly commoner in females.
Slightly commoner to right.
Features mid-way between adolescent
  thoracic and lumbar.

Lumbar

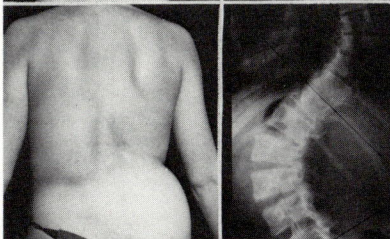

Commoner in females.
80% convex to left.
One hip prominent but no ribs to accen-
  tuate deformity.
Therefore not noticed early, but backache
  in adult life.

Combined

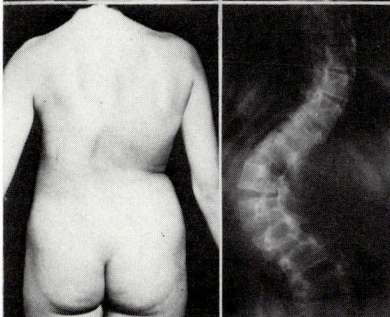

2 primary curves, one in each direction.
Even when radiologically severe clinical
  deformity relatively slight because
  always well balanced.

17.13 FIXED SCOLIOSIS (2) IDIOPATHIC CURVE PATTERNS

The varieties of scoliosis already described between them account for at least 95 per cent of cases seen in scoliosis clinics; the following rare causes are occasionally seen:

SYRINGOMYELIA — In syringomyelia high thoracic scoliosis is common. There is loss of pain and temperature sense, spastic weakness, trophic changes and often claw hands. Charcot's neuropathy may affect joints, chiefly in the upper limbs.

FRIEDREICH'S ATAXIA— In this rare familial condition scoliosis is common and pes cavus is invariable. It presents between the ages of 5 and 15 years with increasing clumsiness, ataxia, tremor and slurred speech.

DYSTROPHIES — In many bone dystrophies and malformation syndromes there may be an associated scoliosis; examples are osteogenesis imperfecta and Marfan's syndrome.

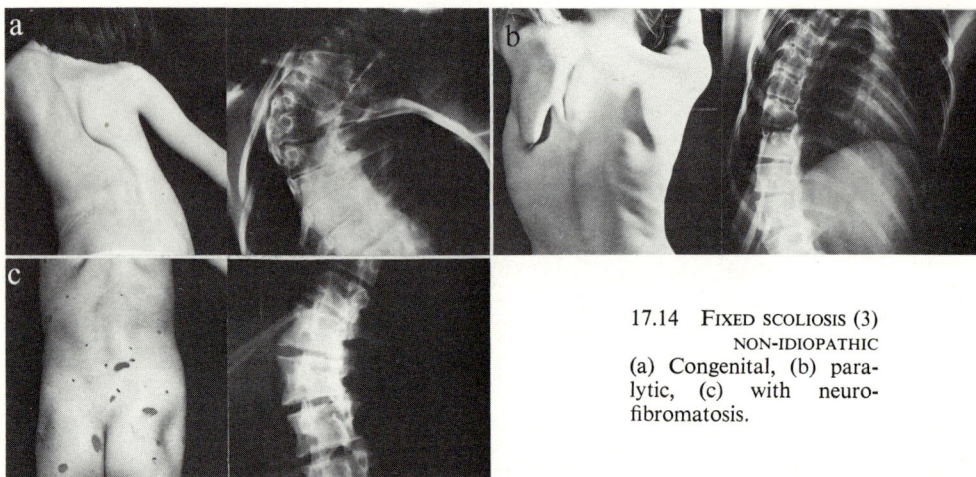

17.14   FIXED SCOLIOSIS (3)
NON-IDIOPATHIC
(a) Congenital, (b) paralytic, (c) with neurofibromatosis.

SYMPTOMS

Deformity is usually the presenting symptom, and the age of onset is important; high curves are likely to be noticed earlier and to become severe. Lumbar curves and combined curves may pass unnoticed until an adult presents with backache.

SIGNS

Most patients with idiopathic scoliosis are young adolescent girls. Patients should be examined for skin pigmentation, inequality of leg length, muscle weakness or neurological disorder. The heart and lungs should be examined because: (a) Some patients with congenital heart disease also have thoracic scoliosis. (b) An increasing thoracic curve causes progressive decrease in the vital capacity (occasionally cor pulmonale develops aged 30–40 years). The local signs are as follows.

LOOK — With thoracic scoliosis not only is the spine obviously deviated from the midline, but the rotation causes the rib angles to protrude; these may be sufficiently prominent to justify the term 'razor-back'. In front the chest looks flattened on one side, and with high curves the shoulders are not symmetrical. In the lumbar spine the most obvious feature is that one hip sticks out.

FEEL — The deviated spinous processes and prominent rib angles can be felt.

MOVE — When the patient bends forward the curve becomes more obvious; this is the diagnostic sign of fixed (as distinct from mobile) scoliosis, and is due to the vertebral rotation.

X-RAYS — X-ray films reveal any congenital anomalies and are also used to measure the angle of curvature (that is the angle between unwedged discs at each end of the primary curve).

TREATMENT

Prognosis is the key to treatment: the aim is to prevent severe deformity. With paralytic and idiopathic curves (the commonest varieties) the younger the child and the higher the curve the worse is the prognosis. Congenital curves are hard to predict and need careful watching in the early stages. Neurofibromatosis carries a bad prognosis and nearly always requires operation.

A period of preliminary observation may be needed before deciding between conservative and operative treatment. At 3-monthly intervals the patient is examined, photographed and x-rayed so that the curve can be measured.

CONSERVATIVE TREATMENT

Supports are useful: (*a*) with mild curves in children approaching spinal maturity, to halt progress until danger has passed; (*b*) with younger children needing operation to hold the curve stationary until aged 10, when fusion is more likely to succeed.

Three kinds are available. (1) A distraction plaster jacket is applied on a Risser frame with traction to the head and pelvis, and a localizer minimizing the rib hump. (2) A Milwaukee brace has adjustable steel supports transferring stress from the occiput to the iliac crests; extending the steels straightens the curve. (3) A Boston brace (for lumbar or thoraco-lumbar curves) is similar, but extends only from the pelvis to the thoracic cage.

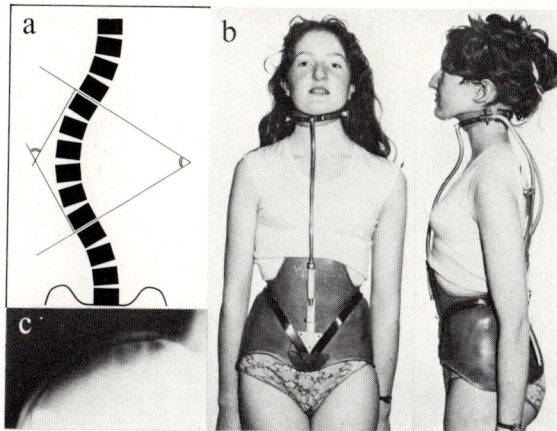

17.15 FIXED SCOLIOSIS (4) CONSERVATIVE TREATMENT
(a) Measuring the primary curve: the disc spaces are wider on the convex side — at each end of the primary curve lines are drawn to show the angle of curvature. (b) A Milwaukee brace. (c) Risser's sign.

OPERATIVE TREATMENT

Operation is indicated with severe curves (70 degrees was considered 'severe', but today's higher standards suggest 50 degrees); it should not be delayed in milder cases likely to progress. High curves, younger patients, paralytic curves and those associated with neuro-fibromatosis usually need operative treatment. With congenital scoliosis, a pre-operative myelogram is essential to exclude diastematomyelia.

CORRECTION AND FUSION

(1) With moderate curves no pre-operative correction is needed. The entire primary curve is cleared of soft tissue, the facet joints denuded of cartilage and the laminae and processes decorticated. A Harrington rod is applied to the top and bottom vertebrae, extended to separate them (thereby reducing the curve) and left in situ as internal fixation. Bone grafts

are applied over the entire area and the wound is closed. After a few days the patient is allowed up in a well-fitting plaster which is worn for at least 6 months.

(2) With more severe curves some pre-operative correction is desirable. As a preliminary Cotrel's method is useful; an ingenious system of strings and pulleys attached to a head halter enables the supine patient to push with her feet and hands in such a way as to elongate her trunk. Operative fusion (including a Harrington rod) is then performed. Subsequently a plaster jacket is applied, preferably with a posterior window over the concavity, and an inflatable bag over the convexity.

A more powerful method of pre-operative correction is halo-pelvic traction, but complications are not uncommon. A metal hoop (the halo) is screwed to the outer table of the skull and a second hoop anchored by transfixing screws to the pelvis; the two hoops are gradually racked apart via connecting steel rods. The child walks about in this apparatus, and it is retained for the first few post-operative weeks until replaced by plaster. Alternatively halo-femoral traction may be used: the patient is treated on a Stryker bed, with traction applied through the halo and counter-traction through femoral skeletal pins.

(3) Dwyer's technique is particularly useful for lumbar and thoraco-lumbar curves, especially paralytic. A series of wedges is excised, each including an intervertebral disc and the adjoining vertebral end-plates. Staples and screws are fixed to the vertebral bodies and through the screw heads a cable is inserted. Tightening the cable closes the vertebral wedges and straightens the curve.

OTHER METHODS

(1) Growth control by excising growth discs on the convex side has been used, but is unreliable.

(2) Electrical devices to stimulate the muscles on the convex side are being tried.

(3) Excision of the rib hump as a cosmetic procedure is occasionally worth considering; but a special silhouette x-ray must first be taken to ensure that the hump consists of ribs and not laminae.

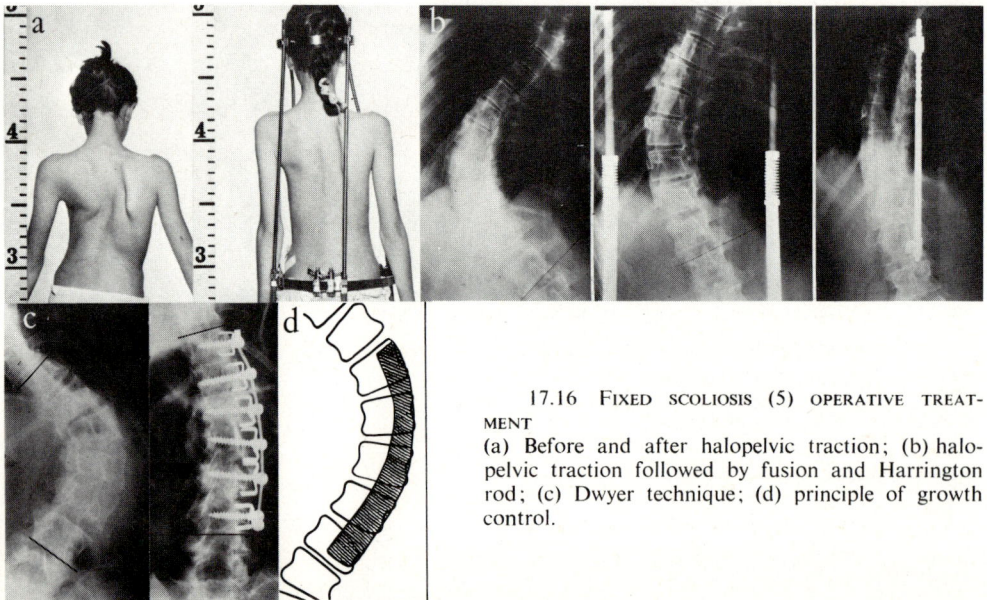

17.16 FIXED SCOLIOSIS (5) OPERATIVE TREATMENT
(a) Before and after halopelvic traction; (b) halo-pelvic traction followed by fusion and Harrington rod; (c) Dwyer technique; (d) principle of growth control.

KYPHOSIS

CLASSIFICATION

MOBILE KYPHOSIS — Mobile kyphosis may be (a) postural; (b) associated with muscle weakness; or (c) compensatory to lumbar lordosis. Mobile deformities are not in themselves important, though they may in later life cause backache. They are correctable either by the patient's own muscular efforts or by the surgeon.

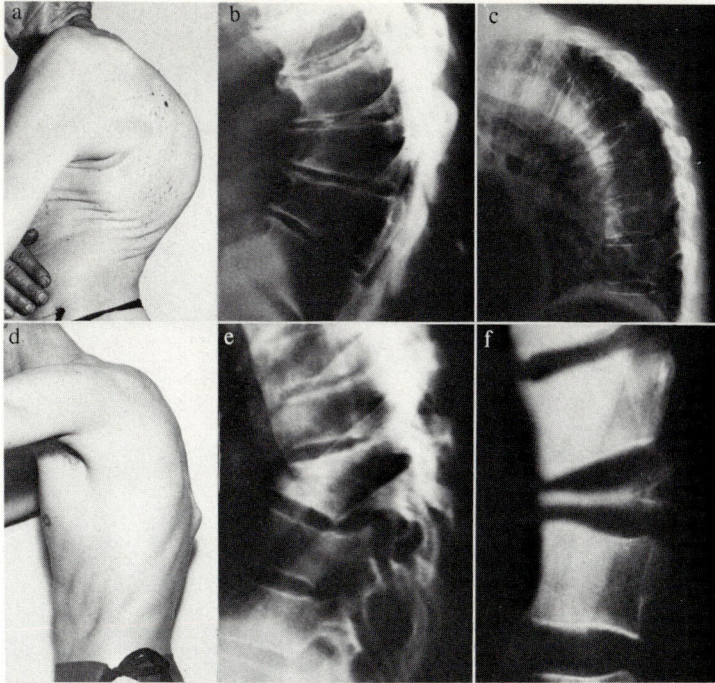

17.17 KYPHOSIS
AND KYPHOS
(a, b) Old Scheuermann's disease (c) senile kyphosis.

(d, e) Small kyphos due to tuberculosis.
(f) Calvé's disease.

Postural — Postural kyphosis is common, and associated with other postural defects, such as flat feet. It occurs most often in adolescents, in women after childbirth, and with obesity. The treatment is posture training, exercises and dieting.

Muscle weakness — Weakness of the trunk muscles, as in muscle dystrophies and poliomyelitis, is often associated with lumbar lordosis and thoracic kyphosis.

Compensatory — Gross hip deformity, such as congenital dislocation or fixed flexion, is accompanied by excessive lumbar lordosis which is balanced by thoracic kyphosis.

FIXED KYPHOSIS — The following varieties occur: (*a*) Scheuermann's disease (page 212); (*b*) ankylosing spondylitis (page 213); (*c*) senile kyphosis (page 215). Some bone dystrophies are associated with kyphosis, but this is not the presenting feature (*see* Chapter 6).

A fixed kyphosis cannot be corrected by the patient or the surgeon; it is balanced by a lumbar lordosis unless the lumbar spine also is stiff, as in ankylosing spondylitis or senile kyphosis.

ANGULAR KYPHOSIS (KYPHOS) — Forward angulation may be (*a*) congenital; (*b*) tuberculous; (*c*) following a fracture (which may be pathological); or (*d*) due to Calvé's disease. A kyphos is always fixed. The distinction between a sharp angular kyphos and a smooth kyphosis is of the utmost help in diagnosis.

In congenital kyphos vertebral bodies are partly missing or fused anteriorly. Progressive deformity is inevitable and operative correction (from the front or the back) is needed.

In Calvé's disease, a rare condition which is probably the sequel to an eosinophilic granuloma, one vertebral body becomes flattened but the disc spaces remain normal. A child develops back pain and an angular kyphos. Clinical recovery occurs after a few months rest.

AGE OF ONSET — In children, a congenital cause is likely; in adolescents, kyphosis is usually postural or due to Scheuermann's disease; in young adults, ankylosing spondylitis is an important cause; in the elderly, senile kyphosis, pathological fractures and Paget's disease must be considered; at all ages, tuberculosis must be excluded.

RIGID KYPHOSIS OF ADOLESCENCE (Scheuermann's Disease)

The cause of this condition is unknown. Scheuermann used the term osteochondritis because the epiphyseal plates are irregularly ossified. Schmorl drew attention to the function of the cartilage plates in transmitting pressure evenly and suggested that a defect in them threw undue strain on the anterior portion of the vertebral bodies. Lambrinudi suggested that when a patient flexes, the epiphyseal plates may be damaged if hip flexion is limited by tight hamstrings.

CLINICAL FEATURES

The parents notice that the child, an otherwise fit teenager, is becoming increasingly round shouldered. The patient may complain of backache, and has the following local signs.

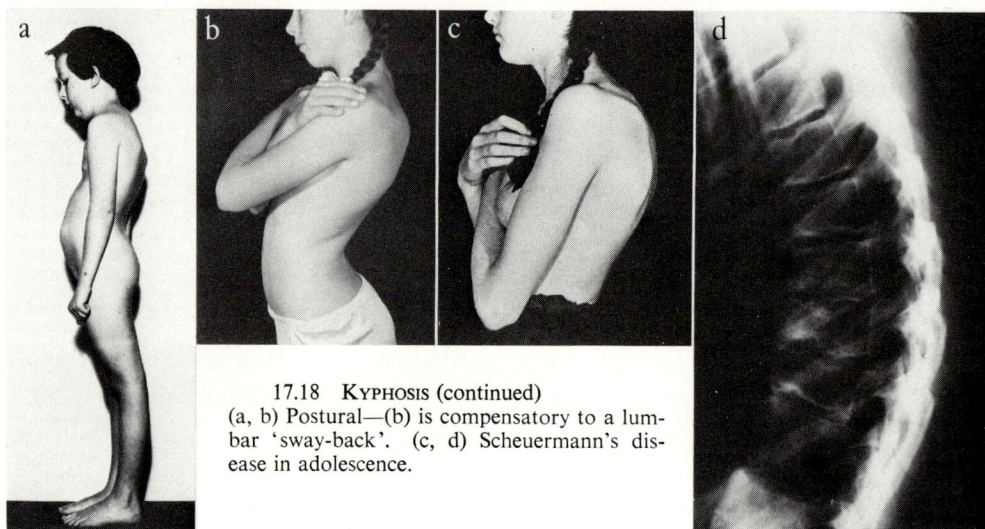

17.18 KYPHOSIS (continued)
(a, b) Postural—(b) is compensatory to a lumbar 'sway-back'. (c, d) Scheuermann's disease in adolescence.

LOOK — A smooth thoracic kyphosis is seen and may be severe. Below it is a compensatory lumbar lordosis.

FEEL — No abnormality can be felt.

MOVE — The deformity cannot be corrected by the patient or the surgeon. Lumbar spine movements are normal. Straight-leg raising is often limited to 60 degrees by tight hamstrings.

X-RAY — The bodies of several adjacent vertebrae, usually Th. 6–10, are wedged; that is, narrower in front. They may contain small translucent areas (Schmorl's nodes). The epiphyseal plates appear fragmented, especially anteriorly.

DIFFERENTIAL DIAGNOSIS

Postural kyphosis is common in adolescence. It is painless, and the deformity is correctable by the patient's own efforts if properly instructed. The curve is a long one and other postural defects are common. The x-ray appearance is normal.

Tuberculosis produces an angular kyphos. X-rays show destruction of at least two adjacent vertebrae with narrowing of the intervening disc and often a paravertebral abscess.

TREATMENT

AMBULANT TREATMENT—This is indicated if there is little pain and the deformity is not severe. The patient is taught to stand as well as possible. Any slight ache disappears within 12 months. A Milwaukee brace is useful for severe cases.

RECUMBENT TREATMENT — Recumbency on a flat bed or a posterior plaster shell is rarely indicated and only if pain is severe, deformity considerable and spinal growth not yet complete. When pain disappears the patient is allowed up wearing a brace by day and sleeping in the plaster shell at night.

ANKYLOSING SPONDYLITIS

Ankylosing spondylitis is much commoner in the relatives of patients than in the rest of the population; the genetic factor may be the histocompatibility antigen HLA-B27 which is present in over 90 per cent of patients though in less than 10 per cent of the population as a whole. It may be significant that some cases of Reiter's disease progress to a picture indistinguishable from ankylosing spondylitis; and atypical forms of the disease occur with psoriasis and ulcerative colitis.

PATHOLOGY

Little is known of the pathology. In synovial joints the early changes are similar to those of rheumatoid arthritis; but around the sacro-iliac joints, where the disease often seems to start, there is apparently a true osteitis. The most characteristic changes are in the spine: the intervertebral discs are at first replaced by vascular connective tissue, and then undergo ossification which particularly affects the periphery of the annulus fibrosus and the intervertebral ligaments.

SYMPTOMS

The commonest presenting symptoms are pain and stiffness in the lumbar spine and buttocks. Sometimes the pain has a sciatic radiation but, unlike the sciatica of disc prolapse, it may alternate from side to side. The onset is insidious and at first the symptoms are intermittent, usually worse on getting up. In at least 10 per cent of patients, however, the earliest feature is a polyarthritis which is asymmetrical and chiefly affects large joints in the lower limbs. Vague chest pains and painful heels are less common, but malaise, fatigue, and loss of weight are usual during phases of activity.

SIGNS

The disease usually begins between the ages of 15 and 35 and is much commoner in men than women. In at least half the patients the process stops before significant deformity has occurred and these patients are not much disabled. But the disease may pursue a long course over many years, with phases of activity during which additional areas become affected; and it may not burn itself out until the entire spine and several large joints have stiffened.

While the disease is active the patient looks unwell, the sedimentation rate is raised and there is often slight anaemia. Iritis occurs in 25 per cent of patients. The local signs are as follows:

LOOK — A severely affected patient stands in a characteristic way; the back forms one continuous curve from sacrum to head and the knees are bent to maintain balance. Even in milder cases the normal lumbar lordosis is usually absent.

FEEL — Sometimes there is tenderness over the manubrio-sternal joint, iliac crests and symphysis pubis.

MOVE — The lumbar spine is stiff but the unwary may be misled by mobile hips. Chest expansion is permanently and grossly reduced—a diagnostic feature. Sacro-iliac springing is painful in active phases. The limb joints, especially the hips and sometimes other large joints, may be stiff. Small joints are unaffected. Except during active phases of the disease, attempted movement is not painful.

X-RAY — The earliest changes are seen in the sacro-iliac joints: the joint line becomes blurred and irregular with surrounding sclerosis; the joint space gradually diminishes and in time is obliterated. Similar changes occur in the symphysis pubis and the manubrio-sternal joints. In the spine the vertebral bodies lose their normal slight anterior concavity and look unusually 'square'; their borders are well-defined or even sclerosed and the interior architecture lost; calcification of the intervertebral ligaments completes the classical picture of a 'bamboo' spine. Other joints may be obliterated.

TREATMENT

REST AND EXERCISE — Although ankylosing spondylitis is an inflammatory disorder there is no evidence that rest is beneficial. On the contrary exercises appear to help and, although strenuous activities should be avoided, swimming, walking and similar pursuits should be encouraged. A course of physiotherapy including back exercises, deep breathing and joint mobilization may be helpful. It is important to try to prevent kyphosis and the patient should sleep on a hard bed with only one pillow; a back brace may occasionally be advisable.

DRUGS — Salicylates may be adequate for the mild case. Phenylbutazone (not more than 400 mg daily) is remarkably effective; side effects, however, are not uncommon and probably indomethacin (25 mg t.d.s.) should be tried first. Steroids are not indicated, except perhaps with severe iritis.

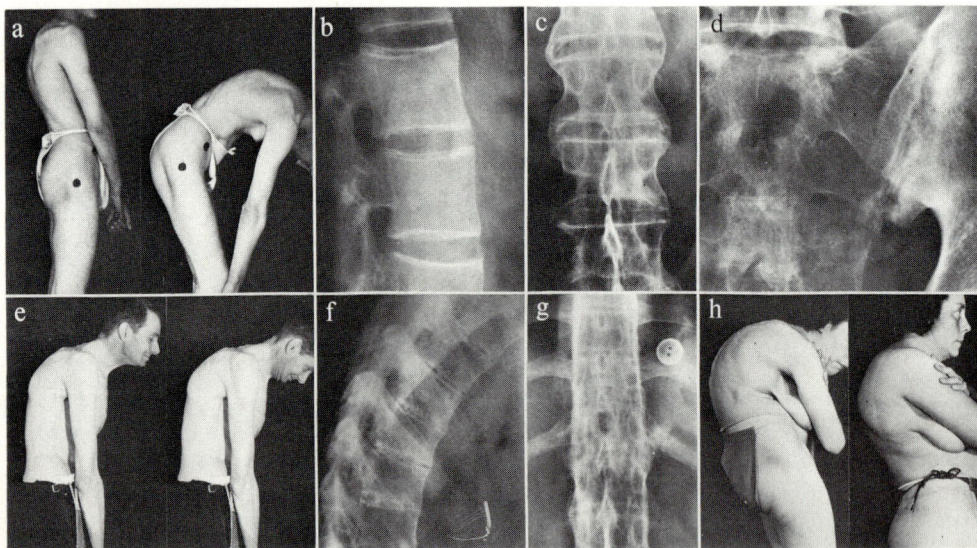

17.19 ANKYLOSING SPONDYLITIS
(a) Back stiffness without deformity in a mild case; (b, c) early calcification of spinal ligaments; (d) fuzziness of the sacro-iliac joint.
(e) Advanced case with kyphosis and gross stiffness (the patient is bending forward as far as he can).
(f, g) 'Bamboo' spine.
(h) Before and after osteotomy of the lumbar spine.

RADIOTHERAPY — Although an excellent palliative, radiotherapy does not restore mobility and the dangers are considerable. It leads to a higher incidence of leukaemia, and in young women it is impossible to irradiate the sacro-iliac joints without risking genetic effects or sterility. Consequently, except for peripheral joints, radiotherapy is not justified unless pain is considerable and is unrelieved by a long course of drugs.

OPERATIONS—If both hips are stiff total replacement is very rewarding. If kyphosis is so gross that the patient cannot see in front of him, osteotomy of the mid-lumbar spine is feasible; but hip replacement, by abolishing fixed flexion, often makes the more dangerous spine operations unnecessary.

KYPHOSIS IN THE ELDERLY

Kyphosis may begin in an elderly person in a variety of conditions.

TRUE SENILE KYPHOSIS — Degeneration of intervertebral discs probably produces the gradually increasing stoop characteristic of the ageing. The disc spaces become narrowed and the vertebrae slightly wedged. There is little pain unless osteoarthritis of the facet joints is also present.

SENILE OSTEOPOROSIS — The patients, usually women, are thin and kyphotic ('dowager's hump'). There is widespread osteoporosis and the discs indent the soft vertebral bodies, which become biconcave. There may be pain, and pathological fractures are common (see page 82).

PAGET'S DISEASE — Considerable kyphosis occurs because of bone softening. There is usually evidence of Paget's disease (such as thick bent bones) elsewhere. The affected vertebrae are enlarged, and show coarse trabeculation.

PATHOLOGICAL FRACTURE IN MALIGNANT DISEASE — Usually the affected vertebra is the site of a secondary deposit and collapses with slight trauma. There is a kyphos and x-rays show that only the vertebral body (or bodies) is affected.

TREATMENT

The deformity itself requires treatment only if it is painful. A walking stick relieves the patient from the strain of forcing himself to stand upright. Heat and analgesics are soothing. A corset is often prescribed but is either too short to be effective or too high to be tolerated.

Senile osteoporosis may benefit from dietary treatment (page 83), and pain due to a carcinomatous deposit is often relieved by radiotherapy.

DISORDERS OF INTERVERTEBRAL DISCS

The nucleus pulposus is normally under tension and surrounded by a fibrous annulus which, in turn, is held in place by ligaments. The disc space may be *too wide* because the bones are abnormally soft and the tense discs bulge into them, becoming biconvex. The main causes of soft bone are dysplasias, nutritional deficiencies, endocrine disorders and senile osteoporosis.

On the other hand, the space may be *too narrow* because disc material has degenerated or has been 'displaced'. Degeneration occurs in senile kyphosis. 'Displacement' may be (a) prolapse of disc substance into the vertebral canal, which is the commonest cause of narrowing and is nearly always immediately above or below the sixth cervical or fifth lumbar vertebra; (b) extrusion around the periphery which occurs in spondylosis; or (c) protrusion into the vertebral bodies which occurs in Scheuermann's disease, causing Schmorl's nodes.

LUMBAR DISC PROLAPSE
CAUSAL FACTORS

INJURY — A lifting strain with the back bent may tear the posterior longitudinal ligament so that the tense disc bulges backwards. The annulus also may be torn and through the tear nuclear material is squeezed out; the torn annulus sometimes hinges into the vertebral canal. If a tear does not heal further prolapse is likely with trivial strains, such as coughing while the back is bent.

INCREASED TENSION — The nucleus may absorb fluid, swell and either bulge the annulus or burst through it. Fluid absorption occurs in some physical illnesses, and animal experiments suggest that it also occurs with emotional stress.

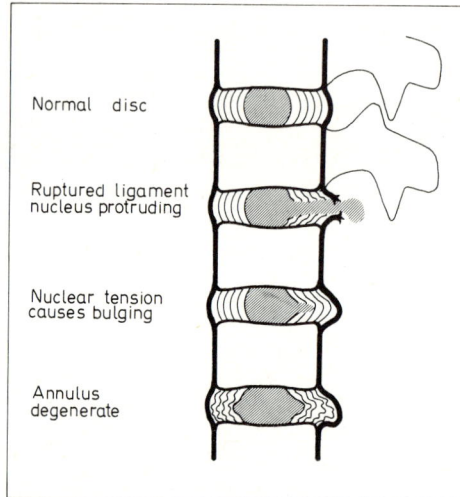

17.20 LUMBAR DISCS (1) PATHOLOGY OF PROLAPSE Pressures on discs are considerable (5–15 kg/cm²); they are least when lying, more standing, still more sitting, and most when lifting.

DEGENERATION — As it ages, the disc loses elasticity, partly because of physicochemical changes in the collagen fibres, and partly because its fluid content decreases (desiccation). The weakened disc is unable to resist body weight and is liable to bulge.

PATHOLOGY

Prolapsed disc material, whether a bulging annulus or a herniated nucleus, may press on dura mater (causing backache) or on nerve roots (causing backache or sciatica or both). The prolapse is nearly always immediately below or above the fifth lumbar vertebra. At first pressure may increase because of oedema. As this subsides the prolapsed material may shrink or slip back into place. If it remains prolapsed it may in time be absorbed or become adherent to root sheaths. Long-standing prolapse disturbs the mechanics of the facet joints.

17.21 LUMBAR DISCS (2) PATHOLOGY OF PAIN A prolapsed disc may press on the dura or on the nerve roots.

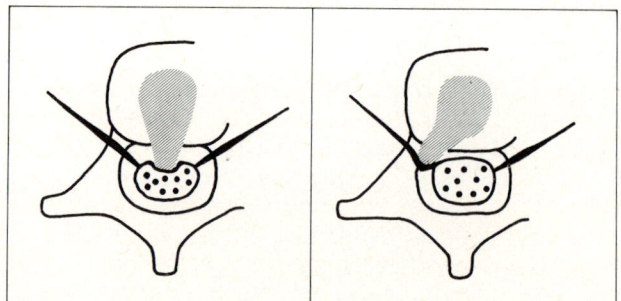

SYMPTOMS

FIRST ATTACK — The first attack is often sudden in onset and occurs while lifting or stooping, though sometimes pain is slight at first but increases over the next few hours. The patient may be fixed bent and has backache ('lumbago'); sometimes sciatica follows soon after, and both are made worse by straining. Usually these symptoms subside in a few days or weeks.

SUBSEQUENT ATTACKS — Subsequent attacks also may be sudden in onset, but often follow a trivial event such as coughing. The patient may complain of backache, of sciatica or of both; his pain is made worse by straining or stooping. Sciatic pain is usually felt in the buttock and radiates to the posterior thigh, outer calf and sometimes the toes. There may also be paraesthesia in this distribution and (rarely) weakness.

BETWEEN ATTACKS — Between attacks the patient may be completely normal, or may have a 'lame back' which he is afraid to subject to stress.

SIGNS

The patient is usually a healthy adult. General examination shows no abnormality; this point must be stressed because if he has lost weight or is in any way unfit a diagnosis of prolapsed disc is almost certainly wrong.

SIGNS IN THE BACK — Between attacks the back may be normal. The signs during an attack are as follows.

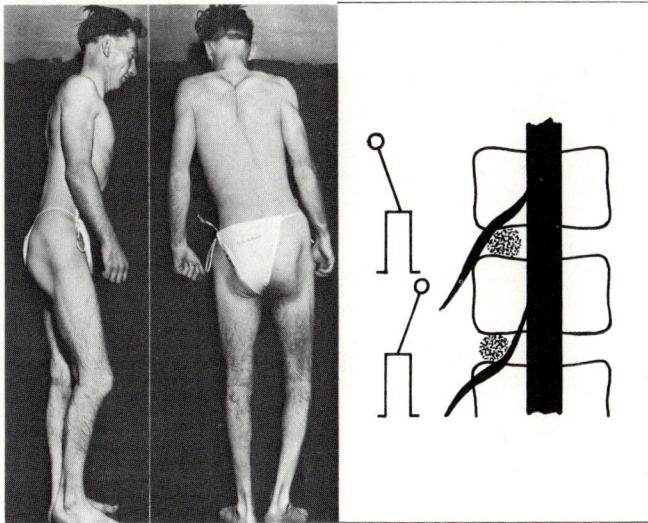

17.22 LUMBAR DISCS (3) CLINICAL FEATURES
The acute disc may present with a tilt forwards and sideways.
Paracaudal prolapse often causes tilt to the same side, pararadicular prolapse to the opposite side.

LOOK — There may be deformity in two planes: slight forward tilt obliterating the lumbar lordosis; and lateral tilt, sometimes called 'sciatic scoliosis'.
FEEL — There is often tenderness in the midline of the low back and in the buttock.
MOVE — With acute lumbago all movements are limited for a day or two, and the muscles are in spasm. Later, movement is limited only in some directions, usually forward flexion and lateral flexion to either side, or sometimes extension. Full movement in any one direction is important for it strongly suggests a purely mechanical derangement.

SIGNS IN THE LEG(S) — During an attack there may be evidence of root pressure in one or both legs.   (Rarely, a large central prolapse causes urinary disturbance.)

ROOT STRETCHING — With sciatic nerve-root irritation straight-leg raising is diminished and painful, and pain is increased by foot dorsiflexion; leg raising with the knee bent is painless and unrestricted.   Femoral nerve-root irritation causes pain on knee flexion with the patient prone (i.e. with the hip extended).

SENSATION — This may be impaired, especially along the outer thigh, calf and foot.

MOTOR — There may be weakness, especially of the long extensor or flexor muscles of the hallux, and sometimes of the gluteal muscles.

REFLEXES — The ankle jerk may be diminished.   (The knee jerk is affected only rarely and when the disc prolapse is higher than usual.)

X-RAY

X-rays of the lumbo-sacral spine are essential; their chief purpose is not to show a diminished space, but to exclude bone disease or deposit.   The antero-posterior view may show a tilt.   The lateral view often shows a diminished disc space, but a normal space does not exclude a small disc prolapse (even a small prolapse can produce severe symptoms).

Myelography can demonstrate the prolapse as a filling defect and is indicated when the diagnosis is uncertain.   Radiculography is valuable for low discs.

Localization of prolapse — The exact site of a prolapse is difficult to determine, but the following points may help.

Central prolapse (directly backwards) may produce backache and bilateral leg signs. Paracaudal prolapse (in the axilla of the root) causes pain which is made worse when the patient bends sideways away from the painful leg.   Para-radicular prolapse (lateral to the root) causes pain which increases when he bends sideways towards the affected leg.

Postero-lateral prolapse below the fifth lumbar vertebra presses only on the first sacral

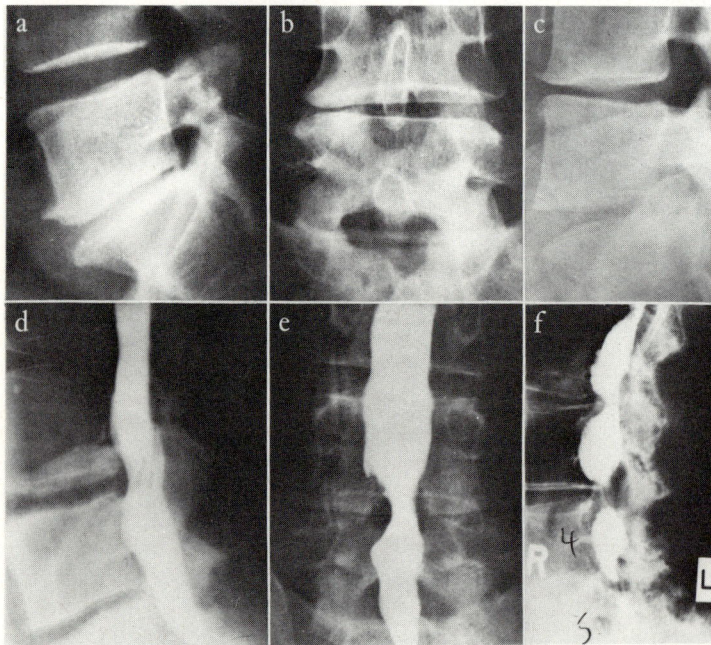

17.23   LUMBAR DISCS
(4) X-RAYS
(a) Diminished disc space at L.5/S.1; (b, c) at L.4/L.5, with tilt at this level in the AP view.

(d, e) The defect in this myelogram suggests disc protrusion.   (f) Spinal stenosis.

root.   It is likely to produce pain and paraesthesia along the outer thigh, leg and foot; weakness of the flexor hallucis longus muscle; and a diminished ankle jerk.

Postero-lateral prolapse of the disc above the fifth lumbar vertebra may press on the first sacral or fifth lumbar root or both.   It may produce pain and paraesthesia situated more antero-medially; weakness of the extensor hallucis longus muscle; a marked sideways tilt of the back; and cross-leg pain, that is, raising the good leg produces pain down the other.

X-ray — As a guide to the level of prolapse a diminished disc space on x-ray is unreliable. A previous prolapse may have narrowed the space and if the material has been absorbed it no longer causes symptoms.

DIFFERENTIAL DIAGNOSIS

The fit patient with backache and sciatica is nearly always suffering from a prolapsed disc; especially if episodes of pain are punctuated by intervals of normality. When the patient is unfit suspicion must be alerted to more serious disorders; especially if the backache is not associated with sciatica, or is constant rather than intermittent.

It follows that in all cases a careful history, a detailed general examination and x-rays are the minimum requirement.   Where the slightest diagnostic doubt exists further investigation is essential, including rectal or vaginal examination, a sedimentation rate and a full blood count.   The following are some of the disorders which must be excluded:

TUBERCULOSIS (page 200) — The patient is unfit, the sedimentation rate raised and x-rays shows a narrow disc space with adjacent bone destruction.

NON-TUBERCULOUS OSTEOMYELITIS — Brucellosis and low-grade pyogenic infections resemble tuberculosis, with chronic backache, vague ill-health, a raised sedimentation

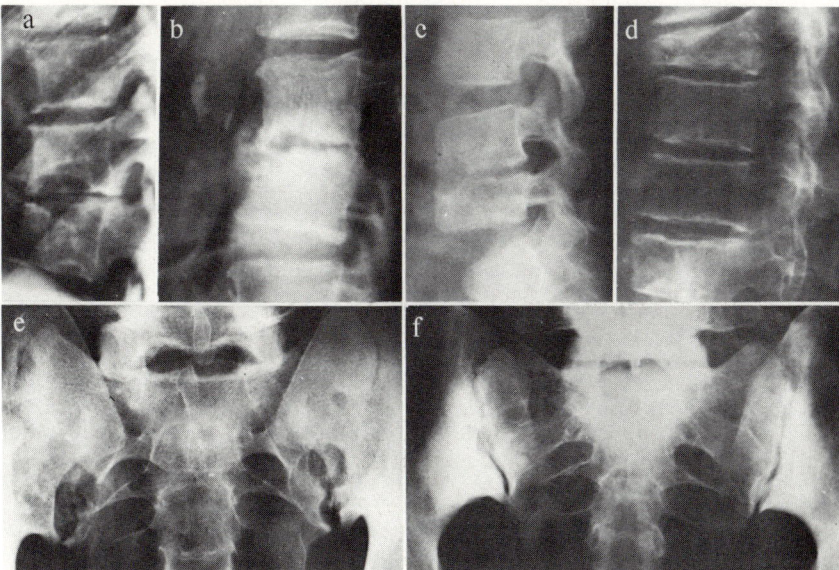

17.24   LUMBAR DISCS (5) DIAGNOSIS
(a) Tuberculosis; (b) acute osteomyelitis — note the sclerosis which developed within a few weeks; (c) discitis.   (d) Here, unlike the previous three, the disc spaces are normal — the bodies are not — these are secondary deposits.   (e) Bilateral sacro-iliac tuberculosis; (f) osteitis condensans ilii, which is probably symptomless.

rate and radiological bone destruction.   But often only one vertebra is involved and the disc spaces may remain normal.   Blood examination, aspiration, or biopsy may be needed to establish the diagnosis.

Acute pyogenic osteomyelitis is quite different.   The patient becomes rapidly ill with high fever, severe back pain and often severe root pain.   The x-rays at first show no abnormality; after 2–3 weeks bone destruction is seen.   If antibiotic treatment is prompt and effective the patient recovers and the x-rays show sclerosis.

DISCITIS — In children, this presents with backache or leg pain (Menelaus, 1964). The child is unwell and has limited back movement. X-rays at first show narrowing of the disc space, then scalloping of bone on each side, and finally obliteration of the space with bony fusion.   Bed rest and antibiotics are effective.   In adults (Kemp, 1973), paraplegia may occur, necessitating operative decompression.

ANKYLOSING SPONDYLITIS (page 213) — A young, slightly unfit adult, presents with backache and stiffness.   X-rays show no bone destruction or disc narrowing, but woolly sacro-iliac joints and, later, calcified spinal ligaments.

SACRO-ILIAC DISEASE — The slight displacement beloved of osteopaths is probably mythical, and the radiological density of multipara (osteitis condensans ilii) does not cause symptoms.   Apart from ankylosing spondylitis and related disorders, the only important sacro-iliac disease is tuberculosis.   The patient presents with back pain, a buttock abscess or associated urogenital tuberculosis.   X-rays show widening of the joint or a large cavity.   Treatment is by rest and chemotherapy; later it is worth excising necrotic material and inserting bone grafts.

TUMOURS — Vertebrae are a favourite site for secondary deposits; hence the importance of a detailed general examination.   If bone destruction shows on x-ray then it involves a vertebral body—not the disc, nor two adjacent bodies.   Primary bone tumours as well as tumours of the cord or roots must also be considered.   If the x-ray is inconclusive a bone scan may be justified.

TREATMENT

Heat and analgesics soothe, and exercises strengthen the muscles; but there are only three ways of treating the prolapse itself.

REST

Bed — With a severe attack the patient should go to bed with boards placed under the mattress to stop it sagging.   He should, with a severe first attack, remain in bed for 3 weeks.

Corset — If the attack is less severe, or the patient cannot go to bed, a corset is worn. It may be made of plaster, polythene or canvas reinforced with steels.

Modified activity — If the attack is trivial he is advised to avoid stooping or lifting.

'REDUCTION'

Traction — Skin traction applied to one leg or to the pelvis is useful; even if traction does not open up the disc space, it certainly enforces rest.   If the patient cannot stay in hospital, a traction table is a fairly effective alternative; the pelvis and chest are racked apart for 20 minutes daily.

Manipulation — Manipulation is sometimes successful, especially with an attack of recent onset, but it should be avoided if there is sciatica.

Other methods — It is claimed that procaine (0·5 per cent solution) injected epidurally into the sacral canal may help to 'reduce' a prolapse; at least 50 ml, and often much more, is injected.   Another method being tried experimentally is to inject 2 mg of chymopapain into the disc space; the enzyme is said to dissolve the nucleus pulposus but to have no effect on the annulus, ligaments or nerve tissue.   Oral chymotrypsin also is being tried.

17.25   LUMBAR DISCS
        (6) TREATMENT
(a) Exercises; (b) corset;

(c) manipulation; (d) epidural
injection.

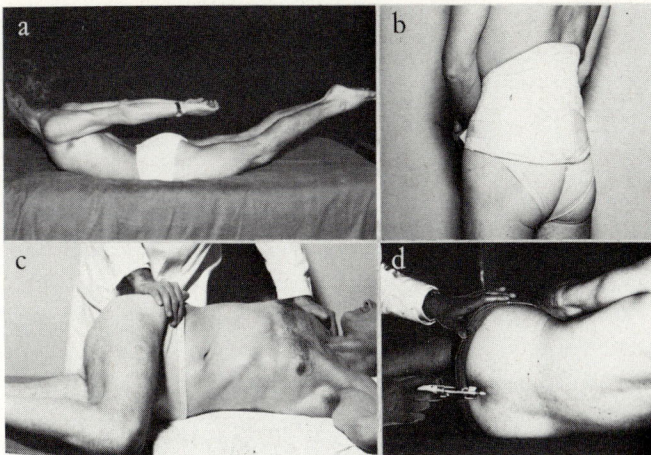

REMOVAL

Operative removal effects lasting cure in only 80 per cent of cases; therefore it is indicated only if attacks are severe, disabling, recurrent, and persisting in spite of conservative treatment.   In rare cases, bladder disturbance demands emergency operation.

Methods — The following methods may be used.

Laminectomy — Through a midline incision the laminae are exposed, the muscles being stripped off them with wide chisels and held by self-retaining retractors.   Half of the fifth lamina on the side with most recent pain is nibbled off and the ligamentum flavum dissected away.   The dura and root are gently retracted and the lumbo-sacral disc inspected.   If prolapsed, bulging or unduly soft, the entire disc is plucked out piecemeal with pituitary forceps.   If no prolapse is seen, the nerve root is explored.

The disc above must be inspected even when a lesion has already been found, for both may be prolapsed.   Unless a lesion consistent with the clinical findings has been demonstrated, cure is unlikely.

Fenestration — An interlaminar approach may be adequate, but if a tumour is suspected, laminectomy is advisable.

Disc removal and spine fusion — With evidence of instability (*see* below) disc removal followed by spine fusion has theoretical advantages; the combined procedure is simpler through an anterior approach.

Rehabilitation — After recovery from a prolapsed disc or its removal, the patient is shown how to lift by bending at the hips rather than the spine, taught exercises to restore suppleness and power, and advised to sleep on a firm mattress.

NOTE ON THORACIC DISC PROLAPSE.   Because this is rare it is diagnosed late.   Patients usually present, not with backache, but with symptoms in one or both limbs (weakness, heaviness, pain, numbness or coldness), or with girdle pain.   Neurological features are usual and, strikingly, when back pain develops, signs of cord compression rapidly follow. X-rays may show disc calcification, but myelography is essential.   Lateral rhachotomy is probably the safest method of decompression.

LUMBAR SPONDYLOSIS

Discs degenerate with age and lose their normal elasticity (*see* page 216).   With the pressure of body weight disc material extrudes round the periphery; posteriorly it may adhere to nerve root sheaths, elsewhere it may calcify, producing lipping. Degenerative changes may also develop in the facet joints, producing a true osteoarthritis.

SYMPTOMS

Backache is usually gradual in onset and eased by rest. Pain may also be felt in the groin or buttocks. Sometimes acute attacks of backache or sciatica supervene if more disc material prolapses.

SIGNS

The patient is over the age of 40 and fit in himself.

LOOK — The appearance is usually normal.

FEEL — Often tender areas are felt in the back or buttocks.

MOVE — All lumbar movements are limited and may be painful at their extremes. There may also be leg signs of nerve root pressure.

X-RAY — Several disc spaces are diminished, with lipping at the corners of the vertebral bodies. So-called traction osteophytes, which project horizontally forwards 2 mm above and below a disc, are thought to indicate segmental instability. The facet joints may be narrowed and irregular. (Identical changes may occur without any symptoms.)

TREATMENT

Heat and massage are soothing and manipulation occasionally helps, but a stiff lumbar corset, limiting extremes of movement, is the most effective treatment. Spinal fusion is rarely·indicated.

SPINAL STENOSIS

The spinal canal may be congenitally small and symptoms develop where it is further narrowed in later life by disc protrusion, spondylolisthesis, osteophytes, inflammatory products or a tumour. The patient, almost always male, aged over 40, complains of difficulty in walking, with weakness, heaviness and paraesthesia of the legs. Bending forward helps and, with severe stenosis, he may have to sit after walking 100 yards (intermittent claudication of the cauda equina). Another possible presentation is with atypical sciatica, involving one leg, made worse by activity with no pain on coughing or straining. A myelogram may appear normal when the back is flexed, but extension will produce either a break up in the column of dye or a complete block at L.4/5, this being the level most severely affected. Decompression relieves the symptoms.

SPONDYLOLISTHESIS

Spondylolisthesis means forward shift of the spine. The shift is nearly always between L.4 and L.5, or between L.5 and the sacrum. Normal laminae and facets constitute a locking mechanism which prevents each vertebra from moving forwards on the one below. Forward shift (or slip) occurs only when this mechanism has failed. Three varieties are described:

Dysplastic (20 per cent) — The superior sacral facets are congenitally defective; slow but inexorable forward slip leads to severe displacement.

Degenerative (25 per cent) — Degenerative changes in the facet joints and the discs permit forward slip (nearly always at L.4–5) despite intact laminae.

Isthmic (50 per cent) — Usually the lamina is in two pieces (spondylolytic) with a gap in the pars inter-articularis; occasionally, however, the lamina is intact, but is attenuated and elongated. It is difficult to exclude a genetic factor because spondylolisthesis often runs in families, and is commoner in certain races, notably Eskimos; but the incidence increases with age, so an acquired factor probably co-exists. This acquired factor is almost certainly stress; the repeated falls of the toddler, or the continual stress imposed in later life by the upright posture might well be the damaging forces.

The remaining 5 per cent of cases comprise traumatic spondylolisthesis following a single major injury, and pathological spondylolisthesis due to bone disease or neoplasm.

PATHOLOGY

When the pars interarticularis is in two pieces, the gap is occupied by fibrous tissue; behind the gap the spinous process, laminae and inferior articular facets remain as an isolated segment. With stress the vertebral body and superior facets in front of the gap may subluxate or dislocate forwards, carrying the superimposed vertebral column; the isolated segment maintains its normal relationship to the sacral facets. When there is no gap the pars interarticularis is elongated or the facets are defective.

With forward slipping there may be pressure on the dura mater and cauda equina, or on the emerging nerve roots; these roots may also be compressed in the narrowed intervertebral foramina. Disc prolapse is liable to occur.

SYMPTOMS

In children the condition is painless but the mother may notice the unduly protruding abdomen. In adolescents and adults backache is the usual presenting symptom; it is often intermittent, coming on after exercise or strain. Sciatic pain may occur in one or both legs.

Spondylolysis, and even a well-marked spondylolisthesis, may be discovered incidentally during routine x-ray examination.

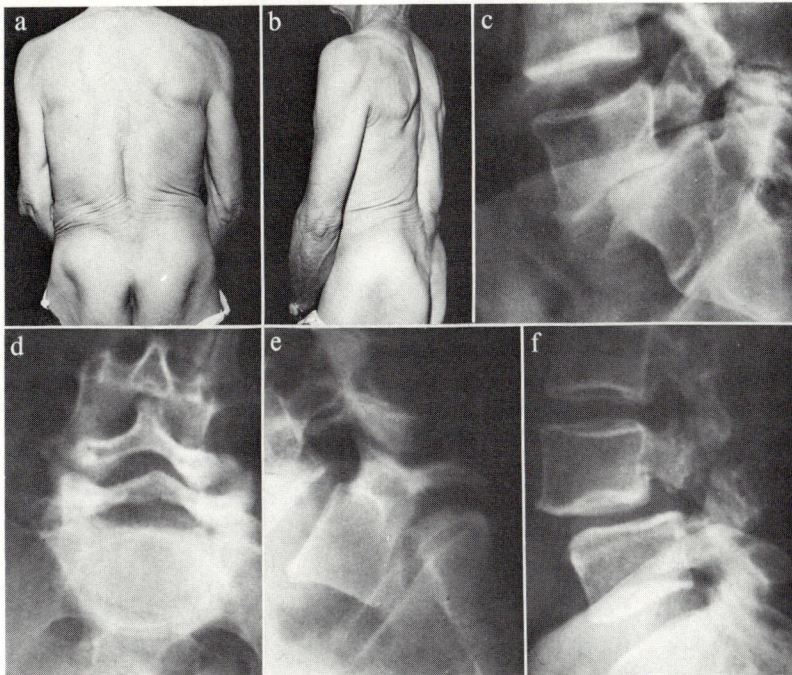

17.26 SPONDYLOLISTHESIS (1)
(a, b) The transverse loin creases, short lumbar spine and long sacrum are characteristic. (c) Forward slip of L.5 on S.1; the AP view (d) shows the 'bow'; (e) gross forward slip of L.5 on S.1; (f) forward slip of L.4 on L.5.

SIGNS

Dysplastic and degenerative spondylolisthesis are commoner in females, the isthmic variety in males. Degenerative spondylolisthesis rarely presents below the age of 40 years; the other varieties at any time from childhood onwards.

There may be signs of root pressure in one or both legs (page 218). The back signs are as follows:

LOOK — The buttocks look curiously flat, the sacrum appears to extend to the waist, and transverse loin creases are seen. The lumbar spine is on a plane in front of the sacrum and is too short. Occasionally there is a lumbar scoliosis.

FEEL — A 'step' is felt when the fingers are run down the spinous processes.

MOVE — Often movements are normal unless there has been a recent 'attack'; but occasionally the lumbar spine is almost rigid.

X-RAY — The antero-posterior view shows that the upper border of the fifth lumbar vertebra is too low, on a level with the transverse processes. Lateral views demonstrate any forward shift, a gap in the lamina, elongation of the lamina, or defective facets. Oblique views may show the laminae and the gap more clearly.

TREATMENT

Conservative treatment is indicated (*a*) if the patient is no longer young and symptoms are not disabling; or (*b*) there is doubt whether the symptoms arise directly from the slip or are due to an associated disc prolapse. It consists of bed rest during an acute attack and a supporting corset between attacks.

Operative treatment is indicated if (*a*) at any age the symptoms are disabling; (*b*) in the young adult with even moderate symptoms. Three methods are available.

DIRECT REPAIR — Buck (1970), who regards the bony gap as a fatigue fracture, advises direct repair. Through a posterior approach the gap is thoroughly rawed, then fixed by chip grafts and a screw; both sides are fixed. The method applies only where there is a gap and slipping is not severe; its advantage is that no movement whatsoever is sacrificed.

POSTERIOR FUSION — To prevent further slipping of the fifth lumbar body on the sacrum, the spinous process of L.5 must be fixed (by bone grafts), not to the sacrum, but to the spinous process of L.4; but if intertransverse grafting is done the slipped vertebra is fixed to the one below. This apparently baffling paradox is solved by studying the skeletal structures.

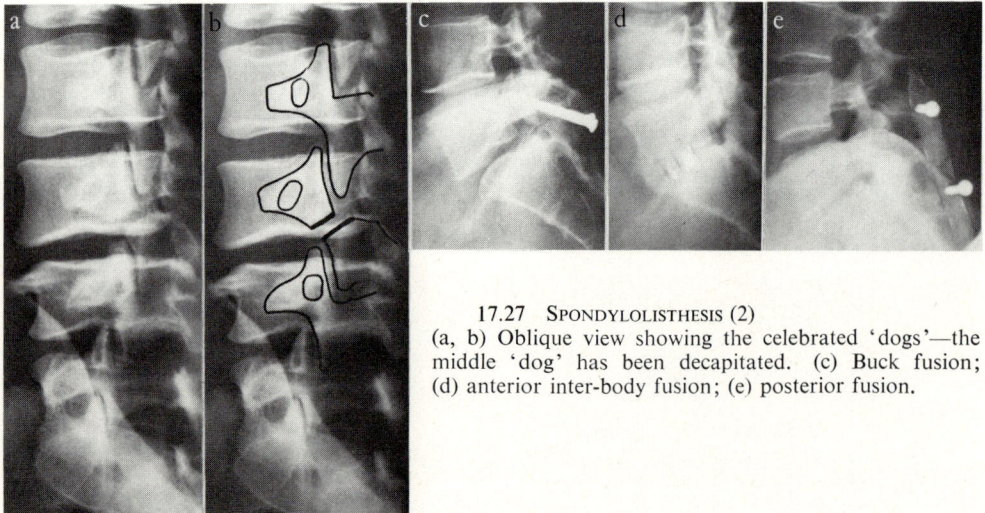

17.27 SPONDYLOLISTHESIS (2)
(a, b) Oblique view showing the celebrated 'dogs'—the middle 'dog' has been decapitated. (c) Buck fusion; (d) anterior inter-body fusion; (e) posterior fusion.

ANTERIOR FUSION — The disc between the forwardly slipped vertebra and the one below is removed and one or more bone grafts used to fix the bodies together. Freebody (1971), who reports excellent results, advises a transperitoneal approach with careful dissection of the pre-sacral nerve.

NOTE ON POST-TRAUMATIC SPONDYLOLISTHESIS

The patient found to have spondylolysis or spondylolisthesis after recent back injury (usually hyperextension), may have fractured a lamina, or merely have strained the fibrous tissue of a pre-existing lesion. If doubt exists (and it usually does) a plaster jacket is worn for three months; the recent fracture may join spontaneously. If union does not occur the assumption is that spondylolisthesis was present before injury and treatment is along the lines already indicated.

CAUSES OF BACKACHE

There are many causes of backache and it is useful to group them.

INJURY

(a) *Twisting force*, causing muscle injury (sometimes with a fractured transverse process).

(b) *Lifting strain*, causing ligament injury: (i) posterior longitudinal ligament injury, permitting a prolapsed disc; (ii) interspinous ligament injury, causing a 'sprung back'.

(c) *Crushing force*, causing bony injury (compression fracture).

In all these the onset is sudden, after strain or violence; the patient is otherwise fit, and the x-ray appearance is normal or shows a fracture.

'DEGENERATION'

The back is mechanically unsound and joint degeneration has developed because of some underlying structural fault as follows.

(a) *Congenital*; for example, scoliosis, spina bifida.

(b) *Acquired*; for example, scoliosis, spondylolisthesis, kyphosis (thoracic kyphosis often gives lumbar pain because this area is constantly under strain to keep the patient upright).

(c) Due to *lumbar spondylosis*.

In all these conditions the onset is gradual, though often there is a history of previous back trouble; the pain is worse after strain and better after rest; the patient has no general illness; and x-rays show lipping of the vertebral bodies and may reveal the deformity.

SPINAL DISEASE

(a) *Inflammation* — the most important chronic inflammatory conditions are tuberculosis and ankylosing spondylitis. Pyogenic osteomyelitis is rare but may present acutely.

(b) *Tumours* — The most common tumour is a secondary vertebral deposit. Other tumours may involve the cord, meninges or nerve roots. Vertebral haemangioma is often symptomless.

(c) *Paget's disease*.

In all these conditions the onset is not sudden or with violence; the patient may have other evidence of disease, and x-rays often reveal the cause.

DISEASE ELSEWHERE

Backache is common in non-spinal conditions as follows.

(a) *Any acute febrile illness*; for example, influenza.

(b) *Disorders of abdominal viscera*; for example, the stomach, duodenum, pancreas and urogenital tract.

(c) *Disorders, including carcinoma and pre-sacral malignant deposits, of the pelvic viscera*; for example, the uterus, ovaries, bladder and rectum. (Hence the importance of rectal and vaginal examination.)

In all these conditions the onset is not sudden or with violence; there is other evidence of disease; and x-rays of the spine itself are normal.

'IDIOPATHIC'

There are so many patients in whom the cause of backache is never found that various unconvincing explanations have been put forward.   The following are examples.
(*a*) *Fibrositis and myofasciitis.*
(*b*) *Sacro-iliac strain.*
(*c*) *Osteitis condensans ilii.*
These are grist to the mill of the osteopath.

CAUSES OF SCIATICA

INFLAMMATION

Rarely, in sciatica, there is a true neuritis (often a polyneuritis) which may be (*a*) *toxic*; for example alcoholic or diabetic neuritis; or (*b*) '*infective*'; as in 'focal sepsis', rheumatism, syphilis, and other conditions.

In all these conditions the onset is not sudden, the patient is unfit, and the nerve itself is tender.

COMPRESSION OF NERVE ROOTS

(*a*) *In the vertebral canal* compression is usually due to a prolapsed disc, occasionally to tuberculous material or to a tumour of the cauda equina or meninges.

(*b*) *In the intervertebral foramen* compression may arise from a tumour of the root, a lymphadenomatous deposit or because of narrowing of the foramen in spondylolisthesis.

(*c*) *In the pelvis or buttock* compression may arise from an abscess, if very large, or a tumour if impacted or adherent to the root.

In all these stretching the nerve is painful.   A prolapsed disc is much the most common cause, and also the most innocuous.

'REFERRED'

Pain may be referred from an area of '*fibrositis*' in the back or buttock.   Fibrositic pain is recurrent and often barometric.

In this condition there are tender areas on which pressure may also provoke sciatic pain; local anaesthesia abolishes both the local and the referred pain.   The patient is otherwise fit, though other fibrositic or rheumatic affections may coexist.   The x-ray appearance of the spine is normal.

Suggestions for further reading

Benson, M. K. D. and Byrnes, D. P. (1975). ' The Clinical Syndromes and Surgical Treatment of Thoracic Intervertebral Disc Prolapse.' *J. Bone Jt Surg.* **57B,** 471

Bradford, D. S. *et al.* (1975). ' Scheuermann's Kyphosis.' *J. Bone Jt Surg.* **57A,** 439

Buck, J. E. (1970). ' Direct Repair of the Defect in Spondylolisthesis.' *J. Bone Jt Surg.* **52B,** 432

Fitzgerald, J. A. W. and Newman, P. H. (1976). ' Degenerative Spondylo-listhesis.' *J. Bone Jt Surg.* **58B,** 184

Freebody, D., Bendall, R. and Taylor, R. D. (1971).   'Anterior Transperitoneal Lumbar Fusion.' *J. Bone Jt Surg.* **53B,** 617

Hodgson, A. R. and Yau, A. (1969). 'Surgical Approaches to the Spinal Column.' In *Recent Advances in Orthopaedics,* Ed. by A. Graham Apley. London; Churchill

Hoppenfeld, S. (1967). *Scoliosis.* London; Pitman

James, J. I. P. (1976). *Scoliosis* 2nd ed. Edinburgh: Livingstone

Journal of Bone and Joint Surgery (1968) **50A**, 382–428—Symposium: Complications of Lumbar Disc Surgery, Prevention and Treatment by Various Authors. Instructional Course Lectures

— (1968) **50A**, 167–210—Symposium: Low Back and Sciatic Pain by Various Authors. Instructional Course Lectures

Kemp, H. B. S. *et al.* (1973). 'Pyogenic Infections Occurring Primarily in Intervertebral Discs.' *J. Bone Jt Surg.* **55B**, 698

McCulloch, J. A. (1977). 'Chemonucleolysis.' *J. Bone Jt Surg.* **59B**, 45

Mehta, M. H. (1972). 'The Rib-Vertebra Angle in the Early Diagnosis Between Resolving and Progressive Infantile Scoliosis.' *J. Bone Jt Surg.* **54B**, 230

Menelaus, M. B. (1964). 'Discitis.' *J. Bone Jt Surg.* **46B**, 16

Nelson, M. A. (1973). 'Lumbar Spinal Stenosis.' *J. Bone Jt Surg.* **55B**, 506

Newman, P. H. (1973). 'Surgical Treatment for Derangement of the Lumbar Spine.' *J. Bone Jt Surg.* **55B**, 7

Newman, P. H., and Stone, K. H. (1963). 'The Etiology of Spondylolisthesis.' *J. Bone Jt Surg.* **45B**, 1, 39

Seddon, H. J. (1976). 'The Choice of Treatment in Pott's Disease.' *J. Bone Jt Surg.* **58B**, 393

Winter, R. B., Moe, J. H. and Wang, J. F. (1973). 'Congenital Kyphosis.' *J. Bone Jt Surg.* **55A**, 223

Wynne-Davies, R. (1975). 'Infantile Idiopathic Scoliosis.' *J. Bone Jt Surg.* **57B**, 138

CHAPTER 18

THE HIP JOINT

EXAMINATION OF THE HIP

SYMPTOMS

The four common symptoms of hip disorder are pain, which is in front rather than in the buttock and radiates to the knee; limp, which is often Trendelenburg in type; deformity, especially shortening; and stiffness.

The age of onset of symptoms often suggests the diagnosis: 0–5 years—congenital dislocation; 5–10 years—Perthes' disease; 10–15 years—slipped epiphysis; 20–40 years—osteoarthritis due to previous disorder; over 40 years—osteoarthritis (idiopathic), or ununited fracture of the femoral neck. Tuberculosis of the hip may occur at any age.

SIGNS WITH THE PATIENT LYING ON HIS BACK

LOOK

Skin — Scars or sinuses may be seen.

Shape — Asymmetry, swelling or wasting is observed

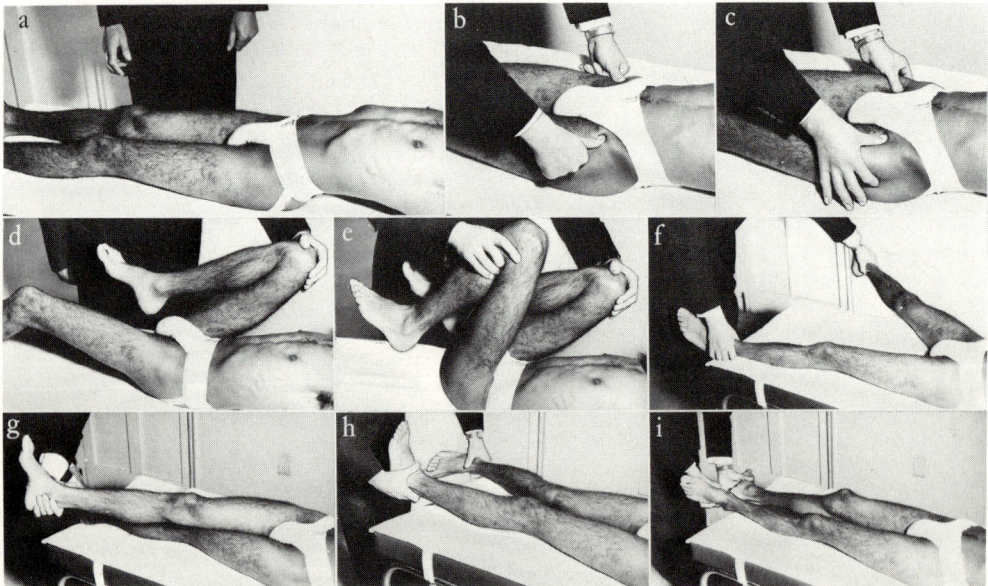

18.1 EXAMINATION OF THE HIP (1) WITH THE PATIENT SUPINE
(a) Looking at the patient: his legs and pelvis are square with the couch: the lordosis indicates fixed flexion of the hip. (b) Feeling the anterior superior iliac spine. (c) Locating the top of the great trochanter. (d) Flexing the right hip causes the left to lift off the couch (fixed flexion). The left hip also has limitation of (e) flexion, (f) abduction, (g) adduction, (h) internal rotation, and (i) external rotation.

Position — There may be deformity or shortening (see later).

FEEL

Skin — The joint is too deep for excessive warmth to be detected.

Soft tissues — Synovial thickening and fluid are not detectable in the hip. Muscle bulk and tautness should be tested; but this is best done with the patient prone.

Bones — The method used for comparing the height of the trochanters is used in palpation. With the thumbs anchored against the anterior superior iliac spines, the middle fingers palpate each greater trochanter. With the fingers pressing against the trochanters, the thumbs are moved medially in an attempt to feel the head of the femur; if the head is not in its socket, the thumb sinks in too far. Occasionally tenderness is elicited.

MOVE

To test extension the sound hip is flexed until any lumbar lordosis is obliterated; if by this manœuvre the affected thigh is raised from the couch, then extension is shown to be limited (such limitation is by custom referred to as 'fixed flexion').

Flexion of the hips is compared by flexing both simultaneously to their limit.

To test abduction both anterior superior iliac spines must first be level. The sound hip is then abducted until the pelvis starts to move; it is left in the abducted position while the affected hip in turn is abducted until the pelvis starts to move. In this way the difference in abduction of the two hips is easily seen.

Adduction is compared by moving each hip in turn and watching the pelvis for movement.

To test rotation both legs are lifted by grasping them at the ankles; they are then rotated first internally then externally. The patellae are observed as an index of the degree of rotation. Alternatively, rotation can be tested with the hip and knee flexed 90 degrees.

Shortening — Shortening of the lower limb is analysed as follows.

Is it real or apparent? — Real shortening means that the leg really is short; apparent shortening that the leg appears short. A patient with fixed adduction deformity of the hip has to hitch up the pelvis on that side to avoid having his legs crossed; this makes the leg appear short.

Shortening is measured with the patient flat on the couch, his legs together and, if possible, with the legs at right-angles to a line joining both anterior superior iliac spines. If this position is possible, there is no fixed adduction or abduction deformity. Any shortening is real. Its amount can be judged by noting the discrepancy between the two heels. Real shortening is measured from the anterior superior iliac spine (the tape must be anchored firmly against its inferior aspect) to the bottom of the medial malleolus.

If the legs cannot be placed at right-angles to the pelvis there is fixed deformity. With the common adduction deformity, apparent shortening is present; again, its amount can be gauged by the discrepancy between the heels. Apparent shortening is measured from any point in the midline of the trunk (such as the xiphisternum) to the medial malleolus. To measure real shortening in the presence of fixed deformity, however, it is necessary first to place the unaffected leg in a position of deformity comparable to that of the affected leg.

Is it above or below the knee? — Both knees are flexed while the heels remain together on the couch. It is then obvious whether shortening is in the femur or tibia.

Is it above or below the greater trochanter? — With a thumb pressed firmly against each anterior superior iliac spine, the surgeon gropes with his middle fingers for the top of each greater trochanter. With the hands in this position, it is easy to estimate elevation of one trochanter. More formal methods of estimation are: (a) to draw Nélaton's line, which runs from the anterior superior iliac spine by the shortest route to the ischial tuberosity; with the hip flexed and adducted the line normally crosses the top of the greater trochanter; or (b) to construct Bryant's triangle, in which a vertical line is drawn from the anterior superior iliac spine to the couch, and a perpendicular drawn from this line to the top of the trochanter; by comparing the length of the perpendicular at each hip, trochanteric elevation can be measured.

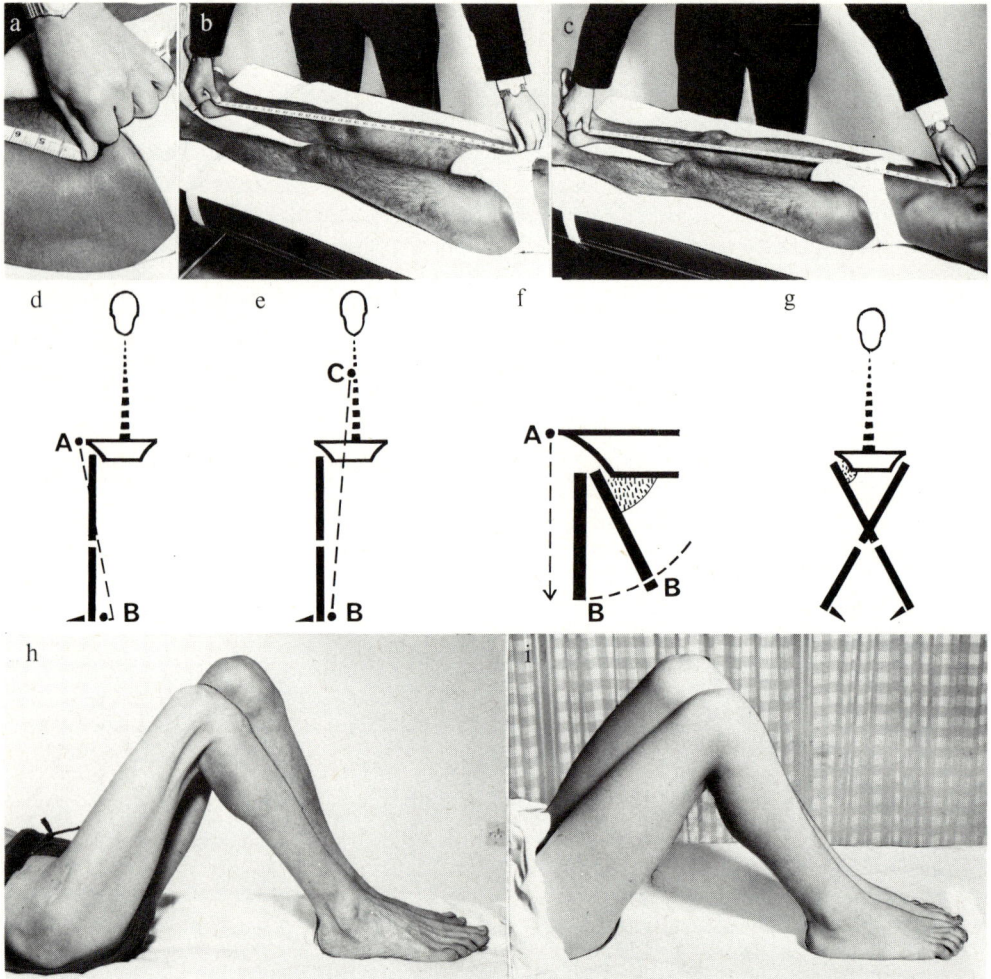

18.2 EXAMINATION OF THE HIP (2) LEG LENGTH
(a) The thumb holds the tape measure pressed up against the anterior superior iliac spine. The photograph (b) and the diagram (d) show measurement of real length (A–B); the photograph (c) and diagram (e) measurement of apparent length (C–B). Diagram (f) shows that when the hip is fixed in adduction measurement of length gives a false reading; to compensate for this the good leg must be placed in the comparable position (g) for measurement.
(h, i) Providing the heels are exactly level, bending the knees immediately shows whether shortening is above or below the knee.

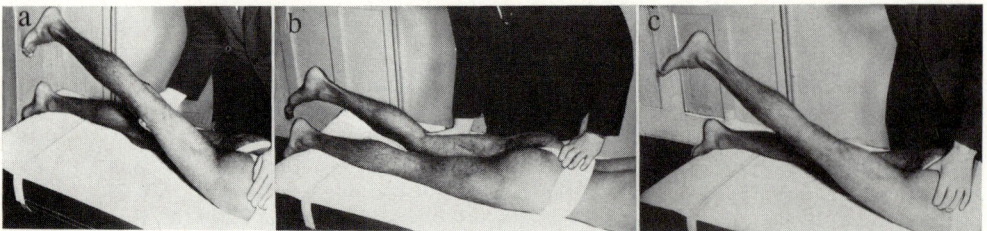

18.3 EXAMINATION OF THE HIP (3) WITH THE PATIENT PRONE
(a) Extension of the good hip is full; in the affected leg (b) it is limited. (c) Testing power in the glutei.

SIGNS WITH THE PATIENT LYING ON HIS FACE

LOOK — Scars, sinuses or wasting are noted.

FEEL — Muscle bulk and tautness are most easily assessed when the patient is prone.

MOVE — Extension of the two hips is most accurately compared with the patient lying on his face. Rotation also can be assessed prone by first flexing both knees.

SIGNS WITH THE PATIENT STANDING

(1) The patient is asked to lift his bad leg by bending his hip and knee. The weight-bearing hip, which is the normal one, abducts and the pelvis consequently rises on the unsupported side.

(2) The patient is asked to lower the bad leg and lift the good one. He is now taking weight through the affected hip and, if there is a positive Trendelenburg sign, the pelvis drops on the unsupported side (that is, the 'sound side sags').

(3) He is observed while walking, then running, then hopping.

TRENDELENBURG'S SIGN — Normally each leg bears half the body weight. When one leg is lifted (as in normal walking) the other takes the entire weight. As a result the trunk has to incline towards the weight-bearing leg. This is achieved by the hip abductors; their insertion is fixed and the pull is exerted on their origin (the ilium).

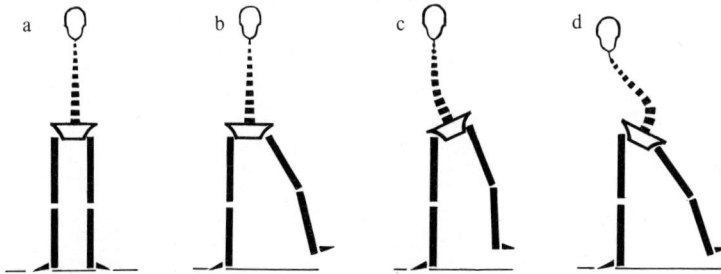

18.4 EXAMINATION OF THE HIP (4) WITH THE PATIENT STANDING
Standing on both legs (a) half the body weight is transmitted through each. When one leg is lifted what happens? (b) is impossible — no additional weight has been transferred to the supporting leg; (c) is the normal — all the weight is passing through the supporting leg because the pelvis has tilted; (d) is a positive Trendelenburg — the supporting hip is faulty: abduction cannot occur — the trunk and shoulder must move right across to transfer weight to the supporting leg.

Consequently the pelvis tilts, rising on the side not taking weight. When this mechanism fails Trendelenburg's sign is positive. The pelvis drops instead of rising on the unsupported side, and this occurs if (*a*) the abductors are weak, as in poliomyelitis or muscle dystrophies; (*b*) there is insufficient room for abduction, as in coxa vara where the trochanter meets the pelvic wall before the pelvis can tilt sufficiently; (*c*) the hip is dislocated so that the muscles have no stable fulcrum, as in congenital or pathological dislocations; (*d*) the femoral neck is fractured so that the lever system is not intact; or (*e*) if it hurts the patient to put the abductors into action, as in inflammatory conditions.

X-RAY

With the antero-posterior view it is always an advantage to have both hips on the same film. The bone density and architecture on the two sides can be compared, as well as the hip joints themselves; any difference in the size, shape or position of the two femoral heads is important. With a normal hip Shenton's line, which continues from the inferior border of the femoral neck to the inferior border of the pubic ramus, looks smooth; any interruption in the line suggests a mechanical disorder.

Lateral films are important in nearly all juvenile disorders and in some adult ones; they are more difficult to read and it helps in orientation to remember that the lesser trochanter projects posteriorly.

CONGENITAL DISLOCATION OF THE HIP

CAUSAL FACTORS

GENETIC — The familial incidence of congenital hip dislocation has long been recognized; clearly it is linked with the relatively high frequency in certain geographic areas (e.g. North Italy) where inter-marriage is common.   It is now known that two separate genetic factors are involved: (1) joint laxity (of dominant inheritance) which accounts for most of the cases diagnosed in the first week of life; and (2) acetabular dysplasia (of polygenic inheritance) which accounts for those diagnosed late.   Probably three-quarters of the early cases with lax joints recover spontaneously; that is, hips which were dislocatable do not remain so.

ENVIRONMENTAL — Shortly before delivery the mother secretes a ligament-relaxing hormone.   If this crosses the placental barrier any tendency to joint laxity is enhanced.   This accounts for the rarity of dislocation in premature babies (born before the hormones reach their peak) and possibly for the relative infrequency in boys (in whom male hormones counteract the female).

Intra-uterine mal-position (especially a breech position with extended legs) favours dislocation; this is linked with the higher incidence in first-born babies, because in them spontaneous version is less likely.

In the post-natal period racial customs influence the frequency.   Dislocation is commoner in Lapps and North American Indians who swaddle their babies tightly with the hips fully extended; and is rare in Hong Kong Chinese and in some African groups where the baby's hips are not extended and may indeed be kept abducted.

PATHOLOGY

With a dislocated hip, the acetabular roof is defective.   On its lateral aspect the acetabulum is underdeveloped; it is too shallow and its roof slopes too steeply.   After weight-bearing a false acetabulum develops above the original fossa.   The bony nucleus of the femoral head appears later than on the normal side and remains smaller; the cartilaginous head, however, is large.   The dislocation is always posterior and, as the head rides upwards, the slope of the pelvis pushes it laterally. The femoral neck is usually short and is often excessively anteverted.

The capsule, unlike that in traumatic dislocation, remains intact.   In time it becomes hour-glass in shape, developing an isthmus where it is crossed by the psoas muscle.   The cartilaginous labrum is often unduly large and folded into the acetabulum; the infolded portion (the limbus) constitutes an obstacle to reduction.   The ligamentum teres is often unduly thick.   In time the muscles arising from the pelvis become adaptively shortened.

SYMPTOMS

Before the baby starts walking an observant mother may spot asymmetry, a clicking hip, or difficulty in applying the napkin because of limited abduction. Contrary to popular belief late walking is not a marked feature; nevertheless dislocation must be excluded. After walking starts asymmetry is more obvious and now limp also becomes apparent.

Nearly all the above symptoms refer to unilateral dislocation. Bilateral dislocation rarely presents early, because there is no asymmetry and the characteristic waddling gait is mistaken by the parents for normal toddling.

SIGNS

Dislocation is much more common in girls than in boys, the left hip is more often affected than the right, and occasionally there are other congenital anomalies, such as a calcaneo-valgus foot.

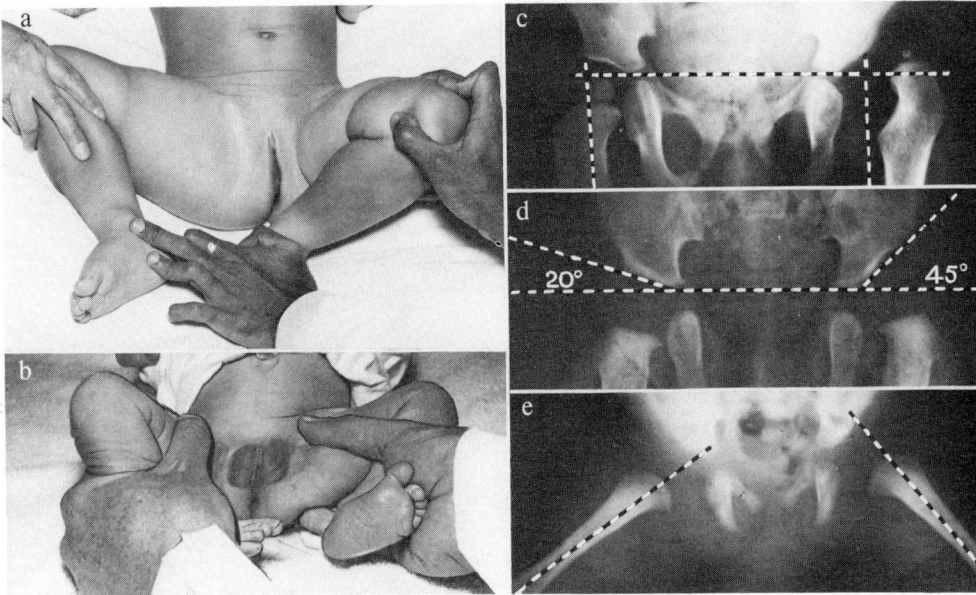

18.5 CONGENITAL HIP DISLOCATION (1) EARLY SIGNS
(a) Ortolani's test; (b) Barlow's test. (c) Perkins' lines; (d) acetabular angle; (e) von Rosen's lines.

LOOK — The skin creases are asymmetrical; in this connection it is the groin creases which are the significant ones. The pelvis looks a little wider on the affected side, the leg may be rotated outwards a little, and it looks slightly short.

In bilateral dislocation there is no asymmetry but the pelvis is abnormally wide on both sides, and there is a perineal gap.

FEEL — The head cannot be felt in its socket.

MOVE — Abduction is decreased; this is most obvious in flexion. The flexed hip of a young baby should abduct almost to a right angle. In congenital dislocation it often stops halfway; but if pressure is then applied to it there is a clunk as the dislocation reduces and then the hip abducts fully (Ortolani's 'jerk of entry'). Another valuable test is Barlow's: the surgeon holds the upper femur between his middle finger on the great trochanter and his thumb in the groin; by levering the femoral head in and out of the acetabulum dislocation is demonstrated. These important signs indicate a reducible dislocation and should be sought in every new-born baby; later they are not obtainable. Obviously decreased abduction without a clunk suggests irreducible dislocation.

When the child can stand, a positive Trendelenburg sign and gait are detectable.

X-RAY — In older children the dislocation is obvious. Before the bony nucleus of the head is well developed diagnosis is facilitated by drawing Perkins' lines (a horizontal through the triradiate cartilages and verticals from the outer edge of each acetabulum; the head normally lies medial to the vertical and below the horizontal lines). Alternatively, the increased acetabular angle due to the defective roof can be measured. In newborn babies Von Rosen's method is probably the best: a film is taken with both hips abducted 45 degrees and internally rotated; the line of the femoral shaft is produced upwards and on the dislocated side strikes the pelvis above the top of the acetabulum.

Before commencing treatment an arthrogram may be useful; and occasionally lateral views are taken to measure anteversion of the neck.

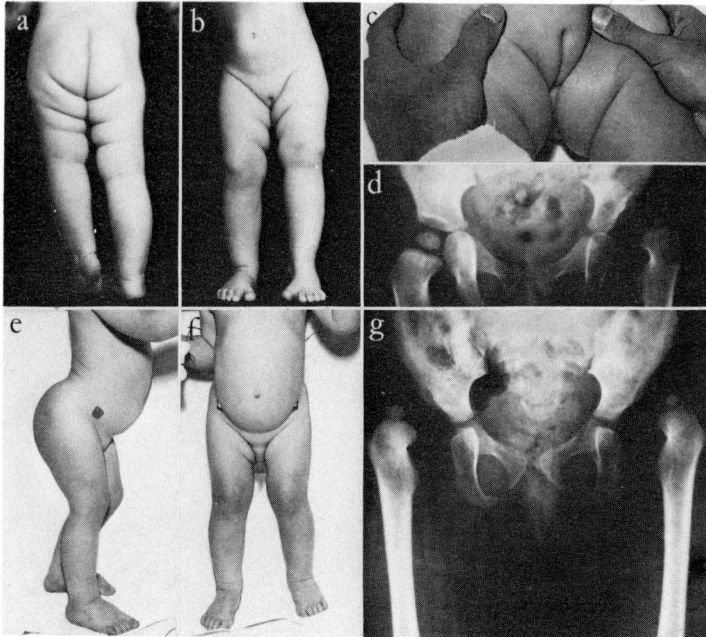

18.6 CONGENITAL HIP DISLOCATION (2) LATE SIGNS
Unilateral dislocation of left hip: (a, b) asymmetry, (c, d) the head is not in the socket.

Bilateral dislocation: (e, f) lordosis and a perineal gap, (g) both hips obviously dislocated.

DIFFERENTIAL DIAGNOSIS

OTHER CAUSES OF LATE WALKING — These include mental backwardness, spina bifida and cerebral palsy. Many late walkers are otherwise normal and do later walk normally. Nevertheless the hip should be x-rayed if walking has been unduly delayed.

OTHER CAUSES OF A PAINLESS LIMP SINCE INFANCY — The most important are as follows.
Infantile coxa vara — Congenital dislocation is simulated except that the head can be felt in its socket and the x-ray appearance is distinctive.
Pathological dislocation — There is a history of illness in infancy and a scar; x-rays show absence of the femoral head.
Poliomyelitis — Trophic changes are present and evidence of paralysis. Moreover the head is in its socket, although paralytic dislocation can occur.

TREATMENT BEFORE WEIGHT-BEARING

Weight-bearing begins long before walking; it begins with crawling when the baby is only a few months old. Before then, treatment is simple and the prognosis excellent. Von Rosen at Malmö and Barlow at Salford have both convincingly demonstrated that routine post-natal examination enables dislocation to be diagnosed, and that treatment at this early age gives consistently excellent results. Much unnecessary crippling disability could be prevented if their methods were followed everywhere.

The hip with a positive Barlow or Ortolani sign is dislocatable, but may become normal without treatment. To avoid unnecessary splintage many surgeons (by no means all) advocate waiting three weeks. If either sign is then still positive the hip is abducted fully (no anaesthetic is needed) and so reduced. Both hips are held in abduction by means of a polyurethane foam pillow or a pliable aluminium splint until, after a few months, x-rays show a good acetabular roof. If the hip is irreducible the treatment advocated in the next group is applied.

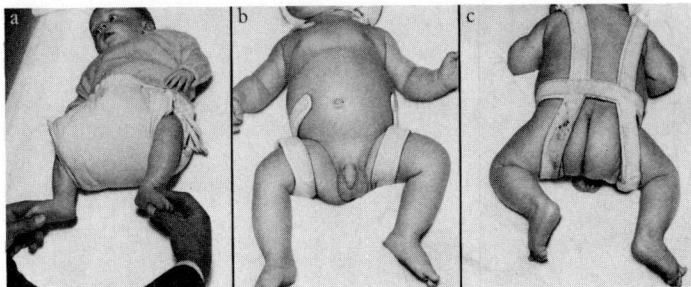

18.7 CONGENITAL HIP DISLOCATION (3) CLOSED TREATMENT BEFORE WEIGHT-BEARING
(a) Abduction napkin;
(b, c) von Rosen splint.

TREATMENT AFTER WEIGHT-BEARING BUT BELOW THE AGE LIMIT

The prognosis in this group is rather less satisfactory, and many different techniques of treatment are available; but the principle does not vary—the hip must be reduced and held reduced until it is stable.

REDUCE

Closed reduction — This is the ideal, but manipulation endangers the blood supply to the femoral head. To minimize this risk traction is applied, preferably to both legs on a vertical frame. Abduction is gradually increased until, by three weeks, the legs are widely separated. This manoeuvre alone (aided if necessary by adductor tenotomy), may be sufficient to achieve stable, concentric reduction. If not, the gentlest manipulation under anaesthesia at this stage may succeed and is probably not harmful.

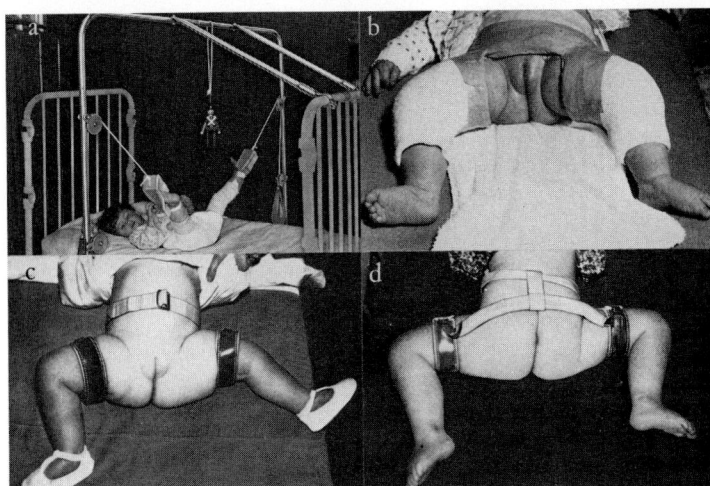

18.8 CONGENITAL HIP DISLOCATION (4) CLOSED TREATMENT AFTER WEIGHT-BEARING
(a) Vertical traction with abduction gradually increased; (b) plaster;

(c, d) Denis Browne splint.

Open reduction — If reduction feels unstable, or x-ray shows that it is not concentric, an arthrogram is performed.   This may reveal an infolded limbus; if so, open reduction and limbectomy is advisable.   But if no obstruction is revealed the hip is splinted (*see below*) and re-assessed after a few weeks; by then it may be concentric.

HOLD

Splintage — The concentrically reduced hip is held in plaster for six weeks; both hips are included.   Salter (1969) has shown that the frog position formerly used (90 degrees adduction, 90 degrees flexion) is potentially harmful and ' appropriate only to frogs '; he advocates the ' human position ' with the hips flexed more than 90 degrees but abducted much less.   After six weeks the plaster is replaced by a Denis Browne splint — a splendid device which prevents adduction but allows movement (and indeed walking — of a sort).   Within 12 months (often less) x-rays may show a concentric femoral head with a normal acetabular roof; if so, splintage is discarded.

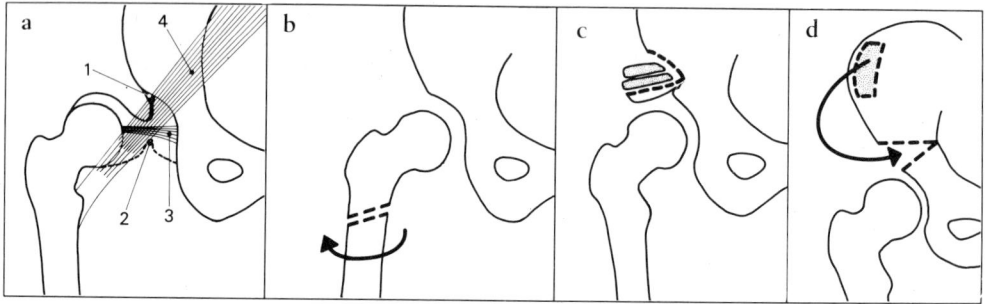

18.9   CONGENITAL HIP DISLOCATION (5) OPERATIVE TREATMENT
(a) Obstructions to closed reduction: 1. inverted limbus, 2. hour glass constriction of capsule, 3. thick ligamentum teres, 4. tight psoas. (b) Rotation osteotomy; (c) shelf operation; (d) innominate osteotomy.

Operation — But if, after 12 months of splintage, the head is not correctly placed or is partly uncovered, operation is needed.   The hip may look satisfactory only when rotated medially; the treatment then is subtrochanteric osteotomy.   The hip is left pointing in its stable direction, but the leg below the osteotomy is de-rotated until the foot points forward; internal fixation is reinforced by plaster.

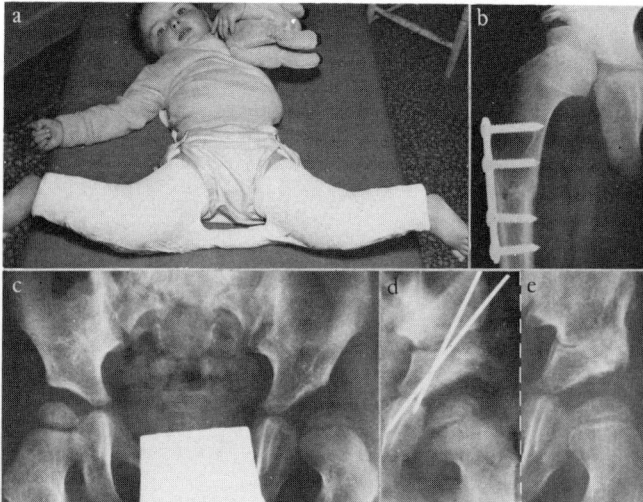

18.10   CONGENITAL HIP DIS-LOCATION (6) OPERATIVE TREATMENT (continued)
(a) Reduced open, but stable only in medial rotation—six weeks later (b) de-rotation osteotomy.

(c) Reduced open, but head poorly covered; (d, e) innominate osteotomy.

If the medially rotated hip does not look satisfactory on x-ray, osteotomy alone is of no value. The hip which is still considerably displaced, or even dislocated, must be opened. Removal of a mechanical obstacle, such as a large limbus or a thick ligamentum teres, may permit reduction; the hip is then held by plaster in its most stable position (nearly always medial rotation), and de-rotation osteotomy performed six weeks later. But if the head, though reduced, is still poorly covered, it should be provided with a bony roof; a shelf operation is one method, but innominate osteotomy (Salter, 1961) is better. Whatever operation is needed the hip is subsequently held in plaster until radiologically satisfactory.

TREATMENT ABOVE THE AGE LIMIT

The term 'age limit' implies that above a certain age reduction of the dislocation is unwise. The force needed for reduction damages the hip so much that pain and stiffness are likely to develop within a few years.

With unilateral dislocation the age limit is about six years. The untreated hip is mobile; the patient limps but has no pain until middle life. This is the justification for non-intervention. A contrary view (a minority opinion but gaining ground) advocates reduction even above the age limit; the possible techniques include capsular arthroplasty (Colonna), innominate osteotomy (Salter) and pelvic osteotomy (Chiari). The leg is restored to its correct length and, should pain develop, the technical problems of operating are much reduced because the head is in its socket.

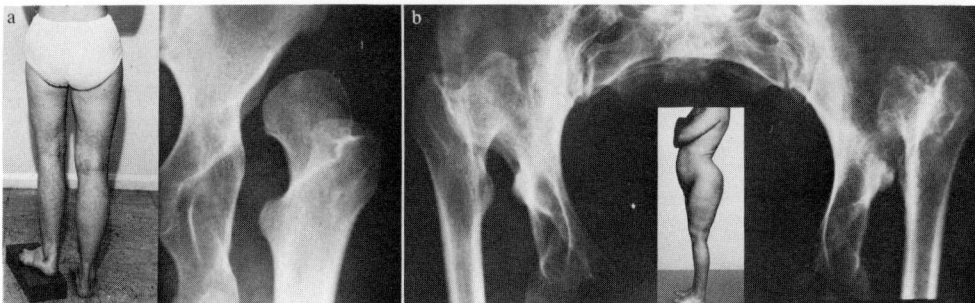

18.11 CONGENITAL DISLOCATION OF THE HIP (7) ABOVE THE AGE LIMIT
(a) Unilateral dislocation in a young adult. (b) Bilateral dislocation — this patient had no symptoms till aged 40 when she presented with backache.

With bilateral dislocation the age limit is about four. It is lower because the risk of intervention is doubled, and because partial failure leads to asymmetry. Two short legs are better than one. The untreated patient waddles through life until, at the age of 40 or 50, she develops backache (a sequel to the lumbar lordosis). Unhappily this is difficult to manage; a corset is a placebo, but bilateral total hip replacement in the absence of reasonable acetabulae is a formidable undertaking.

SUBLUXATION OF THE HIP

For normal weight transmission the hemispherical femoral head must be contained within a hemispherical socket. If the acetabulum is dysplastic the lateral part is sloping instead of being nearly horizontal and containment is inadequate. The hip is, in effect, subluxed; the femoral head (often too big) is not displaced upwards like a dislocation, but stands away too far laterally. Acetabular dysplasia, a familial disorder of polygenic inheritance, may result in subluxation or dislocation; and (see page 236) the unsuccessfully treated dislocation ends as a subluxation.

In either case weight transmission is faulty and early degeneration follows. These patients develop painful and progressive osteoarthritis in their twenties; the remedy is early diagnosis.

CLINICAL FEATURES

All hips should be examined soon after birth. Diagnosis is less obvious than with dislocation because there is neither shortening nor a click; but abduction in flexion is limited and this should always alert suspicion. The same sign is detected when an observant mother brings the child because she has noticed asymmetrical creases or difficulty in applying napkins. X-rays at this age are not easy to read; the bony nucleus of the femoral head does not appear before the age of about six months, but the acetabular angle shows that the roof is too sloping.

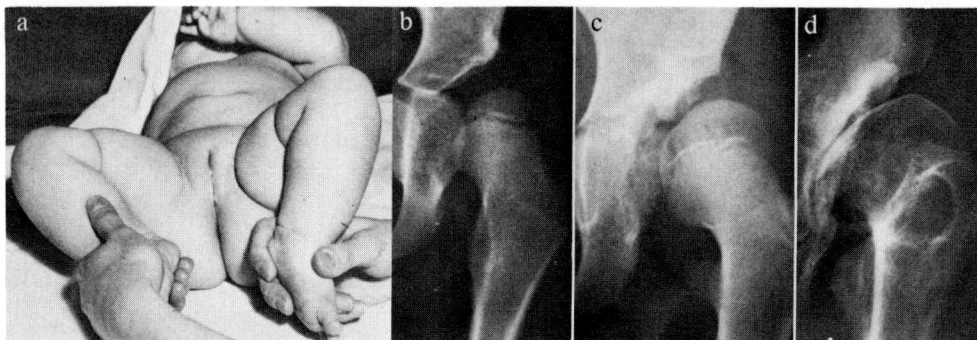

18.12 CONGENITAL SUBLUXATION OF THE HIP
(a) The cardinal physical sign; (b) x-ray in childhood; (c) in adolescence; (d) degeneration in early adult life.

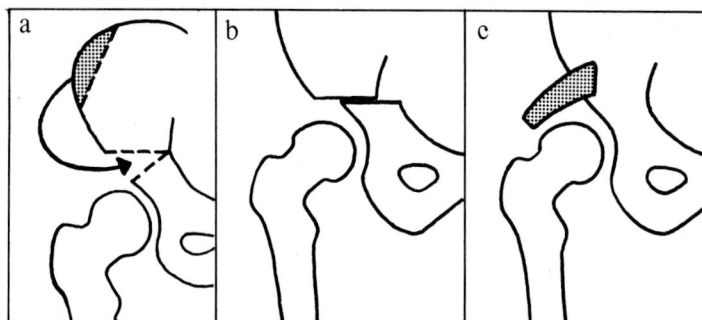

18.13 CONGENITAL SUBLUXATION — TREATMENT
(a) Salter's innominate osteotomy; (b) Chiari's pelvic osteotomy; (c) giant shelf.

Bilateral subluxation is even more likely to be missed. Napkin difficulty is greater but there is no asymmetry. Clinical experience is needed to appreciate that both hips have limited abduction in flexion, and radiological awareness to notice that both acetabulae are too sloping.

TREATMENT

The infant under a year old often responds to closed treatment similar to that for dislocation. A vertical frame is used; skin traction is applied to both legs which are gradually separated. When abduction is full a Denis Browne splint is applied; it is worn until, after a few months, the acetabular roof looks normal.

If the femoral head remains poorly covered, or if the child is more than a year old, operation is needed. A varus femoral osteotomy may be enough to produce a congruent joint under the age of about two. In the older child it is better to provide a good acetabular roof by Salter's innominate osteotomy, Chiari's pelvic osteotomy, or by constructing a massive shelf.

PATHOLOGICAL DISLOCATION OF THE HIP

In infancy the femur may be infected via the umbilicus or via femoral vein puncture; at this age the growth disc is no barrier and infection readily involves the femoral head and the joint. In older children acute osteomyelitis usually affects the metaphysis; but since this is intracapsular again the joint is readily attacked. If the infection is unchecked the head and neck of the femur may be destroyed and a pathological dislocation result. The pus may escape and, when the child recovers, the sinus heals. The hip signs then resemble those of a congenital dislocation, but the tell-tale scar remains and on x-ray the femoral head is completely absent.

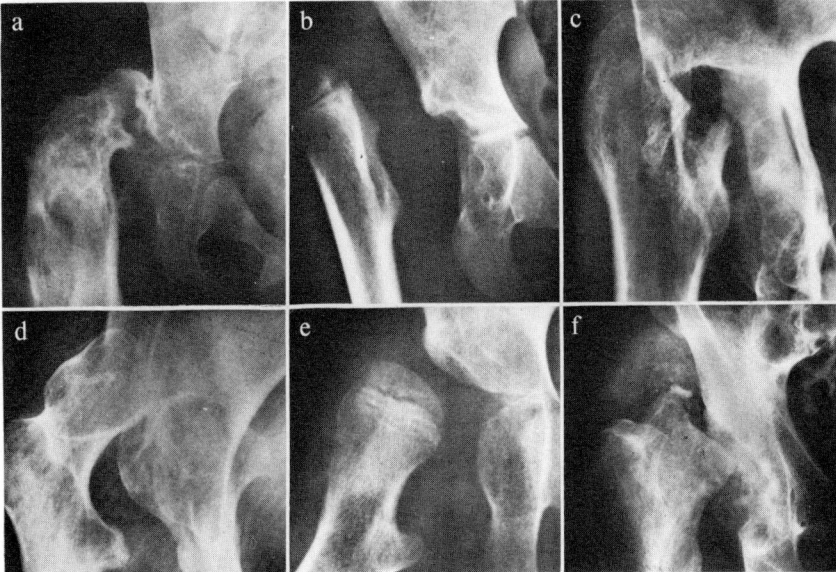

18.14 ACQUIRED NON-TRAUMATIC HIP DISLOCATIONS
(a) Acute suppurative arthritis following osteomyelitis of the femoral neck. (b) Acute suppurative arthritis in infancy has resulted in complete disappearance of the femoral head and neck. (c) Pathological dislocation in tuberculosis. (d) Unbalanced paralysis in polio has led to dislocation. (e) Similar appearance in cerebral palsy. (f) Charcot's disease.

Even in the acute stage diagnosis is not easy. The ill child who cries when the hip is moved presents little problem; but some of these children have immuno-deficiency and in them the signs are deceptively slight despite severe bone destruction (Lloyd-Roberts, 1975). Aspiration under anaesthesia is often necessary. Even if pus is withdrawn immediate arthrotomy is still advisable (Paterson, 1970); a piece of capsule and synovium is excised, antibiotic instilled and the wound closed without drainage. Systemic antibiotics are given and the hip is splinted (preferably in a Denis Browne splint) for 3 months.

THE IRRITABLE HIP

The patient with an irritable hip (the term 'irritable' is non-specific) presents with pain and limp. Both are usually intermittent, following activity. The pain is felt in the groin or front of the thigh, sometimes reaching as far as the knee. Slight wasting may be detectable, but the cardinal sign is that the extremes of all movements are limited, and the attempt to produce them is painful.

A thorough general examination and x-rays are the first steps in management. The patient is put to bed without delay, and skin traction applied to the affected leg. Blood investigations are instituted and every effort is made to establish the diagnosis. The following conditions must be considered:

Transient synovitis — The cause is unknown and the irritability subsides quickly. X-rays are normal and investigations negative.

Tuberculosis — In its early stages tuberculosis presents as an irritable hip. The patient may be unwell, the sedimentation rate raised and the Heaf test positive. X-rays may show general rarefaction of the hip or a bone abscess.

Chronic synovitis — A chronic synovitis of rheumatoid type is indistinguishable from early tuberculosis without a positive serum latex test or biopsy. Other joints usually become affected later.

Perthes' disease — The child is aged 5 to 10 years, is well, and the irritability subsides fairly quickly. Abduction in flexion is the movement most restricted, and x-rays show increased density of the head with an increased joint space.

Slipped epiphysis — The gradual type may present with an irritable hip. Age and build are characteristic and the x-ray appearance is diagnostic, providing a lateral view also is taken.

TUBERCULOSIS OF THE HIP

The disease process may start as a synovitis, or as an osteomyelitis in the bone of the acetabulum, femoral head or neck. Once arthritis develops, destruction is rapid.

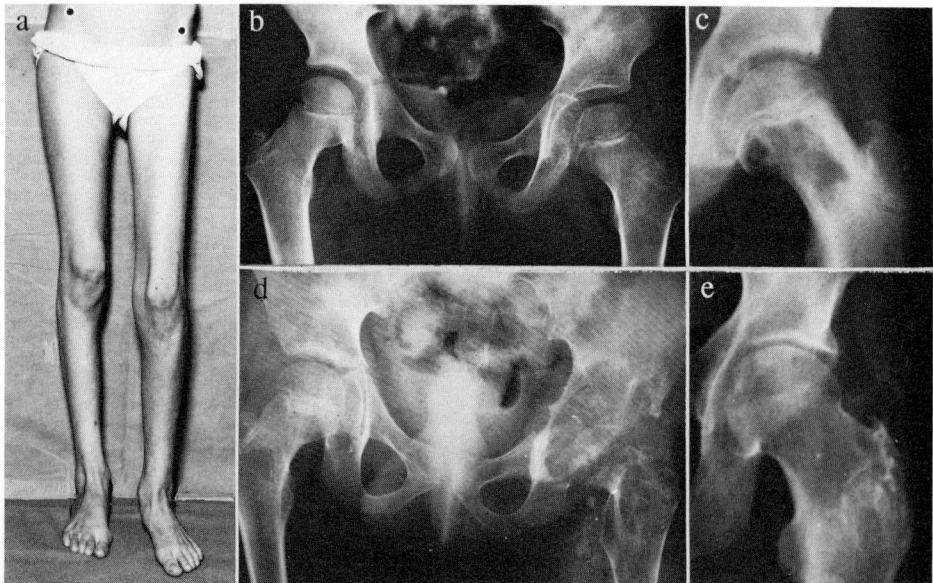

18.15 HIP TUBERCULOSIS (1) ACTIVE
(a) Apparent lengthening in early disease of the left hip. (b) Synovitis of left hip.
(c) Osteomyelitis of the femoral neck. (d) Florid arthritis. (e) Trochanteric infection — this rarely extends to the joint.

Muscle spasm presses the femoral head against the acetabulum, which is soft and appears to enlarge upwards (wandering acetabulum). The femoral head may also be destroyed, permitting pathological dislocation. Healing usually leaves a long unsound fibrous joint with considerable limb shortening and deformity.

CLINICAL FEATURES

The patient, usually a child, limps a little and complains of slight ache in the groin or thigh; later, pain is more severe and may wake the child from sleep.

With early disease (synovitis or osteomyelitis) the joint is held slightly flexed and abducted, and extremes of movement are a little limited and painful; but until x-ray changes appear the hip is merely 'irritable' and diagnosis is difficult. If arthritis supervenes the hip becomes flexed, adducted and medially rotated, muscle wasting becomes obvious, and all movements are grossly limited by pain and spasm.

The first x-ray change is general rarefaction but with a normal joint space and line; the femoral epiphysis may be enlarged or a bone abscess visible; with arthritis, in addition to the general rarefaction, there is destruction of the acetabular roof or the femoral head, usually both; the joint may be subluxed or even dislocated. With healing the bones re-calcify.

Early disease may heal leaving a normal or almost normal hip; but if there has been arthritis the usual result is an unsound fibrous joint. The leg is scarred and thin; shortening is often severe because many factors contribute—adduction deformity,

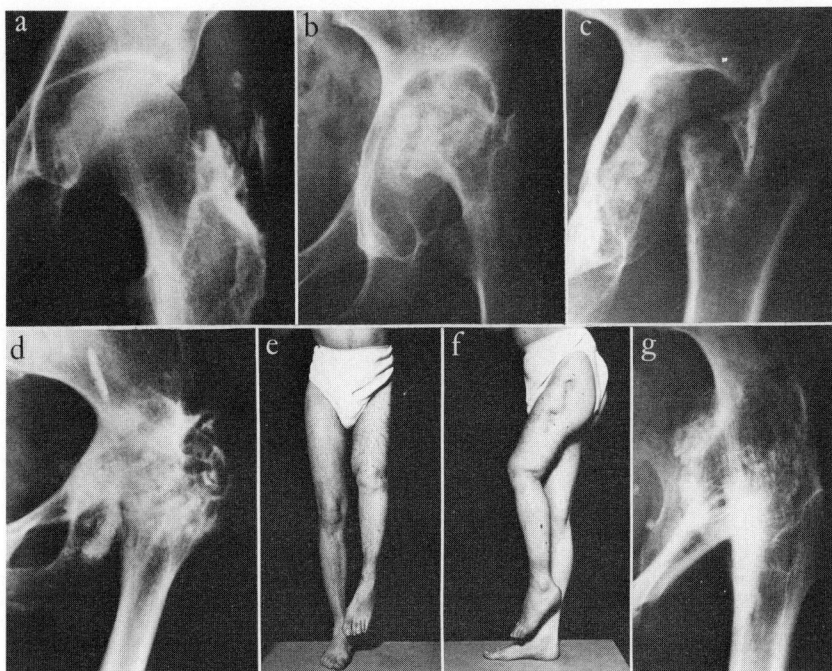

18.16 HIP TUBERCULOSIS (2) HEALING AND AFTERMATH
(a) Healed trochanteric disease with the hip joint still normal. (b) Healing arthritis with gross enlargement of the acetabulum. (c) Healing arthritis with large acetabulum and destruction of the head. (d) Joint destruction with considerable calcification in the aftermath stage; and (e, f) appearance of the hip in this patient — note the gross shortening. (g) A patient in whom secondary infection was followed by bony ankylosis.

bone destruction, damage to the upper femoral epiphysis and occasionally premature fusion of the lower femoral epiphysis.

TREATMENT

Anti-tuberculous drugs are, of course, essential (page 35). Skin traction is applied and, for a child, a double abduction frame may be used. An abscess in the femoral neck is best evacuated; if, after 6–8 weeks an arthritis is not settling, joint 'débridement' is performed.

As the disease settles traction is discontinued and the patient is got up: non-weight-bearing with crutches if the joint has been preserved, weight-bearing in an abduction plaster if it has been destroyed.

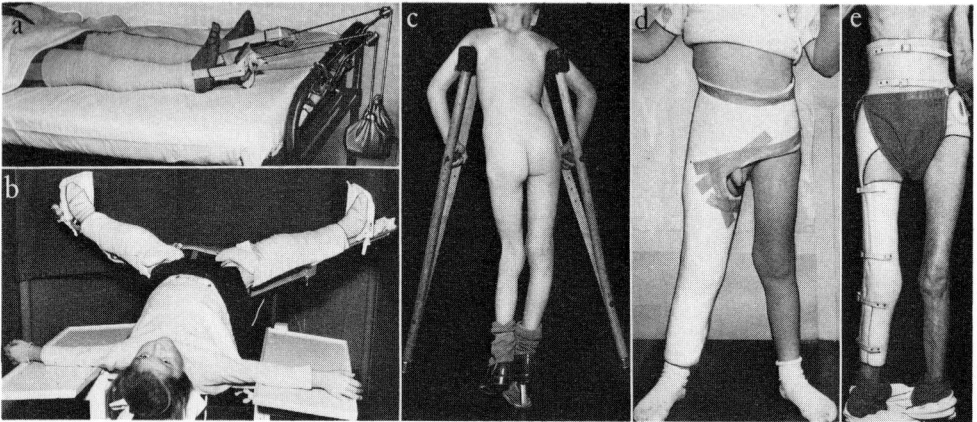

18.17 HIP TUBERCULOSIS (3) CLOSED TREATMENT
(a) In the active stage the adult is usually treated with skin traction; (b) a child being treated on a Pyrford double abduction frame. (c) The disease has been arrested early — weight-bearing is avoided by using a patten and crutches. (d) The disease has been arrested late — weight-bearing is permitted but the hip held in plaster; (e) later, a removable polythene spica may be sufficient.

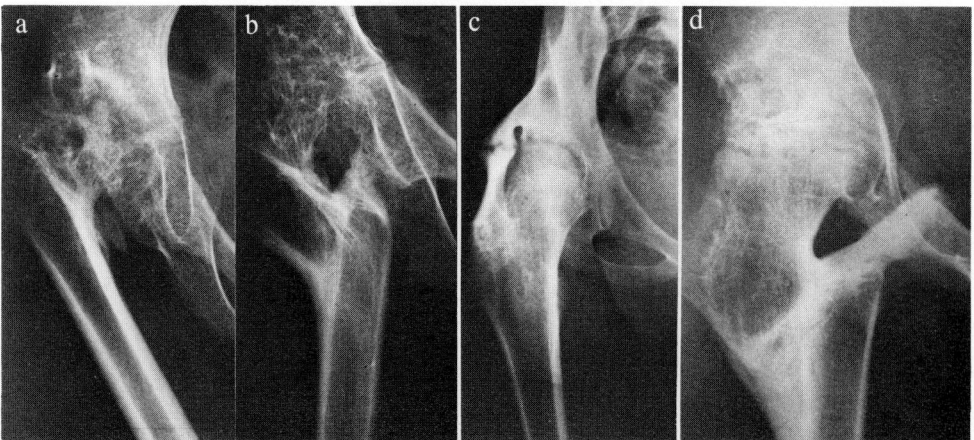

18.18 HIP TUBERCULOSIS (4) OPERATIVE TREATMENT
(a, b) Before and after osteotomy in the late healing stage. (c) Attempted ilio-femoral arthrodesis has failed — the graft is not in compression. (d) Brittain's combined osteotomy and arthrodesis has succeeded (the Norwich V-arthrodesis is sometimes preferred).

For the aftermath of tuberculous arthritis a raised shoe and a removable splint may be useful; in addition three operative procedures are available:

Osteotomy — Subtrochanteric osteotomy is useful to correct deformity and to increase apparent length; a full-length hip spica is needed for at least 3 months. Sometimes an unsound hip becomes sound after osteotomy.

Arthrodesis — Arthrodesis, preferably extra-articular, is the method of choice for unsoundness and instability. A bone graft may be slid up from the greater trochanter (Hibbs), turned down from the ilium (Wilson), or bridged from the ischium to the femur (Trumble).

Osteotomy combined with arthrodesis (Brittain) — This is probably the best method of all. Subtrochanteric osteotomy is performed, and through the gap an ischio-femoral graft is inserted. The shaft is then abducted and plaster applied, and retained for about 6 months.

PERTHES' DISEASE (Coxa plana; Pseudccoxalgia)

CAUSE
The femoral head becomes partly or wholly avascular. The cause is not definitely known, but a logical explanation is emerging; the picture is of a precipitating cause operating against an anatomical background.

THE BACKGROUND — For the first three or four years of life the predominant blood supply to the femoral head is from metaphyseal vessels which cross the future growth plate; a further supply comes from lateral epiphyseal vessels, but virtually none through the ligamentum teres. From the age of three or four the growth disc blocks the metaphyseal supply; after the age of seven or eight the artery of the ligamentum teres is fully developed; between these ages the head may depend upon the lateral epiphyseal vessels and its blood supply is precarious.

THE PRECIPITATING CAUSE — Probably this is an effusion into the hip joint; Kemp (1971) has shown experimentally that ischaemia can be produced in this way. The effusion could follow trauma, of which there is a history in over half the cases; a non-specific infection, or transient synovitis, could explain others. Recent studies strongly suggest that one incident of ischaemia (infarction) is not enough to cause Perthes' disease; two or more are needed.

OTHER THEORIES — As usual with an ill-understood disorder, metabolic, endocrine and constitutional factors have been blamed, with little or no foundation.

PATHOLOGY

The pathological process takes $2\frac{1}{2}$–4 years to complete and can be conveniently studied in serial x-rays.

THE FEMORAL HEAD DIES (AVASCULAR NECROSIS) — Ischaemia affects all or part of the femoral head; the avascular part looks dense on x-ray and does not grow; the cartilaginous envelope surrounding it, however, continues to enlarge (perhaps because it is independently nourished by synovial fluid). The growing cartilage is not being occupied by growing bone, hence the apparent increase of joint space.

THE DEAD HEAD IS REPLACED (CREEPING SUBSTITUTION) — Blood vessels grow in through the neck; the metaphysis, being hyperaemic, becomes soft and looks rare on x-ray. The soft bone squashes easily (hence the thick neck) and bends easily (hence the slight coxa vara). Possibly localized hyperaemia explains the occasional cystic appearance in the metaphysis.

When the blood vessels reach the femoral head, the dead bone is absorbed piecemeal. The bone therefore appears rarefied (in patches or all over). The new vessels to the head enter from the periphery, which revascularizes first; consequently the shape of the head is further distorted. Eventually new bone of normal density and architecture is deposited, but the head remains permanently flat.

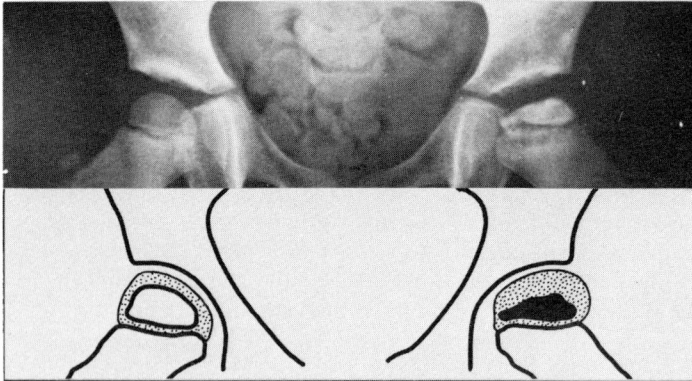

18.19   PERTHES' DISEASE (1)
The joint space increases because the cartilage of the epiphysis continues to grow while the bony nucleus does not.

CLINICAL FEATURES

There are no general symptoms.   The local symptoms are limp and ache, often slight and intermittent; indeed, once the irritable stage has passed, pain is distinctly unusual.   The contrast between paucity of symptoms and gross x-ray changes is striking.

The usual age is 5–10 years (rarely 2–18) but often the bone age is less.   The condition is four times commoner in boys and is sometimes bilateral.   Some 4 per cent of patients have an associated urogenital anomaly.   In other respects the patient is fit, and the local signs are as follows.

18.20   PERTHES' DISEASE (2)
Serial x-rays over a period of five years.   Despite radiological severity the clinical signs are usually slight, but abduction in flexion is nearly always limited (inset).

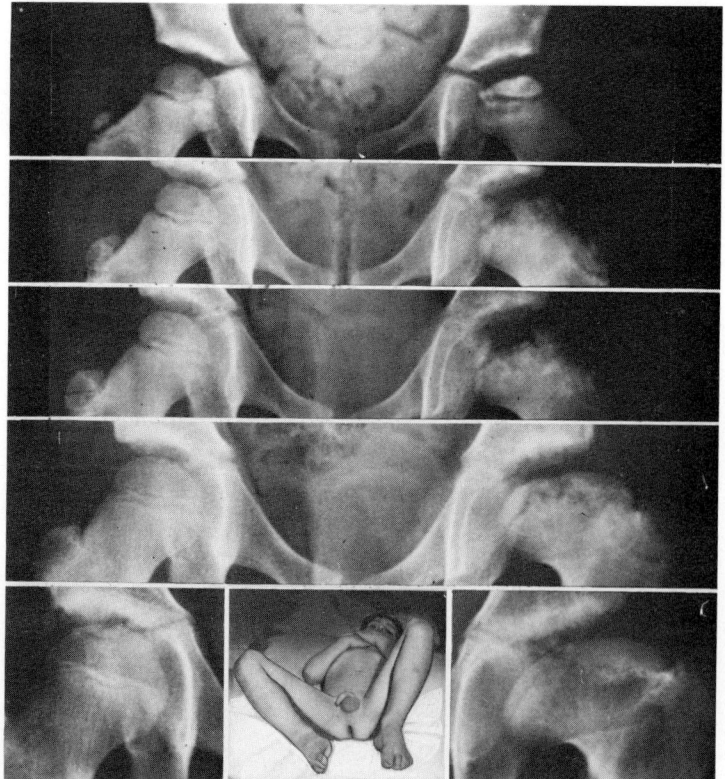

LOOK — There may be slight wasting and trivial shortening, but often the appearance is almost normal.

FEEL — The greater trochanter is only slightly elevated and is more prominent than on the normal side. The neck may feel slightly thick.

MOVE — If the patient is seen early in the disease, the hip is irritable and all movements are slightly diminished. Usually, however, there is no irritability; abduction, especially in flexion, is nearly always diminished and so is medial rotation. Other movements are often full and painless.

X-RAY — From the outset, the joint space looks increased and the head 'stands away' too far laterally. The ischaemic areas of the femoral head show increased density, at first granular, then more uniform. Flattening and patchy fragmentation follow. The picture is extremely variable because it depends on how far the pathological process has progressed in each individual area, and on how much of the head is involved. The neck becomes wide and sometimes there is a band of rarefaction at the metaphysis or even a cystic appearance with surrounding sclerosis.

Catterall (1972) has, on radiological grounds, classified the cases into four groups. In group 1 only half the head is necrotic and no collapse occurs; in group 2 slightly more than half the head is involved, but the remaining viable portion prevents collapse; in group 3 most of the head, and in group 4 all of it, is ischaemic, so that collapse may be severe.

DIFFERENTIAL DIAGNOSIS

The irritable hip of early Perthes' disease must be differentiated from other causes of irritability; the child's fitness, the increased joint space and the patchy bone density are characteristic. In transient synovitis the x-ray is normal. In Morquio–Brailsford disease, cretinism, multiple epiphyseal dysplasia, sickle-cell disease and Gaucher's disease, the femoral heads may be flat and irregular; but usually they are not dense and other diagnostic features are apparent.

TREATMENT

AVAILABLE METHODS

(1) *Traction* — As long as the hip is irritable the child should be in bed with skin traction applied to the affected leg.

(2) *Avoiding weight* — Once irritability had subsided it was formerly the practice to get the child up, but with some device (e.g. a leg sling or a caliper) to prevent weight-bearing. The assumption was that ischaemic bone was crushed by weight transmission. Evidence is accumulating to refute this assumption. Probably weight-bearing in itself is harmless and the attempt to relieve it should be abandoned.

(3) *'Containment'* — The femoral head should be contained within the acetabulum; lateral displacement ('standing away') adversely affects the result. Containment can be achieved: (*a*) by holding the hips widely abducted, in plaster or in a removable splint (ambulation, though awkward, is just possible, but the position must be maintained for at least a year); or (*b*) by operation, either a varus osteotomy of the femur (which may give a little shortening) or by an innominate osteotomy of the pelvis; after operation plaster is worn until the osteotomy has united (2–3 months) after which the child is allowed free.

PROGNOSIS AND CHOICE OF METHOD

The sequel to deformity of the femoral head is osteoarthritis. The more misshapen the head the worse the outlook, although even with considerable deformity significant symptoms are unlikely to develop before middle life. The factors which influence the choice of method are as follows.

(1) *Age* — The younger the better; the child under five nearly always does well and, once irritability has subsided, no treatment is needed.

(2) *Severity* — Catterall's groupings, though helpful, are less useful as guides to treatment than the concept of the ' head at risk '. The radiological features of such a femoral head are: (*a*) It is subluxed laterally and partially uncovered; (*b*) there is a translucent area in the lateral part of the epiphysis; (*c*) specks of calcification are seen lateral to the epiphysis and (*d*) the metaphyseal reaction is severe.

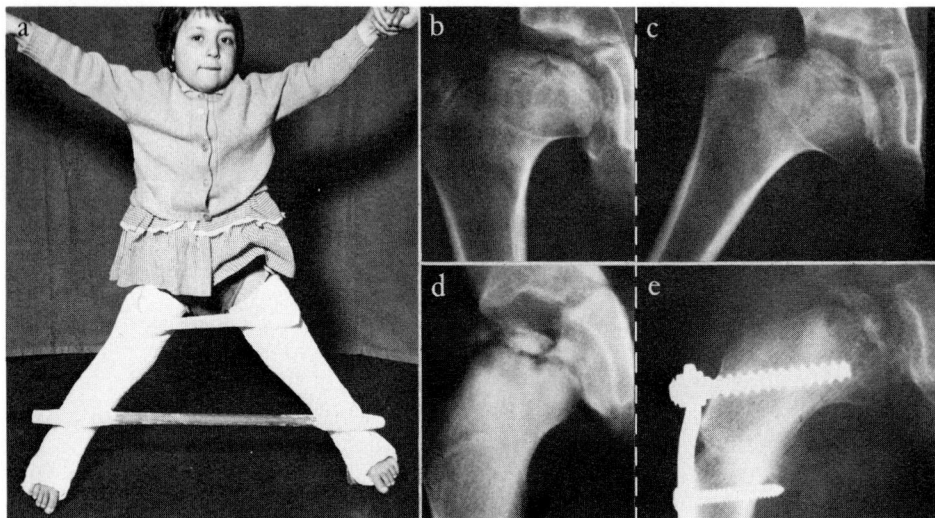

18.21 PERTHES' DISEASE (3) TREATMENT
Broomstick plaster (a) can achieve containment of the head (b, c). Similar containment after osteotomy (d, e).

Femoral osteotomy (varus-rotation type) is advised if the head is ' at risk ', but only if severe deformity has not already occurred (Lloyd-Roberts, 1976); severe deformity implies that acetabular adaptation has already taken place and any disturbance in position is likely to precipitate early degeneration.

(3) *Philosophy* — Long term statistics are not available and the choice of treatment must be influenced by the surgeon's philosophy. Once the child is past the stage of irritability he has no symptoms, only an abnormal x-ray. Symptoms of osteoarthritis are unlikely before middle life and may never develop. Consequently a case for treatment by ' supervised neglect ' certainly exists.

Nevertheless, treatment by containment frequently gives a much better x-ray appearance, which may imply that osteoarthritis can be postponed or even possibly prevented. I am almost persuaded that severe cases with persistent pain, or the head markedly ' at risk ', merit containment; and to me, osteotomy, in which treatment is completed within 3 months, is preferable to prolonged splintage.

SLIPPED EPIPHYSIS

In adolescents the upper femoral epiphysis may become displaced at the growth disc, resulting in coxa vara. This condition is termed 'slipped epiphysis'. The slipping occurs gradually in 70 per cent of cases, and suddenly in 30 per cent. The cause and pathology are similar in both varieties.

CAUSE

A slipped epiphysis resembles a pathological fracture. Trauma may be the precipitating cause, but an underlying abnormality predisposes to slipping.

TRAUMA — This is undoubtedly a factor because (*a*) there is often a history of hip 'sprains'; (*b*) sometimes a gross slip is seen immediately following a fall; and (*c*) during growth the femoral growth disc becomes increasingly oblique, and is thus more liable to displacement with injury.

UNDERLYING ABNORMALITY — An underlying abnormality is strongly suggested because (*a*) the slipping occurs gradually in 70 per cent of cases; (*b*) it often becomes bilateral and the second side may slip even while the patient is in bed undergoing treatment for the first; and (*c*) the disorder occurs just before puberty, many of the patients show evidence of endocrine imbalance and the pituitary fossa on x-ray is sometimes small.

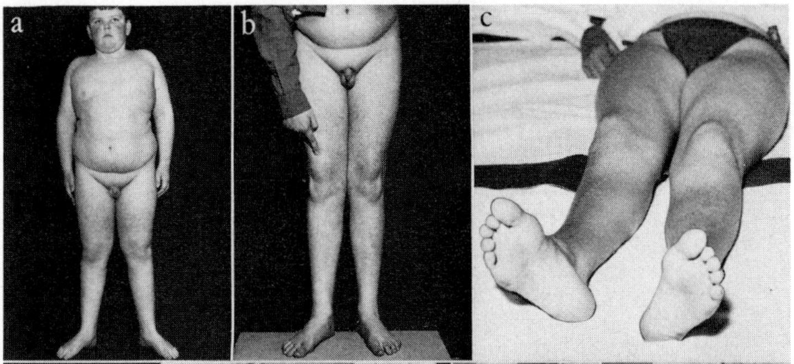

18.22 SLIPPED EPIPHYSIS (1) CLINICAL FEATURES (a) The build is unmistakable; (b) this patient complained of pain only in the knee—note (c) the lateral rotation.

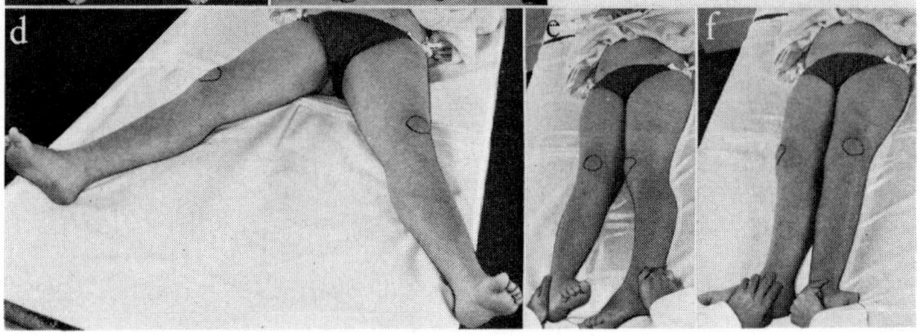

Another patient showing (d) diminished abduction, (e) diminished medial rotation, and (f) increased lateral rotation.

PATHOLOGY

The nature of the underlying abnormality is not known with certainty. The following hypothesis, based on animal experiments, is plausible.

Shortly before puberty, growth hormones stimulate the growth disc to produce much additional cartilage in preparation for the pre-puberty growth spurt. The sex hormones normally play a part in converting this additional cartilage to bone; if they fail to keep pace, there is too much unossified cartilage which is unable to resist the stress imposed by the increase in body weight. Consequently, during walking and standing, the shaft of the femur will tend to drive upwards, and when the patient is lying in bed, the weight of the leg will tend to make the shaft roll outwards.

GRADUAL SLIP

SYMPTOMS

Even with 'gradual slip' there is a history of injury in half the cases. Pain, sometimes in the groin, but often only in the thigh or knee, is the presenting symptom.

It is regarded as a sprain; often, and unfortunately, it is disregarded. It soon disappears only to recur with further exercise. Limp also occurs early and is more constant.

SIGNS

The disorder is slightly commoner in boys than in girls. In boys the average age of onset is 15, in girls it is 12 and is rare after menstruation has started. Two-thirds of the patients are unduly fat and sexually underdeveloped; the other third may be tall, thin and sexually normal. The local signs are as follows.

LOOK — In the earliest stage the appearance is normal, but the patient is rarely seen until significant slipping has occurred and deformity is perceptible. The leg then is laterally rotated and is half to one inch short. Slight wasting is not uncommon.

FEEL — The greater trochanter may be higher and more posterior than that of the unaffected hip.

MOVE — The joint is sometimes irritable with a little diminution of movement in all directions, but the most constant and diagnostic limitations are of abduction and medial rotation. The more definite the slip, the more are these two movements limited.

Muscle bulk is often reduced and a Trendelenburg sign and limp may be present.

X-RAY — In the antero-posterior view, even when slipping is trivial, changes are apparent. The growth disc is too wide and too 'woolly' on its metaphyseal side. A line drawn along the superior surface of the neck remains superior to the head instead of passing through it (Trethowan's sign). In a normal hip the posterior acetabular margin cuts across the medial corner of the upper femoral metaphysis; with slipping the entire metaphysis is lateral to the posterior acetabular margin (Capener's sign). With further slipping, the upward displacement of the shaft and neck becomes more apparent.

In the lateral view, deformity is usually obvious from the beginning. The head and neck are angulated on each other so that there is a forward bow.

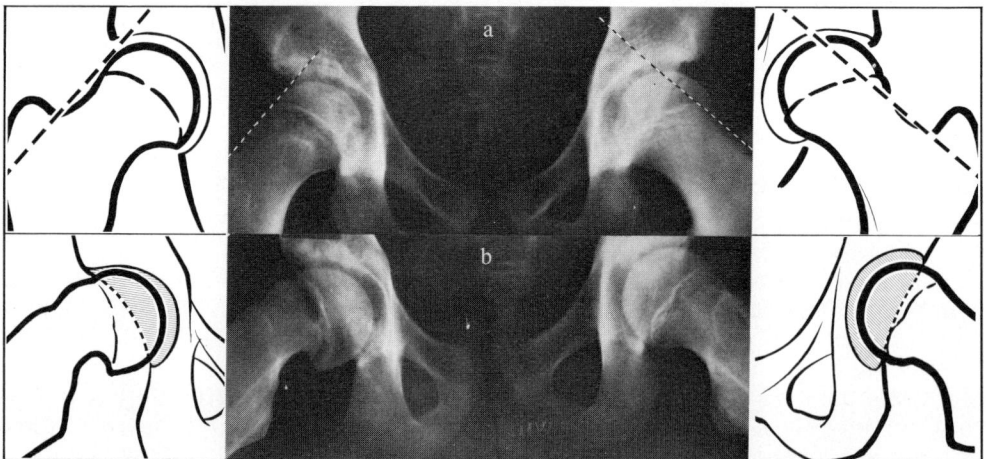

18.23 SLIPPED EPIPHYSIS (2) X-RAYS
(a) Antero-posterior and (b) lateral views of early slipped epiphysis right hip. The upper diagrams show Trethowan's line passing just above the head on the affected side, but cutting through it on the normal. The lower diagrams show Capener's sign: the femoral head is apparently extruded from the acetabulum on the affected side, but contained within it on the normal.

Pre-slipping stage — A pre-slipping stage has been postulated. However, it seems unlikely that the condition could present clinically without slight displacement, and a lateral x-ray shows even the smallest slip.

TREATMENT

With modest displacement (less than $\frac{1}{3}$ slip) reduction is not attempted. Under x-ray control the epiphysis is fixed where it is, using at least 3 threaded pins. If operation is to be delayed, traction is useful in preventing further slip.

With unacceptable displacement reduction is desirable, but traction is ineffective and manipulation is dangerous (the blood supply to the femoral head, already reduced by the slip, may be still further impaired). Open reduction is theoretically ideal, but has a fairly high complication rate (from avascular necrosis or chondrolysis). The safest procedure is to fix the head in its displaced position with 3 pins and to compensate for the displacement by an osteotomy when the epiphysis has joined (usually within a few months). Griffith (1976) has shown that the epiphysis rotates downwards and backwards around the curved upper surface of the metaphysis: he has designed an ingenious ' geometric flexion osteotomy ' to correct the deformity. The alternative is an immediate subtrochanteric osteotomy, designed to make the growth disc more horizontal; a laterally-based wedge of bone is excised, rotation also is corrected and the new position held in an abduction plaster or by internal fixation.

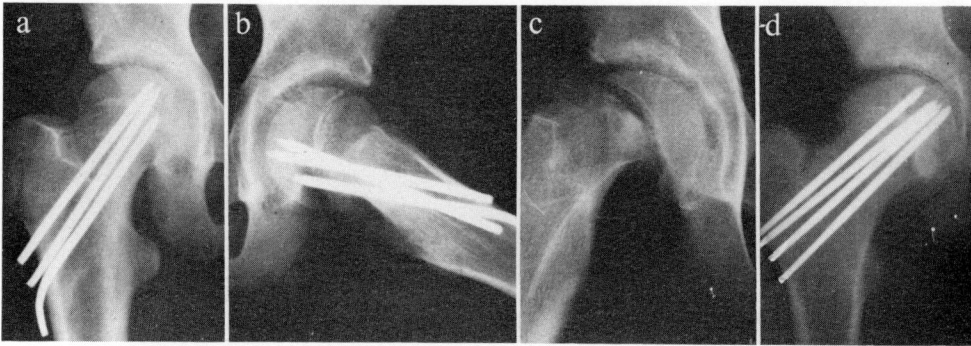

18.24 SLIPPED EPIPHYSIS (3) TREATMENT
(a, b) Minimal slip — no reduction has been attempted, but further slip prevented by 3 Moore's pins. (c, d) A sudden slip has been reduced by manipulation, and fixed in position.

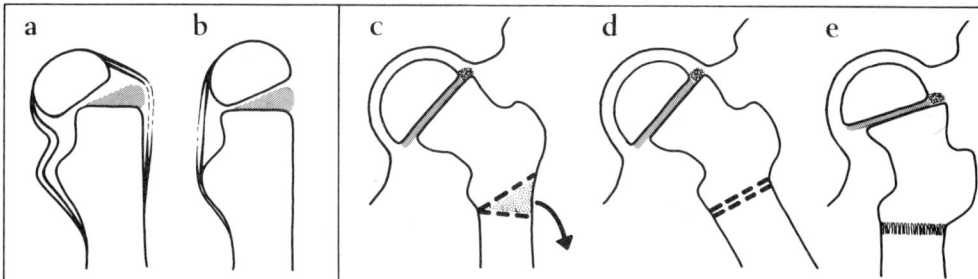

18.25 SLIPPED EPIPHYSIS (4) TREATMENT (continued)
(a) The head has slipped backwards off the neck, new bone has formed and the anterior blood vessels are stretched or torn; (b) if the head is dragged into position over this new bone, the remaining posterior vessels are endangered. In (c) — an AP view — the deformity has been left but a lateral wedge of bone has been excised lower down; (d) the leg is held abducted until the osteotomy joins; (e) when the leg returns to its correct position the growth disc becomes more horizontal.

SUDDEN SLIP

The term is misleading. Almost certainly gradual slipping occurs first; then, following a fall, there is severe displacement or even complete separation. The signs are those of a fractured neck of femur. Traction or gentle manipulation, though ineffective with gradual slip, may restore a sudden slip to the pre-injury position. If so, the epiphysis is fixed with threaded pins. But reduction may be spurious (an illusion created by altered rotation of the limb), and even gentle manipulation may be hazardous; consequently some surgeons advocate the same treatment as for a gradual slip, namely, immediate fixation without attempted reduction, followed by trochanteric osteotomy (if needed) when the epiphysis has closed.

SEQUELS TO SLIPPED EPIPHYSIS

COXA VARA — If displacement has not been reduced, the epiphysis fuses in its deformed position. The patient limps, but the condition is painless until osteoarthritis later develops. The leg is short and laterally rotated; the trochanter is too high and too posterior; and abduction and medial rotation remain permanently limited, whereas adduction and lateral rotation may be greater than normal. A Trendelenburg sign and limp are often present. X-rays show the coxa vara, often with a downward 'step' from the femoral neck on to the head. Osteotomy should be performed to relieve symptoms and in the hope of preventing osteoarthritis.

AVASCULAR NECROSIS — Death of the femoral head is an important complication. Formerly common, the incidence has been reduced by: (a) avoiding forcible manipulation; and (b) using threaded pins in preference to a bulky trifin nail.

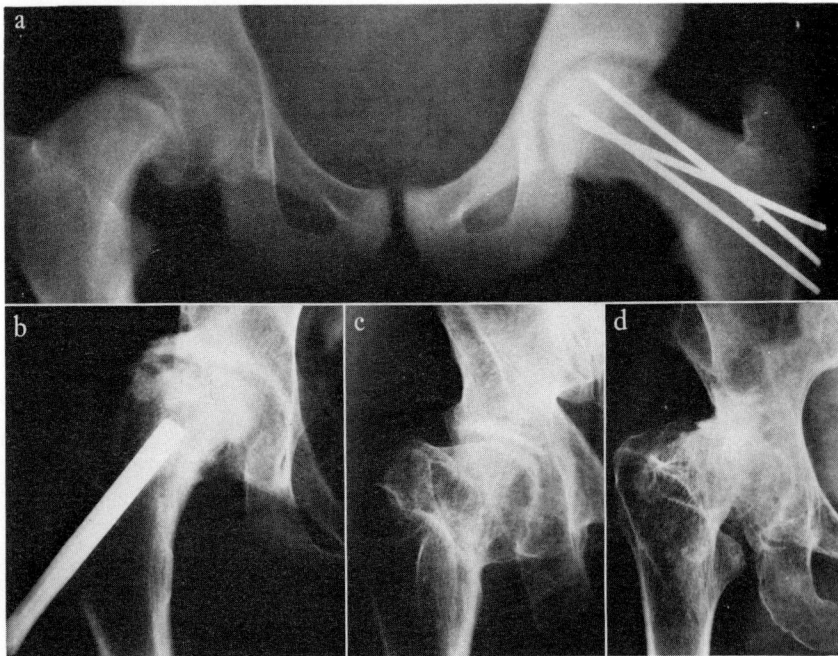

18.26 SLIPPED EPIPHYSIS (5) SEQUELS
(a) The left side had been pinned — now the right has slipped — the patient should be warned of this possibility. (b) Avascular necrosis after trifin nailing — this type of fixation has now been abandoned. (c) Mal-union in an untreated patient. (d) Osteoarthritis aged 45 followed mal-union.

CHONDROLYSIS — The femoral head is not dense but rarefied, and the joint space becomes much narrower. The hip becomes very stiff. Relief of weight-bearing may lead to restoration of the joint space, but movement does not often return.

OSTEOARTHRITIS — Early osteoarthritis is a likely sequel if displacement has not been reduced, and inevitable if there has been avascular necrosis.

BILATERAL SLIPPING — The parents should be warned that, up to 2 years after a slipped epiphysis, slipping may occur at the other hip. This happens in 15–30 per cent of cases and is commoner in patients with endocrine abnormality.

COXA VARA
In coxa vara the angle between the neck and shaft of the femur is diminished. The normal is 160 degrees in a child, decreasing to 130 degrees in adult life.

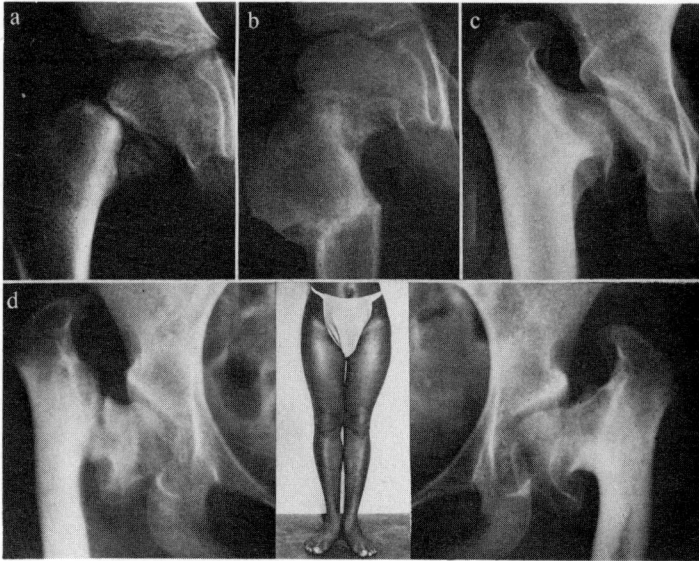

18.27 INFANTILE COXA VARA
(a) Growth disc too vertical and triangle of bone on under surface of neck; (b) abduction osteotomy should be performed early; otherwise (c) the shaft migrates upwards. (d) Bilateral infantile coxa vara — untreated — only a few inches of leg separation was possible.

CONGENITAL (INFANTILE) — The epiphyseal line is too vertical; with stress the shaft is gradually but inevitably pushed upwards. The condition is painless and presents as a short leg in infancy; clinically it is distinguishable from congenital dislocation by the fact that the head is in the socket. X-ray shows that the epiphyseal line is too vertical, and in the infant there is also a separate triangle of bone in the inferior portion of the metaphysis (Fairbank's triangle). Subtrochanteric osteotomy is necessary. If bilateral, the condition may not be seen until a young adult presents with osteoarthritis. Sometimes congenital coxa vara is associated with a congenitally short or bowed proximal shaft of femur (page 73).

ACQUIRED — Coxa vara can develop only if the neck bends (because it is soft) or if it breaks.
Bone softening — Bone softening may produce coxa vara in children (rickets, bone dystrophies and possibly Perthes' disease); in adults (osteomalacia); and in the elderly (osteoporosis and Paget's disease).

At any age, tuberculosis or pyogenic infection may soften bone and lead to coxa vara, but the deformity is overshadowed by the causal condition.

Fracture — Fracture may produce coxa vara in children (through a solitary cyst); in adolescents (slipped epiphysis); and in the elderly (mal-union of a trochanteric fracture).

OSTEOARTHRITIS
(*See also* Chapter 5)

CAUSES

Osteoarthritis of the hip is liable to develop in a relatively young adult as the sequel to congenital subluxation or dysplasia, Perthes' disease, coxa vara or following injury. In the older patient osteoarthritis may supervene on rheumatoid arthritis, or following injury (fracture or dislocation), especially when the femoral head becomes avascular. Avascular necrosis also occurs without injury (page 46).

Another precursor of osteoarthritis is protrusio acetabuli (Otto pelvis). This usually affects females and develops soon after puberty; at this stage there are often no symptoms though movements are limited. X-rays show the sunken acetabulum which may form as much as two-thirds of a sphere instead of the normal half.

Even when no cause is apparent it should be sought; minor degrees of slipped epiphysis probably account for some cases previously labelled ' primary ' (Murray, 1965).

PATHOLOGY

The pathology is described in detail on pages 46–48, but may be summarized as follows.

ARTICULAR CARTILAGE AND BONE — At the pressure area (top of the femoral head and acetabular roof) the articular cartilage is worn away, becoming thin and rough. The underlying bone becomes dense, hard, and sometimes cystic. At the non-pressure area the cartilage becomes thicker; it may ossify giving lipping and osteophytes.

SYNOVIAL MEMBRANE AND CAPSULE — Some synovial hypertrophy may occur. The capsule becomes thick and fibrosed. The hip is an 'extreme range' joint and, as the fibrous tissue shrinks, extension and abduction (which are needed in walking) are soon restricted. Symptoms therefore appear early and often become severe.

CLINICAL FEATURES

Pain radiates from the groin to the knee. At first it occurs when movement follows a period of rest; later it is more constant, more severe and sometimes disturbs sleep. Stiffness at first is also noticed only after rest; later it increases progressively until putting on socks and shoes becomes difficult. Limp is often noticed early and the patient may say his leg is getting shorter.

The patient is usually fit in himself and, unless there has been previous hip disorder, is aged over 50. The signs in the hip are as follows.

LOOK — The leg lies laterally rotated and appears short because of fixed adduction. There is also fixed flexion.

FEEL — The greater trochanter is slightly elevated and too posterior.

MOVE — Movements are diminished, but within a limited range are painless. The restriction is asymmetrical: abduction, extension and medial rotation are lost early and are the most restricted; their opposites are lost late and are less restricted.

Muscle wasting (chiefly of the glutei) is detectable but usually not severe.

True shortening is slight, but apparent shortening amounts to an inch or two.

X-RAY — At the pressure area (superiorly) the joint space is decreased and the bone sclerosed; acetabular sclerosis, whose shape has inspired the French term ' sourci ' may

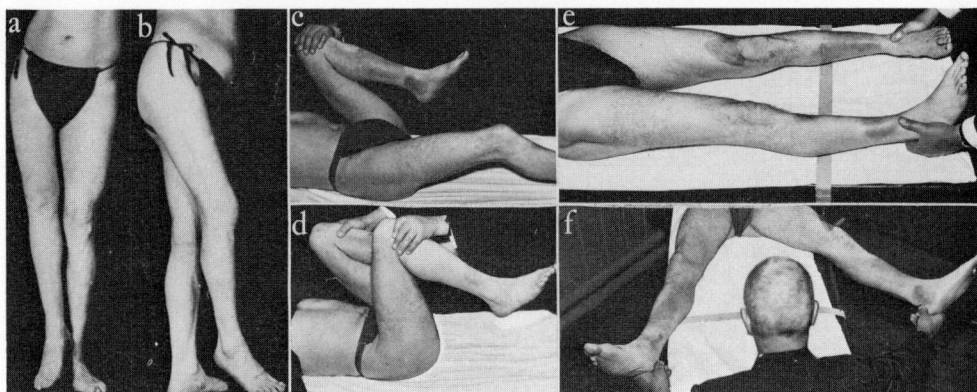

18.28 OSTEOARTHRITIS (1) SIGNS
The right hip is affected. (a, b) Apparent shortening with deformity. (c) Fixed
flexion. (d, e, f) Limitation of flexion, medial rotation, and abduction.

be the first sign. Elsewhere the joint space is not decreased, but lipping and osteophytes
may be seen. There may also be cysts in the femoral head and thickening of the under
side of the neck.

Note — The above description applies to the commonest type of osteoarthritis. In
a less common variety (probably secondary to low-grade inflammation) flexion
and extension are somewhat limited but other movements virtually absent; fixed
flexion is the only deformity, and the x-ray shows uniform ' concentric ' diminution
of joint space.

18.29 OSTEOARTHRITIS
(2) X-RAYS
(a) The common 'eccen-
tric' loss of joint space;
(b) cysts like these are
often associated with
pain; (c) 'concentric'
type of degeneration.

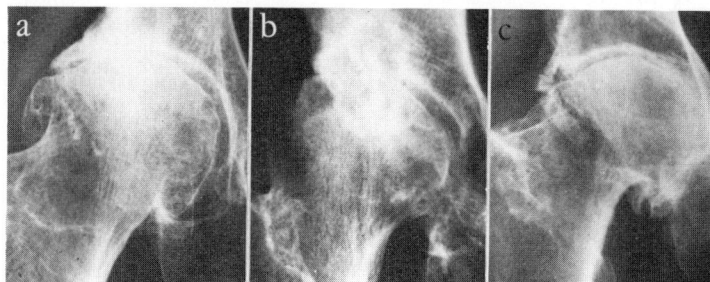

CONSERVATIVE TREATMENT (page 49)

Warmth is soothing and may be applied by rubbing in liniments, using a hot-water
bottle or electric pad at night, by radiant heat or by short-wave diathermy. The
patient is encouraged to try to preserve movement by non-weight-bearing exercises.
In early cases a manipulation under anaesthesia (accompanied by a hydrocortisone
injection) is often useful; the patient should try to preserve the increased range
obtained.

OPERATIVE TREATMENT

There are three main operations: osteotomy, arthrodesis and arthroplasty.
Osteotomy, if performed early, can arrest the degenerative process, or may even
reverse it so that the joint space re-forms and cysts heal. Arthrodesis is now rarely

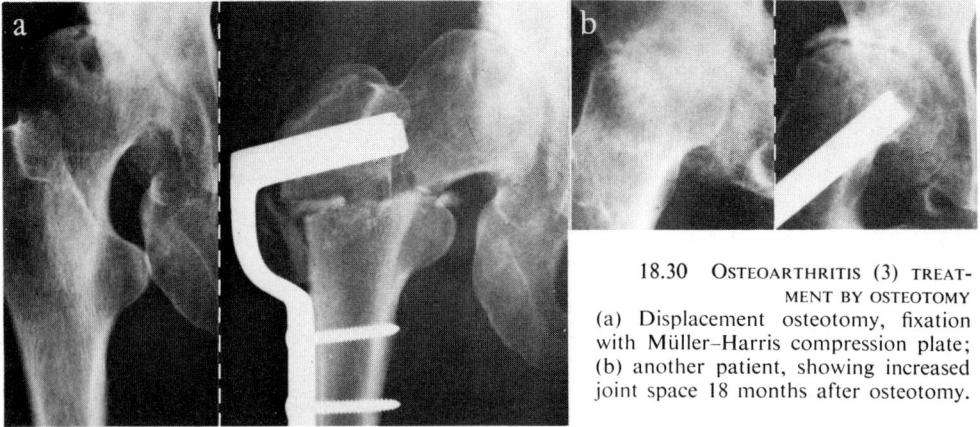

18.30 OSTEOARTHRITIS (3) TREAT-
MENT BY OSTEOTOMY
(a) Displacement osteotomy, fixation
with Müller–Harris compression plate;
(b) another patient, showing increased
joint space 18 months after osteotomy.

performed. The tide of opinion is against it, despite its great advantages in the young (*see below*). Arthroplasty, and especially total joint replacement, is much the most popular operation in those who are no longer young.

OSTEOTOMY — This is best performed early (before collapse of the head), in the hope that the disease will regress. Even when performed late it often reduces pain (especially pain at rest), it allows deformity to be corrected and some movement to be retained; but if movement is considerably limited before operation then the joint may become even stiffer afterwards. The femur is divided just above the lesser trochanter; fixed flexion is corrected, and the shaft abducted, brought to neutral rotation and its upper end shifted medially. Although the corrected position can be held in plaster, internal fixation is better, and a compression device is often used.

ARTHRODESIS — Arthrodesis is the only certain way to achieve total and permanent freedom from pain. Providing the 'compensating' joints (lumbar spine, knee and opposite hip) are fully mobile the patient has no pain, little limp, can walk long distances, run, and play vigorous games. The techniques of arthrodesis are illustrated in Fig. 11.2 and on page 255.

ARTHROPLASTY — Arthroplasty is theoretically the ideal treatment, and nowadays this virtually means total hip replacement. Cup arthroplasty is still occasionally used in a youngish patient, but as a remedy for osteoarthritis, femoral head replacement alone has been abandoned.

The technique and complications of total hip replacement are described on pages 132–135.

EXPOSURE OF THE HIP

Anterior (*Smith–Petersen*) *approach* — The patient lies on his back with a small sandbag under the affected buttock and a large one under the knee. The skin is incised from the anterior superior iliac spine upwards along the iliac crest for one-third of its length, and downwards for 12 cm towards the lateral side of the patella. The deep fascia is incised in the same line. The abductor muscles are detached from the lateral aspect of the iliac crest and the abdominal muscles from its medial aspect. From both aspects the muscles are separated subperiosteally by gauze dissection and a pack is left in to control oozing. The plane between the sartorius muscle medially and the tensor fascia lata laterally is deepened, preserving the lateral cutaneous nerve of the thigh. Retracting these muscles exposes the rectus femoris on the lateral side of which a leash of circumflex vessels is divided between ligatures. The rectus is then detached from the anterior inferior iliac spine and retracted medially with the psoas, exposing the hip capsule. To expose the

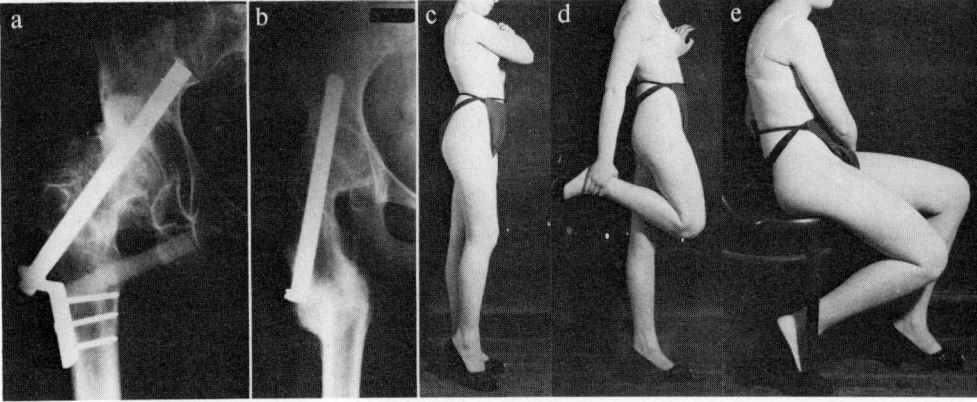

18.31 OSTEOARTHRITIS OF THE HIP (4) TREATMENT BY ARTHRODESIS
(a) Norwich V technique. (b) Pyrford arthrodesis with osteotomy; (c-e) patient
after Pyrford arthrodesis; (c) standing posture, (d, e) show why it is important for
the lumbar spine and knee to be fully mobile with an arthrodesed hip.

femoral head, the capsule is incised parallel to the neck. If dislocation is required the
capsule is divided in front and the femur rotated laterally.

Lateral approaches — Charnley, for his low-friction arthroplasty, advocates a lateral
approach with the patient supine. A 25 cm skin incision is made in the line of the
femur; its upper limit is at the level of the anterior superior iliac spine. The deep fascia
and ilio-tibial tract are divided, exposing the greater trochanter. The anterior capsule
of the hip is exposed by defining the interval between tensor fascia lata and the gluteus
medius and minimus. The capsule is incised in the line of the femoral neck, but not
excised. The greater trochanter is osteotomized about 1 cm above the attachment of the
vastus lateralis aponeurosis and turned upwards with its attached muscle and capsule.
The hip is now dislocated by adduction.

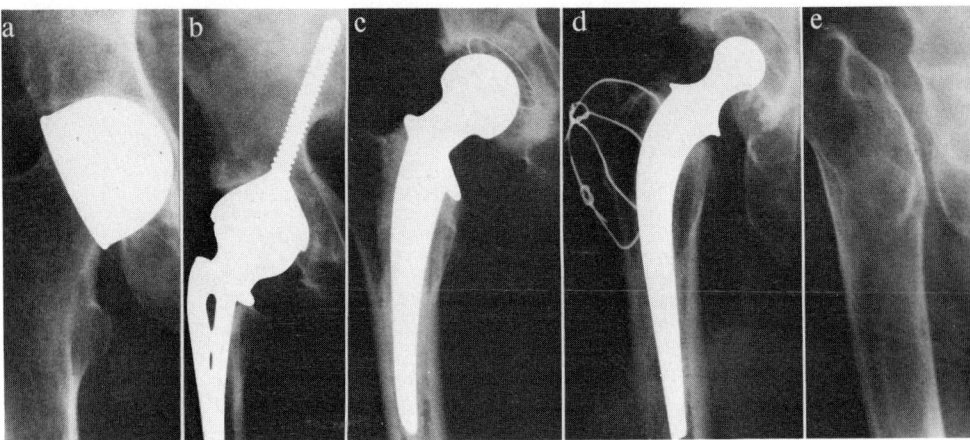

18.32 OSTEOARTHRITIS (5) TREATMENT BY ARTHROPLASTY
(a) Smith–Petersen cup, sometimes used in young patients. Total hip replacements:
(b) Ring; (c) McKee; (d) Charnley. Girdlestone's operation (e) has gained a new
lease of life as a salvage procedure.

For the McKee–Farrar hip replacement an antero-lateral approach is used. The patient is supine and the skin incision runs from the iliac crest (just behind the anterior superior spine) downwards and backwards to the greater trochanter, and then along the line of the upper femoral shaft. The interval between tensor fascia lata and the gluteus medius and minimus is developed, and by retraction the anterior hip capsule is exposed. It is thoroughly excised and the hip is dislocated by adduction and lateral rotation.

Posterior approach — The patient lies slightly prone of the full lateral position. The curved incision is centred over the greater trochanter, extending down the line of the femur for 10 cm, and for the same distance upwards and backwards towards the posterior superior iliac spine. In the line of the incision, the sheet composed above of gluteus maximus fibres and below of the ilio-tibial band is split: the posterior flap of this layer overlies the sciatic nerve. The small lateral rotators of the hip (pyriformis, obturators, gemelli and, if necessary, quadratus femoris) are divided near their insertions into the femur, turned back to expose the posterior part of the hip capsule, and used to protect the sciatic nerve. After capsulectomy, the hip may be dislocated by medially rotating the thigh. This approach is quicker than the anterior and lateral approaches, but access to the acetabulum is somewhat limited. It is not suitable for cup arthroplasty, but is excellent for prosthetic replacement. After operation the hip is stable to lateral rotation forces and the patient can usually be allowed up after a few days.

Suggestions for further reading

Catterall, A. (1972). 'Coxa Plana.' In *Modern Trends in Orthopaedics—6*, Ed. by A. Graham Apley. London: Butterworths

Charnley, J. (1972). 'The Long-term Results of Low-Friction Arthroplasty of the Hip Performed as a Primary Intervention.' *J. Bone Jt Surg.* **54B**, 61

Colton, C. L. (1972). 'Chiari Osteotomy for Acetabular Dysplasia in Young Subjects.' *J. Bone Jt Surg.* **54B**, 578

Griffith, M. J. (1976). 'Slipping of the Capital Femoral Epiphysis.' *Ann R. Coll Surg. Engl.* **58**, 34

Kemp, H. B. S. *et al.* (1971). 'Recurrent Perthes' Disease.' *Br. J. Radiol.* **44**, 675

Lloyd-Roberts, G. C. (1975). 'Some Aspects of Orthopaedic Surgery in Childhood.' *Ann R. Coll. Surg. Engl.* **57**, 1, 28

Lloyd-Roberts, G. C., Catterall, A. and Salamon, P. B. (1976). 'A Controlled Study of the Indications for and the Results of Femoral Osteotomy in Perthes' Disease.' *J. Bone Jt Surg.* **58B**, 31

Maurer, R. C. *et al.* (1970). 'Acute Necrosis of Cartilage in Slipped Capital Femoral Epiphysis.' *J. Bone Jt Surg.* **52A**, 39

McKee, G. K. and Watson-Farrar, J. (1966). 'Replacement of Arthritic Hips by the McKee-Farrar Prosthesis.' *J. Bone Jt Surg.* **48B**, 2, 245

Murray, R. O. (1965). 'The Aetiology of Primary Osteoarthritis of the Hip.' *Br. J. Radiol.* **38**, 810–824

Paterson, D. C. (1970). 'Acute Suppurative Arthritis in Infancy and Childhood.' *J. Bone Jt Surg.* **52B**, 474

Salter, R. B. (1961). 'Innominate Osteotomy in the Treatment of Congenital Dislocation and Subluxation.' *J. Bone Jt Surg.* **43B**, 518

Salter, R. B., Smith, W. J., Ponseti, I. V. and Ryder, C. T. (1966). Separate Articles on the treatment of dislocated hips in older children. *J. Bone Jt Surg.* **48A**, 7, 1390 *et seq.*

Salter, R. B. and Kostuik, J. (1969). 'Avascular Necrosis of the Femoral Head as a Complication of Treatment for Congenital Dislocation of the Hip in Young Children.' *Canadian J. Surg.* **12**, 44

Solomon, L. (1976). 'Patterns of Osteoarthritis of the Hip.' *J. Bone Jt Surg.* **58B**, 176

Wynne-Davies, R. (1970). 'Acetabular Dysplasia and Familial Joint Laxity: Two Etiological Factors in Congenital Dislocation of the Hip.' *J. Bone Jt Surg.* **52B**, 704.

CHAPTER 19

THE KNEE JOINT

EXAMINATION OF THE KNEE

Both knees are compared, and a man should have his trousers, shoes and socks off. It must be remembered that pain in the knee may be referred from the hip. Like the hip, the knee is examined in three distinct stages.

SYMPTOMS

The five common symptoms are pain, swelling, stiffness, mechanical disorders (such as locking, giving way, clicking), and limp.

SIGNS WITH THE PATIENT LYING ON HIS BACK

LOOK
Skin — The colour of the skin and any sinuses or scars are noted.
Shape — Wasting, swelling or lumps are observed.
Position — The knee may be held flexed, hyperextended, valgus or varus.

FEEL
Skin — Increased warmth is detected either by comparing the two knees or, better, by noting the temperature gradient of the affected limb.
Soft tissues — Any swelling or lumps must be examined. Swelling of the suprapatellar pouch may be due to fluid (when fluctuation, a patellar tap, or the bulge test can be elicited); or blood (which has a doughy feel); or thickened synovium (the edge of which is easily palpated). The bulk and tautness of the quadriceps muscle are estimated and, if necessary, the circumference of the two thighs is compared.
Bones — To identify the bony points and to localize tenderness, the knees should be flexed, if possible to 90 degrees. The joint is then palpated systematically with both thumbs: first the femoral condyles, then the tibial condyles and joint line, and finally the ligamentous attachments.

MOVE
Flexion and extension — Normally the knee flexes until the calf meets the ham, and extends completely with a snap; even slight loss of extension, or 'springiness' on attempting it, is important.
Abduction and adduction — These movements are virtually absent with the knee straight. Any laxity or pain on attempting angulation is noted.
Rotation — This is tested first with the patient's hip and knee flexed to 90 degrees and with one hand steadying and feeling the knee, and the other rotating the foot; rotation is then repeated with the knee in varying degrees of flexion. In McMurray's test, the knee is rotated in varying degrees of flexion while being subjected to an abduction force. There may be pain, or a click, or the cartilage may be felt to protrude.

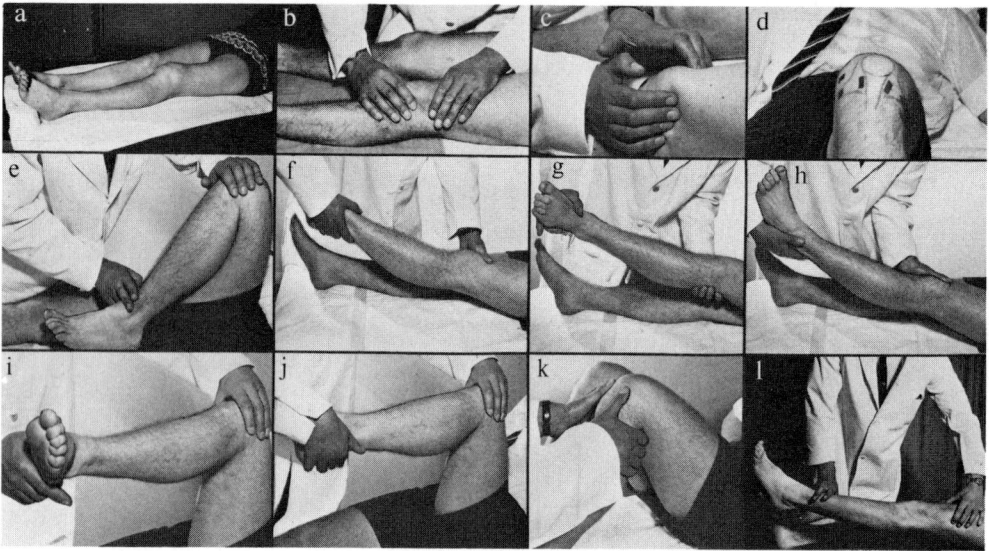

19.1 EXAMINATION OF THE KNEE (1)
(a) Looking at both knees — the left is swollen and the thigh wasted; (b) testing for
fluid by cross fluctuation; (c) feeling for synovial thickening; (d) the points which
should be palpated for tenderness.
Testing movements: (e) flexion, (f) extension, (g) abduction, (h) adduction. Lateral
rotation (i), medial rotation (j) and antero-posterior glide (k) are tested with the
knee bent; (l) testing quadriceps power. (Alternative methods are shown in Fig.
1.2 on page 3 and Fig. 19.11 on page 268).

Antero-posterior glide — The patient's hips are flexed 45 degrees and his knees 90 degrees.
The surgeon sits on the patient's feet and with both hands rocks the tibia backwards and
forwards; this test is repeated with the leg in medial and lateral rotation.

SIGNS AT THE PATELLO-FEMORAL JOINT

This joint is more often at fault than is commonly supposed. It is worthwhile
devoting special attention to it while the patient is still lying on his back.

LOOK — The appearance is usually normal.

FEEL — The size, shape and position of the patella are noted. Sometimes there is
tenderness around the edges of the patella and a portion of the articular surface can be
readily felt if the patella is pushed first medially then laterally.

MOVE — With the knee straight and the patella compressed against the femur, the patella
is moved from side to side and up and down. This 'patellar friction' test is positive if
painful grating occurs, indicating articular cartilage degeneration.

The 'apprehension' test is tried.   With one hand the patella is pushed laterally while
the other hand is used to flex the patient's knee.   If the patient has recurrent dislocation,
this movement is vigorously resisted.

SIGNS WITH THE PATIENT LYING ON HIS FACE

LOOK — Scars or swellings are noted.

FEEL — Any lump is palpated.

MOVE — The knee is flexed to 90 degrees and rotated while a compression force is applied;
this, the grinding test, reproduces symptoms if a meniscus is torn. Rotation is then
repeated while the leg is pulled upwards with the surgeon's knee holding the thigh down;

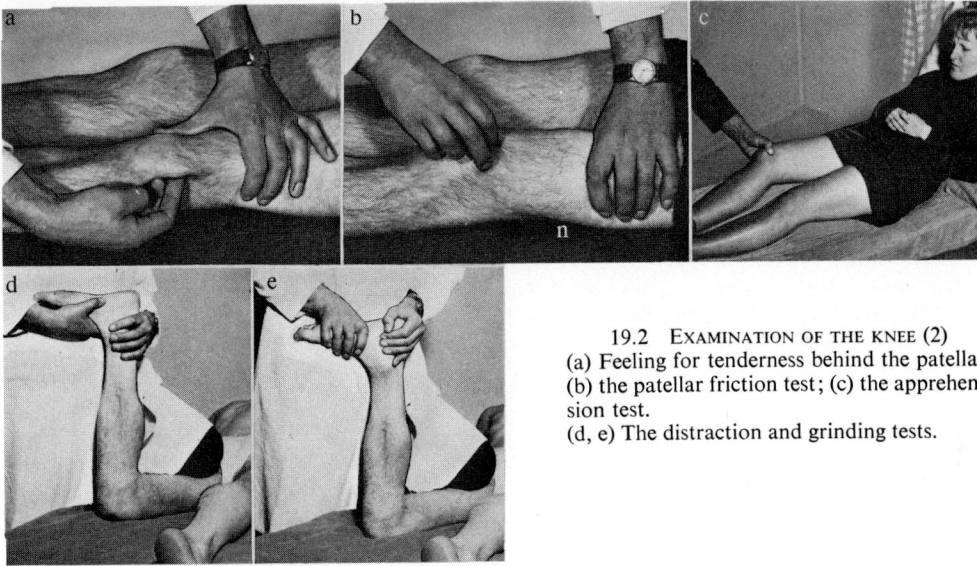

19.2 EXAMINATION OF THE KNEE (2)
(a) Feeling for tenderness behind the patella;
(b) the patellar friction test; (c) the apprehension test.
(d, e) The distraction and grinding tests.

this, the distraction test, produces increased pain only if there is ligament damage (Apley, 1947).

X-RAY

Antero-posterior, lateral and sometimes patello-femoral (or skyline) views are needed. It is worth while inspecting the tibio-femoral joint first, then the patello-femoral joint as a separate entity. When a loose body is seen, its origin should be sought; it should not be confused with a fabella, which lies on the lateral side and behind the line joining the femur to the tibia. Arthrography is useful in doubtful meniscal or ligament injuries.

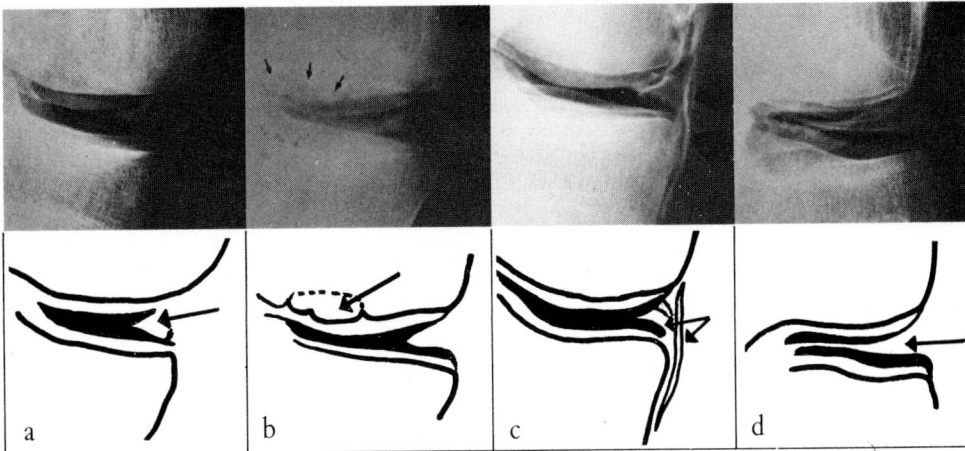

19.3 ARTHROGRAPHY
Double contrast technique. (a) Left knee — torn medial meniscus; (b) left knee — osteochondritis dissecans of medial femoral condyle; (c) left knee — torn medial meniscus with tear of medial collateral ligament; (d) right knee — discoid lateral meniscus. (By courtesy of Dr. J. Pemberton and Dr. M. J. Simmons.)

ARTHROSCOPY

Arthroscopy is useful: (1) to establish or refine the accuracy of diagnosis; (2) to help in deciding whether to operate, or to plan the operative approach with more precision; (3) to observe and record photographically the progress of a knee disorder. Arthroscopy is not a substitute for clinical examination; a detailed history and meticulous assessment of the physical signs are indispensable preliminaries and remain the sheet anchor of diagnosis.

Technique — Full asepsis in an operating theatre is essential. The patient is anaesthetized and a thigh tourniquet applied. Saline is injected into the joint and, through a tiny skin incision, the trochar and cannula introduced. Penetration of synovium is recognized by the flow of saline when the trochar is withdrawn. A fibreoptic viewer, light source and irrigation system are attached. All compartments of the joint are now systematically inspected; with some models limited biopsy is possible. Before withdrawing the instrument saline is squeezed out. A skin stitch is inserted and a firm bandage applied. Unless operative exposure has followed, the patient may leave hospital within a few hours.

DEFORMITIES OF THE KNEE

KNOCK KNEE (Genu Valgum)
CAUSES

IDIOPATHIC — This is much the commonest. It is almost invariably bilateral and is so common in young children that it may almost be considered normal.

OTHER VARIETIES — Many other conditions may be associated with knock knee. These include: (1) *bone softening*, occurring in rickets (especially delayed rickets and renal rickets), in bone dysplasias, and with rheumatoid arthritis; (2) *bone injury*, with epiphyseal damage, or following a fractured lateral tibial condyle; (3) *thinned cartilage*, when osteoarthritis predominantly affects the lateral half of the joint; and (4) *stretched ligaments*, in association with Charcot's disease, with paralytic deformities, and when a patient walks on a fixed adducted hip.

SYMPTOMS

With idiopathic knock knee deformity is the only symptom. In the other varieties there may also be symptoms due to the underlying cause.

SIGNS

IDIOPATHIC — Idiopathic knock knee usually appears at the age of 2–3 years and nearly always recovers by the age of 6. Other postural deformities such as flat foot may co-exist but these children are normal in all other respects.

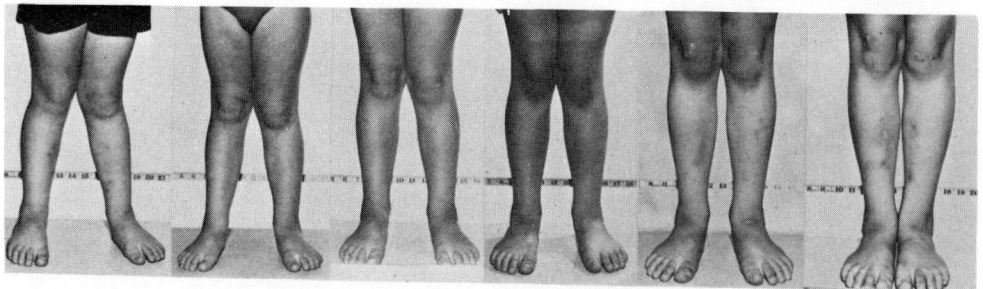

19.5 GENU VALGUM
Idiopathic knock knee — natural history without treatment.
Age 3 years 3½ 4 5 6 7.

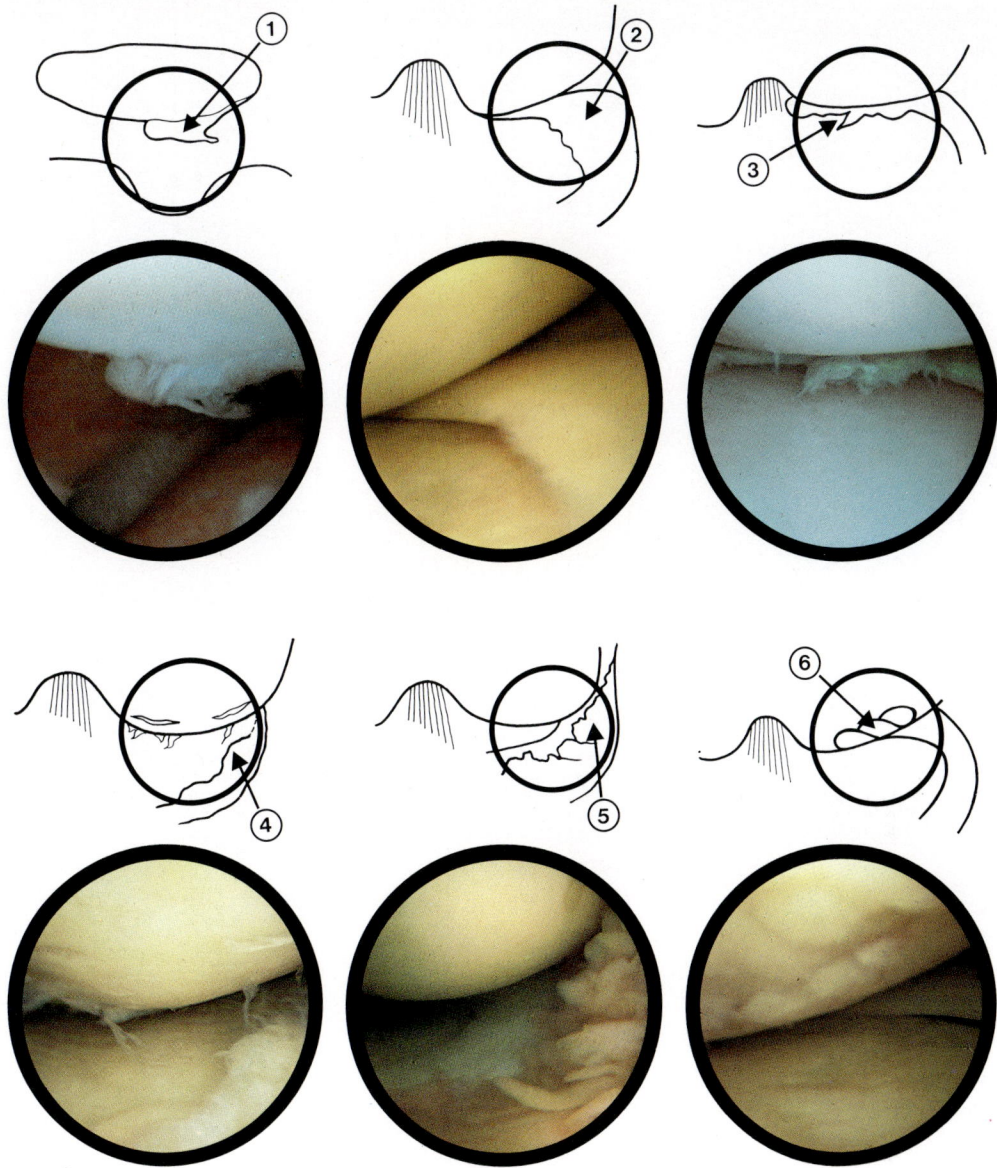

19.4 ARTHROSCOPY
In each case the view is of the right knee from the lateral side. (1) Chondromalacia patellae; (2) Normal medial meniscus; (3) Torn medial meniscus; (4) Degenerate medial meniscus and osteoarthritic femoral condyle; (5) Rheumatoid synovium; (6) Osteochondritis dissecans medial femoral condyle.

To estimate the amount of knock knee the patient is placed supine and the surgeon holds the legs.   They are rotated until the patellae face the ceiling and brought together until the inner sides of the knees touch each other.   The distance between the malleoli is then measured.

The joints are in all other respects normal to examine.   There is no swelling, tenderness or limitation of movement.   The x-rays also are normal (except that the lower femoral epiphysis may be somewhat sloping) and, indeed, x-ray films are unnecessary in this condition.   If, however, the deformity exceeds 10 cm or the knock knee is unilateral then x-rays are essential.

OTHER VARIETIES — In all these there may be general or local signs of the underlying abnormality.   Thus with renal rickets the child is usually anaemic and the knee deformity often develops rapidly in adolescence; with bone dystrophies and dysplasias other deformities may co-exist and the x-ray is usually diagnostic; with osteoarthritis movements are limited and painful.   Charcot's disease is characterized by joint laxity, bone destruction and calcified masses in the capsule.

TREATMENT

IDIOPATHIC — The child is seen at 3-monthly intervals and progress recorded.   The parents should be told that the legs will grow straight; almost invariably the condition requires no treatment.   Raising the inner side of the heels by an eighth of an inch may help to relieve strain on the ankles and helps to set the mother's fears at rest.

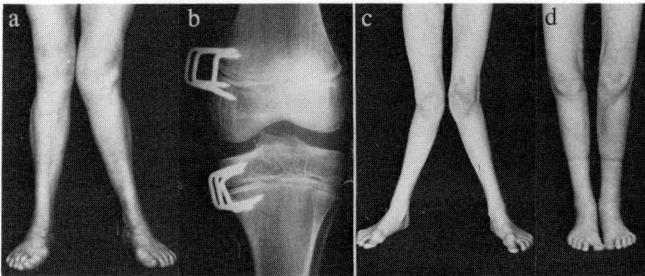

19.6 GENU VALGUM
Only rarely does knock knee persist: (a, b) an adolescent treated by stapling; (c, d) before and after bilateral osteotomy for severe deformity.

Splints were used extensively in the past.   Whether worn only at night or continuously, they are ineffective, unnecessary, and psychologically harmful.

In the rare cases of severe deformity persisting after the age of 10 years, correction is possible by (a) stapling the inner side of the knee epiphyses (the staples are removed when the knee has grown slightly varus); or (b) supracondylar osteotomy after growth is complete.

OTHER VARIETIES — Knock knee due to delayed rickets or dystrophy may require osteotomy but it is important first to exclude renal rickets because operation may provoke a uraemic crisis.   Knock knee following a fractured lateral tibial condyle rarely needs treatment; surprisingly, osteoarthritis does not follow.   Following epiphyseal damage osteotomy may be necessary, and when knock knee is associated with osteoarthritis the pain and deformity can be treated by low femoral osteotomy.   With Charcot's disease a caliper is usually necessary.

BOW LEGS (Genu Varum)
CAUSES

IDIOPATHIC — Some babies are born with slight bow legs, or develop the deformity while wearing napkins. These children nearly all grow straight.

OTHER VARIETIES — Other conditions which may be associated with bow legs include: (1) *bone softening*, occurring in rickets, and with Paget's disease; (2) *bone injury*, with epiphyseal injuries, and sometimes following fractures of the upper tibia; (3) *thinned cartilage*, in association with osteoarthritis; and (4) *stretched ligaments*, which may account for the bow legs of jockeys. A special variety, common in the West Indies, is tibia vara (Blount's disease) in which the postero-medial part of the proximal tibial epiphysis fails to grow normally.

SYMPTOMS

Deformity is the only symptom. In women, bow legs are considered ugly. When osteoarthritis supervenes, there is pain.

SIGNS

LOOK — The patient should be lying supine, the knees extended, the patellae facing the ceiling and the medial malleoli touching each other. The distance between the knees can then be measured; if more than 5 cm further investigation is needed.

FEEL — Usually no abnormality can be felt.

MOVE — There is full painless range, but, in adults who have had bow legs for many years, osteoarthritis is likely to be present.

X-RAY — This may show an oblique upper tibial epiphysis or occasionally evidence of an underlying cause.

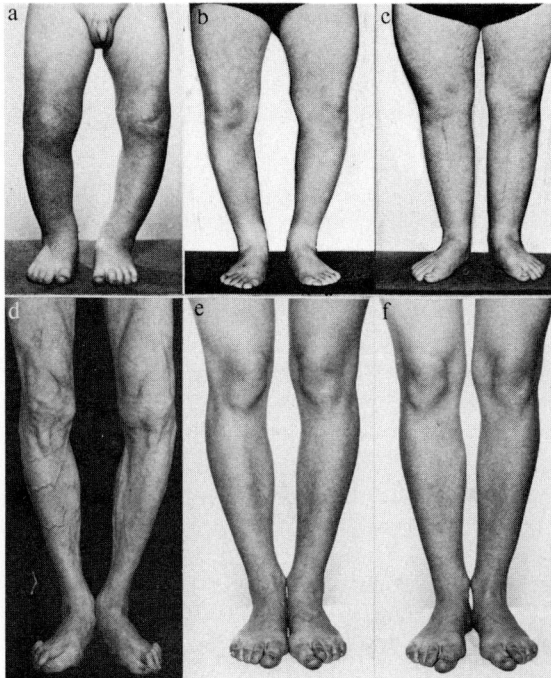

19.7 BOW LEGS
(a) Infantile, which usually recovers spontaneously.
(b) In this older child deformity persisted and osteotomy was performed (c).

(d) Bow leg in osteoarthritis.
(e) 'Apparent' bow legs due to internal rotation of the femora—(f) shows that when the patellae face forwards the deformity disappears.

DIFFERENTIAL DIAGNOSIS

The child with idiopathic bow legs may be brought up because of an intoe gait, which is more marked if there is an associated tibial torsion making the feet turn inwards.   Not uncommonly, however, the child with intoe gait is found to have no deformity of the knees or tibiae, but the hips rotate inwards much more than they do outwards.   This altered arc of rotation rarely needs treatment; only if severe and persistent should osteotomy be considered.

TREATMENT

Idiopathic bow legs usually recover, and in any case splints are probably of no value.   If bow legs persist beyond childhood operation is desirable, both for cosmetic reasons and to prevent osteoarthritis.   There are three methods: (*a*) closed osteoclasis of the tibia; (*b*) stapling the lateral side of the lower femoral epiphysis; or (*c*) upper tibial osteotomy.

HYPEREXTENSION OF THE KNEE (Genu Recurvatum)

CAUSES

1. CONGENITAL — A child may be born with considerable hyperextension of the knee due to abnormal intra-uterine posture; spontaneous recovery usually occurs.   Very rarely gross hyperextension is the precursor of true congenital dislocation of the knee.

2. LAX LIGAMENTS — Prolonged traction, especially on a frame, or holding the knee hyperextended in a plaster, may over-stretch ligaments leading to permanent hyper-extension deformity.   Ligaments may also become over-stretched following chronic or recurrent synovitis, the hypotonia of rickets, the flailness of poliomyelitis, or the insensi-tivity of Charcot's disease.   Generalized laxity of ligaments is described on page 7.

3. BONE INJURY — Epiphyseal injury may result in faulty growth, and a mal-united fracture also may lead to hyperextension deformity.

CLINICAL FEATURES AND TREATMENT

The symptoms and signs depend largely upon the underlying condition.   In itself, the hyperextension may be symptomless and may be accompanied by no other abnormal signs; but other evidence of ligamentous laxity should be sought, the patello-femoral joint examined for recurrent dislocation, and the knees x-rayed for bony abnormality.   If treatment is needed the possibilities are a caliper, soft tissue reconstruction (*see* page 114), or bone carpentry.

SWELLING OF THE KNEE

TRAUMATIC SYNOVITIS

Injury stimulates the synovial membrane to produce excess fluid.   When the fluid is synovial, with little or no blood, swelling is rarely obvious until several hours after injury.   The patient complains, not only of swelling, but of pain and weakness.

SIGNS

LOOK — A swelling extends from the joint into the suprapatellar pouch but not beyond it.

FEEL — The swelling is cold, fluctuant, and often a patellar tap can be elicited.

MOVE — Usually movements are as normal as the quantity of fluid permits. If the injury is recent, muscle tautness is lost.

X-RAY — Fluid in the joint may push the patella forwards so that in the lateral view it is too far from the femur.

TREATMENT

Quadriceps exercises are essential. If the muscles are allowed to waste, the knee loses stability and is easily resprained; a vicious circle is thereby set up. A crêpe bandage helps to control the swelling and is comforting.

The patient should be up and walking, but may need a back splint until he has regained muscle control; that is, until he can lift the straight leg against resistance.

NON-TRAUMATIC SYNOVITIS

Without injury, the knee may become swollen either gradually or rapidly, and the swelling may be transient, or chronic, or intermittent. Causes include.

INFLAMMATION — This group comprises acute (pyogenic or 'transient') and chronic (rheumatoid or tuberculous) inflammation.

DEGENERATION — In this group are osteoarthritis (including patello-femoral osteoarthritis) and Charcot's disease.

DOUBTFUL CAUSES — This group includes villous synovitis and recurrent synovitis.

SIGNS

There may be general signs of the underlying cause. The local signs, other than swelling in the suprapatellar pouch, vary with the cause.

In acute suppurative arthritis the joint is held flexed, feels hot and tender, movement is prevented by spasm, and the x-ray appearance is at first normal.

In transient synovitis there is slight wasting, a little increased warmth and tenderness, limitation of extremes of movement, and a normal x-ray appearance.

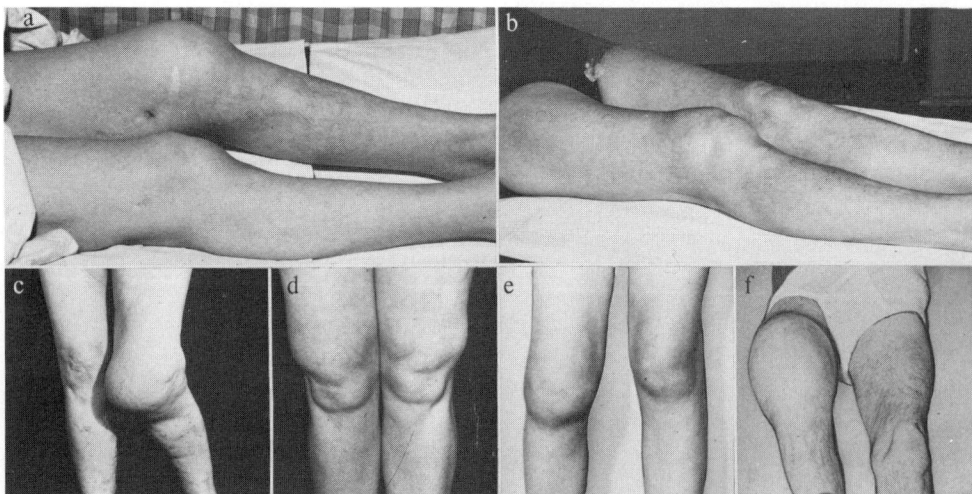

19.8 SWOLLEN KNEES
Some causes of chronic swelling in the absence of trauma—(a) Tuberculous arthritis.
(b) Rheumatoid arthritis. (c) Charcot's disease. (d) Villous synovitis. (e) Haemophilia. (f) Malignant synovioma.

In chronic inflammations due to tuberculosis or rheumatoid arthritis wasting is marked, there may be warmth and tenderness, movement is restricted and x-rays show generalized rarefaction.

In osteoarthritis wasting is slight, the joint is not warm, tenderness is usually localized, movement limited at extremes, and x-rays show diminution of joint space at the pressure area with underlying sclerosis and often lipping.

In Charcot's disease the joint is grossly swollen and deformed, neither warm nor tender, has abnormal painless mobility and x-rays show bone destruction and calcification in the capsule.

In villous synovitis there is gross synovial thickening, but often no warmth or tenderness, a surprisingly good range of movement and a normal x-ray appearance. Middle-aged women are particularly affected and sometimes both knees are grossly swollen. The folds of synovium may be pinched and bleed, so that the condition (thought to be a chronic inflammation) is sometimes called pigmented villo-nodular synovitis. Only rarely is synovectomy indicated.

HAEMARTHROSIS

In the absence of injury haemarthrosis is rare: it occurs in haemophilia (page 53) and occasionally in osteochondritis dissecans (page 56).

Following severe injury the joint may rapidly fill with blood and synovial fluid. The swelling becomes obvious within an hour or two and pain is often considerable.

SIGNS

LOOK — The joint is held flexed and the suprapatellar pouch is swollen.

FEEL — The knee feels warm, tense and tender; later it feels 'doughy'.

MOVE — Movement is painful and restricted and the quadriceps muscle cannot tauten.

X-RAY — There may be a fracture into the joint.

TREATMENT

The joint should be aspirated under aseptic conditions. If a ligament injury is suspected examination under anaethesia is helpful and may indicate the need for operation; otherwise a crêpe bandage is applied and the leg cradled in a back splint.

Quadriceps exercises are practised from the start. The patient may get up when he is comfortable, retaining the back splint until muscle control returns.

TUBERCULOSIS OF THE KNEE (see Chapter 4)

The blood-borne infection settles in synovium or in bone; the metaphysis or epiphysis of the femur or tibia may be affected, very rarely the patella. This early stage may heal by resolution or may progress to arthritis. After arthritis, healing can only occur by fibrosis, and a fairly short fibrous ankylosis is common. As the joint is superficial, sinuses are likely to develop.

CLINICAL FEATURES

Limp and ache are early symptoms; later there is swelling and stiffness with night cries and increasing deformity. In the active stage the signs are as follows.

LOOK — With early disease (synovitis or osteomyelitis) the joint is held slightly flexed and is a little swollen; muscle wasting makes the swelling more obvious. With late disease (arthritis) the joint is more flexed, wasting is gross and sinuses may be seen.

FEEL — The skin feels warm and a little fluid is sometimes detectable. With synovial infection the membrane feels thick and its attachments tender. With osteomyelitis there

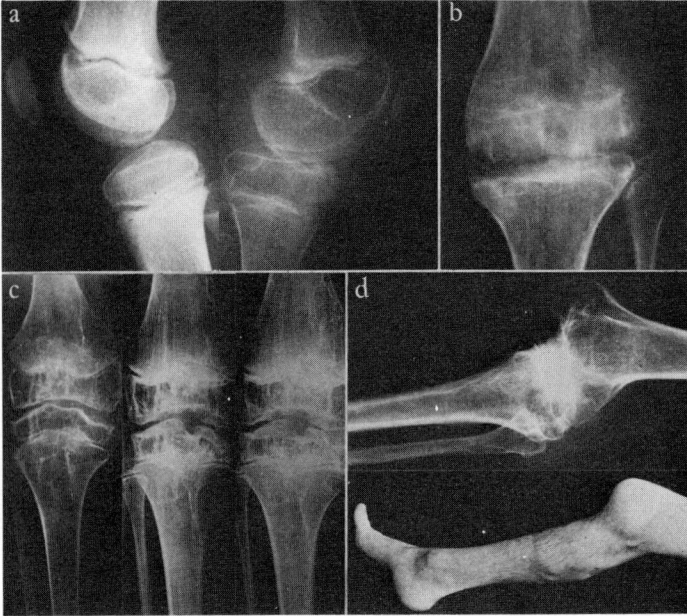

In synovitis (a) the bones are rare and the epiphyses enlarged compared with the normal side; (b) arthritis.

(c) Series showing healing with re-calcification, but with joint destruction. (d) The aftermath of arthritis.

may be tenderness over the bone focus. With an arthritis the soft tissues feel thick, 'doughy', and diffusely tender.

MOVE — With early disease the joint is 'irritable', that is movement in all directions is slightly limited and attempting to force an extreme of range is painful. With an arthritis movements are grossly restricted by spasm.

X-RAY — There is general rarefaction but so long as the articular cartilage is undamaged the joint space and line remain normal. With synovial infection the epiphyses may be enlarged, and with osteomyelitis a bone focus is seen. Once arthritis has developed the joint space is reduced and the line irregular.

As the disease heals, any pain subsides; the patient looks and feels well, and the joint is no longer warm or tender. X-rays show re-calcification. If the disease is arrested early, movement gradually returns; otherwise a varying degree of stiffness remains, and the fibrous joint, being unsound, may increasingly deform, and may give pain.

DIFFERENTIAL DIAGNOSIS

If treatment is to be effective, tuberculous synovitis must be diagnosed promptly and the most important conditions from which it must be distinguished are transient synovitis, and chronic synovitis of rheumatoid type presenting at a single joint. Both are common at the knee; whenever synovitis persists despite rest, or recurs with activity, further investigations are needed, including a full blood count, chest x-ray, serum latex test and, if necessary, a synovial biopsy.

TREATMENT

ACTIVE STAGE — Apart from general treatment (*see* page 35), the essentials are as follows.
Rest — A Thomas' bed knee splint is used.
Traction — Skin traction is applied and the tapes tied to the foot of the Thomas' splint.

19.10 TUBERCULOSIS OF THE KNEE (2)

TREATMENT

(a) Active disease—traction on a Thomas' splint.

Healing disease—(b) weight-relieving caliper; (c) patten and crutches; (d) removable polythene splint.

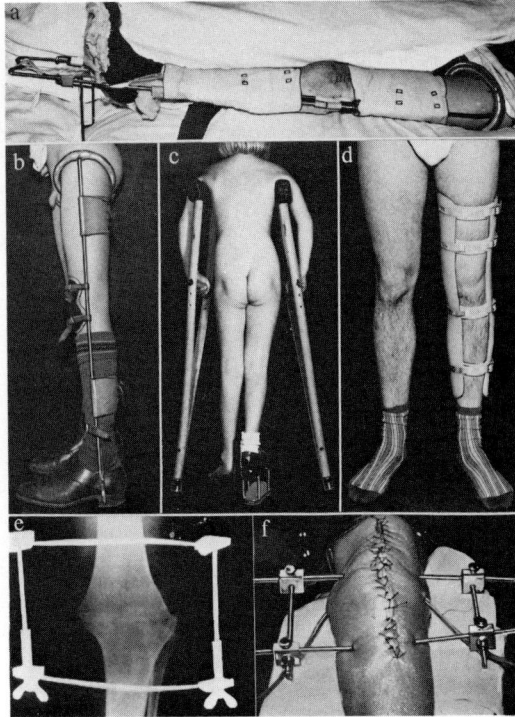

(e, f) Arthrodesis in the aftermath stage (Charnley's method).

Clearance — A bone abscess in the tibia should be evacuated. In the femur this is less advisable because the joint may become infected by the operation. With synovitis or arthritis a clearance operation should be considered if, after 6–8 weeks of rest and chemotherapy, progress is not satisfactory; the careful evacuation of dead and diseased material often accelerates healing.

HEALING STAGE — If the disease is arrested early, the patient is gradually allowed free, and got up wearing a weight-relieving caliper during the day. Gradually the caliper is left off, but frequent observation is essential. If the disease is arrested late, the aim is stiffness in the straight position. The patient is got up in a plaster tube or weight-bearing caliper, for which a removable polythene splint is later substituted.

AFTERMATH — An unsound joint is best arthrodesed. In children the operation is usually postponed until growth is almost completed.

Charnley's compression technique — The synovium and patella are excised and the bone ends sawn across. Steinmann pins are inserted transversely into the femur and tibia and the skin sutured. The pins are connected at their outer ends by clamps which are tightened firmly to compress the bone ends together. A protective plaster back slab is usually added. The clamps are tightened daily. After 4 weeks the pins are removed and a plaster tube applied. At 3 months union is sufficiently sound for splintage to be discarded.

LIGAMENT INJURIES

MECHANISM

The fully extended knee is stable, partly because the femoral condyles fit into the tibial condyles (deepened by the menisci), but chiefly because the capsule and ligaments are taut: in this position sideways tilt, antero-posterior glide and rotation cannot occur. The straight knee may sustain ligamentous injury as a result of hyper-extension or of a force applied from either side, but such injuries are rare.

Most ligament injuries occur while the knee is bent, relaxing the capsule and ligaments, and permitting rotation. The damaging force may be a straight thrust (e.g. a dashboard injury forcing the tibia backwards) or, more commonly, a combined rotation and impact injury to the bent weight-bearing knee as in a football tackle. A wide variety of complex injuries may result (O'Donoghue, 1973; Hughston, 1976); it is best to picture a damaged segment (of capsule and ligaments) rather than individual torn ligaments.

CLINICAL FEATURES

The history is misleading and the signs deceptive. Partial tears are easy to diagnose, but complete tears are often missed — for three reasons. (1) The story (of a sports injury, fall, or road accident), is always imprecise, unless an onlooker can describe it. More important, it seems perverse: thus, with a complete tear (in which nerve fibres also are torn) the patient has little or no pain, and can usually walk or even run in comfort (though he cannot pivot); with a partial tear the knee is painful and the patient lame. (2) Swelling also is worse with partial tears, because haemorrhage remains confined within the joint; with complete tears the ruptured capsule permits leakage and diffusion. (In either case it comes on within an hour or two — much sooner than the effusion of a torn meniscus.) (3) With a partial tear attempted movement is painful; the abnormal movement of a complete tear is painless or prevented by spasm.

The signs in the acute stage are as follows:

LOOK — Abrasions suggest the site of impact, but bruising is more important and indicates the site of damage.

FEEL — The doughy feel of a haemarthrosis distinguishes ligament injuries from the fluctuant feel of the synovial effusion of a meniscus injury. Tenderness localizes the lesion, but the sharply-defined tender spot of a partial tear (usually medial and 2·5 cm above the joint line) contrasts with the diffuse tenderness of a complete one.

MOVE — Partial tears permit no abnormal movement, but the attempt causes pain. Complete tears permit abnormal movement which sometimes is painless. To distinguish between the two is critical because their treatment is totally different; so if there is doubt, examination under anaesthesia is mandatory.

The important movements are: (a) sideways tilting, examined first with the knee straight, then at 30 degrees of flexion; (b) antero-posterior glide, tested with the leg neutral, then laterally rotated, then medially; and (c) rotation of the flexed knee in both

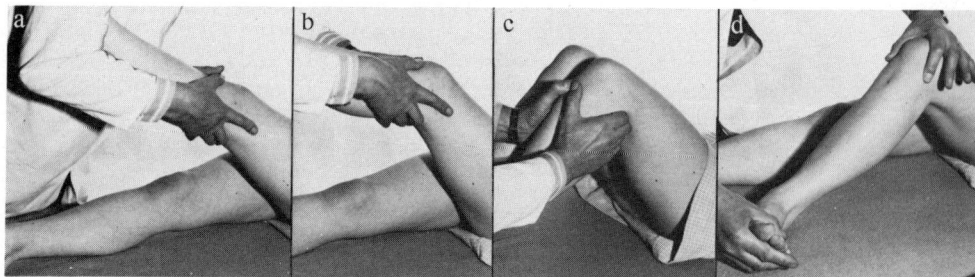

19.11   KNEE LIGAMENTS
Grips used in examination for abnormal movements. (a) Sideways tilting with the knee straight, and (b) with the knee flexed; (c) antero-posterior glide; (d) rotation of the flexed knee.

directions. Undoubted increase of any of these movements (as compared with the normal knee) is an indication for operation.

X-RAY — Plain films may show that the ligament has avulsed a small piece of bone, the medial ligament usually from the femur, the lateral ligament from the fibula, the cruciate ligament from the tibial spine. Stress films demonstrate if the joint hinges open on one side.

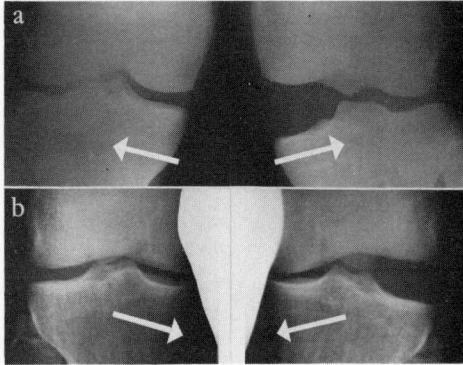

19.12 LIGAMENT INJURIES
Strain films show (a) complete tear of medial ligament, left knee; (b) complete tear of lateral ligament, left knee. In both, the anterior cruciate also was torn.

TREATMENT

PARTIAL TEARS — The intact fibres splint the torn ones and spontaneous healing will occur. The hazard is adhesions, so active exercise is prescribed from the start, facilitated by aspirating a tense effusion and injecting local anaesthetic into the tender area. Weight-bearing is permitted but the knee is protected from rotation or angulation strain by a heavily padded bandage or a posterior splint. A complete plaster cast is unnecessary and disadvantageous; it inhibits movement and prevents weekly re-assessment — an important precaution if the occasional error is to be avoided.

COMPLETE TEARS — In theory healing can occur providing the torn ends are closely apposed and held still in plaster, But the prospects of success are poor. Operation is wiser and affords the best chance of avoiding future instability. The guiding principles are: (1) operate early (the earlier the better and certainly within 14 days); (2) use a generous incision (if posterior structures also are torn and access inadequate, a second, posterior incision helps); (3) repair every torn structure tightly and, if possible, by re-attachment to bone (staples, or sutures through drill holes are useful); (4) protect the repair in an above-knee plaster with the knee 40 degrees flexed (the leg should be medially rotated if medial structures mainly are involved, laterally rotated with lateral damage).

COMPLICATIONS

ADHESIONS — If the knee with a partial ligament tear is not actively exercised, torn fibres stick to intact fibres and to bone. The knee ' gives way ' with catches of pain; localized tenderness is present and pain on abduction and lateral rotation. The obvious confusion with a torn meniscus can be resolved by the grinding test (page 258), or by manipulation and injection under anaesthesia, which is usually curative. Occasionally an abduction injury is followed by calcification near the upper attachment of the medial ligament (Pellegrini-Stieda's disease).

INSTABILITY — The knee gives way and is unreliable. The instability is progressive and eventually degeneration follows. Stabilization is desirable, but late operation only occasionally succeeds and may not last; so conservative treatment is important. Vigorous quadriceps excercises are essential; they are an indispensable preliminary to operation and may allow the patient to lead a normal life even without operation. With the addition of an external brace games may be possible.

If symptoms are unacceptable or a higher athletic standard is demanded, then stabilization must be considered; but if the patient also has a torn meniscus, it should be removed before embarking on more major procedures. Once stabilization is decided upon, the detailed anatomy of individual ligaments can be ignored; ligament repair is no longer feasible and the aim is to prevent abnormal movements.

Backward subluxation (straight or rotatory) cannot be prevented; nor can old cruciate ligament tears be repaired (though prosthetic replacements are being tried). Lateral hinging and forward rotatory subluxations can sometimes be prevented by tightening lax structures, re-inforcing them and, where possible, also providing an alternative control mechanism.

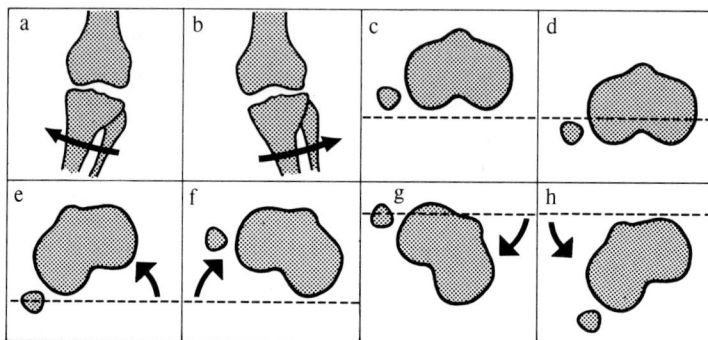

19.13   KNEE LIGAMENTS—INSTABILITY
Top row: Straight subluxations: (a) Tilting into varus (b) into valgus; (c) forward shift: (d) backward.
Bottom row: Rotatory subluxations of tibia: (e) Medial condyle forward; (f) lateral condyle forward; (g) medial condyle backward; (h) lateral condyle backward.

For lateral hinge — The lax medial structures can be tightened by re-attaching the upper end more proximally or the lower end more distally. The repair can be re-inforced by re-routing the semitendinosus tendon over the medial femoral condyle, or by advancing semimembranosus forwards.

For forward subluxation of the medial tibial condyle — This rotatory instability is often associated with lateral hinge. The same structures are therefore tightened, but the lower end is also moved forward, or the upper end backwards. A pes anserinus transplant provides additional and dynamic control; the lower two-thirds of the tendon group is detached, reflected upwards and sutured to the patellar ligament.

For forward subluxation of the lateral tibial condyle — With this rotatory instability tightening lax structures by re-attachment may be possible. A so-called pivot shift operation provides additional control; a strip of fascia lata is detached proximally, looped under the lateral ligament, then threaded through and sutured to the lateral intermuscular septum.

In all cases an above-knee plaster with the knee 40 degrees flexed and the tibia rotated so as to relieve tension is worn for 8 weeks. An arduous period of rehabilitation follows; during the early weeks a brace is a wise precaution.

MENISCUS LESIONS

TORN MEDIAL MENISCUS

The meniscus is split along its substance by a force grinding it between the femur and tibia. In the young, this can only occur when (*a*) weight is being taken; (*b*) the knee is flexed; and (c) there is a twisting strain; hence the frequency in footballers and miners. In middle life, when fibrosis has restricted mobility of the meniscus, tears occur with relatively little force.

The initial split may be in the anterior horn, posterior horn, or both (bucket-handle type). The torn portion may displace and become jammed between femur and tibia, blocking extension. Further injuries may extend the tear or cause secondary tears. Recurrent displacement leads to osteoarthritis.

A meniscus is avascular and is incapable of repair (unless the tear is peripheral). After excision, partial regeneration may occur, but the new 'meniscus' has a blood supply.

SYMPTOMS

An accurate history is all-important.

THE ORIGINAL INJURY — Only a twisting force to the bent knee while it is taking weight can split the meniscus. Following injury, there is pain on the inner side, sometimes locking and, within a few hours, swelling. Apparent recovery may occur. It is important to realize that, in patients aged 40 or more, the original injury may be apparently trivial.

FURTHER INCIDENTS — With relatively little force, the knee periodically gives trouble. With each attack, the patient may complain of locking (an unreliable symptom), unlocking (sudden unlocking is pathognomonic of a mechanical block), 'something moving', a click, or pain on the inner side, often with a click.

Locking — The term 'locking' is unfortunate, because a locked door is immovable, whereas a locked knee will flex but not extend. Moreover, the patient speaks of 'locking' when his knee is too painful to move, whereas to the surgeon locking means that extension is blocked mechanically. With a torn meniscus, usually only the last few degrees of extension (or rarely only of flexion) are prevented.

BETWEEN INCIDENTS — Between incidents, the knee is normal, unless the quadriceps muscle is wasted or a bucket-handle tear is in the intercondylar fossa.

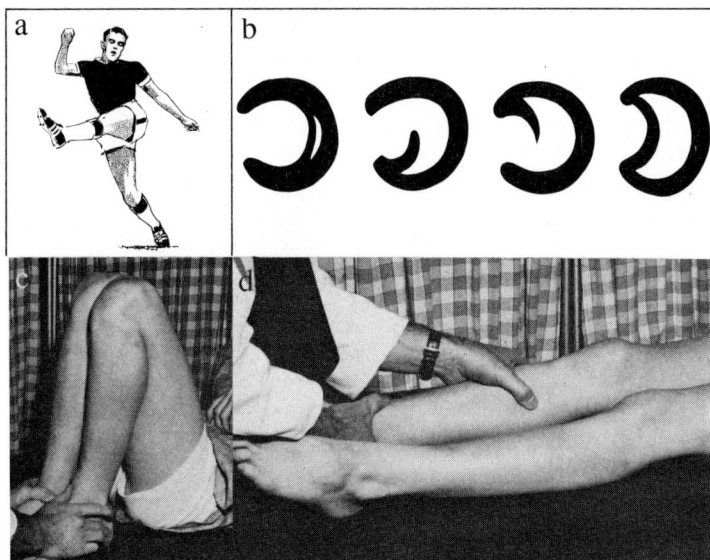

19.14 TORN MEDIAL MENISCUS
(a) The meniscus is torn by a twisting force with the knee bent and taking weight; (b) the initial split may extend; (c) a locked knee flexes fully but (d) lacks full extension.

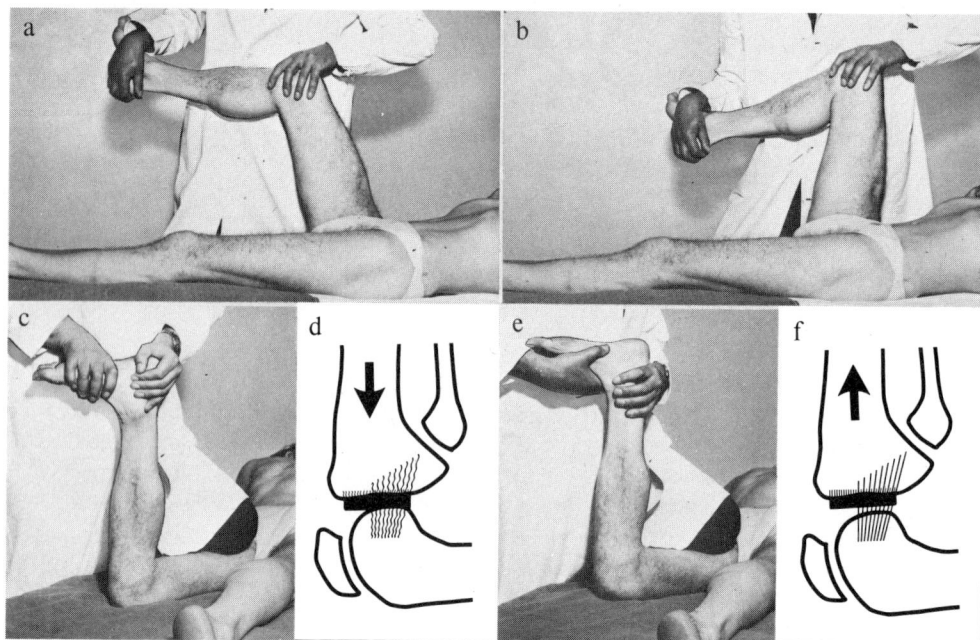

19.15   Torn medial meniscus — special tests
(a, b) McMurray's test is performed at varying angles of flexion.   (c, d) The grinding test relaxes the ligaments but compresses the meniscus — it causes pain with meniscus lesions.   (e, f) The distraction test releases the meniscus but stretches the ligaments and causes pain if these are injured.

SIGNS

About half the patients are fit young men; a few are young women indulging in 'manly' pastimes; the remainder (in whom the onset is often with trivial injury) are aged 40 or more.

The local signs depend upon how soon after an attack the patient is seen and whether the joint is still locked.

IF THE JOINT IS LOCKED — The joint is held flexed, but usually only 10–20 degrees.   The medial joint line is tender and there is some fluid.   Full extension is impossible; the attempt provokes pain and the surgeon feels an elastic resistance.   Flexion is almost full and usually painless.   Lateral rotation with the knee flexed may hurt.

IF THE JOINT IS NOT LOCKED — Soon after an attack the signs are the same as when the joint is locked except that extension is full.

ONCE AN ATTACK HAS SUBSIDED — Tenderness and pain on rotation may completely disappear.   Diagnosis rests upon the history, aided by special tests; namely, McMurray's test and the grinding test.

POSTERIOR HORN TEAR — A torn posterior horn rarely causes locking, and presents with a less definite history and less definite signs.   Tenderness is more posterior and the special tests often helpful.

X-RAY — The plain x-ray appearance is normal; arthrography may reveal the tear.

DIFFERENTIAL DIAGNOSIS

It is first necessary to make sure that (*a*) the lesion is mechanical and not inflammatory; and (*b*) the hip is normal, because hip pain is often referred to the knee. Once these two possibilities have been excluded the diagnosis is from the following:

OTHER CAUSES OF TRUE LOCKING

Loose bodies — The original history is different and the attacks variable in character. A loose body may be palpable and is often visible on x-ray.

Recurrent dislocation of the patella — The locking is more dramatic and throws the patient to the ground. The joint may be tender on the medial side. Attempts to reproduce the dislocation are painful and resisted.

Fracture — A fractured tibial spine (page 436) may be missed on x-ray. The joint cannot be fully extended but the history is unlike that of a torn meniscus and tenderness is in front.

ATTACKS OF 'PSEUDO-LOCKING'

Ligament injuries — The coronary fibres attaching the medial meniscus to the tibia may be damaged by a twisting injury. If adhesions develop, there are recurrent attacks of giving way, followed by pain and tenderness on the medial side. As with a meniscus injury, rotation is painful; but unlike a meniscus injury the grinding test gives less pain, and the distraction test more pain. Coronary ligament sprains can usually be cured by manipulation followed by exercises.

Chondromalacia patellae — Young adults complain that the knee gives way, especially on stairs. Pressing the patella against the femur with the knee straight, then moving it up and down and from side to side, reproduces the pain.

Fat-pad injuries — It is conceivable that an enlarged infrapatellar fat pad or a synovial fringe may become pinched on movement, producing sudden twinges of pain and giving way. Tenderness is not over the meniscus and there may be evidence of osteoarthritis.

TREATMENT

CONSERVATIVE — Conservative treatment is indicated in the following circumstances. (*a*) The patient is seen after the original injury and the joint is not locked. It is then justifiable to hope that the tear is peripheral and can repair. The knee is held straight in a plaster back slab for 4 weeks. Quadriceps exercises are practised. (*b*) Attacks are infrequent, not disabling, and the patient is willing to abandon those activities which provoke them.

MANIPULATIVE — Manipulation (if necessary under anaesthesia) is indicated if a joint is locked, but operation is inconvenient. The joint is rotated in varying degrees of flexion. Sometimes spurious unlocking is achieved because the torn fragment slips into the intercondylar fossa. Further symptoms are then inevitable.

OPERATIVE — Operation is indicated (*a*) if the joint cannot be unlocked, and (*b*) if symptoms arc recurrent. The meniscus should be excised, not only to cure the symptoms, but to prevent repeated damage to articular cartilage.

Technique of meniscectomy — A thigh tourniquet is applied and the patient lies on his back with the knee bent to 90 degrees over the end of the table. The skin incision may be transverse and directly over the meniscus (if the diagnosis is certain) or obliquely downwards and laterally (to avoid the infrapatellar branch of the saphenous nerve) if there is the slightest doubt. The capsule is defined, incised transversely just above the meniscus and undercut for ease of suture. The synovium is incised and when the meniscus is seen, the incision is extended transversely just above it. Fluid is mopped away and the joint carefully inspected.

The anterior horn is separated from the tibia by cutting first vertically, then horizontally, and the freed portion held in Kocher's forceps while the anterior attachment to the tibia is cut off. A retractor is placed in the medial side of the joint and the front of the meniscus is pulled laterally. The attachments to the tibia and to the medial ligament are carefully divided under direct vision until the whole meniscus can be displaced into the centre of the joint. The attachment to the posterior tibial spine is then divided, taking care to avoid the cruciate ligaments, and the meniscus is removed. (If the posterior horn is accidentally left behind it can be excised through a separate postero-medial incision; but the chances of disability following two incisions are as great as if the posterior horn is left.)

For closure, the knee is first straightened, the synovium sutured with continuous catgut (for haemostasis), the capsule with interrupted catgut, and the skin with wire or silk. A pressure bandage is applied and the tourniquet removed. Quadriceps exercises are started next day. Stitches are removed on the tenth day and the patient alowed to get up when he can lift the straight leg against resistance.

OTHER MENISCUS LESIONS

IMMOBILE MENISCUS

Degenerative fibrosis may limit the normal excursion of the medial meniscus on the tibia. The patient, usually aged 40–60 years, complains of aching and sometimes of swelling. The joint is tender over the meniscus and rotation is painful. The condition resembles an early osteoarthritic knee, but the x-ray appearance is normal. Heat, massage and deep frictions sometimes produce relief. Manipulation under anaesthesia accompanied by local hydrocortisone injection often helps. Meniscectomy cures the symptoms but is rarely necessary.

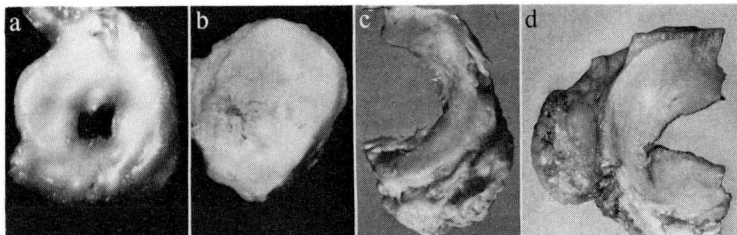

19.16 OTHER MENISCUS LESIONS
Whereas tears are much more common on the medial side, discoid meniscus and cysts are much more common on the lateral. (a) Partial and (b) complete discoid lateral meniscus; (c) cyst of lateral, and (d) of medial meniscus. These examples are all from left knees.

TORN LATERAL MENISCUS

The lateral meniscus is less likely to tear than the medial because its attachments permit freer mobility. An injury is followed by attacks of pain and giving way, but rarely locking. Tenderness is on the lateral side and rotation, especially medial, is painful. If the symptoms warrant, the meniscus should be excised.

DISCOID LATERAL MENISCUS

In the foetus the meniscus is not semilunar but disc-like; if this shape persists, symptoms are likely. A young patient complains that, without any history of injury, the knee gives way and 'thuds' loudly. A characteristic clunk may be felt at 110 degrees as the knee is bent and at 10 degrees as it is being straightened. The meniscus should be excised.

MENISCUS CYSTS

Pathologically, cysts of the menisci are probably traumatic in origin and not degenerative or neoplastic as formerly supposed; synovial cells become displaced into the vascular area between meniscus and capsule and there multiply. The trauma is usually minor and often forgotten, but months or years later the patient complains of ache or a lump. The ache is localized and intermittent, often worse soon after going to bed and sometimes after activity. The lump also may appear to be intermittent, so that for months at a time there may be no symptoms.

The lateral meniscus is much more often cystic than the medial, and the patient, usually an adult male, presents with a characteristic lump on the outer side of the knee. The lump is hard, almost bony, often just below the joint line, and most easily seen with the knee slightly flexed. Rotation may be painful and the grinding test positive. Medial meniscus cysts when they do occur are larger and softer.

If the symptoms warrant operation the meniscus should be removed; excising the cyst alone is inadequate because recurrence is likely.

EXTENSOR MECHANISM LESIONS

STRAINS, AVULSIONS AND RUPTURES

Resisted extension of the knee may tear the extensor mechanism. The patient stumbles on a stair, catches his foot while walking or running, or may only be kicking

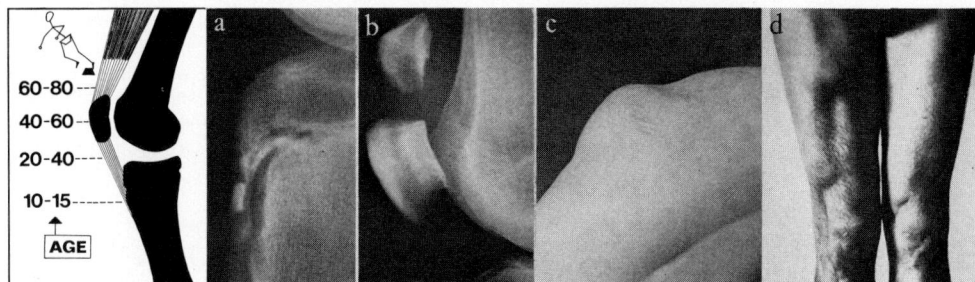

19.17 EXTENSOR MECHANISM LESIONS
These follow resisted action of the quadriceps; they usually occur at a progressively higher level with increasing age (diag.).
(a) Schlatter's disease — the only one which usually does not follow a definite accident; (b) gap fracture of patella; (c) ruptured quadriceps tendon (note the suprapatellar depression); (d) ruptured rectus femoris causing a lump with a hollow below.

a muddy football. In all these incidents, active knee extension is prevented by an obstacle. The precise lesion varies with the patient's age. In the elderly, the injury is usually above the patella; in middle life, the patella fractures; in young adults the patellar ligament can rupture. In adolescents, the upper tibial apophysis is occasionally avulsed; much more often it is merely 'strained'.

BELOW THE PATELLA

OSGOOD-SCHLATTER'S DISEASE — This condition is common. Although often called osteochondritis, it is nothing more than a traction injury of the apophysis into which part of the patellar tendon is inserted (the remainder is inserted on each side of the apophysis and prevents complete separation).

There is no history of injury and sometimes the condition is bilateral. A young adolescent complains of pain after activity, and of a lump. The lump is bony and tender and its situation in an adolescent is diagnostic. Sometimes active extension of the knee against resistance is painful and x-rays may show fragmentation of the apophysis.

Spontaneous recovery occurs and usually it is sufficient to restrict such activities as cycling and soccer. If symptoms persist a plaster tube is applied with the knee straight and is worn for 2 months. Occasionally symptoms persist and removal of a piece of cartilage or bone from the deep surface of the tendon is then worth while.

FRACTURE-SEPARATION OF UPPER TIBIAL EPIPHYSIS (*see* page 437) — This condition is uncommon. The displacement must be reduced under anaesthesia and held reduced in a plaster tube with the knee straight for 6 weeks.

AROUND THE PATELLA

Three lesions occur: transverse fracture of the patella; avulsion of the quadriceps tendon; and rupture of the patellar ligament. In all three the joint is swollen and held slightly flexed; a gap may be palpable and the patient is unable to lift his leg with the knee straight. The essential treatment is the repair of the extensor mechanism.

TRANSVERSE FRACTURE OF PATELLA (*see also* page 439).—This, the commonest lesion, occurs in middle life. The fractured patella may be repaired or excised, but the essential is reconstitution of the extensor mechanism, including repair of the lateral expansions which are always torn. A plaster back slab is applied, in which the patient soon gets up. This support is needed until powerful active extension is regained, usually about 6 weeks; meanwhile non-weight-bearing exercises assist in regaining flexion.

AVULSION OF QUADRICEPS TENDON — Avulsion from the upper border of the patella occurs in elderly people and is sometimes bilateral. Operative repair is essential and the after-care is as for a fratured patella. Sometimes avulsion of the tendon is only partial and no operation is then needed.

RUPTURE OF PATELLAR LIGAMENT — This occurs in young adults. Sometimes the ligament is avulsed from the lower pole of the patella. Operative repair is necessary and the after-care is the same as for a fractured patella.

ABOVE THE PATELLA

RUPTURE OF RECTUS FEMORIS — This lesion occurs in the belly of the rectus femoris muscle well above the knee. Usually the patient is elderly and, as the tissues are degenerate, suture is not feasible. The avulsed muscle fibres retract and form a characteristic lump, which becomes more obvious and harder when the muscle is put into action. Function is usually good, so that no treatment is required.

Occasionally a similar injury, but at the musculo-tendinous junction, occurs in young athletes. If it is diagnosed early, suture is probably advisable, or athletic prowess is likely to be reduced.

RECURRENT DISLOCATION OF PATELLA

CAUSES

LAX LIGAMENTS—In generalized joint hypermobility (page 7) the knees hyperextend, and recurrent patellar dislocation is common.
WEAK MUSCLES — Following reduction of a traumatic patellar dislocation the muscles must be exercised vigorously; otherwise, weakness (especially of vastus medialis) facilitates recurrence.

ANATOMICAL ABNORMALITIES — With normal ligaments and muscles dislocation is prevented by a bony ridge on the lateral femoral condyle. This checking mechanism fails if the ridge is poorly developed, if the patella is too small or too high, or if the knee hyperextends. Genu valgum also favours dislocation because the line of quadriceps pull exerts a lateral force on the patella.

PATHOLOGY

Dislocation is always to the lateral side. The capsule on the medial side of the patella is torn and, if it fails to unite properly, lateral laxity persists. Repeated dislocation damages the contiguous surfaces of patella and femoral condyle; degenerative changes follow which may result in flattening of the condyle, so facilitating further dislocations.

SYMPTOMS AND SIGNS

Sudden attacks occur without injury. The knee gets stuck (though often only momentarily) in a much more flexed position than with meniscus injuries, and the patient is thrown to the ground. The patella always dislocates laterally; but the patient may think it has displaced medially because the uncovered medial femoral condyle shows as a lump. Between attacks the patient has no symptoms.

Young adults, usually females, are affected, and the condition may be bilateral. If the knee is seen while the patella is dislocated, diagnosis is obvious. The signs between attacks are as follows.

LOOK — Usually the appearance is normal, but the knee may hyperextend.

FEEL — The patella may be too small or too high.

MOVE — Full painless range of the knee is present, but one special test is nearly always positive: try to push the patella laterally while flexing the knee; this is painful and is vigorously resisted. (The term 'apprehension test' has been coined because the patient fears that dislocation will recur.)

After repeated dislocations, moving the patella against the femur may produce painful grating, indicating that chondromalacia (see below) has supervened.

X-RAY — The appearance is usually normal.

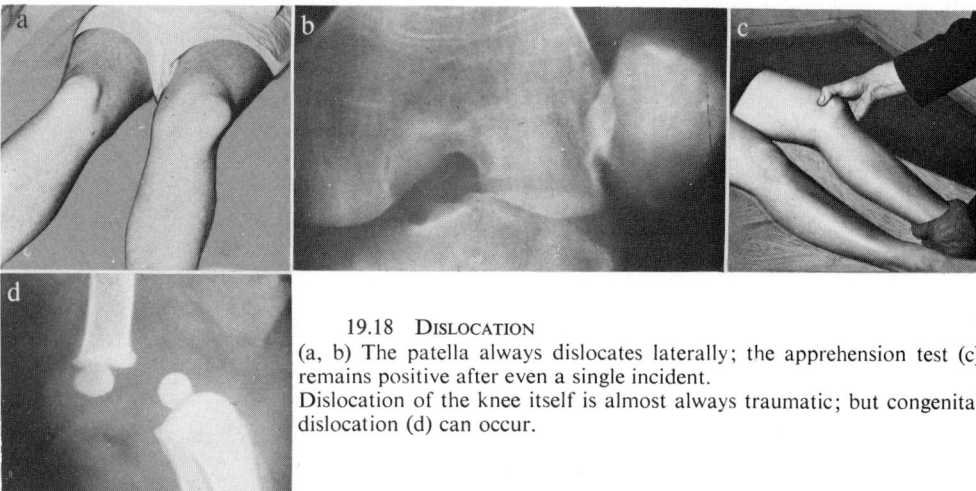

19.18 DISLOCATION
(a, b) The patella always dislocates laterally; the apprehension test (c) remains positive after even a single incident.
Dislocation of the knee itself is almost always traumatic; but congenital dislocation (d) can occur.

TREATMENT

The first time a patella dislocates it should be reduced, temporarily rested in a plaster back slab and the quadriceps muscle vigorously and repeatedly exercised.

Once dislocation has recurred, treatment is operative. Two operations give good results—re-alignment and patellectomy: with either the capsule lateral to the patella should be incised ('released') and the medial capsule tightened by reefing. Re-alignment, which leaves a big scar, is indicated if the articular cartilage of the patella is normal; otherwise patellectomy, which leaves an almost invisible scar, is preferred. With manifest chondromalacia it is feasible to combine both procedures at the one operation.

RE-ALIGNMENT — The patellar ligament with the segment of bone into which it is inserted is freed and re-attached further medially and further distally. Alternatively, the lateral half of the patellar ligament is detached, threaded through the medial half and re-attached more medially and distally. Either procedure prevents dislocation, but if chondromalacia is already present it may progress and subsequent patellectomy will be required.

PATELLECTOMY — The patella is excised and the resulting gap repaired. Chondromalacia is now impossible, but the repaired tendon itself occasionally dislocates, and then subsequent re-alignment as above is necessary. Either operation is therefore sometimes the precursor of the other.

OTHER VARIETIES OF DISLOCATION — Apart from traumatic and recurrent dislocation, there are two kinds: (1) congenital, in which, throughout life, the patella is laterally placed; and (2) habitual, in which dislocation occurs every time the knee is bent.

RECURRENT SUBLUXATION

Recurrent subluxation of the patella is probably more common than usually supposed. The apprehension test is usually positive and chondromalacia may supervene. Treatment is the same as for recurrent dislocation.

CHONDROMALACIA PATELLAE

CAUSE AND PATHOLOGY

The articular cartilage of the patella may be damaged by a single injury, by friction against a ridge on the medial femoral condyle, or by recurrent displacement (subluxation or dislocation); even without displacement a faulty line of quadriceps pull might cause damage. These possibilities alone, however, do not adequately explain the frequency of patello-femoral pain in teenagers, often with no relevant

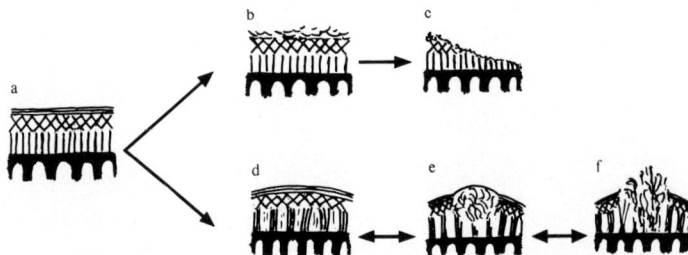

19.19 CHONDROMALACIA PATELLAE — GOODFELLOW'S HYPOTHESIS
(a) Normal. (b) Surface flaking, and (c) fibrillation, are stages of superficial degeneration which is painless. (d) Early fasciculation, (e) blister formation and (f) late fasciculation are all stages of deep degeneration, which is painful. (By courtesy of J. Goodfellow *et al*., and of the Editor of the Journal of Bone and Joint Surgery.)

history and no abnormal signs; nor the fact that, while most recover spontaneously, a few persist and progress. For these a rational hypothesis is suggested by the work of Goodfellow *et al.* (1976).

Two contrasting kinds of articular cartilage degeneration are postulated: superficial and deep. The superficial is painless; the surface looks dull with flaking and fibrillation; it does not heal and after very many years may lead to osteoarthritis. Deep degeneration is painful; the surface looks normal, though it feels spongy and later a blister or cauliflower-like excrescence may be seen; it often heals spontaneously but occasionally pain persists and progresses until relieved by operation. Fig. 19.19. shows the suggested sequence of events.

SYMPTOMS AND SIGNS

Only occasionally is there a history of injury. Usually the patient complains of attacks of pain, especially on stairs, and of occasional swelling. Later, the knee tends to give way, but true locking does not occur unless there are loose bodies.

Young adults, especially females, are affected.

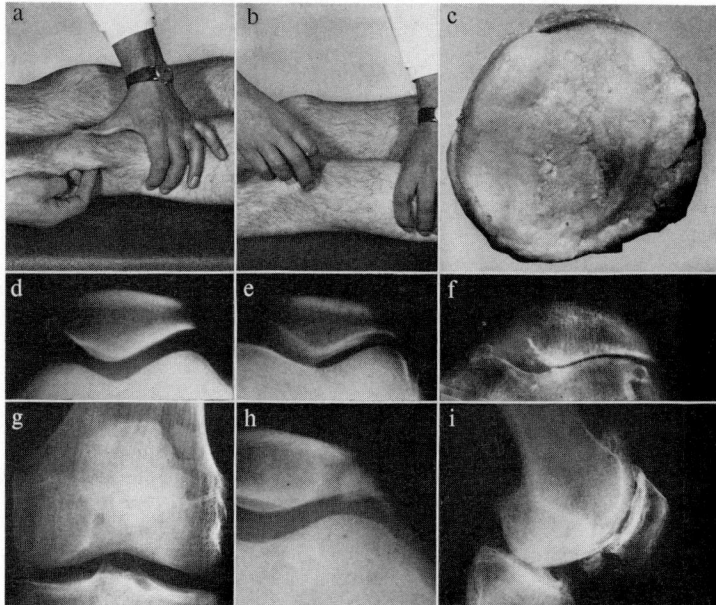

19.20 CHONDROMALACIA PATELLAE
(a) Tenderness behind the patella; (b) pain on patellar friction (c) well marked chondromalacia.

Sky-line views: (d) normal joint, (e) early degeneration, (f) late degeneration.

(g) Bipartite patella which may cause symptoms if (h) the small fragment is out of step; (i) gross osteoarthritis of patello-femoral joint.

LOOK — Slight swelling due to fluid may occasionally be seen; otherwise the appearance is normal.

FEEL — Sometimes there is tenderness of the patellar margin or of its articular surface (which is not difficult to feel if the patella is pushed sideways).

MOVE — Usually knee movements are full and painless, but when the patella is pressed against the femur and is moved (the patellar friction test), there is painful grating.

X-RAY — At first the appearance is usually normal, although tomograms may reveal patellar cysts. Later the patello-femoral joint space narrows and still later osteoarthritic changes appear.

TREATMENT

The patient is advised to avoid violent activity but encouraged to practise non-weight-bearing exercises. Short-wave diathermy also appears to help some patients, but this may be coincidence because spontaneous recovery is not uncommon.

If symptoms are excessively prolonged, or if patellar signs are manifest, operation must be considered. Goodfellow excises the affected disc of articular cartilage; while more likely to succeed than 'shaving' (i.e. paring the surface smooth with a knife), this operation is not yet established. Other possible procedures include: (1) lateral release, i.e. incising the lateral capsule in the hope of correcting faulty alignment; (2) combining lateral release with medial capsule reefing; (3) combining both with transferring part or all of the patellar tendon further medially; (4) levering the front of the upper tibia forwards (Maquet, 1976) thereby lifting the patella away from the femur; and (5) patellectomy. The multiplicity of operations indicates the unsatisfactory state of our knowledge.

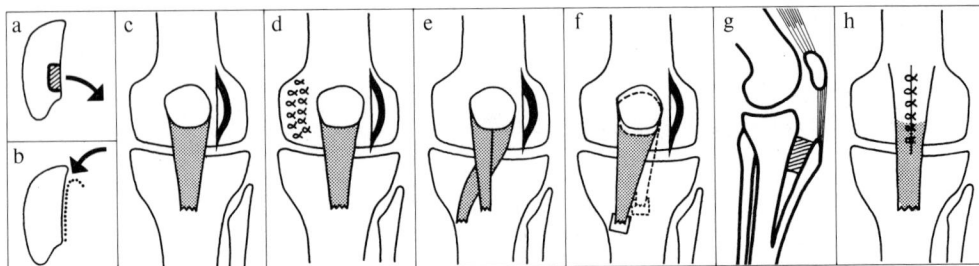

19.21 CHONDROMALACIA PATELLAE — TREATMENT
(a) Excision of diseased area; (b) ' shaving '; (c) incision of lateral capsule (release); (d) lateral release and medial reefing; (e) release and transfer of part of tendon (Goldthwait); (f) release and transfer of entire extensor insertion (Hauser); (g) tibial tubercle advancement; (h) patellectomy.

CONTRACTURE OF THE QUADRICEPS

The quadriceps muscle may become fibrosed and shortened because of congenital disorders, or as a result of repeated injections into the muscle. The vastus intermedius is most commonly involved and the child presents with progressive loss of knee flexion. If the vastus lateralis and ilio-tibial tract are involved, habitual dislocation of the patella is the usual sequel. Division of the affected muscle is necessary in either case.

OTHER DISORDERS OF THE KNEE

BURSAE

PRE-PATELLAR BURSITIS (HOUSEMAID'S KNEE)

An uninfected bursitis is due not to pressure but to constant friction between skin and patella. It occurs in carpet layers and miners but rarely in housemaids, who use vacuum cleaners. The swelling is circumscribed and fluctuant, but the joint itself is normal. Treatment consists of firm bandaging and kneeling is avoided; occasionally aspiration is needed. In chronic cases the lump is best excised.

Infection (possibly due to foreign body implantation) results in a warm, tender swelling. Treatment is by rest, antibiotics and, if necessary, aspiration or incision.

INFRAPATELLAR BURSITIS (CLERGYMAN'S KNEE)

The swelling is superficial to the patellar ligament, being more distally placed than pre-patellar bursitis because one who prays kneels more uprightly than one who scrubs. Treatment is similar to that for pre-patellar bursitis. Occasionally the bursa is affected in gout or syphilis.

SEMI-MEMBRANOSUS BURSA

The bursa between the semi-membranosus and the medial head of the gastrocnemius may become enlarged in children or adults. It presents usually as a painless lump behind the knee, more obvious with the knee straight. The lump is fluctuant but the fluid cannot be pushed into the joint, presumably because the muscles compress and obstruct the normal communication. The knee joint is normal. Occasionally the lump aches and if so it may be excised through a transverse incision.

Two other swellings behind the knee may be confused with an enlarged semi-membranosus bursa.

POPLITEAL CYST — This follows synovial rupture or herniation, so that the joint itself is abnormal; it may be osteoarthritic (the term Baker's cyst is then used) or, more commonly, rheumatoid. The lump is in the mid-line and fluctuates, but is not tender. It may diminish following aspiration and injection of hydrocortisone; excision is not advised,

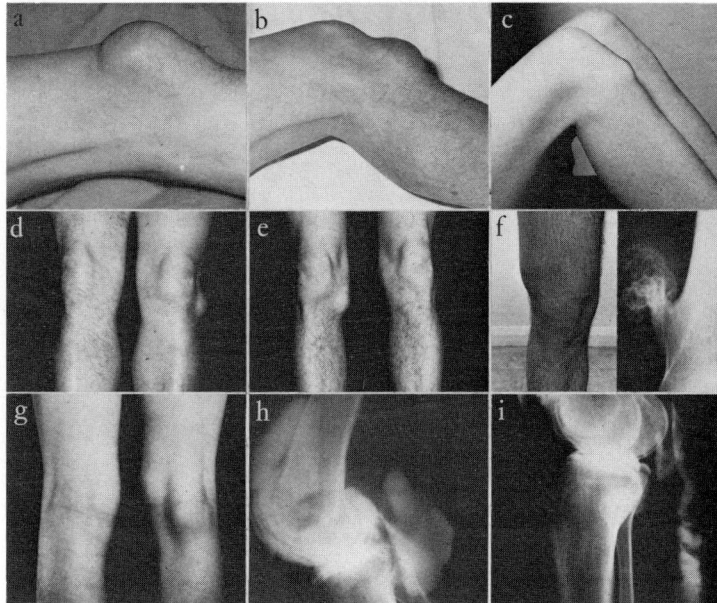

19.22 LUMPS ROUND THE KNEE
In front: (a) prepatellar bursa; (b) infrapatellar bursa; (c) Schlatter's disease.

On either side: (d) cyst of lateral meniscus; (e) cyst of medial meniscus; (f) cancellous osteoma.

Behind: (g) semimembranosus bursa; (h) arthrogram of popliteal cyst; (i) leaking cyst.

because recurrence is common unless the underlying condition also is treated (e.g. by synovectomy).

The cyst may leak or rupture; fluid then tracks down the calf which becomes swollen and tender, mimicking a calf vein thrombosis.

POPLITEAL ANEURYSM — This is the commonest limb aneurysm and is sometimes bilateral. Pain and stiffness of the knee may precede the symptoms of peripheral arterial disease so that it is essential to examine any lump behind the knee for pulsation.

LOOSE BODIES

CAUSE AND PATHOLOGY

INJURY — A piece of bone and cartilage may be broken off by a single definite injury. Osteochondritis dissecans (see page 56) may be traumatic in origin.

DEGENERATION — In osteoarthritis small osteophytes may break off and in Charcot's disease large loose bodies are common.

INFLAMMATION — Small fibrinous loose bodies may occur in chronic inflammatory conditions, but in these the underlying disorder is the dominant feature.

IDIOPATHIC — A synovial villus may hypertrophy, forming at its tip a fibrous nodule which may calcify and sometimes becomes detached. Occasionally a wide area of synovium is similarly affected, a condition known as chondromatosis, or (if the loose bodies calcify) osteochondromatosis. Numerous nodules and loose bodies develop; as many as 700 have been removed from a joint.

SYMPTOMS AND SIGNS

Loose bodies may be symptomless. The usual complaint is of attacks of pain and of sudden locking without injury. The joint gets stuck in a position which varies from one attack to another. Sometimes the locking is only momentary and usually the patient can wriggle the knee until it suddenly unlocks.

In adolescents, a loose body is usually due to osteochondritis dissecans, rarely to injury. In adults, osteoarthritis is the most frequent cause.

Only rarely is the patient seen with the knee still locked. Sometimes, especially after the first attack, there is synovitis or there may be evidence of the underlying cause. A pedunculated loose body may be felt; one which is truly loose tends to slip away during palpation.

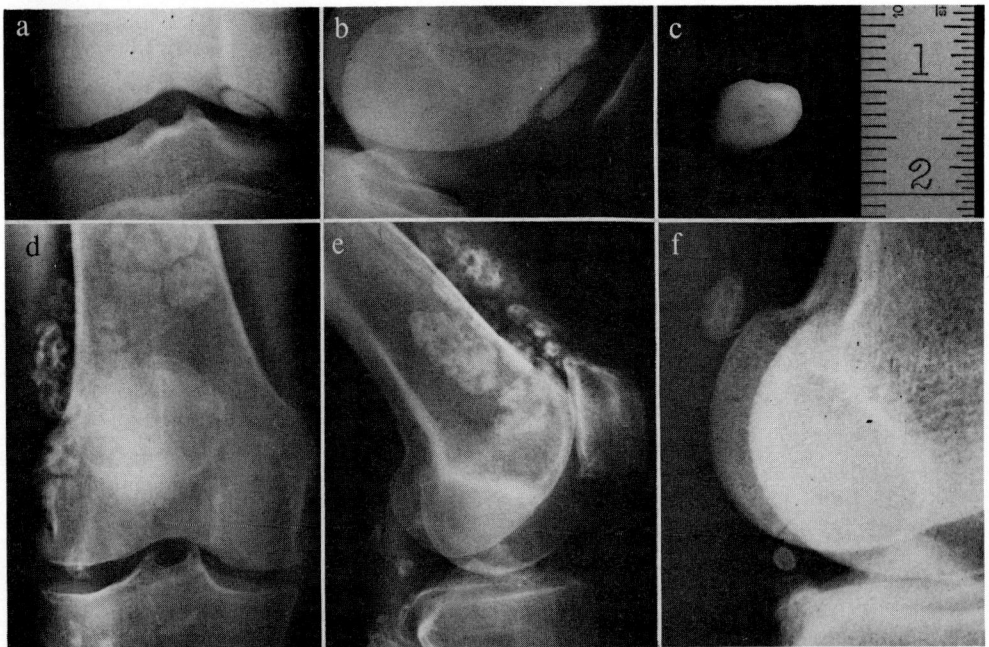

19.23 LOOSE BODIES IN THE KNEE
(a, b) Splitting osteochondritis — and (c) the loose body which was removed. Only one or two loose bodies form in this condition, but in synovial osteochondromatosis (d, e) they are numerous.
Which is the loose body in (f)? Not the large one (which is a fabella), but the small lower one opposite the joint line.

X-RAY — Most loose bodies are radio-opaque.   The films also show any underlying joint abnormality.

TREATMENT

A loose body causing symptoms should be removed unless the joint is severely osteoarthritic.   Operation should not be lightly undertaken, for the loose body may be difficult to find without wide exposure.

OSTEOCHONDRITIS DISSECANS (*see also* page 56)

The likeliest cause is trauma, probably an osteochondral or subchondral fracture which remains un-united.   It may be significant that, in full flexion, the patella makes contact with the classical site.

The convex lower aspect of the medial femoral condyle is usually affected, rarely the lateral condyle, and still more rarely the patella.   An area of softened articular cartilage together with an underlying ovoid piece of bone becomes demarcated from the femoral condyle.   Later, the segment becomes partly detached and finally broken off to form a loose body (sometimes two or three).   A crater remains, at the periphery of which the cartilage is undermined.

SYMPTOMS AND SIGNS

The patient may present with intermittent ache, or swelling.   Later, there are attacks of giving way, followed by swelling, and the knee is 'unreliable'; later still true locking may occur.

The patient is fit and usually aged 15–20 years.   (There is a rare familial type in which several joints are involved.)

Soon after an attack of giving way or locking, the signs of synovitis or haemarthrosis are present.   In addition, however, there is tenderness localized to the medial aspect of the medial femoral condyle, which is almost diagnostic.

X-RAY — At first, a fragment of bone is seen to be separated from the rest of the femur by a clear zone.   Later, the fragment may be hinged on one side and project into the joint.   Still later, there is a loose body, and its site of origin is visible.

TREATMENT

Before the fragment has separated spontaneous healing can probably occur, and the patient is merely taken off games for a few months; but healing is uncertain and, except in the very earliest cases, operation is probably wiser.   If the fragment is partly detached, or even slightly loose, it is best removed (although pinning it back has been advocated); after removal the crater is cleaned out and its base drilled to promote the formation of fibrocartilage.

OSTEOARTHRITIS OF THE KNEE

CAUSES

Osteoarthritis of the knee does not often follow a single injury unless this has resulted in considerable incongruity.   The oft-repeated injury of recurrent subluxation or dislocation, however, frequently, gives rise to patello-femoral osteoarthritis. In the tibio-fibular joint degeneration may result from the traumatic effects of a torn meniscus or a loose body; osteochondritis dissecans is liable to lead to osteoarthritis partly because the loose body inflicts articular damage and partly because the femoral condyle is irregular. Osteoarthritis may also follow chronic inflammation, especially rheumatoid arthritis.

Genu varum is often a precursor of osteoarthritis; moreover if osteoarthritis develops in a previously straight knee varus deformity may then follow. Valgus deformity and osteoarthritis are less often associated.

PATHOLOGY

The process appears to start in the articular cartilage. At the pressure area the cartilage becomes rough, fibrillated and thinned, and pieces flake off; beneath it the bone may be sclerosed. At the non-pressure areas the articular cartilage proliferates and calcifies, giving osteophytes which occasionally break off as loose bodies.

The synovial membrane often proliferates and excess fluid is formed.

CLINICAL FEATURES

Pain is the leading symptom, worse after use, or (if the patello-femoral joint is affected) on stairs. After rest, the joint feels stiff and it hurts to ' get going ' after sitting for any length of time. Swelling is common, and giving way or locking may occur. With time, the pain and swelling tend to increase, though remissions may occur.

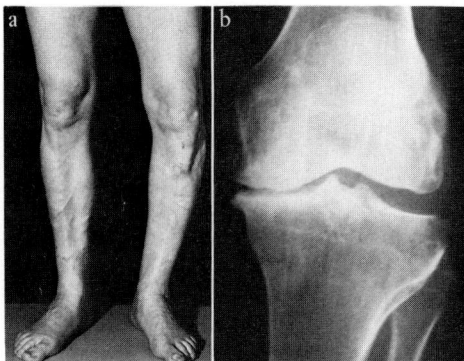

19.24 OSTEOARTHRITIS OF THE KNEE
(a, b) Varus deformity and degeneration on the medial side.

The patient is a fit adult, and the local signs are as follows:

LOOK — There may be swelling and slight wasting of the quadriceps muscle. Varus deformity is common, but occasionally the knee is valgus.

FEEL — Except during an exacerbation, there is little fluid and no warmth; nor is the synovial membrane thickened. The articular margins may be tender.

MOVE — Extremes of movement are usually slightly limited, and attempts to produce them are painful. If the patella is firmly pressed against the femur and then moved, pain is usually elicited.

X-RAY — The joint space is diminished, at the patello-femoral joint or the tibio-femoral joint or both. The true extent of tibio-femoral narrowing is best demonstrated by a weight-bearing film. Medial narrowing usually predominates, but occasionally lateral. Lipping and osteophytes are often seen and there may be loose bodies.

CONSERVATIVE TREATMENT

If pain is not severe, conservative treatment is used. A useful first step, especially in early cases, is to manipulate the joint under anaesthesia (trying to restore full range) and to inject hydrocortisone; then to retain the increase and strengthen the knee by quadriceps exercises and faradism. Analgesics are prescribed, and warmth (e.g. by massage, radiant heat, short-wave diathermy or a bandage) is soothing.   The patient is encouraged to use a stick, but will rarely tolerate a removable splint.

OPERATIVE TREATMENT

OSTEOTOMY — When painful osteoarthritis is associated with varus deformity high tibial osteotomy is valuable.   One method is to excise the upper 3 cm of the fibula, remove a laterally-based wedge of tibia and hold the straight leg in plaster till union has occurred.

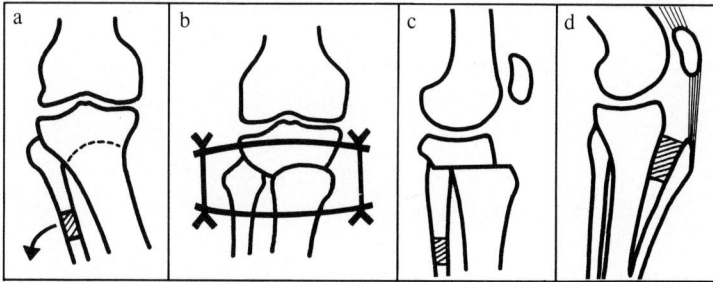

19.25 OSTEOARTHRITIS — TREATMENT BY OSTEOTOMY (after Maquet)
(a, b) Before and after ' barrel-stave ' osteotomy for osteoarthritis with varus. This may be combined with (c) if patello-femoral osteoarthritis is also present. (d) Another method of treating patello-femoral osteoarthritis.

Maquet (1976) has devised a curved high tibial osteotomy in which no bone is excised and precise correction is controlled with transfixing pins; moving the lower fragment forward at the same time relieves patello-femoral pain.   Low femoral osteotomy is used when the deformity is valgus, but the results are less satisfactory.   Double osteotomy (low femur and upper tibia) has been advocated, especially when degeneration is secondary to rheumatoid arthritis (Benjamin, 1969).

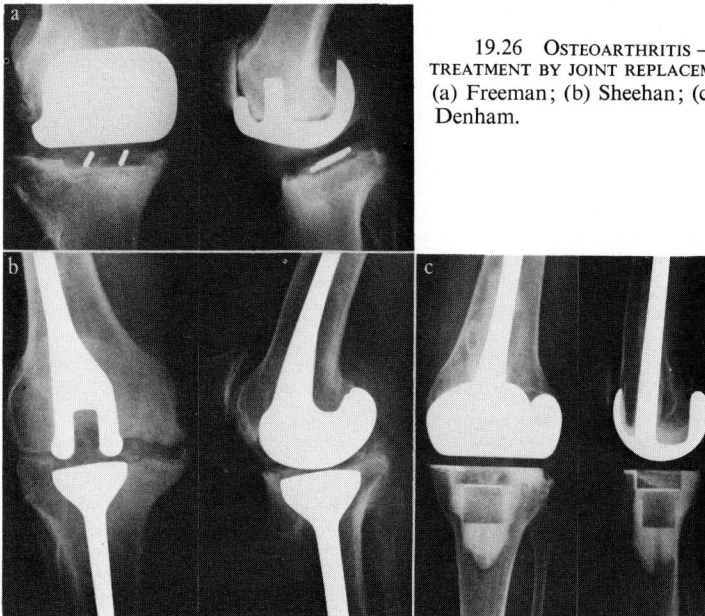

19.26 OSTEOARTHRITIS — TREATMENT BY JOINT REPLACEMENT
(a) Freeman; (b) Sheehan; (c) Denham.

ARTHRODESIS — This is the only certain method of affording complete and permanent relief, but a stiff knee is a great nuisance because the leg sticks out in buses. The operation is therefore indicated only when severe pain is unrelieved by conservative measures. A short period in a plaster tube before operation enables the patient to decide if the relief of pain is worth the inconvenience.

ARTHROPLASTY — Patellectomy is, in effect, an arthroplasty of the patello-femoral joint; and when this section is mainly affected, patellectomy is worth considering. Total replacement of the knee is not uncommonly used for rheumatoid disease, but less often for osteoarthritis when osteotomy is usually preferred. The indications and technique are discussed on page 135.

ARTHROTOMY — This is undertaken when a loose body causes repeated locking. ' House-cleaning ' (removing osteophytes, excising torn menisci and drilling damaged articular cartilage) has been advocated.

CHARCOT'S DISEASE (see also page 52)
CAUSE AND PATHOLOGY

Probably trauma to an insensitive joint is the immediate cause; the underlying cause is nearly always tabes. Destruction of bone is rapid and leads to instability. Loose pieces of bone break off into the joint. There is gross enlargement of the joint, with a thick but stretched capsule, ragged hypertrophy of the synovial membrane, and increased fluid. Large calcified masses form in the capsule.

CLINICAL FEATURES

The onset is usually insidious, but progress is sometimes rapid. Swelling is gross and if it increases rapidly there may be temporary oedema and reddening of the skin. Instability is the most important symptom. Pain is usually absent, though tabetic lightning pains may occur.

The patient is tabetic, and usually aged over 40 years.

LOOK — The joint is enormously swollen, and often grossly deformed.

FEEL — The joint feels like a bag of bones and fluid, but is not warm or tender.

MOVE — Movement is increased and abnormal mobility (such as hyperextension and lateral wobble) is present. The joint can be moved painlessly into almost any position.

X-RAY — The joint is usually subluxed, bone destruction is obvious and there are irregular calcified masses in the joint and in the capsule.

TREATMENT

A caliper is worn because of the instability. A course of penicillin may relieve lightning pains and possibly arrest degenerative changes. Arthrodesis is feasible but demands a meticulous technique (Drennan, 1971).

Suggestions for further reading

Aichroth, P. (1971). 'Osteochondritis Dissecans of the Knee.' *J. Bone Jt Surg.* **53B,** 440, 448

Apley, A. Graham (1947). 'The Diagnosis of Meniscus Injuries: Some New Clinical Methods.' *J. Bone Jt Surg.* **29,** 171

— (1960). 'The Patello-femoral Joint: Methods of Diagnosis, Clinical Disorders and their Treatment.' *Postgrad. Med. J.* **36,** 36

— (1964). Editorial: 'Intelligent Kneemanship.' *Postgrad. Med. J.* **40,** 519

Benjamin, A. (1969). 'Double Osteotomy for the Painful Knee in Rheumatoid Arthritis and Osteoarthritis.' *J. Bone Jt Surg.* **51B,** 694

Bentley, G. (1970). 'Chondromalacia Patellae.' *J. Bone Jt Surg.* **52A,** 221

Bose, K. and Chong, K. C. (1976). 'Clinical Manifestations and Patho-mechanics of Contracture of the Extensor Mechanism of the Knee.' *J. Bone Jt Surg.* **58B,** 478

Drennan, D. B. *et al.* (1971). 'Important Factors in Achieving Arthrodesis of the Charcot Knee.' *J. Bone Jt Surg.* **53A,** 1180

Goodfellow, J. *et al.* (1976). 'Patello-Femoral Joint Mechanics and Pathology.' *J. Bone Jt Surg.* **58B,** 287 and 291

Helfet, A. J. (1974). *Disorders of the Knee.* Philadelphia; Lippincott

Hughston, J. C. (1976). 'Classification of Knee Ligament Instabilities.' Part I p. 159, Part II p. 173

Jackson, J. P. *et al.* (1969). 'High Tibial Osteotomy for Osteoarthritis of the Knee.' *J. Bone Jt Surg.* **51B,** 88

Jackson, J. P. and Waugh, W. (1974). 'The Technique and Complications of Upper Tibial Osteotomy.' *J. Bone Jt Surg.* **56B,** 236

Maquet, P. G. J. (1976). *Biomechanics of the Knee.* Berlin, Heidelberg, New York; Springer-Verlag

Nicholas, J. A. (1973). 'The Five-One Reconstruction for Anteromedial Instability of the Knee.' *J. Bone Jt Surg.* **55A,** 899

O'Donoghue, D. H. (1973). 'Reconstruction for Medial Instability of the Knee.' *J. Bone Jt Surg.* **55A,** 941

Slocum, D. B. and Larson, R. L. (1968). 'Pes Anserinus Transplantation.' *J. Bone Jt Surg.* **50A,** 226

Smillie, I. S. (1974). *Diseases of the Knee Joint.* Edinburgh and London; Churchill-Livingstone

CHAPTER 20

THE ANKLE AND FOOT

EXAMINATION OF THE ANKLE AND FOOT

SYMPTOMS

The most common presenting symptoms are pain, deformity and swelling. It is important to know whether standing or walking provokes the symptoms and whether shoe pressure is a factor.

SIGNS WITH THE PATIENT STANDING AND WALKING

The patient, whose lower limbs should be exposed from the knees downwards, stands first facing the surgeon, then with his back to the surgeon.

LOOK — The legs, ankles, feet and toes are systematically inspected. Particular points to observe are the colour of the skin, and any swelling or deformity.

FEEL — Palpation is postponed until the patient is sitting.

MOVE — The patient is asked to stand on tip toes, then to walk normally and finally to walk on tip toes.

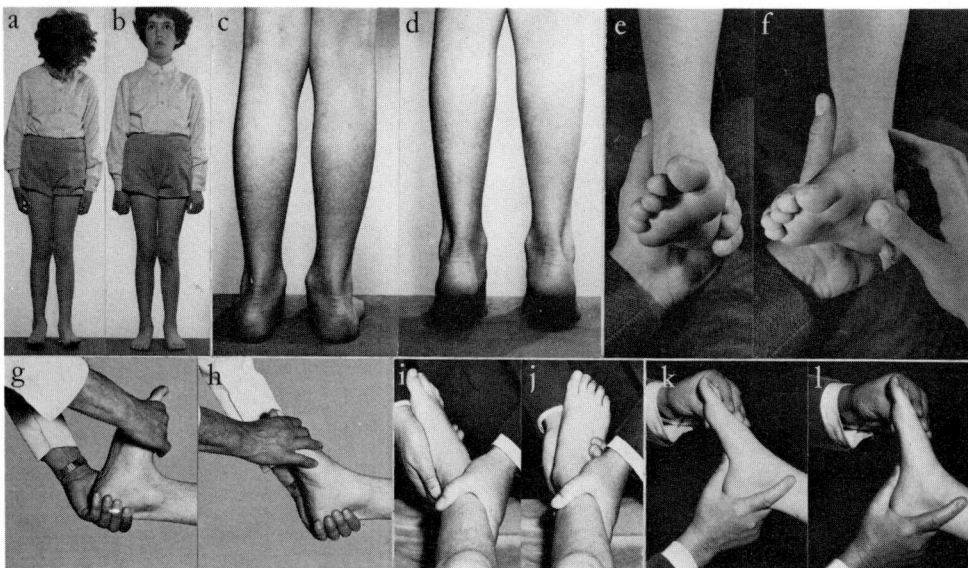

20.1 EXAMINATION OF THE FOOT

The patient examined standing, instinctively looks at her feet; this throws her off balance (a); she should look straight ahead (b).   Next the feet are examined from behind (c) and on tiptoe (d); then held on the surgeon's lap with the heel square to see if the forefoot is varus (e), and to feel for tenderness (f). Ankle dorsiflexion (g) and plantar-flexion (h) are examined; then subtalar inversion (i) and eversion (j). Finally (k, l) mid-tarsal movements are tested.

SIGNS WITH THE PATIENT SITTING OR LYING

The patient is next examined lying on a couch, or it may be more convenient if he sits opposite the surgeon and places his feet on the surgeon's lap.

LOOK — The heel is held square so that any foot deformity can be assessed. The sole and toes should be inspected for callosities.

FEEL — The skin temperature is assessed and the pulses are felt. If there is tenderness in the foot it must be correctly localized, for its site is often diagnostic. Any swelling, oedema or lumps must be examined. Sensation may be abnormal.

MOVE — The foot can be regarded as a series of joints which should be examined methodically:

Ankle joint — With the heel grasped in the left hand and the midfoot in the right, dorsiflexion and plantar flexion are tested.

Subtalar joint — Grasping the heel alone, inversion and eversion are examined.

Midtarsal joint — The heel is held still with one hand while the other moves the tarsus up and down and from side to side.

Toes — Movement at the metatarso-phalangeal and interphalangeal joints is tested.

SHOES — The shoe may be deformed or show uneven wear.

X-RAY APPEARANCES

Antero-posterior and lateral views of the ankle and foot joints are examined in the routine way. Standing films, strain films and special views are sometimes needed.

CLUB FOOT

TALIPES EQUINOVARUS

CAUSAL FACTORS

Genetic and environmental factors are involved. The genetic factor is the larger and the disorder is of polygenic inheritance. The main environmental factor is uterine pressure. Denis Browne showed that the legs of a baby with talipes can, soon after birth, be folded in such a way as to reproduce the uterine position in which pressure deformed the feet; dimples at convexities, also presumably due to pressure, are confirmatory. Animal experiments suggest that intra-uterine compression unduly immobilizes the limbs and this causes deformity. Drugs constitute another environmental factor; thus talipes was one of the many deformities found in thalidomide babies.

PATHOLOGY

The talus points downwards (equinus), the calcaneum faces inwards (varus) and the forefoot is adducted. At first this faulty position may be the only abnormality, but not uncommonly adaptive changes are already present at birth. The soft tissues of the calf and the tibialis anterior and posterior appear to be too short and they fail to grow normally. The bones also show structural changes, either at birth, or developing later, especially if the condition is untreated: the foot does not grow to its normal size; the neck of the talus becomes too long; the calcaneum is too small, is tilted downwards, points inwards and faces inwards; and the navicular lies on the medial aspect of the talus. Even after treatment the foot is liable to be short and stubby.

CLINICAL FEATURES

Deformity is the only symptom in infancy. Painful callosities develop years later if the deformity remains uncorrected.

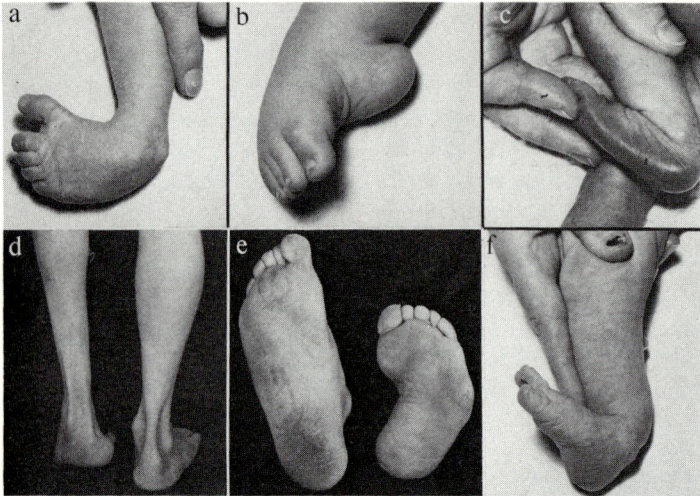

20.2 CONGENITAL TALIPES
(a, b) Two feet showing the classical deformities. (c) Testing for talipes— this foot is normal.

(d, e) Old untreated club foot.
(f) Calcaneo-valgus deformity (the hip should be tested for dislocation).

Boys are affected twice as often as girls. The deformity is bilateral in one-third of cases. Associated congenital deformities, especially spina bifida, should be sought. The local signs are as follows.

LOOK — The calf may be thin. Equinus deformity is seen at the ankle, varus deformity at the subtalar joint, and adduction at the midtarsal joint.

FEEL — Palpation is of little value.

MOVE — The deformities are fixed and cannot be passively corrected. Although the feet of a normal baby may lie naturally in an equinovarus position, they can be passively dorsiflexed until the toes touch the front of the leg.

X-RAY — Films showing the shape and position of the talus may be useful in assessing treatment.

DIFFERENTIAL DIAGNOSIS

Equinovarus deformity occurs also in the following conditions:

POLIOMYELITIS — The foot is cold and blue, and there is usually evidence of paralysis.

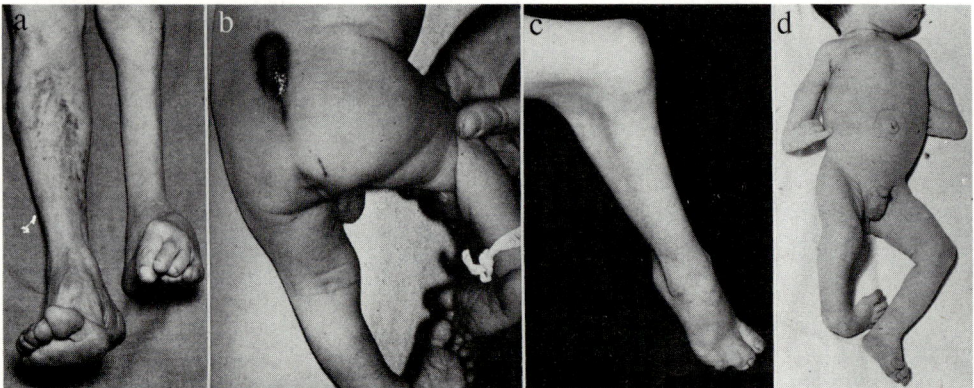

20.3 OTHER CAUSES OF CLUB FOOT
(a) Old polio; (b) spina bifida; (c) arthrogryposis multiplex congenita; (d) multiple deformities in a thalidomide baby.

SPINA BIFIDA — There may be altered sensation in the foot, and trophic changes. The back must always be inspected in any patient with club foot.

ARTHROGRYPOSIS MULTIPLEX CONGENITA (*see* page 7).

TREATMENT

The essentials of treatment are to overcome the deformity fully, then to hold the corrected position until it is stable. There seem to be two clinically distinct varieties of idiopathic talipes: 'easy' and 'resistant' (Attenborough, 1966). The easy cases respond readily to stretching and strapping alone. Resistant cases respond poorly and then only to manipulation which is dangerously forcible; in them, early operation is advisable so that manipulations (followed by strapping) can be gentle. In resistant cases the calf is usually thin, and the heel small and high.

STRETCHING AND STRAPPING — Treatment begins within 2 or 3 days of birth. Without anaesthesia the foot is firmly but gently moulded, each aspect of the deformity being corrected in turn, until finally the foot is in calcaneo-valgus position with the forefoot abducted. Correction is held by adhesive strapping, with felt protecting the skin at points of pressure. The process is at first repeated weekly, and within 3–6 weeks it has usually become apparent whether the case is easy or resistant.

OPERATION — The resistant case is best operated on at 3–6 weeks. Through a medial incision the tendo achillis is elongated and the foot invertors, plantar flexors and plantar fascia inspected; tight structures (tibialis posterior seems to be the commonest) are elongated or divided.

Whether or not operation was needed stretching and strapping continues, but now the process may only need to be repeated at fortnightly or even longer intervals. Treatment must continue for many months and it is probably safer to continue strapping until the child is ready to begin walking. Even then it may be wise to bandage the feet to a Denis Browne splint at night, and it is essential to examine the child at frequent intervals for several years.

LATER OPERATIONS — If the previous methods have failed and the patient is less than 5 years old, open division of the contracted soft tissues is necessary for correction. The tendo achillis is elongated. Two incisions are then made on the inner side of the foot, one on each side of the neurovascular bundle. Through each incision soft tissues on the concave aspect of the deformity are divided under direct vision. When the foot

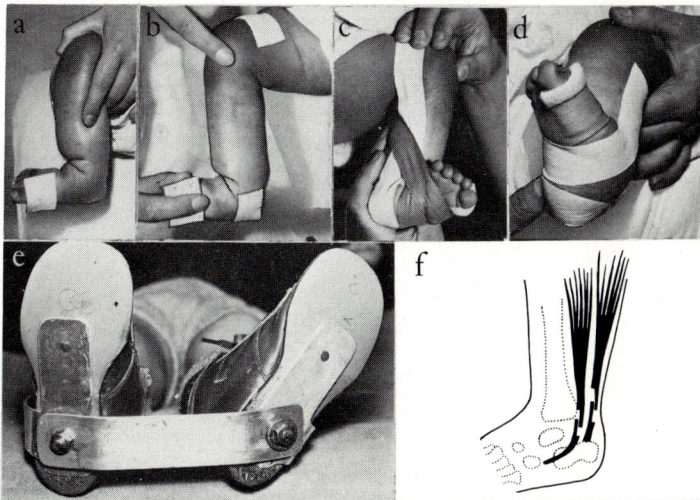

20.4 TREATMENT OF CONGENITAL TALIPES
(a–d) Manipulation and strapping;

(e) Denis Browne night shoes.
(f) Very early operation.

easily falls into a corrected position, the skin is sutured and an above-knee plaster is worn for 6 months (Perkins, 1961).

Over the age of about 5 years, club foot is always associated with structural bone deformities and correction is impossible without bone carpentry. Evans (1961) advised release of the contracted soft tissues on the medial side, combined with excision of a lateral segment of bone including the calcaneo-cuboid joint. If varus deformity predominates calcaneal osteotomy is a valuable procedure (Dwyer, 1963). Over the age of 10 years the best operation is probably a wedge tarsectomy, in which the detailed anatomy of the foot is ignored and a wedge of bone based on the lateral side is removed. All these operations can be combined with elongation of the tendo achillis and are followed by immobilization in plaster.

OTHER VARIETIES OF TALIPES

Talipes calcaneus (the foot dorsiflexed) is common and often associated with valgus deformity. The deformity usually disappears spontaneously but, if it is severe or persistent, correction is easily and quickly obtained by manipulation and splintage. With calcaneovalgus deformity it is important to exclude congenital dislocation of the hip.

Sometimes the only deformity is an adducted forefoot, which may also be corrected by manipulation and splintage. Less than 10 per cent need operation: up to the age of 4 years dividing the capsules and ligaments of all the tarso-metatarsal joints seems to permit good realignment; for older children the possibilities are Evans' procedure (see above) or osteotomy of all five metatarsals.

THE ANKLE AND SUBTALAR JOINTS

Giving way may be due to adhesions following a sprain, to recurrent subluxation of the ankle, or to recurrent dislocation of the peroneal tendons. These conditions are

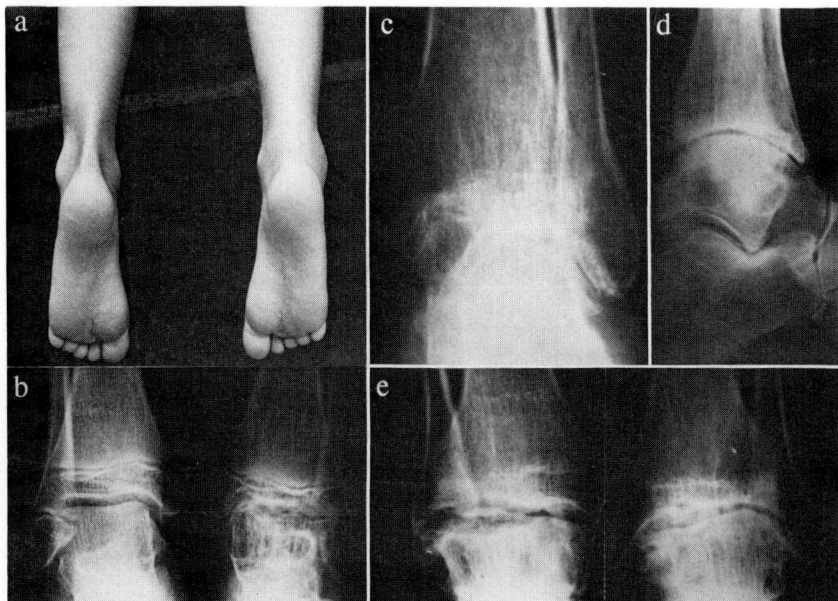

20.5 ANKLE DISORDERS
(a) Tuberculous arthritis with swelling (best seen from behind), wasting of the calf, and (b) joint destruction. (c) Rheumatoid arthritis. (d) Osteoarthritis (following old fracture). (e) Bilateral degenerative changes in haemophilia.

described on page 448. It should not be forgotten that badly-made high-heeled shoes may be unstable and also may cause giving way.

Pain and swelling usually go together and often are associated with *stiffness*. Except when the symptoms are post-traumatic (or post-plaster) in origin, the following causes should be considered.

RHEUMATOID ARTHRITIS

This is the commonest cause of chronic pain and swelling; indeed, bilateral involvement of the subtalar or ankle joints is almost invariably due to rheumatoid disease. The clinical features and treatment are described in Chapter 3.

Bilateral swelling without pain may be due to cardiac or renal disorders. If these can be excluded, and in unilateral cases, the possibility of a lymphatic cause must be considered.

TUBERCULOUS ARTHRITIS

This begins as a synovitis or as an osteomyelitis and, because walking is painful, may present before true arthritis supervenes. The ankle is swollen and the calf markedly wasted; the skin feels warm and movements are restricted. Sinus formation occurs early. X-rays show generalized rarefaction, sometimes a bone abscess and, with late disease, narrowing and irregularity of the joint space.

In addition to general treatment (Chapter 4) a removable splint is used to rest the foot in neutral position. If the disease is arrested early, the patient is allowed up non-weight-bearing in a caliper; gradually he resumes weight, then discards the caliper. Following arthritis, weight-bearing is harmless, but stiffness is inevitable and usually arthrodesis is the best treatment.

OSTEOARTHRITIS

This may be the sequel to an imperfectly reduced fracture, to osteochondritis dissecans with loose body formation, or to repeated bleeding with haemophilia. Osteoarthritis of the ankle does not necessarily cause symptoms, because extremes of range are not required with normal use; only occasionally is operation (arthrodesis) needed.

THE HEEL

RUPTURED TENDO ACHILLIS

Probably rupture occurs only if the tendon is degenerate (avascular). Consequently most patients are aged over 40. While pushing off (running or jumping), the calf muscle contracts; but the contraction is resisted by body weight and the tendon ruptures. The patient feels as if he has been struck just above the heel, and he is unable to tiptoe. Soon after the tear occurs, a gap can be seen and felt 5 cm above the insertion of the tendon. Plantarflexion of the foot is weak and is not accompanied by tautening of the tendon. Where doubt exists, Simmonds' test is helpful: with the patient prone, the calf is squeezed; if the tendon is intact, the foot is seen to plantarflex; if the tendon is ruptured the foot remains still.

DIFFERENTIAL DIAGNOSIS

'INCOMPLETE' TEAR — This is uncommon, but is frequently diagnosed in error. The mistake arises because, if a complete rupture is not seen within 24 hours the gap is difficult to feel; moreover the patient may be able to stand on tiptoe (just), by using his long toe flexors. A correct diagnosis of incomplete tear is seldom possible without operation; if it can be made probably a raised heel and reasonable caution are adequate.

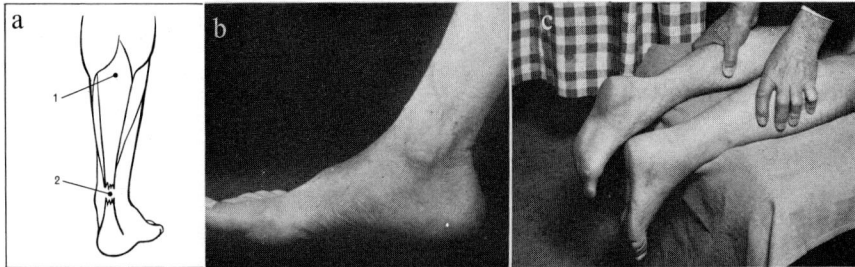

20.6 THE TENDO ACHILLIS
(a) The soleus may tear at its musculo-tendinous junction (1), but the tendo-achillis itself ruptures 4 cm above its insertion (2). (b) The depression seen in this picture at the site of rupture later fills with blood. (c) Simmonds' test: both calves are being squeezed — only the left foot plantar-flexes — the right tendon is ruptured.

TEAR OF SOLEUS MUSCLE — A tear at the musculo-tendinous junction causes pain and tenderness halfway up the calf. This recovers with the aid of physiotherapy and raising the heel of the shoe.

TORN PLANTARIS TENDON — This does not occur.

TREATMENT

If the patient is seen early, the ends of the tendon may approximate when the foot is passively plantarflexed. If so, plaster is applied with the foot in equinus and is worn for eight weeks. A shoe with a raised heel is worn for a further six weeks. Operative repair is probably safer, but an equinus plaster for eight weeks and a heel raise for a further six weeks are still needed.

PAINFUL HEEL

The causes of pain in the region of the heel may conveniently be classified according to the age group in which they commonly occur.

CHILDREN

Sever's disease (apophysitis) usually occurs in boys of about 10 years of age. It is not a 'disease' but a mild traction injury. Pain and tenderness are localized to the tendo achillis insertion. The x-ray report usually refers to increased density and fragmentation of the apophysis, but this appearance is probably normal and often the painless heel looks exactly similar. The heel of the shoe should be raised a little and strenuous activities restricted for a few weeks.

ADOLESCENTS

In girls aged 15–20 years, a calcaneal knob (often bilateral) is common. The postero-lateral portion of the calcaneum is too prominent and the shoe rubs on it, causing pain. If attention to footwear does not help, the knob should be gouged away or removed with bone nibblers.

YOUNG ADULTS

Bursitis just above the insertion of the tendo achillis may result from ill-fitting footwear, especially in young women and army recruits. Localized pain and tenderness occur. Pain is relieved by removing the stiffener from the heel of the shoe.

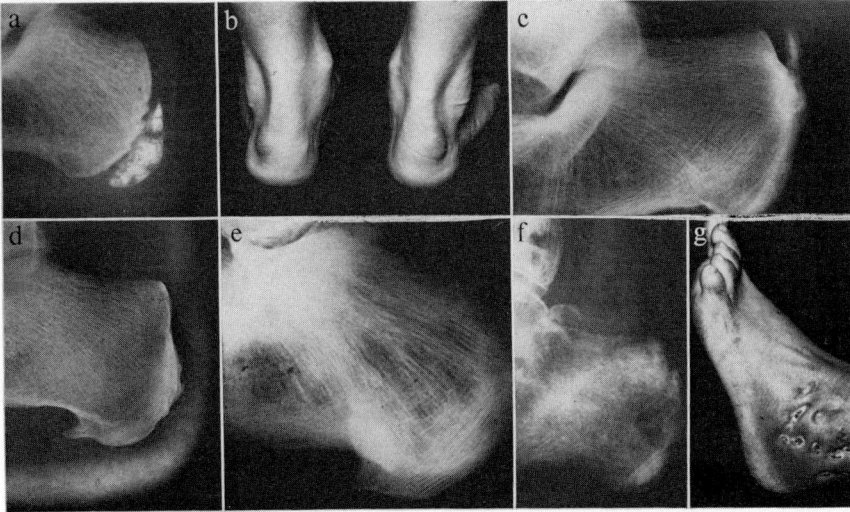

20.7 HEEL DISORDERS
(a) Sever's disease — the apophysis is dense and fragmented. (b) Bilateral heel knobs. (c) Achillis bursitis, in this case with calcification. (d) 'Policeman's heel' — both heels had spurs but only one side was painful. (e) Paget's disease. (f, g.) Tuberculosis of the calcaneum.

Acute plantar fasciitis is said to occur with acute infection, particularly gonorrhoea. Pain and tenderness are localized to the undersurface of the front of the calcaneum. The underlying cause should be treated and the painful area protected from pressure.

OLDER ADULTS

'Policeman's heel' is common in patients aged 40–60. It is sometimes called plantar fasciitis, but neither cause nor pathology is known. The only abnormal physical sign is localized tenderness beneath the calcaneum. A pad is made to transfer pressure away from the tender area. An injection of hydrocortisone occasionally helps. The pain slowly subsides in 6–12 months, and only rarely is division of the plantar fascia indicated.

A bony spur projecting forwards from the under surface of the calcaneal tuberosity is sometimes seen on x-ray. Even when associated with a painful heel, it probably has no significance.

Paget's disease sometimes affects the calcaneum, causing deep-seated aching which is resistant to treatment. Following a fractured calcaneum, pain on the lateral aspect is not uncommon.

CHRONIC BONE INFECTION

At any age, the calcaneum may be the site of chronic bone infection. A Brodie's abscess has a well-defined margin with surrounding bone sclerosis, whereas a tuberculous infection shows widespread rarefaction and the abscess margin is ill-defined.

THE ARCH

FLAT FOOT

Body weight is normally transmitted through two columns, with the medial border of each foot raised from the ground like the arch of a bridge. The height of the arch may be normally low or normally high, but the term 'flat foot' implies that the apex of the arch has collapsed inwards.

Terminology in flat foot is confused. Thus, the terms 'pes planus', 'valgus foot' or 'pronated foot' are simply anatomical descriptions: as the arch collapses its apex drops and shifts medially; the heel becomes valgus and the foot pronates at the subtalar–midtarsal complex. The terms 'unstable', 'hypermobile' or 'postural' flat foot are descriptions of a common physiological predisposing factor; and terms like 'foot strain' and 'rigid flat foot' describe sequels to the deformity.

CAUSES

ANATOMICAL — Five groups of anatomical peculiarities predispose to flat foot; their frequent inheritance explains the familial incidence.

Limb rotation — The entire limb may be externally rotated, or the leg only may be rotated from the knee downwards. In either case, the patient stands like Charlie Chaplin and the line of body weight, which should come between the first and second metatarsal bones, falls too far medially. As the body moves forwards its weight therefore tends to make the arch collapse.

Genu valgum — At the knee there may be genu valgum. In this, which is common in children, again the body weight is taken too far medially.

Equinus deformity — At the ankle there may be equinus deformity. If the tendo achillis is short, the foot is unable to dorsiflex above the right angle in walking without the tendon taking a short cut. Consequently the arch collapses inwards.

Varus deformity — During walking, weight comes on to the forefoot; if this is varus, the medial border is forced downwards and medially, resulting in flat foot.

Congenital — This is rare, except with myelomeningocele. The foot is valgus and 'boat-shaped', being convex downwards (rocker foot) and very stiff. X-rays show the calcaneum in equinus; the talus is almost vertical and its head is dislocated.

PHYSIOLOGICAL — The bony arch of the foot is potentially unstable. It is bound together by ligaments, but these are capable of resisting short-term stress only; even an anatomically perfect foot will rapidly become flat unless there are muscles of good bulk and tone to support it (e.g. paralytic flat foot).

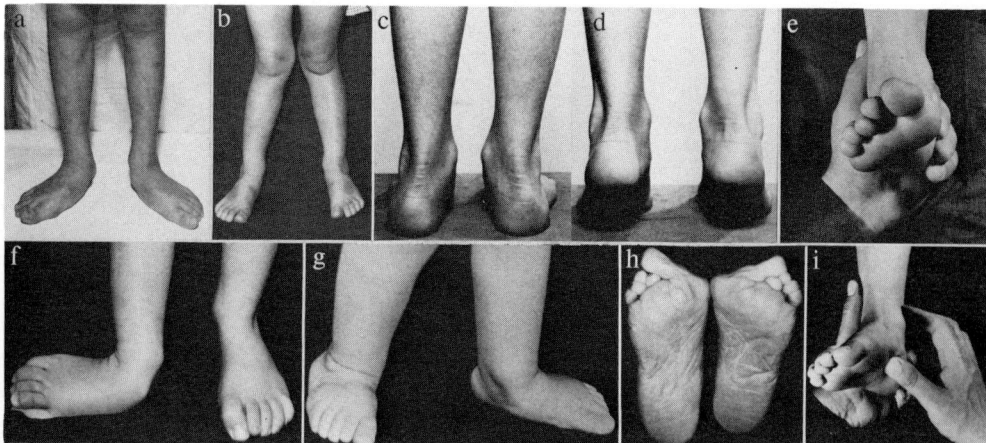

20.8 FLAT FOOT (1) CAUSAL FACTORS
Flat foot may be associated with anatomical faults (upper row), or with physiological faults (lower row). (a) External rotation of the legs; (b) knock knees; (c) a tight tendo-achillis — note that standing on tiptoe (d) restores the arch; (e) a varus forefoot. (f) Paralytic flat foot from old polio; (g) infantile flat foot; (h) middle-aged splay foot; (i) tenderness in temporary flat foot (foot strain).

Infantile flat foot — Until an infant has learnt to control the balancing muscles, the foot collapses on weight-bearing. Sometimes the infantile lack of control persists long after walking, and consequently the foot remains flat for years.

Postural flat foot — The posture of many children is poor. They stand with a thoracic kyphosis, a lumbar lordosis and the pelvis tilted forwards. The gluteal, leg and foot muscles share in the generalized poor muscle tone and flat foot may result.

Middle-aged flat foot — In middle age muscles tend to become flabby. The housewife not only stands for long periods of time but is likely to put on weight. She gets less support just when she needs more. Flat foot is one of the results; subsequent joint degeneration may lead to stiffness.

Temporary flat foot — During prolonged illness in bed the muscles lose their bulk and tone, and on resumption of weight bearing the feet may rapidly become flat; the ligament damage causes pain and tenderness ('acute foot strain').

CLINICAL FEATURES

Often there are no symptoms; but the school doctor may 'complain' that the feet look flat, or the mother that the shoes wear badly. Pain is not a feature except (*a*) with acute foot strain following prolonged recumbency; (*b*) if joint degeneration has supervened; or (*c*) if secondary forefoot deformities (bunions or curly toes) have developed.

There are rarely any general signs, although with severe flat foot the back and the central nervous system should be examined. The local signs are as follows.

LOOK — The legs are inspected for abnormal rotation and for knock knee. Then the feet themselves are examined; if the arch has collapsed the tuberosity of the navicular is unduly prominent. From behind, the heel is seen to be valgus (the tendo achillis angulates laterally), but the deformity usually disappears when standing on tiptoe.

The patient now sits, and each foot is examined in turn while the surgeon holds it with the heel square. It is then possible to see if the forefoot is varus and to assess any associated toe disorders.

FEEL — The foot is palpated for tenderness: first under the arch, then at the midtarsal region, and finally at the forefoot.

MOVE — With the heel still held square and the knee straight, movements are tested. First the ankle: does it dorsiflex above a right angle? If there is a tight tendo achillis, dorsiflexion does not occur without the heel moving into valgus. The subtalar, midtarsal and metatarso-phalangeal joints are each examined in turn to determine their range of movement.

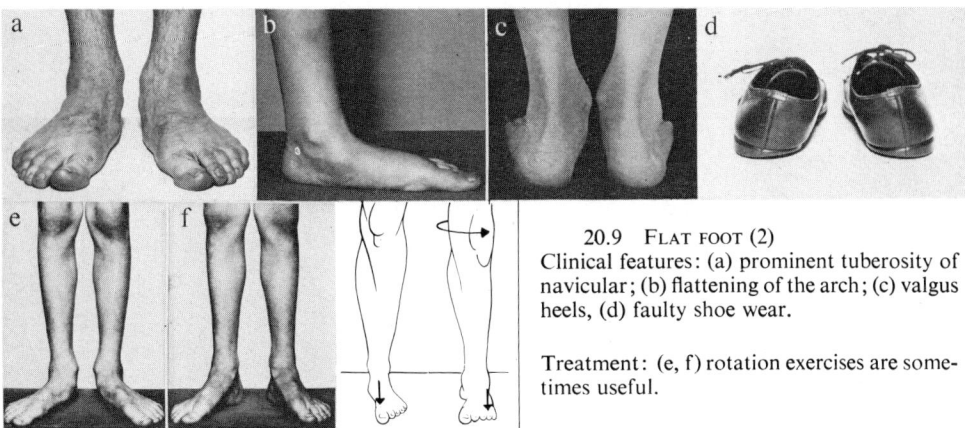

20.9 FLAT FOOT (2)
Clinical features: (a) prominent tuberosity of navicular; (b) flattening of the arch; (c) valgus heels, (d) faulty shoe wear.

Treatment: (e, f) rotation exercises are sometimes useful.

TREATMENT

In the vast majority of cases flat foot is painless and no treatment is required. Exercises may strengthen the muscles, and supports may prop up the arch; the middle-aged patient with pain sometimes finds the combination comforting, but it does not restore the arch to normal. Children with painless flat foot are certainly best left untreated. The mother, who often demands treatment, should be told that the arch may develop during growth, but that treatment does not influence the outcome; supports or heel seats are justified only if experience shows that their use cuts down wear and tear on shoes.

Only two kinds of flat foot, both rare, need treatment: congenital flat foot and acute foot strain. Acute foot strain is painful, but the only requirement is a period of rest combined with graduated exercises and a temporary support. With congenital flat foot, however, reduction of the talar dislocation is essential. It is probably best to operate through a postero-medial incision, first elongating the tendo achillis and excising the navicular bone; the talus is then reduced, the tibialis anterior implanted into its neck and the reduction held with a Kirschner wire and plaster (Colton, 1973).

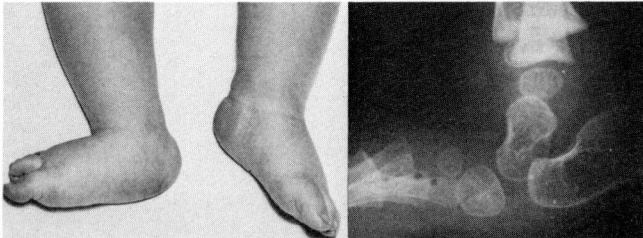

20.10 FLAT FOOT
(3) CONGENITAL
Note the 'rocker bottom' foot and the vertical talus.

SPASMODIC FLAT FOOT

The term is a misnomer: the foot is not flat, nor is the disorder spasmodic; but the foot is everted and the muscles are in spasm. The likeliest cause is an anatomical abnormality, for in many cases an abnormal bar of bone can be demonstrated joining the calcaneum to the talus or to the navicular; the term tarsal coalition is used but the bar is not necessarily complete. The flaw presumably leads to a faulty pattern of movement at the remainder of the subtalar-midtarsal complex; hence the pain and spasm. Relatives of affected patients often show tarsal coalitions on x-ray, but in them symptoms are rare (Leonard, 1974).

SYMPTOMS AND SIGNS

Pain is the presenting symptom. The condition usually occurs between the ages of 12 and 16 years, is twice as common in boys, and is often bilateral.

LOOK — The foot is held everted and the peroneal and extensor tendons can be seen standing out in spasm under the skin.

FEEL — There may be diffuse tenderness around the tarsus.

MOVE — Ankle movements are normal. Subtalar joint movement is grossly restricted and often painful; even if no spasm was previously visible, attempted movement provokes it. Midtarsal movements also are restricted.

X-RAY — An abnormal bar of bone may be seen although special views are sometimes needed to demonstrate it.

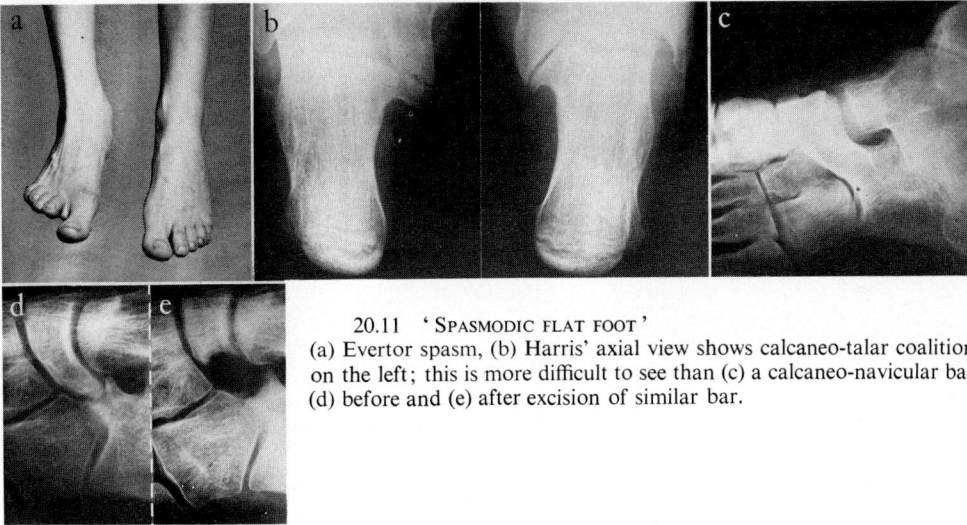

20.11 'SPASMODIC FLAT FOOT'
(a) Evertor spasm, (b) Harris' axial view shows calcaneo-talar coalition
on the left; this is more difficult to see than (c) a calcaneo-navicular bar;
(d) before and (e) after excision of similar bar.

TREATMENT

CONSERVATIVE — A walking plaster is applied with the foot in its normal position (an
anaesthetic may be necessary). The plaster is worn for at least 6 weeks. An outside
iron and inside T-strap can then if necessary be worn for a further 3 months.

OPERATIVE — A calcaneo-navicular bar can be excised and sometimes normal movement
is restored. If this fails, or with a talo-calcaneal bar, the pain can be relieved by a triple
arthrodesis.

PAINFUL TARSUS

In children, pain in the midtarsal region is rare; one cause is Köhler's disease
(osteochondritis of the navicular). The bony nucleus of the navicular becomes dense
and fragmented. The child, under the age of 5, has a painful limp, and a tender

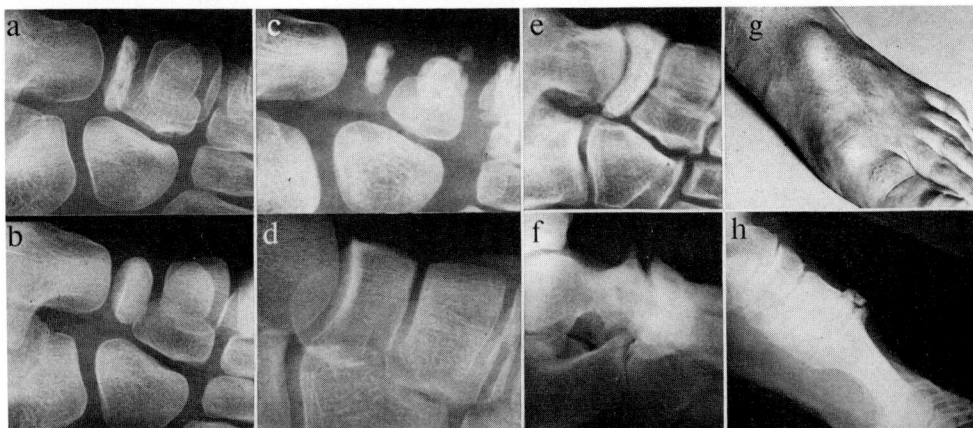

20.12 PAINFUL TARSUS
(a) Köhler's disease compared with (b) the normal foot below. (c) Another example
of Köhler's disease and (d) below, the same foot fully grown — it has become normal.
(e) Brailsford's disease, the adult equivalent of Köhler's disease. (f) Degeneration
of the talonavicular joint. (g, h) The 'over-bone' at the first cuneiform-metatarsal
joint.

warm thickening over the navicular.   The condition resembles tuberculosis, but there is no wasting and movements are full.   If the foot is strapped, and activity restricted for a few weeks, symptoms disappear.   The foot eventually becomes completely normal clinically and radiologically.   A comparable condition occasionally develops in middle-aged women (Brailsford's disease); the navicular becomes dense, then altered in shape, and later the mid-tarsal joint may degenerate.

In adults, especially if the arch is high, a ridge of bone sometimes develops on the adjacent dorsal surfaces of the medial cuneiform and the first metatarsal ('the over-bone').   A lump can be seen which feels bony and may become bigger and tender if the shoe presses on it.   If shoe adjustment fails to provide relief the lump may be bevelled off.

PES CAVUS
CAUSES
MUSCLE IMBALANCE — The lumbrical and interosseus muscles normally flex the straight toes (that is, they flex the metatarso-phalangeal joints and extend the interphalangeal joints). If these short intrinsic muscles are weak, they are overpowered by the long toe muscles and claw foot and curly toes are produced.

The muscle weakness may be due to neurological disease or to a myopathy.
Often, however, no cause is found and the condition is termed ' idiopathic '.

MUSCLE FIBROSIS — A similar deformity may occur if the intrinsic muscles shorten as a result of fibrosis e.g. following Volkmann's ischaemia.

PATHOLOGY
The deformity resulting from muscle imbalance is a complex one.   At the sub-talar joint there is inversion of the heel.   At the midtarsal joint there is plantaris deformity, that is, the forefoot is plantarflexed, bringing it below its normal level. The metatarso-phalangeal joints are hyperextended.   The interphalangeal joints are flexed.

After a time these deformities become fixed and the foot takes pressure over too small an area of the sole, where painful callosities develop under the metatarsal heads.   There is not enough height in the shoe for the curly toes and callosities develop on their dorsum.

CLINICAL FEATURES
Deformity may be noticed by the mother or the school doctor before there is any pain.   Usually, pain is felt at the site of callosities.   Sometimes there is also a general aching of the foot and calf after exercise.   The ankle may sprain easily because of the varus heel.

Idiopathic pes cavus is first noticed at the age of 8–10 years in an otherwise fit child.   There is often a family history and as a rule both feet are affected.

LOOK — The deformities described are obvious.   The extensor tendons stand out as tight bands under the skin.   Callosities may be visible.

FEEL — The callosities are often tender.

MOVE — The ankle may move normally, but even when it is dorsiflexed the forefoot remains at a lower level than the heel (plantaris deformity).   The subtalar joint is in fixed inversion.   The midtarsal joint is in fixed plantaris and cannot be dorsiflexed.   The metatarso-phalangeal joints are fixed in hyperextension and are often subluxed or dislo-cated.   The interphalangeal joints are fixed flexed.

X-RAY — There is no abnormality of the individual bones. It is important to exclude spina bifida.

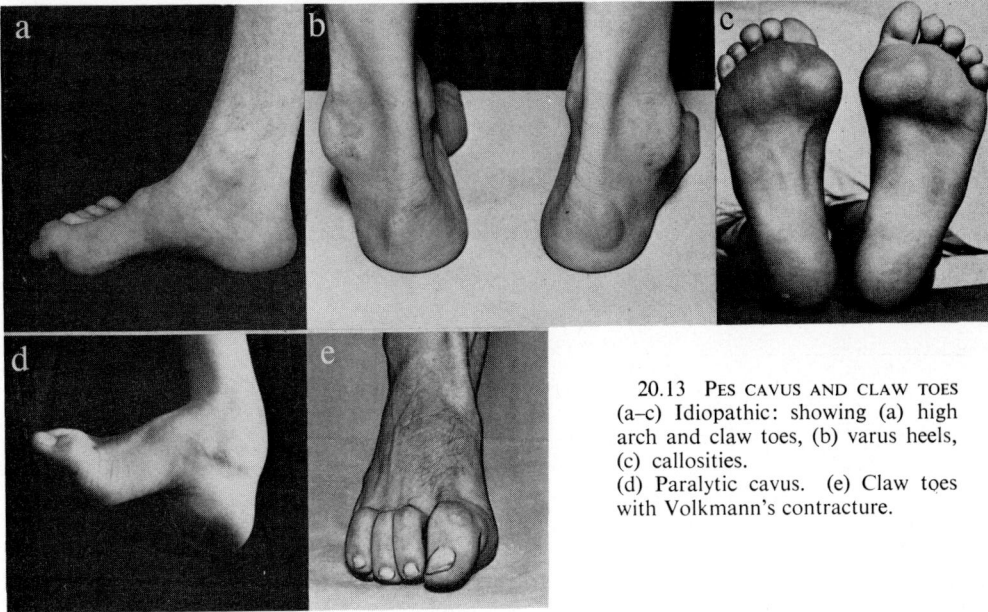

20.13 PES CAVUS AND CLAW TOES
(a–c) Idiopathic: showing (a) high
arch and claw toes, (b) varus heels,
(c) callosities.
(d) Paralytic cavus. (e) Claw toes
with Volkmann's contracture.

DIFFERENTIAL DIAGNOSIS

Before claw foot is labelled as idiopathic the following conditions must be excluded.

NEUROLOGICAL DISORDERS — These include Friedreich's ataxia and spina bifida, in both of which there is other evidence of the cause.

MYOPATHIES — In peroneal muscle atrophy usually the hands also are clawed.

VOLKMANN'S ISCHAEMIA — In Volkmann's ischaemia of the calf there is a history of injury; the claw foot results from contracture of the muscles.

TREATMENT

IN YOUNG CHILDREN — An attempt is made to strengthen the intrinsic muscles by exercises in which the straight toes are taught to flex at the metatarso-phalangeal joints. Great care is necessary to see that the shoes are long enough and the heel low.

Operation may become necessary. Before the toe deformities become fixed the long flexor tendons of the outer four toes are transplanted into the extensor tendons, and the interphalangeal joint of the hallux arthrodesed. This straightens the toes, but if there is much cavus deformity Steindler's operation is performed at the same time: in this the tissues arising from the undersurface of the calcaneum are divided and the foot wrenched until it flattens. The corrected position is held in plaster for at least 6 weeks.

IN ADOLESCENTS — If the toe deformities have become fixed it is best to arthrodese all the interphalangeal joints (so that the long flexors now flex the toes instead of bunching them up) and the long extensors are re-inserted into the metatarsal necks (so that they elevate the forefoot). The outer four toes are held with wires and the hallux with a screw.

When varus deformity of the heel is a prominent feature a calcaneal osteotomy is valuable and can usefully be combined with Steindler's operation.

IN ADULTS — Palliative treatment is usually all that is practicable in adults. A cork or sponge insole is fitted to distribute pressure evenly, and shoes are made specially. The

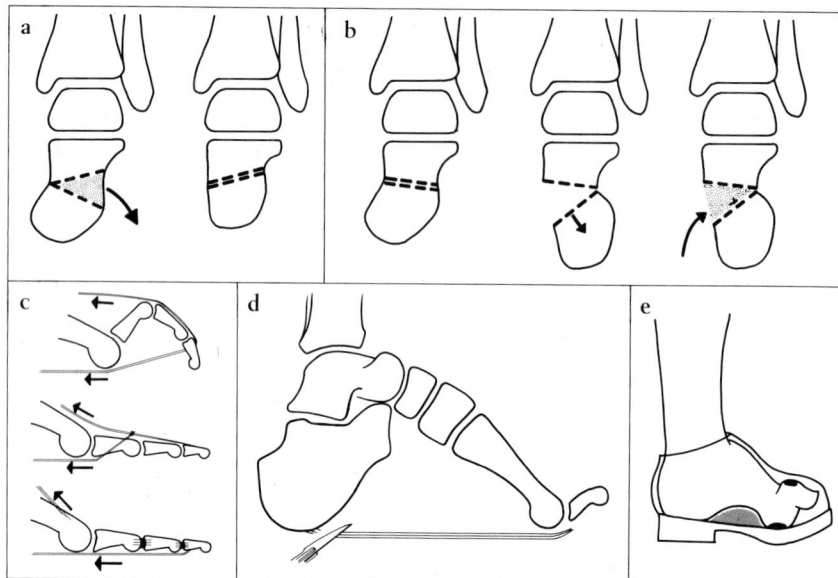

20.14 TREATMENT OF PES CAVUS AND CLAW TOES

Correction of the varus heel by (a) excising a laterally-based wedge of bone; or (b) inserting a medial wedge (Dwyer).

(c) Claw toes due to over-action of the long tendons may be dealt with by transplanting flexor to extensor tendons or by arthrodesing the toe joints and re-attaching the long extensors more proximally. (d) Division of the plantar fascia (Steindler).

(e) Padding and special shoes for the late untreated case.

shoe must be large enough to accommodate the foot, the claw toes and the insole, all without undue pressure. With care and chiropody, most patients can be made comfortable.

THE HALLUX

HALLUX VALGUS

CAUSAL FACTORS

VARUS FIRST METATARSAL — This, usually regarded as the basic deformity, may be congenital or acquired.

Congenital — The condition is often familial, and the first metatarsal is rotated (like a thumb), suggesting an atavistic abnormality. Sometimes, however, the valgus deformity of the toe seems to precede the varus position of the metatarsal.

Acquired — In middle age and with increasing weight, the forefoot splays so that the first metatarsal becomes more varus.

SHOES — Shoes cannot, of course, produce metatarsus varus deformity; but, when that deformity is present, they may force the hallux into valgus, because no modern shoe allows the toe to continue along the line of a varus first metatarsal. The importance of footwear in causing hallux valgus is much disputed; its importance in causing the symptoms is undeniable.

PATHOLOGY

The most obvious feature of the deformity is prominence of the first metatarsal head. This undue prominence results from several factors: (*a*) increased width of the forefoot, with the first metatarsal shaft deviated medially away from the second;

(*b*) the metatarsal head develops a protective bursa (bunion) where the shoe rubs; and (*c*) the proximal phalanx of the hallux is inclined laterally towards the second toe, which is crowded and may become deformed.

Into the gap between the first and second metatarsal heads, the long tendon of the hallux and the sesamoid bones are shifted laterally; once this shift has occurred, the 'bow-stringing' effect tends to increase the toe deformity.

CLINICAL FEATURES

Often there are no symptoms, even with gross hallux valgus. Deformity may be the presenting symptom. Pain, if present, may be due to (*a*) an inflamed bunion; (*b*) a hammer toe; or (*c*) an associated wide splay foot (with pain under the metatarsal heads).

Hallux valgus is usually bilateral, and is commonest in the sixth decade and in females. There is a variety, strongly familial and by no means uncommon, which presents in adolescents.

LOOK — The forefoot is too wide. The hallux has a varus metatarsal with too prominent a head, over which there is a bursa; and the proximal phalanx is valgus and often rotated. The extensor tendon can be seen standing out as a tight band. The second toe may overlap the first or underlap it, or be a hammer toe. There may be callosities under the metatarsal heads.

FEEL — The site of tenderness is important and must be accurately localized, for it may influence treatment.

MOVE — The metatarso-phalangeal joint, in spite of deformity, usually has a good range of painless movement.

X-RAY — The varus first metatarsal and the lateral shift of the sesamoid bones are clearly seen.

TREATMENT

ADOLESCENTS — Deformity is usually the only symptom, but the mother is anxious to prevent it becoming as severe as her own. Nothing short of operation can prevent the deformity from increasing.

It is possible to correct varus deformity of the first metatarsal by an osteotomy near its base, and to maintain correction by inserting into the osteotomy a wedge of bone removed from the prominent metatarsal head; at the same operation the adductor hallucis can be re-inserted into the metatarsal neck (Simmonds, 1960).

A less radical procedure suitable for the older adolescent (or a young adult) is to osteotomize the first metatarsal obliquely through its distal third; the distal portion is displaced laterally and held in position by angulating the toe into varus (Wilson, 1963).

ADULTS — All patients with hallux valgus can be made comfortable by careful attention to footwear. The shoe should be wide and the upper soft. Padding may be used to protect the bunion or a hammer toe. Foot exercises and an anterior platform type of support are useful when there is a splay foot with metatarsalgia.

Surgery is only sometimes successful. Operations in adults with hallux valgus are palliative, and are reserved for patients whose symptoms are not relieved by conservative measures.

Arthroplasty — This is the commonest procedure. It relieves pain due to a bunion but not pain under the metatarsal heads. It usually weakens the foot a little.

Keller's operation — The proximal third of the proximal phalanx is excised, and the prominent portion of the metatarsal head trimmed. This is the most popular operation.

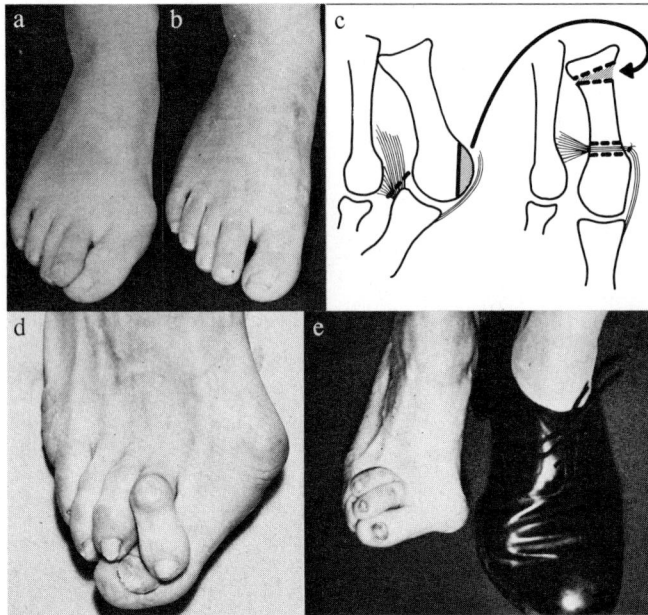

20.15 Hallux valgus (1)
(a, b) Adolescent, before and after operative correction; (c) principles of Simmonds' operation. (d) Severe deformity in middle age. (e) This patient was comfortable in wide shoes — the simplest treatment.

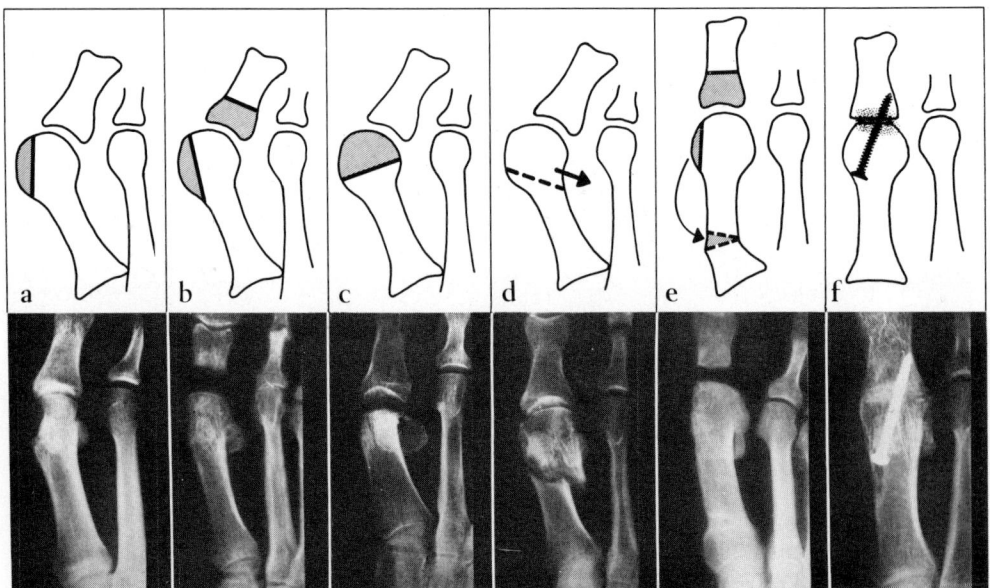

20.16 Hallux valgus (2)
Surgical procedures: (a) Bevelling; (b) Keller's operation; (c) Mayo's operation; (d) Wilson's osteotomy; (e) Keller's operation combined with osteotomy; (f) arthrodesis.

Mayo's operation — The metatarsal head is excised and the prominent portion of the proximal phalanx trimmed. In theory this weakens the foot more than Keller's operation but in practice results are the same.

With either Mayo's or Keller's operation it is often wise to elongate the extensor hallucis tendon and to shorten and straighten the second toe. A plaster toecap with the toe joints straight is sometimes applied and removed after 2 weeks. Foot exercises are then necessary, and supports are sometimes advisable.

Arthrodesis — Arthrodesis abolishes pain, but does not permit of much variation in the height of the heel worn by the patient.

The articular cartilage is removed, deformity corrected and the bones fixed together with a screw or small compression clamps.

Other procedures

Bunionectomy — Excising the bunion with the underlying knob of bone is a simple palliative procedure, but symptoms often recur. Slightly better results may follow if the medial ligament is carefully reconstructed after the operation.

Osteotomy — In patients aged under 50 who have a grossly varus first metatarsal, Keller's operation may be combined with an osteotomy near the metatarsal base. Plaster for 6 weeks is necessary.

HALLUX RIGIDUS
CAUSES

CONGENITAL — If the first metatarsal is short or congenitally elevated, the metatarso-phalangeal joint must hyperextend to allow the ball of the toe to reach the ground. The joint is constantly in an extreme position and therefore liable to degeneration.

ACQUIRED — If the hallux is longer than the second toe, it is liable to be stubbed repeatedly against the toecap of the shoe. A splitting osteochondritis of the first metatarsal head (possibly traumatic in origin) has been described as a cause of hallux rigidus. Another possible precursor is sesamoid chondromalacia.

CLINICAL FEATURES

Pain on walking, especially on slopes or rough ground, is the predominant symptom. Adult males are chiefly affected, but the condition also occurs in adolescents of either sex. It is often bilateral.

LOOK — The hallux is characteristically straight and not valgus. The metatarso-phalangeal joint is knobbly. Often there is a callosity under the medial side of the distal phalanx. The outer side of the sole of the shoe may be unduly worn.

FEEL — The joint feels knobbly and is often tender, especially on its dorso-lateral aspect.

MOVE — At the metatarso-phalangeal joint dorsiflexion is restricted and painful; plantar-flexion may also be limited. Sometimes dorsiflexion at the interphalangeal joint is considerably increased; as a result of this compensatory movement there may be no symptoms.

X-RAY — In adults the x-ray changes are those of osteoarthritis. The joint space is narrowed, there is bone sclerosis and often considerable osteophyte formation.

TREATMENT

ADOLESCENTS — A rockered sole usually abolishes pain and is more comfortable than a metatarsal bar; the 'rocking-horse' motion of the shoe in walking obviates the

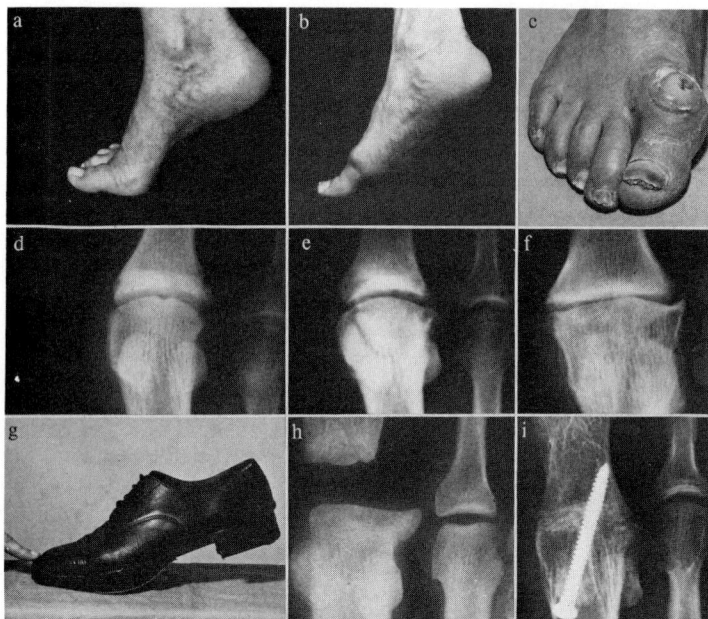

20.17 HALLUX RIGIDUS
(a) In normal walking the hallux dorsiflexes considerably. With rigidus (b), dorsiflexion is limited; a dorsal callosity (c) may develop.

(d) Splitting osteochondritis, or (e) a bipartite sesamoid may be precursors of (f) joint degeneration.

(g) A rocker sole relieves symptoms: operations include Keller's operation (h) and arthrodesis (i).

necessity for dorsiflexion at the metatarso-phalangeal joint. If pain persists, osteotomy of an elevated first metatarsal is worth considering.

ADULTS — A rockered sole often affords complete and permanent relief while the adapted shoe is being worn. Only when pain persists in spite of a rockered sole should operation be considered.

Arthroplasty (Keller's or Mayo's operation) often relieves pain but weakens the foot a little. Joint replacement also usually relieves pain, though movement is not increased much.

Arthrodesis abolishes pain and, as the patients are usually men, variations in the height of heel are not required.

Sometimes a mild hallux rigidus is associated with a large exostosis on the dorsum of the first metatarsal head; if this exostosis is troublesome it may be bevelled off.

OTHER DISORDERS OF THE HALLUX

GOUT (*see* page 22)

Gout often affects the metatarso-phalangeal joint in men. The patient wakes with acute pain and pyrexia. The joint is swollen, hot and acutely irritable. Other evidence of gout is often found.

SESAMOID CHONDROMALACIA

Softening of the articular cartilage on the medial sesamoid may lead to degeneration of the joint between the sesamoid and the first metatarsal head. There is localized pain on walking, and tenderness. If appropriate padding fails to relieve pain, removal of the sesamoid bone is effective.

TOENAIL DISORDERS

The toenail of the hallux may be ingrown, overgrown, or undergrown.

INGROWN — The nail burrows into the nail groove; this ulcerates and its wall grows over the nail, so that the term 'embedded toenail' would be better. The patient is taught

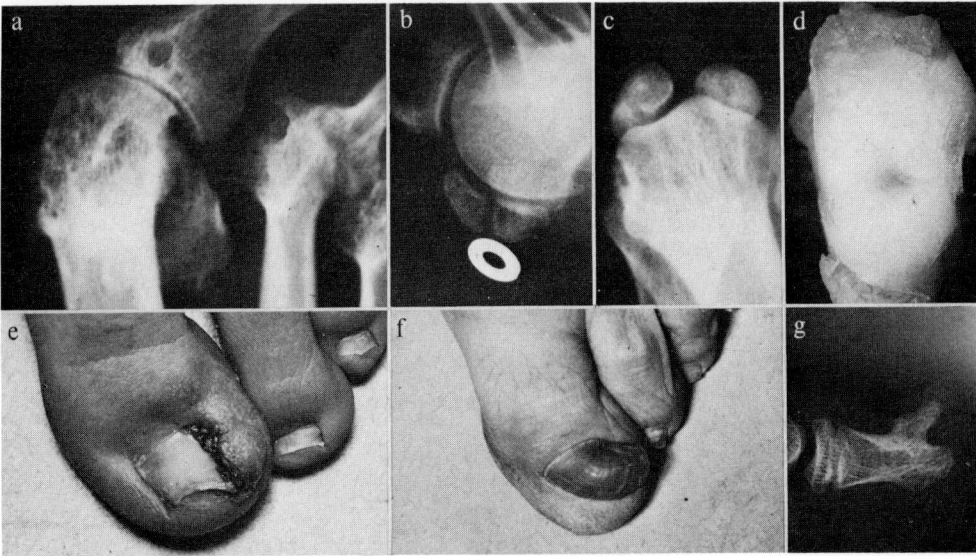

20.18 OTHER DISORDERS OF THE HALLUX
Gout (a) is relatively uncommon. Sesamoid chondromalacia (b, c, d) is relatively common; (b) lateral view of bipartite sesamoid — the marker shows the tender spot; (c) sky-line view of the same patient; (d) the sesamoid has been removed — cartilage degeneration was obvious and the symptoms were relieved.
(e) Ingrown toe-nail; (f) over-grown toe-nail (onychogryphosis): (g) under-grown toe-nail (subungual exostosis).

to cut the nail square, to insert pledgets of wool under the ingrowing edges if necessary, and always to keep the feet clean and dry. If these conservative measures fail, partial or complete removal of the nail may be necessary. It is important to remove the germinal matrix of the nail. Zadik's operation (1950) is usually satisfactory, but in obstinate cases removal of the distal half of the terminal phalanx may be necessary in order to obtain healthy skin cover.

OVERGROWN (ONYCHOGRYPHOSIS) — The nail is hard, thick and curved. A chiropodist can usually make the patient comfortable, but occasionally the nail may need excision.

UNDERGROWN — A subungual exostosis grows on the dorsum of the terminal phalanx and pushes the nail upwards. The exostosis should be removed.

THE METATARSALS AND TOES

METATARSALGIA

This term is used differently by different writers. In its widest sense it simply means pain in the metatarsal region. It is not a disease but a symptom.

Any foot abnormality which results in faulty weight distribution may produce metatarsalgia. The causes are therefore numerous.

DISORDERS OF THE FOOT AS A WHOLE — A splay foot is wide and often associated with hallux valgus and curly toes. It is commonly seen in middle aged women who have put on weight and is in them a frequent cause of metatarsalgia.

A claw foot with claw toes causes pain under the metatarsal heads because weight is taken over too limited an area.

DISORDERS OF INDIVIDUAL TOES — Any of the hallux disorders already described, such as valgus, rigidus, or ingrown toenail is a possible source of pain in the metatarsal region, because of faulty weight distribution.

If any of the other toes is painful or deformed so that it does not take its proper share of weight, pain under its metatarsal head is liable to occur. Thus, hammer toe, claw toes, and curly toes may all produce metatarsalgia.

SPECIAL VARIETIES OF METATARSALGIA

Freiberg's disease — This is a 'crushing' type of osteochondritis of the second metatarsal head (rarely the third). It affects young adults, usually women. A bony lump (the enlarged head) is palpable; it is tender and the affected joint is irritable. X-rays show the head to be wide and flat, the neck thick, and the joint space increased.

Stress fracture — Stress fracture usually affects the second or third metatarsal. It occurs in young adults after unaccustomed activity. The affected shaft feels thick, and tender. The x-ray appearance is at first normal, but later there is fusiform callus around a fine transverse fracture.

Morton's metatarsalgia — This condition is associated with a painful neuroma on a digital nerve. The neuroma occurs at the level of the metatarsal necks just proximal

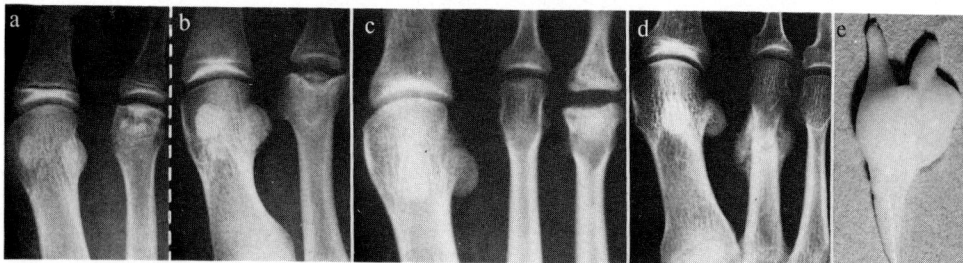

20.19 SPECIAL VARIETIES OF METATARSALGIA
(a, b) Stages in the development of Freiberg's disease; (c) the comparable disorder in the third metatarsal (Köhler's second disease); (d) stress fracture; (e) neuroma excised from patient with Morton's metatarsalgia.

to the division of the digital nerves of the third or fourth clefts. Women aged 40–50 are mainly affected. Sharp intermittent pain shoots into the toes, but is felt only when shoes are worn, possibly because the metatarsal bones are then squeezed together ('compression metatarsalgia'). Tenderness is localized to the neuroma and sensation may be diminished in the affected cleft. An enlarged inter-metatarsal bursa may press on a normal digital nerve producing similar symptoms.

CLINICAL FEATURES

The term 'metatarsalgia' implies pain in the forefoot; deformity is another common symptom.

The age of the patient may suggest the diagnosis. In young adolescents one thinks of idiopathic pes cavus, or acute hallux rigidus; in young adults of Freiberg's disease or a stress fracture; and in older people of splay foot, hallux disorders, curly toes or Morton's metatarsalgia.

LOOK — There may be deformities of the foot as a whole or of the individual toes; callosities may be present. It is important to observe the distribution of weight when the patient stands and when he walks.

The shoes also should be inspected: they may be too short or too long, too narrow or too wide.   The heels may be of unsuitable shape or height.

FEEL — The exact site of tenderness must be found by systematic and careful palpation, which will also disclose the presence of any lumps, or of sensory loss.

MOVE — The foot joints must be examined for pain or limitation of movement.

X-RAY — Freiberg's disease or a stress fracture may be seen.

TREATMENT

This largely depends upon the cause.

CONSERVATIVE — Pads or insoles are used to take pressure from tender areas.   Adequate footwear is provided.   Exercises are given to strengthen the foot muscles.

OPERATIVE — It may be advisable to operate on the hallux or other toes.   If Morton's metatarsalgia does not respond to protective padding, the neuroma is excised through a plantar incision.   If Freiberg's disease remains painful, the metatarsal head is excised through a dorsal incision.   If one (or more) of the middle three metatarsal heads is unduly prominent with a painful callosity, symptoms can be relieved by an oblique osteotomy of the metatarsal shaft (Helal, 1975).

TOE DISORDERS

HAMMER TOE

The metatarso-phalangeal joint is hyperextended, the proximal toe joint fixed flexed, and the distal joint extended.   The second toe on one or both feet is commonly affected.   The toe may have been too long, or the shoes too short, or there may be a hallux valgus.

Corrective strapping is often recommended for children but rarely succeeds.

Operative correction should be deferred until the age of 14; it is then indicated if there is a painful corn on the hammer toe.   The toe is shortened and straightened by excising the joint.   To encourage arthrodesis, the toe is splinted internally with a

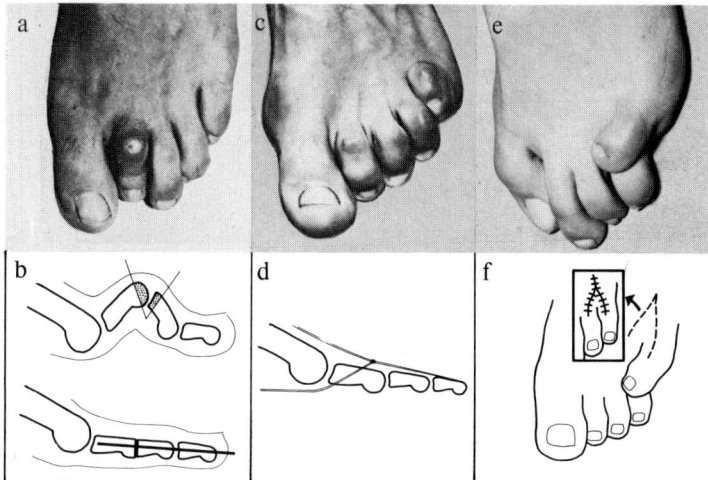

20.20 TOE DISORDERS
(a) Hammer toe, and (b) treatment by excision-arthrodesis. (c) Curly toes and (d) treatment by flexor to extensor transplant. (e) Overlapping fifth toe, and (f) treatment by V–Y plasty.

piece of Kirschner wire, which projects from the tip of the toe. The wire may be left in position for six weeks, or replaced by a collodion splint after three weeks. In older patients excising the proximal phalanx is sufficient.

CURLY TOES

Several toes are affected. As a rule the metatarso-phalangeal joints are hyper-extended and the toe joints flexed. The condition is often bilateral and may be associated with pes cavus deformity. As with many foot deformities there is often a positive family history.

Painful callosities may develop on the dorsum of the toes or under the metatarsal heads. So long as the toes can be passively straightened, surgical correction is possible by transplanting the long toe flexors into the extensors. When the deformity is fixed, if padding and suitable footwear fail to provide relief, the deformed joints should be excised and fused in the straight position.

OVERLAPPING FIFTH TOES

This is a common congenital anomaly. If symptoms warrant, an attempt may be made to straighten the toe by a V-Y plasty, reinforced by transplanting the flexor to the extensor tendon. If this fails, it may be necessary to amputate the toe.

Suggestions for further reading

Attenborough, C. G. (1966) 'Severe Congenital Calipes Equinovarus.' *J. Bone Jt. Surg.* **48B,** 31

Colton, C. L. (1973). 'The Surgical Management of Congenital Vertical Talus.' *J. Bone Jt Surg.* **55B,** 566

Dwyer, F. C. (1963). 'The Treatment of Relapsed Club Foot by the Insertion of a Wedge into the Calcaneum.' *J. Bone Jt Surg.* **45B,** 67

Evans, D. (1961). 'Relapsed Club Foot.' *J. Bone Jt Surg.* **43B,** 722

Helal, B. (1975). 'Metatarsal Osteotomy for Metatarsalgia.' *J. Bone Jt Surg.* **57B,** 187

Leonard, M. A. (1974). 'The Inheritance of Tarsal Coalition and its Relation-ship to Spastic Flat Foot.' *J. Bone Jt Surg.* **56B,** 520

Perkins, G. (1961). *Orthopaedics.* London; Athlone Press

Shephard, E. (1975). 'Intermetatarso-phalangeal Bursitis in the Causation of Morton's Metatarsalgia.' *J. Bone Jt Surg.* **57B,** 115

Simmonds, F. A. and Menelaus, M. B. (1960). 'Hallux Valgus in Adolescents.' *J. Bone Jt Surg.* **42B,** 761

Wilson, J. N. (1963). 'Oblique Displacement Osteotomy for Hallux Valgus.' *J. Bone Jt Surg.* **45B,** 552

Zadik, F. R. (1950). 'Obliteration of the Nail-bed of the Great Toe without shortening the Terminal Phalanx.' *J. Bone Jt Surg.* **32B,** 66

CHAPTER 21

PRINCIPLES OF FRACTURES

The subject of fractures is simplified if it is remembered that bone does not break in a haphazard manner; the varieties of common fractures are limited and their patterns few.

CAUSAL FACTORS AND MECHANISM OF INJURY

The patient who breaks a bone has been subjected to physical force. For the assessment of a fracture it is valuable to consider the amount of the force and the mechanism by which it is transmitted to the bone.

AMOUNT OF FORCE — If the force was insufficient to break normal bone, the fracture is pathological, and further investigation is essential (page 341). Even with normal bone the amount of force determines whether the fracture is complete or not; in children incomplete (greenstick) fractures are common.

MECHANISM OF FORCE — With a direct force the bone breaks at the point of impact; the soft tissues also must be damaged. With an indirect force the bone breaks at a distance from where the force is applied; soft-tissue damage at the fracture site is therefore usually trivial.

An indirect force may be: (a) twisting, which causes a spiral fracture; (b) angulation, which causes a transverse fracture; (c) angulation combined with axial compression, in which the fracture is partly transverse but there is also a separate triangular 'butterfly' fragment; or (d) a combination of twisting, angulation and axial compression, which causes a short oblique fracture (Alms, 1961).

A direct force may be: (a) tapping, which causes a transverse fracture and some skin damage; or (b) crushing, which causes a comminuted fracture often with extensive soft-tissue damage.

The above description applies mainly to the long bones. A cancellous bone, such as a vertebra or the calcaneum, when subjected to sufficient force, sustains a comminuted

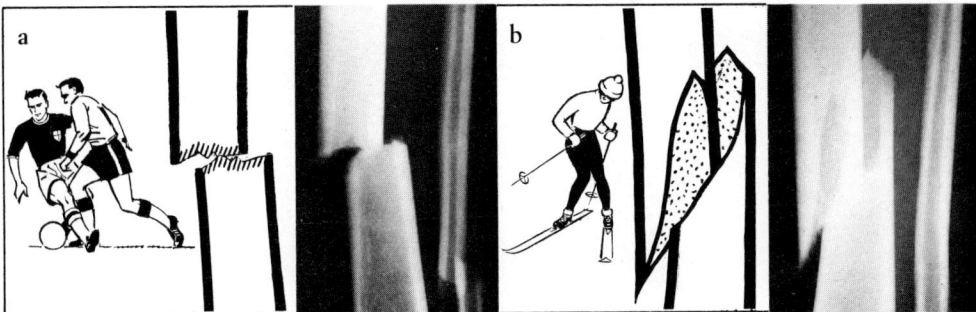

21.1 MECHANISMS OF INJURY (1)
(a) A direct blow causes a transverse fracture; (b) A twisting force causes a spiral fracture.

311

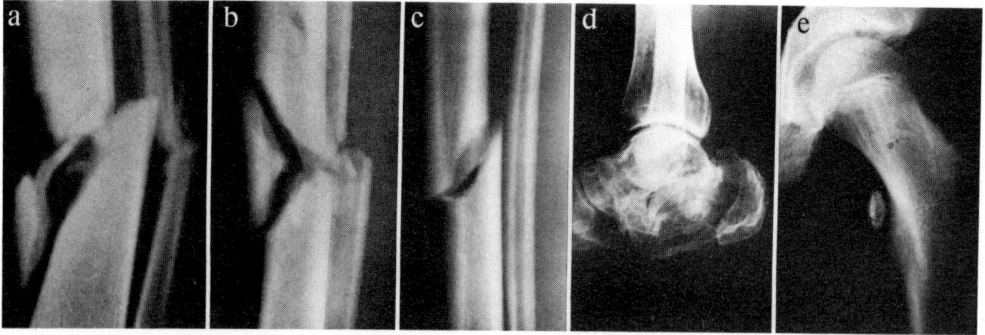

21.2 MECHANISMS OF INJURY (2)
(a) A direct crushing force causes a comminuted fracture with considerable soft tissue damage. (b) Angulation + axial compression causes a 'butterfly' fracture. (c) Angulation + axial compression + rotation causes a short oblique fracture. (d) Cancellous crushing of calcaneum. (e) Avulsion of lesser trochanter apophysis.

crush fracture. At the knee or elbow resisted extension may cause an avulsion fracture of the patella or olecranon; and in a number of situations resisted muscle action may pull off the bony attachment of the muscle.

SYMPTOMS

A fracture is usually followed by pain and loss of function. A pathological fracture may, in addition, have been preceded by pain or by symptoms of an underlying cause (such as a tumour).

GENERAL SIGNS

A broken bone is part of a patient. It is important to look for evidence of: (*a*) shock or haemorrhage; (*b*) associated damage to brain, spinal cord or viscera; and (*c*) a predisposing cause (such as Paget's disease).

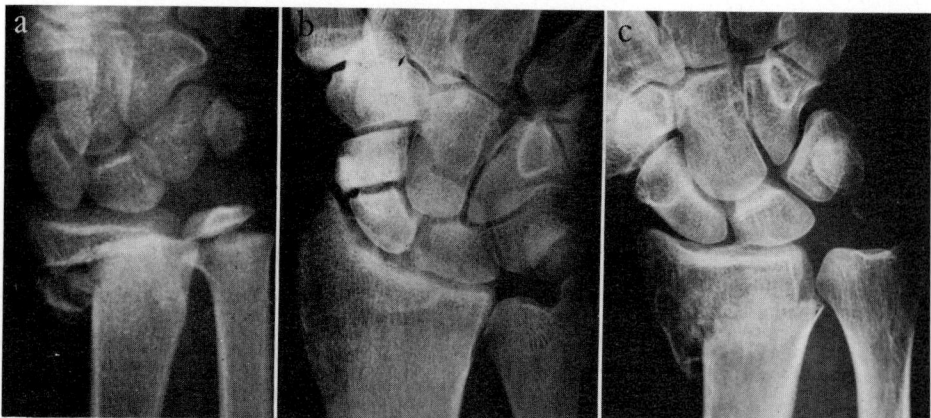

21.3 THE PATIENT'S AGE
Many fractures have a limited age distribution: each of these patients fell on the outstretched hand. (a) Aged 8 — fracture-separation of lower radial epiphysis; (b) aged 30 — fractured scaphoid; (c) aged 60 — Colles' fracture.

LOCAL SIGNS

A possible fracture must be handled gently.   To elicit crepitus or abnormal movement is unnecessarily painful; x-ray diagnosis is more reliable.   Nevertheless the familiar headings of clinical examination should always be considered, or damage to arteries and nerves may be overlooked.

LOOK — Swelling, bruising and deformity may be obvious, but the important point is whether the skin is intact; if the skin is broken, whether from within or without, the fracture is open (compound).

FEEL — There is localized tenderness, but it is necessary also to examine distal to the fracture in order to feel the pulse, and to detect loss of sensation.

MOVE — Crepitus and abnormal movement may be present, but it is more important to ask if the patient can move the joints distal to the injury.

X-RAY — X-ray examination enables a fracture to be accurately described and is essential for medico-legal purposes.   Certain pitfalls must be avoided:

Two views — A fracture or a dislocation may not be seen on a single x-ray film, and at least two views (antero-posterior and lateral) must be taken.

Two occasions — Soon after injury, a fracture (e.g. of the carpal scaphoid) may be difficult to see.   If doubt exists, further examinations must be carried out 10 days later, by which time bone absorption at the fracture site makes diagnosis easier.

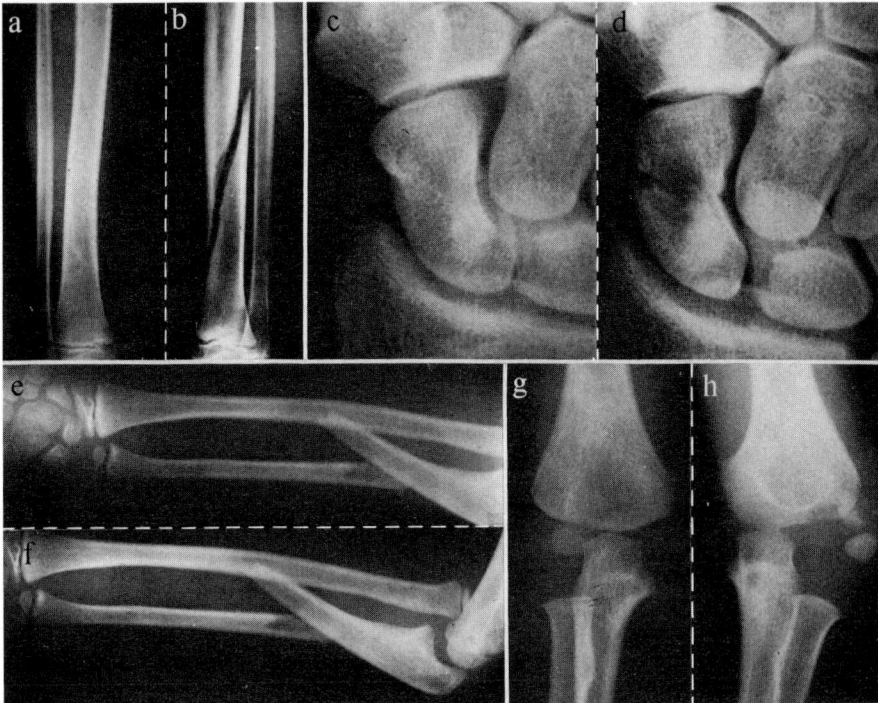

21.4   X-RAY EXAMINATION MUST BE ' ADEQUATE '
(a, b) Two films of the same tibia: the AP fails to show the fracture. (c) Fractured scaphoid not visible on the day of injury, but clearly seen (d) 2 weeks later. (e, f) Monteggia fracture-dislocation: failure to include both joints in forearm fractures (e) may result in a radio-ulnar dislocation (f) being missed. (g, h) Fractured lateral condyle (h) —in a child comparison with the uninjured side (g) is useful.

Two joints — In the forearm or leg one bone may be fractured and angulated. Angulation, however, is impossible unless the other bone also is broken, or a joint dislocated. The joints above and below the fracture must both be included on the x-ray films.

Two limbs — In x-ray of a child's elbow, normal epiphyses may confuse the diagnosis of a fracture, and films of the uninjured elbow are then helpful.

DESCRIPTION

Diagnosing a fracture is usually easy; but the surgeon should also strive to get a mental picture of the nature and direction of the damaging force. To this end accurate description is essential. It is helpful to consider description under three headings: (*a*) situation; (*b*) the line of fracture: whether transverse, oblique or comminuted; and (*c*) the direction of any displacement.

SITUATION — Which bone is broken? Whereabouts in the bone is the fracture? Has the fracture involved a joint surface?

LINE OF FRACTURE — *Transverse:* A transverse fracture is slow to join because the area of contact is small; if the broken surfaces are accurately apposed, however, the fracture is stable to compression. Thus, with an accurately reduced transverse fracture of the tibia, weight-bearing is safe (providing angulation is prevented by plaster).

Spiral: A spiral fracture joins more rapidly because the area of contact is large; it is not, however, stable to compression. Thus, with a spiral fracture of the tibia, early weight-bearing is liable to cause overlap and shortening.

Other varieties: A short oblique fracture has the disadvantages of both spiral and transverse fractures; it is slow to join and unstable to compression. The same is true of the transverse fracture with a separate 'butterfly' fragment.

DISPLACEMENT — Displacement can be resolved into three components:

Shift — Sideways, backwards or forwards shift may occur; there may also be impaction or overlap.

Tilt — Tilt may also be sideways, backwards or forwards.

Twist — Twist may occur in any direction.

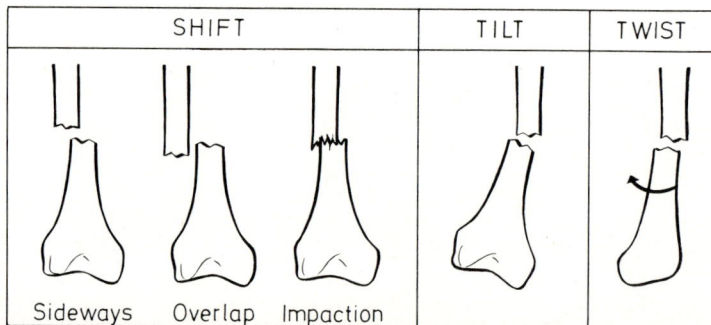

SHIFT			TILT	TWIST
Sideways	Overlap	Impaction		

21.5 FRACTURE DISPLACEMENTS

TREATMENT OF CLOSED FRACTURES

In outline, the treatment of a fracture is as follows.

GENERAL — The sequence of general treatment is: (1) first aid; (2) transport; (3) treatment of shock, haemorrhage or associated injuries.

LOCAL — The sequence of local treatment is: (1) reduce the fracture (by closed manipulation or open operation); (2) hold the fracture reduced (by continuous traction, plaster, or internal fixation); (3) treat the soft tissues (by elevation and exercises).

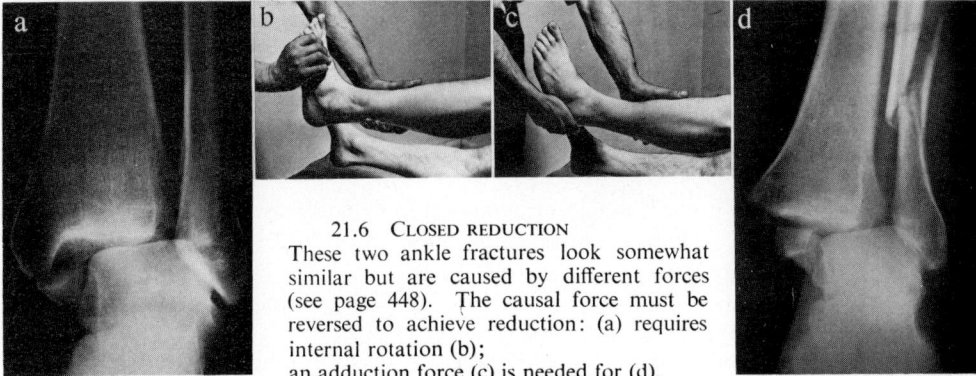

21.6 CLOSED REDUCTION
These two ankle fractures look somewhat similar but are caused by different forces (see page 448). The causal force must be reversed to achieve reduction: (a) requires internal rotation (b); an adduction force (c) is needed for (d).

REDUCE

CLOSED REDUCTION

Accurate reduction by closed manipulation demands a methodical approach. The doctor should first study the x-ray films (thereby deducing the causal force if possible); then, if inexperienced, he should rehearse the manoeuvres needed for reduction. Next, the patient should be appropriately anaesthetized and muscle relaxation assured. The first step in reduction is usually traction along the line of the bone, which is sometimes sufficient to achieve reduction. A force, the reverse of that which

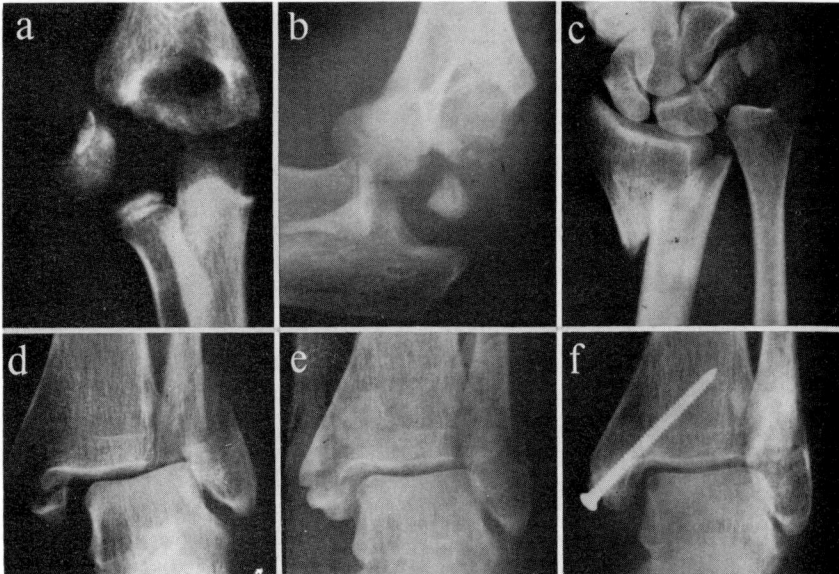

21.7 INDICATIONS FOR OPEN REDUCTION
(a) The elbow was grossly swollen and this fractured lateral condyle could not be reduced by closed manipulation. (b) Similarly this medial epicondyle could be extricated from the joint only by open operation. (c) The sharp fragment of radius had impaled muscle and could not be freed without operation. (d, e, f) This ankle fracture (d) was manipulated closed and the position (e) looks reasonable; but it lacks the accuracy desirable at a joint surface, so open reduction (f) was performed.

caused the fracture, is then applied (for example, for an external rotation Pott's fracture the foot is twisted inwards.)   Reduction must be confirmed by x-ray.

OPEN REDUCTION

Operative reduction is indicated if closed reduction is impossible or insufficiently accurate.

CLOSED REDUCTION IMPOSSIBLE — Closed reduction may fail because (a) a small fragment is unmanageable; (b) a fragment is trapped in a joint; or (c) soft tissues are interposed.

CLOSED REDUCTION INACCURATE — With any fracture accuracy of reduction is desirable; in some it is imperative because (a) fractures involving a joint surface, unless perfectly reduced, are likely to be followed by joint degeneration; and (b) fractures of the radius and ulna in adults, unless perfectly reduced, result in limited rotation.

HOLD REDUCTION

It is important first to consider the need for immobilizing a fracture.   The accepted view is that immobilization is essential; it must be rigidly enforced and uninterruptedly prolonged until union is complete.   Examples widely quoted to support this view are fractures of the carpal scaphoid bone, femoral neck and lower ulna or tibia, which indeed often fail to unite unless immobilized rigidly and uninterruptedly. Consequently, the belief has arisen that 'immobilization causes union', and that 'every fracture needs plaster'.   These assumptions are unjustified; most fractures elsewhere unite whether splinted or not; if unsplinted, however, they may unite in poor position.   In fact, splintage is usually employed to prevent *mal-union* (that is, to hold reduction) and less often to prevent *non-union*.

Three methods of holding reduction are available: continuous traction, plaster splintage and internal fixation.   It should be noted that ' fixation ' (which implies total rigidity) can be achieved only by operating on bone; plaster does not fix the fracture (though it may fix the joints); continuous traction fixes neither bone nor joint but, properly managed, it induces muscle tension which holds the reduction and compresses the fragments together.

21.8 TWO REASONS FOR SPLINTAGE
Fractures such as (a, b, c) must be held immobile or non-union is probable.

Fractures such as (d, e, f) always unite—as these have—but some, such as (e) may need splintage to prevent mal-union.

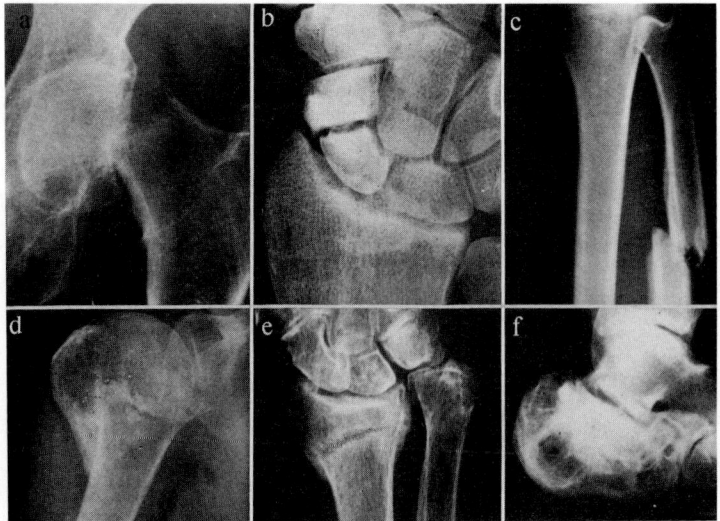

CONTINUOUS TRACTION

As a method of holding reduction, continuous traction is especially useful in spiral fractures of long bones. Traction reduces overlap, the ensheathing effect of the surrounding muscles tends to correct shift, tilt and twist. In transverse fractures excessive traction is liable to pull the ends apart leading to delay or non-union. Whenever traction is employed, the longitudinal muscles crossing the fracture must be exercised regularly and repeatedly.

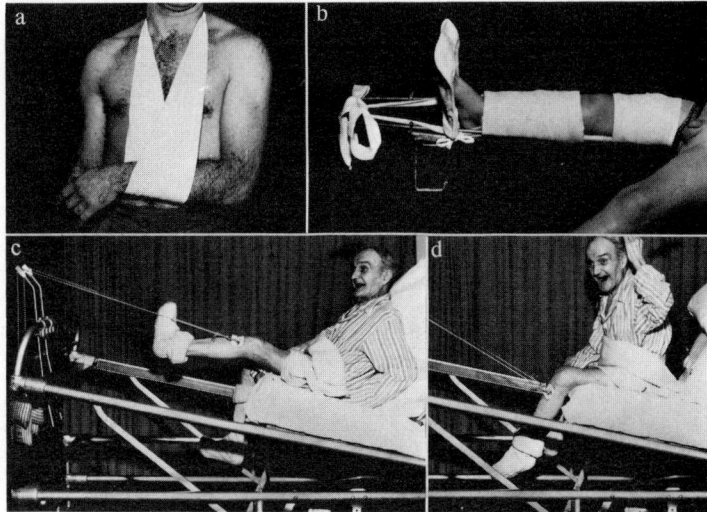

21.9 CONTINUOUS TRACTION
(a) By means of gravity.
(b) Skin traction fixed to the cross piece of a Thomas' splint.

(c, d) Balanced skeletal traction is obviously comfortable: the patient can bend his knee while continuous traction is being maintained.

TRACTION BY GRAVITY ALONE — Traction by gravity alone is used in upper limb injuries. Thus a spiral fracture of the humerus is adequately held by a wrist sling; the weight of the arm provides continuous traction. If the fracture is transverse, a U-shaped plaster slab bandaged on to the arm prevents the fragments from wobbling about too much.

SKIN TRACTION — Skin traction may be used for hip and thigh injuries. Holland strapping, Zopla or one-way-stretch Elastoplast is stuck to the shaved skin and held on by a bandage. The malleoli are protected by Gamgee tissue, and cords or tapes are used for traction.

SKELETAL TRACTION — A Kirschner wire, Steinmann pin or Denham pin is inserted, usually through the upper tibia behind the tibial tubercle for hip and thigh injuries, lower in the tibia or through the calcaneum for tibial fractures. If a pin is used, hooks which can swivel freely are attached, and cords tied to them for applying traction.
Mechanics — Traction must always be opposed by countertraction; that is, the pull must be exerted against something, or it merely drags the patient down the bed.

Fixed traction — The pull is exerted against a fixed point; for example, the tapes are tied to the crosspiece of a Thomas splint and pull the leg down until the root of the limb abuts against the ring of the splint.
Balanced traction — The pull is exerted against an opposing force provided by the weight of the body when the foot of the bed is raised. The cords may be tied to the foot of the bed, or run over pulleys and have weights attached.
Combined traction — A Thomas splint is used. The tapes are tied to the end of the splint and the splint is suspended, or is tied to the end of the bed, which is raised.

PLASTER

TECHNIQUE — After the fracture has been reduced, stockinette is threaded over the limb and the bony points are protected with wool. Plaster is then applied and carefully moulded over the bony points; while the plaster is setting, the surgeon himself should hold the limb. If the fracture is recent, further swelling is likely; the plaster and stockinette are therefore split from top to bottom, exposing the skin. Check x-rays are essential and the plaster may need to be wedged.

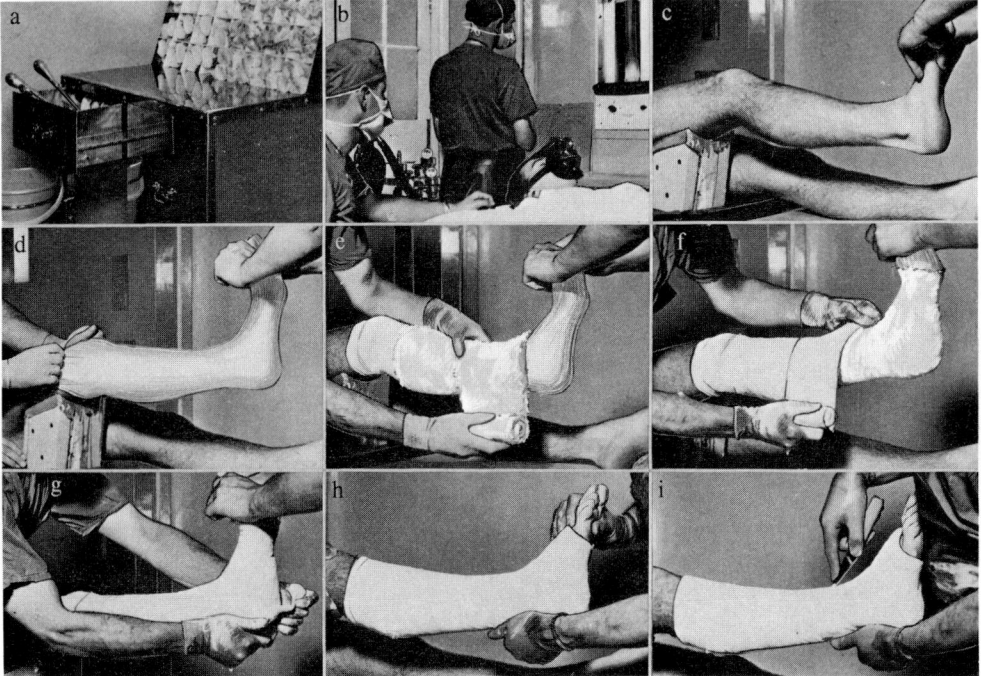

21.10 PLASTER TECHNIQUE

Applying a well fitting and effective plaster needs experience and attention to detail. (a) A well-equipped plaster trolley is invaluable. (b) Adequate anaesthesia and careful study of the x-ray films are both indispensable. (c) For a below-knee plaster the thigh is best supported on a padded block. (d) Stockinette is threaded smoothly on to the leg. (e) For a padded plaster the wool is rolled on and it must be even. (f) Plaster is next applied smoothly, taking a tuck with each turn, and (g) smoothing each layer firmly on to the one beneath. (h) While still wet the cast is moulded away from the bony points. (i) With a recent injury the plaster is then split.

With fractures of the shafts of long bones rotation is controlled only if the plaster includes the joints above and below the fracture. In the lower limb, the knee is usually held slightly flexed, the ankle at a right angle and the tarsus and forefoot neutral (this 'plantigrade' position is essential for normal walking). In the upper limb the position of the splinted joints varies with the fracture. When the fracture is near a joint, usually only that joint is included but the joint above should also be included if rotation cannot otherwise be controlled. Splintage continues until the fracture is consolidated; if plaster changes are needed, check x-rays are essential.

DISADVANTAGES OF PLASTER

The convenience, usefulness and versatility of plaster must not be allowed to obscure its disadvantages, which are considerable. 'Plaster immobilizes the patient but not his fracture'; this aphorism is not always an exaggeration. Plaster is certainly an imprecise method of splintage, whose 'grip' on bone is impeded by intervening muscle and swollen soft tissues. It must extend across and imprison neighbouring joints; otherwise rotation is left uncontrolled. It can itself lead to complications (notably compartment syndromes and skin ulceration) unless expertly applied and supervised.

But above all it leads to stiffness, which has been called the 'fracture disease', though the term 'plaster disease' would be more apt. Post-plaster stiffness has two main causes:

(1) Shaft fractures are associated with haemorrhage and oedema into the surrounding muscles; without repeated exercises (which are inhibited by plaster), the fluid gels, the blood organizes and fibrosis limits muscle excursion.

(2) With fractures into joints, unless perfect position has been restored (a rarity with manipulative reduction), plaster necessarily perpetuates the mal-position.

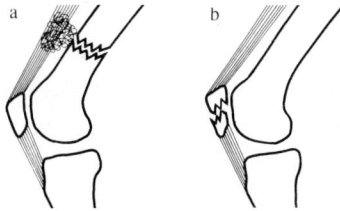

21.11 TWO CAUSES OF STIFFNESS
(a) Fibrosis limiting muscle excursion; (b) mal-union at an articular surface.

The danger of stiffness can be minimized by:

(a) Continuous traction. In shaft fractures a preliminary period of traction enables fluid to be exercised away; once joint movement has been restored plaster can safely be applied. With fractures into joints, the combination of traction with exercises moulds the damaged articular surface to fit the undamaged surface. Moreover it is now known that repeated movement greatly facilitates the repair of damaged cartilage.

(b) Delayed splintage. (See page 320).

(c) Functional bracing. This method (Sarmiento, 1976), originally developed from limb-fitting techniques, is based on the observations that functional activity promotes osteogenesis, and that rigid immobilization is not a prerequisite for fracture healing. First the fracture is 'stabilized', by a few days in plaster for a tibial fracture or a few weeks on traction for a femoral fracture. Then a hinged splint is applied in which functional activity, including movement at all joints, is encouraged. The technique is exacting but rewarding.

INTERNAL FIXATION (*see also* page 139).

Internal metal fixation may be: (a) inlay; for example, by a trifin nail, intramedullary nail, or screws; or (b) onlay, which is always by a plate. Plates should be big and strong and must be screwed to the opposite cortex. The rigidity of fixation can be enhanced by compression techniques (e.g. lag screws, compression plates, tension wiring and external compressors) or by using intramedullary nails which, after the bone has been reamed, fit snugly.

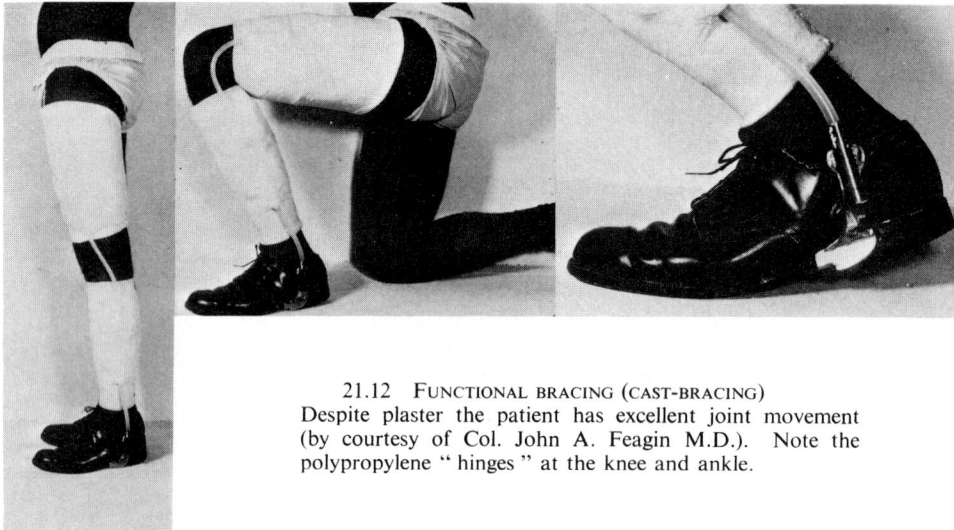

21.12 FUNCTIONAL BRACING (CAST-BRACING)
Despite plaster the patient has excellent joint movement
(by courtesy of Col. John A. Feagin M.D.). Note the
polypropylene " hinges " at the knee and ankle.

INDICATIONS — When a fracture needs to be opened in order to obtain precise reduction (e.g. a fractured medial malleolus, or fractured radius and ulna in an adult), it is reasonable to facilitate after-care by immediate internal fixation. Apart from this, the indications for internal fixation are as follows.

Closed methods impossible — A transverse fracture of the olecranon process, for example, is easy to reduce by closed methods but cannot be held reduced without internal fixation.

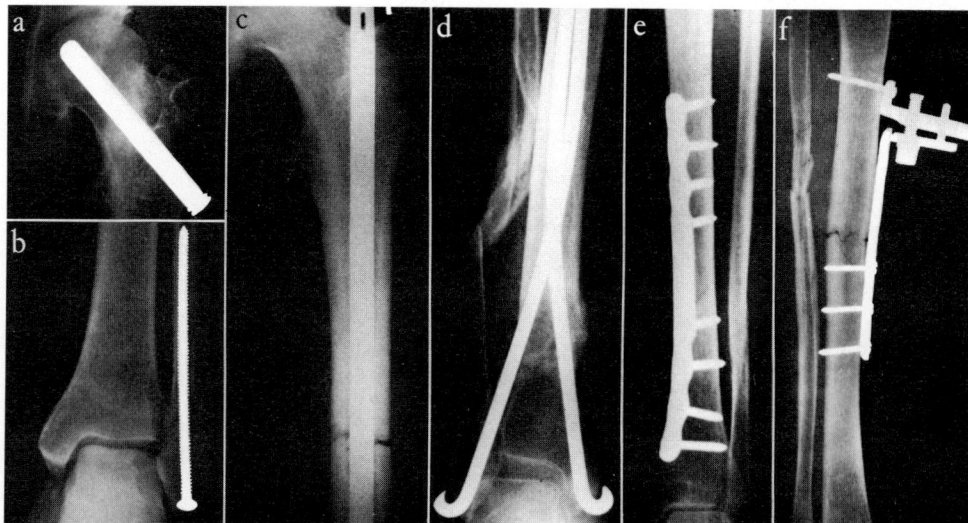

21.13 EXAMPLES OF INTERNAL FIXATION
Inlay techniques: (a) trifin nail (b) intramedullary screw (c) Küntscher nail (d) Rush nails.
   Onlay techniques: (e) plate and screws (f) compression being applied before plating is completed — thus enhancing the fixation.

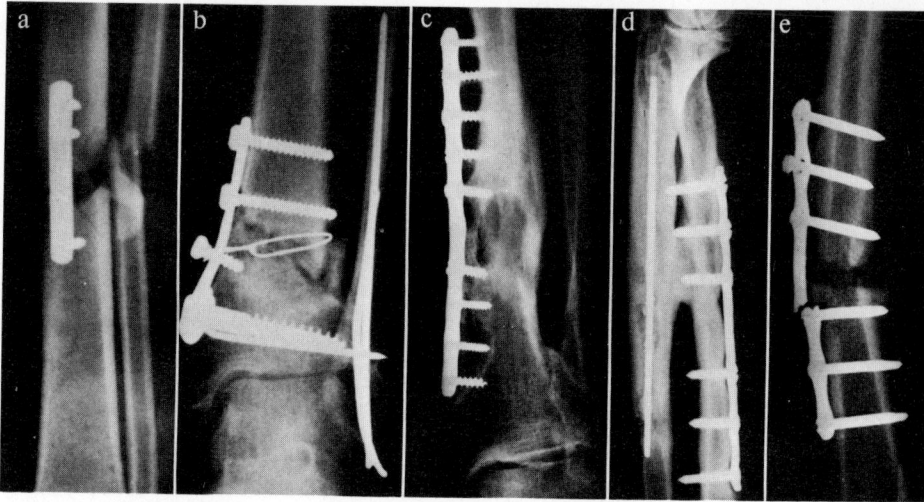

21.14 BAD FIXATION (HOW NOT TO DO IT)
(a) Timidity. (b) Over-exuberance. (c) The screws are too short and the bone infected. (d) Unorthodoxy has resulted in cross-union. (e) Any plate is liable to break unless protected from stress until the fracture has joined.

Closed methods inadequate — A fractured neck of femur (cervical fracture), for example, cannot be adequately held in plaster. Two fractures in one limb are particularly difficult to treat by closed methods; thus, if the femur and the tibia of the same limb are both fractured, one fracture should be neutralized by internal fixation to facilitate closed treatment of the other.

NOTE — Internal fixation is rarely used in children; exceptions are certain elbow fractures (where one or two Kirschner wires may be useful), femoral neck fractures (rare though these are in children) and occasionally forearm fractures or fracture-dislocations.

DELAYED SPLINTAGE — Internal fixation alone is often inadequate and must be supplemented by external splintage. If, for example, a patient walks with a recently plated tibia unprotected by plaster, the plate will break. The disadvantage of plating combined with plaster is that subsequent joint stiffness is often considerable.

To avoid such stiffness, delayed splintage is used: while the patient is in bed after plating, no plaster is used, or at most a removable back slab. Active movements (but not weight-bearing) are encouraged and supervised by a physiotherapist. By the time the stitches are removed, the patient has full range at all joints and is then given a complete plaster. When this is removed, there is little or no stiffness.

A group of Swiss surgeons (A.S.I.F.—The Association for the Study of Internal Fixation) has developed superb instruments and technique for fixing fractures. Their avowed object was to avoid 'the fracture disease', i.e. post-plaster stiffness. The principle is the same as that of delayed splintage, but they often prefer to avoid plaster altogether, relying on the avoidance of stress (e.g. weight-bearing) until union is complete.

EXTERNAL FIXATION

On very rare occasions in the treatment of a fracture plaster may be unwise, internal fixation unsafe and continuous traction inappropriate. This particularly applies to open fractures of the tibia with severe soft tissue damage or in the unconscious patient with cerebral irritation. If arterial repair or skin replacement demand immobility of the fracture, external fixation is a possible method.

21.15 EXTERNAL FIXA-
TION
Open fracture, with severe
skin and soft tissue damage,
reduced and held by ex-
ternal fixation (by cour-
tesy of R. A. Denham
F.R.C.S. whose patient
this was, and whose ap-
paratus is illustrated).

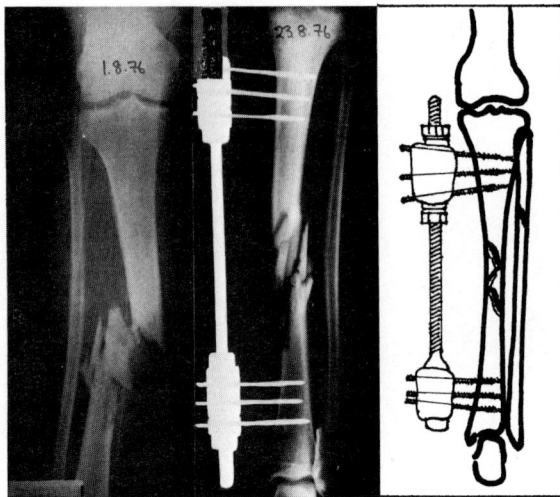

Many appliances are available. Fig 21.15 shows the apparatus devised by R. A. Denham and the following is a brief account of his technique. After wound toilet 3 Denham pins are inserted through healthy skin above the fracture and 3 below it; they must grip the cortex securely. Skeletal traction is applied via the calcaneum (he uses an ice-tong caliper) and the fracture reduced under direct vision. Unless immediate arterial surgery or skin replacement is needed the wound is closed and final adjustments to reduction made under x-ray control. An external compression device is then secured to the pins with acrylic cement. When this has set, the cal-caneal traction is removed and long axis compression applied to the fracture. The fracture is now stable and there is no impediment to subsequent soft tissue surgery.

TIME FACTOR

Repair of a fracture is a continuous process. The fracture haematoma is invaded by capillaries which form organized granulation tissue. Within this, primitive bone-forming cells give rise to chondroblasts and osteoblasts. The chondroblasts secrete phosphatase, and calcium is deposited. The osteoblasts lay down an irregular network of woven bone which gradually replaces the calcified callus. Finally, the woven bone is replaced piecemeal by mature bone in which the lamellae are arranged according to the lines of stress. Any stages into which the repair process is divided are necessarily arbitrary. In this book the terms 'union' and 'consolidation' are used, and they are defined as follows.

Union — Union is incomplete repair; the ensheathing callus is calcified. Clinically the fracture site is still a little tender and, though the bone moves in one piece (and in that sense is united), attempted angulation is painful. X-rays show the fracture line still clearly visible, with fluffy callus around it. Repair is incomplete and it is not safe to subject the unprotected bone to stress.

Consolidation — Consolidation is complete repair; the calcified callus is ossified. Clini-cally the fracture site is not tender, no movement can be obtained and attempted angula-tion is painless. X-rays show the fracture line to be almost obliterated and crossed by bone trabeculae, with well-defined callus around it. Repair is complete and further protection is unnecessary.

21.16 DELAYED SPLINTAGE
This patient's fractured ankle (a) was screwed (b). For the next few days he exercised it actively (c) but took no weight on the leg. When the wound was healed
he walked in a below knee plaster. After 6 weeks the plaster was removed: (d, e)
show the ankle range ten minutes later. Function was rapidly regained — of course
it was! The patient was Professor George Perkins, the pioneer of delayed splintage.

TIME-TABLE — How long does a fracture take to unite and to consolidate? No precise
answer is possible because age, constitution, blood supply, type of fracture and other
factors all influence the time taken.

Approximate prediction is possible and Perkins' time-table is delightfully simple.
A spiral fracture in the upper limb unites in 3 weeks; for consolidation multiply by 2;
for the lower limb multiply by 2 again; for transverse fractures multiply again by 2. A
more sophisticated formula is as follows: A spiral fracture in the upper limb takes
6–8 weeks to consolidate; the lower limb needs twice as long. Add 25 per cent if the

21.17 THE PROCESSES OF REPAIR
(a) Fracture; (b) union; (c) consolidation; (d) bone remodelling. The fracture must
be protected until consolidated; the time required can be roughly forecast from
Perkins' timetable. In children the process is much more rapid: this birth fracture
(e) has a mass of callus (f) in only 19 days.

EXPECTED TIME FOR CONSOLIDATION IN ADULTS (Perkins)

	Spiral Fractures	Transverse Fractures
Upper limb	6 weeks	12 weeks
Lower limb	12 weeks	24 weeks

fracture is not spiral or if it involves the femur. Children of course join more quickly. These figures are only a rough guide; there must be clinical and radiological evidence of consolidation before full stress is permitted without splintage.

TREATMENT OF THE SOFT TISSUES

Whereas a fractured bone may need to be kept still, soft-tissue damage and oedema are best treated by active movement. Here is a dilemma, and different surgeons resolve it by emphasizing one or other aspect of treatment. The fracture itself is of primary importance but the soft tissues must never be neglected. All too often an x-ray appearance is 'treated' instead of the patient.

The objects of soft-tissue treatment are to pump away oedema fluid, to avoid soft tissues sticking together, to prevent muscle wasting and (by exercising the longitudinal muscles crossing a fracture) to compress the bone ends against one another. The essence of soft-tissue treatment may be summed up thus: *elevate and exercise; never dangle, never force.*

ELEVATION

An injured limb usually needs to be elevated; after reduction of a leg fracture, the foot of the bed is raised and exercises begun. If the leg is in plaster the patient is not allowed up until swelling subsides. Then the limb must, at first, be dependent for only short periods; between these periods, the leg is elevated on a chair. The patient is allowed, and encouraged, to exercise the limb actively, but not to let it dangle. When plaster is finally removed, the leg is bandaged and a similar routine of activity punctuated by elevation is practised until circulatory control is fully restored.

Injuries of the upper limb also need elevation. A sling must not be a permanent passive arm-holder; the limb must be elevated intermittently or, if need be, continuously.

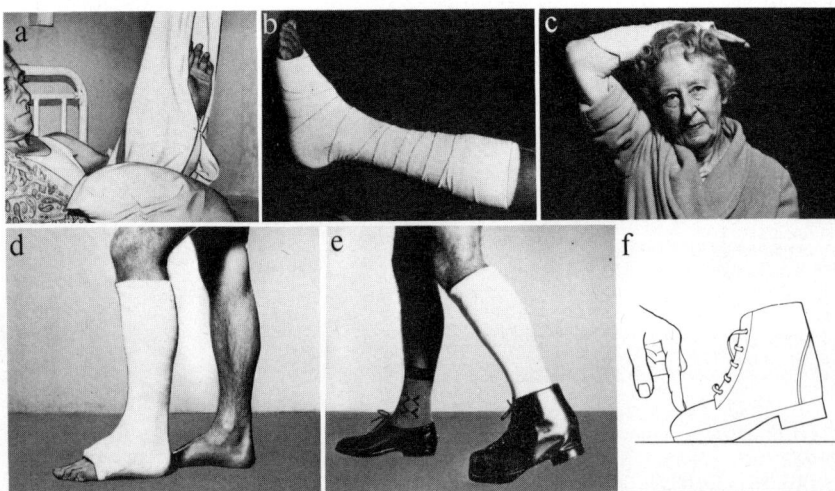

21.18 SOME ASPECTS OF SOFT TISSUE TREATMENT
Swelling is minimized by (a) elevation and (b) firm support. Stiffness is minimized by exercises: this patient(c) with a Colles' fracture is in no danger of a stiff shoulder. To exercise muscles under a plaster is less easy — a walking plaster should be plantigrade (d); an over-boot with rocker action (e, f) facilitates normal walking and muscle activity.

EXERCISES

Passive exercises or forced movements are never permitted in the treatment of fractures. Active exercises, on the contrary, are encouraged and insisted upon.

All unsplinted joints must be used actively from the very start. A patient with a Colles' fracture, for example, must use the fingers, elbow and shoulder as normally as possible.

Joints encased in plaster cannot, of course, be moved, but the muscles passing over them can and must be exercised. A patient with a fractured leg, for example, is fitted with a special boot over the plaster; this boot has a rockered sole to compensate for lack of ankle movement. The patient is then taught to walk, using the normal heel-toe gait so that the long toe muscles are actively exercised. Even if weight-bearing is unsafe and crutches must be used, the patient should still go through the motions of correct walking ('shadow walking').

OPERATION

In closed fractures without complications operation may be indicated for the following reasons:

CLOSED METHODS IMPOSSIBLE — With insensitive skin it is essential to avoid plaster; hence the importance of fixing the spine in patients with traumatic paraplegia.

CLOSED METHODS TOO DIFFICULT — Elderly patients with lower-limb fractures are often best treated operatively to permit early activity.

TIME TOO PRECIOUS — It is often justifiable to treat a pathological fracture through a secondary deposit by internal fixation because the patient may not have long to live and should enjoy activity for as long as possible.

APHORISMS OF FRACTURE TREATMENT

Treat the patient — Do not merely treat the fracture.
Think before you reduce — Is reduction necessary?   Can it be held?
Think before you splint — Splintage is harmful, though often a necessary evil.   Can the muscles or traction hold reduction without a splint?   Are too many joints being splinted?   Are the muscles being actively used?   Is an unreduced fracture into a joint being splinted?   If so, the surgeon is adding insult to injury.
Think before you discard a splint — Is the fracture consolidated?
Never allow passive movement.

SUMMARY OF INDICATIONS FOR OPERATIVE TREATMENT OF FRACTURES

1. Open fractures require urgent operation, namely wound toilet — not internal fixation; the object is to convert them into closed fractures.
2. In closed fractures operation may be indicated: (*a*) to reduce the fracture (open reduction); or (*b*) to hold the fracture reduced (internal fixation); or (*c*) to facilitate treatment of the soft tissues (also internal fixation). With each of these headings the reason for operating may be that closed methods are impossible, or inadequate.

Most of these indications, however, are only relative.   There is always the danger of introducing infection, a surgical disaster.   Operative methods should therefore be avoided unless the aseptic technique of the surgeon, his team and his theatre are all above reproach.
3. The operative treatment of complications is discussed later.

TREATMENT OF OPEN FRACTURES

The word 'open' is preferred to the somewhat old-fashioned word 'compound'. An open fracture is one in which there is skin damage, so that bacteria from without may infect the fracture haematoma. The skin may be cut, or crushed (potential skin loss), or there may be actual skin loss. No matter which, and no matter whether the fracture is open from within or without, it is a surgical emergency.

Treatment begins at the scene of the accident, where the primary objects are to save life and minimize shock; the essentials are morphine, splintage and a dressing. In hospital, anti-shock measures are begun. Further treatment is based on the following considerations: (*a*) bacteria have entered the wound (therefore prophylactic antibiotics and anti-tetanus precautions); (*b*) bacteria may multiply in the wound (therefore wound toilet); and (*c*) more bacteria may enter the wound (therefore wound closure).

WOUND TOILET*

Wound toilet is to remove dead tissue; i.e. tissue which has lost its blood supply. Under general anaesthesia the patient's clothing is removed, while an assistant maintains traction on the limb and holds it still. A sterile pad is placed over the wound and the surrounding skin is cleaned and shaved. The wound itself is then gently cleaned with a harmless detergent. A tourniquet is not used; it would endanger the circulation still further and make it difficult to recognize which structures are devitalized. The tissues are then dealt with as follows.

SKIN — Only the merest sliver of skin is excised from the wound edges; as much skin as possible is spared. The wound often needs to be extended by planned incisions to obtain adequate exposure; once it is enlarged, clothing and other foreign material may be picked out.

FASCIA — Fascia is divided extensively, so that the circulation is not impeded.

MUSCLE — Dead muscle is dangerous, for it provides food for bacteria. Therefore all dead and doubtfully viable muscle is ruthlessly excised.

BLOOD VESSELS — Large bleeding vessels are tied meticulously but, to minimize the amount of catgut left in the wound, small vessels are clamped with artery forceps and twisted.

NERVES — It is usually best to leave a cut nerve undisturbed. If, however, the wound is clean and the nerve ends present without dissection, the sheath is sutured using non-absorbable material for ease of later identification.

TENDONS — As a rule, cut tendons are also left alone. As with nerves, suture is permissible only if the wound is clean and dissection unnecessary.

BONE — The fractured surfaces are gently cleaned and replaced in correct position. Bone, like skin, should be spared, and fragments removed only if they are small and totally detached. Immediate screwing or plating of open fractures is dangerous.

JOINTS — Open joint injuries are best treated by wound toilet, closure of synovium and capsule, and systemic antibiotics; drainage or suction irrigation are used only if contamination is severe.

WOUND CLOSURE

Immediate closure is the ideal, but is dangerous because, as tension rises within the wound, tissues may become avascular, providing food for bacteria, especially anaerobes.

*The word ' débridement ' does not mean removal of débris; it means unbridling, liberating or (in the context of injuries), decompression.

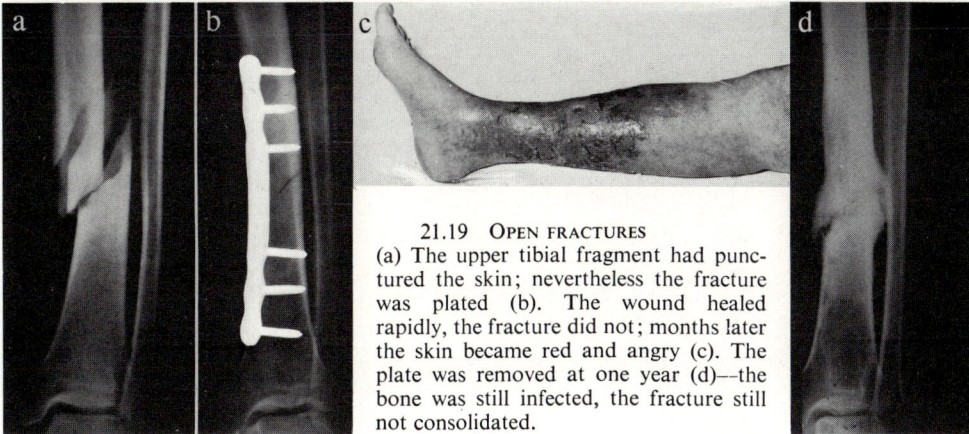

21.19 OPEN FRACTURES
(a) The upper tibial fragment had punctured the skin; nevertheless the fracture was plated (b). The wound healed rapidly, the fracture did not; months later the skin became red and angry (c). The plate was removed at one year (d)—the bone was still infected, the fracture still not consolidated.

If the wound overlies soft tissues, it is best left open, covered with a Vaseline gauze dressing. Closure is postponed until the dangers of tension and infection have passed (delayed primary suture). A wound lying directly over a bone or joint should, if possible, be closed at the primary operation, but provisional cover by split-skin grafts is preferable to suturing with tension. A well-padded plaster is applied, and finally both plaster and wool must be widely split so that skin is visible.

AFTER-CARE

In the ward, the limb is elevated and its circulation carefully watched. Shock may still require treatment. Chemotherapy is continued; if the antibiotic used proves ineffective, the organism is cultured and the appropriate drug substituted.

If the wound has been left open it is inspected at 5–7 days. Delayed primary suture is then often safe, or, if there has been much skin loss, split-skin grafts are applied. If toxaemia or septicaemia persists in spite of chemotherapy, the wound is drained (the only safe treatment if an infected fracture is not seen until 24 hours after injury).

When all reasonable danger of infection has been overcome, definitive treatment of the fracture is carried out.

SEQUELS TO OPEN FRACTURES

SKIN — If there has been skin loss or contracture, grafting may be necessary. When reparative or reconstructive surgery to deeper tissues is required, a full-thickness skin graft is highly desirable.

BONE — Infection may lead to sequestra and to sinuses. Small sequestra should be removed early, but large pieces of bone should not be excised.

Delayed union is inevitable after an infected fracture, but union will occur if infection is controlled and treatment continued for sufficient time.

JOINTS — When an infected fracture communicates with a joint, the principles of treatment are the same as with bone infection, namely drugs, drainage and splintage. The joint should be splinted in the optimum position for ankylosis, lest this occur.

With any open fracture, even if not communicating with a joint, some stiffness is almost inevitable. It can be minimized by slowly increasing active exercises once it is certain that infection has been overcome.

GENERAL COMPLICATIONS OF FRACTURES

SHOCK (*see* page 349)

CRUSH SYNDROME

The crush syndrome may occur if a large bulk of muscle is crushed, as by fallen masonry, or if a tourniquet has been left on too long.   When compression is released, acid myohaematin, from muscle breakdown, is carried in the circulation to the kidney and blocks the tubules.   An alternative explanation is that renal artery spasm occurs and the anoxic tubule cells necrose.

Shock is profound.   The released limb is pulseless and later becomes red, swollen and blistered; sensation and muscle power may be lost.   Renal secretion diminishes and a low-output uraemia with acidosis develops.   If renal secretion returns within a week the patient survives; most patients become increasingly drowsy and die within 14 days.

To avert disaster, a limb crushed severely and for several hours should be amputated.   Thus, if a tourniquet has been left on for more than 6 hours the limb must be sacrificed.   Amputation is carried out above the site of compression and before compression is released.

Once the compression force has been released, amputation is valueless.   The limb must be kept cool and the patient's shock treated.   If oliguria develops, fluid and protein intake are reduced, carbohydrates given (by mouth or into a large vein), protein catabolism reduced (by giving neomycin and an anabolic steroid), and the serum electrolyte balance maintained.   Renal dialysis may be needed.

VENOUS THROMBOSIS AND PULMONARY EMBOLISM

The veins most liable to thrombose are those of the pelvis and lower limbs.   The cause of venous thrombosis is not established.   In the calf veins it may be due to: (*a*) pressure, either against the operating table or mattress, or from a tourniquet or tight bandage, resulting in stasis and possibly intimal damage; (*b*) slowing of the blood flow because of immobility; or (*c*) a raised blood thrombin level, lowered anti-thrombin level and increased number and stickiness of platelets, all of which follow operation or injury.   Thrombosis of the upper thigh veins may be due to an extension of calf vein thrombosis, or it may be primary, especially following sustained excessive flexion of the hip.   In phlebothrombosis (as distinct from thrombophlebitis) the clot is not firmly adherent to the vein wall and emboli may break off and lodge in the lung.   Pulmonary embolism is a complication of venous thrombosis although, in more than half the cases, preceding signs of thrombosis have not been detected.

DIAGNOSIS

With calf vein thrombosis there may be pain and tenderness in the mid-line of the calf, increased warmth, swelling, pain on passive dorsiflexion of the foot (Homan's sign), and slight pyrexia.   Unfortunately clinical features are unreliable; in most patients with vein thrombosis they are negative.   Diagnostic aids include ultrasonic demonstration of obstruction to the venous outflow, and increased uptake of ^{125}I-labelled fibrinogen; most reliable of all is phlebography, which also demonstrates which thrombi are in danger of breaking off to form emboli.

With thrombosis of the thigh veins, pain and tenderness may extend up to the groin and the whole limb becomes swollen.

A small pulmonary embolus causes few symptoms but is a warning that larger emboli may follow.   Signs also are few: specific tests include perfusion scanning, ventilation scanning and selective pulmonary angiography.   Large emboli (which

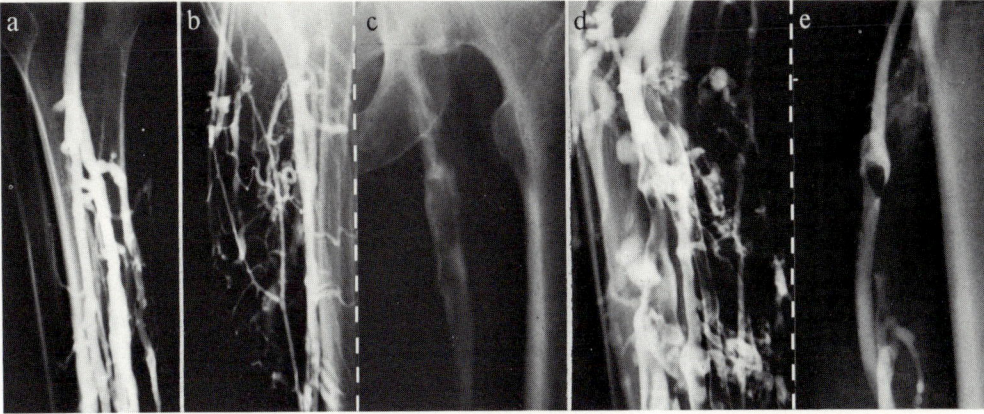

21.20 DEEP VEIN THROMBOSIS — PHLEBOGRAMS
(a, b, c) Patient whose right calf (a) is normal, but whose left calf (b) shows thrombosis; his left femoral vein (c) also is thrombosed; the filling defect is surrounded by contrast on all sides so the thrombosis is potentially mobile, but it does not look recent so the danger is not great. (d, e) Another patient in whom almost every deep calf vein is occupied by thrombus (d) which is fairly recent because the contrast surrounding the filling defect is thin; his thigh (e) shows almost total occlusion of the superficial femoral vein. (By courtesy of Dr. N. W. T. Grieve).

probably originate in the pelvis or thigh) cause pain, haemoptysis and dyspnoea; there is a pleural rub and evidence of lung consolidation. The occasional patient is seized with sudden chest pain, turns pale and falls dead.

PROPHYLACTIC TREATMENT

To await pulmonary embolism and then treat it is dangerous; prophylaxis is far better. Its objects are:

(1) to prevent venous thrombosis from occurring; and (2) once thrombosis has occurred to prevent its extension and thereby reduce the risk of pulmonary embolism. The chief methods of prophylaxis are (1) the avoidance of pressure and stasis; and (2) drugs.

Pressure can be reduced by the use of Sorbo heel pads, and stasis minimized by electrical stimulation of the calf muscles, leg bandaging, pneumatic calf cuffs, and by getting the patient up, or at least moving about in bed, as early as possible.

Prophylactic drugs are indicated for *high risk patients* (those with a history of previous thrombosis, patients who are obese or who have just spent several days in bed, those with malignant disease and those taking contraceptive pills); and under *high risk circumstances* (following pelvic and hip fractures, or before hip operations). The current favourite is low dose heparin (5000 units subcutaneously 2 hours before operation and 8-hourly for 1 week after). Reports suggest that pre-operative inhalation of heparin droplets may prove useful. Less effective prophylaxis is provided by dextran (500 ml of dextran 70 during operation plus 500 ml in the next 24 hours); this is useful when the risk of embolism is only moderate, but there is some risk of bleeding.

TREATMENT OF ESTABLISHED THROMBOSIS AND OF EMBOLISM

ANTICOAGULANTS — These are strongly indicated if pulmonary embolism has already occurred, and with a definite diagnosis of pelvic or thigh vein thrombosis. Calf vein thrombosis is a less definite indication, but the absence of more proximal thrombosis needs to be demonstrated. A tendency to bleed and peptic ulcer are contra-indications.

Heparin given intravenously acts as an anticoagulant within minutes (dose 10,000 units 6-hourly, with protamine as the antidote should bleeding occur). Warfarin (loading dose 30–40 mg) is given orally at the same time and takes 48 hours to act. The heparin is then discontinued and the prothrombin time estimated; this is used to control the subsequent dosage of warfarin (usually given twice daily).

OTHER MEASURES — Vein ligation (to prevent emboli migrating) is not often practised, because emboli do not necessarily come from the obviously affected veins, or even from the clinically abnormal limb; but recurrent pulmonary emboli with x-ray evidence of a loose thrombus is an indication for thrombectomy.

When venous thrombosis has occurred the limb should be supported by a crêpe bandage, elastic bandage or elastic stocking until symptoms have subsided and the limb no longer swells. Streptokinase has been used in the attempt to dissolve the thrombus, but its administration is not without risk of haemorrhage and of anaphylaxis.

If pulmonary embolism has occurred antibiotics are given to prevent lung infection, but it should be remembered that broad-spectrum antibiotics potentiate the action of phenindione (aspirin and phenylbutazone have a similar action).

TETANUS

The tetanus organism flourishes only in dead tissue. It produces an exotoxin which passes to the central nervous system via the blood and the perineural lymphatics from the infected region. The toxin is fixed in the anterior horn cells and thereafter cannot be neutralized by antitoxin.

Established tetanus is characterized by tonic, and later clonic contractions, especially of the muscles of the jaw and face (trismus, risus sardonicus), those near the wound itself, and later of the neck and trunk. Ultimately, the diaphragm and intercostal muscles may be fixed in spasm and the patient dies of asphyxia.

PROPHYLAXIS — Active immunization of the whole population by tetanus toxoid is an attainable ideal. To the patient so immunized booster doses of toxoid are given after all but trivial skin wounding. In non-immunized patients prompt and thorough wound toilet together with antibiotics may be adequate, but if the wound is contaminated, and particularly with delay before operation, then antitoxin is advisable. Horse serum carries a considerable risk of anaphylaxis and human antitoxin (A.T.G.) should be used. The opportunity is taken to initiate active immunization with toxoid at the same time.

TREATMENT — With established tetanus intravenous antitoxin (again human for choice) is advisable. Heavy sedation and relaxant drugs may help; endotracheal intubation and controlled respiration are employed for the patient with respiratory and swallowing embarrassment.

FAT EMBOLISM

Following bony injury, chylomicrons (the normal minute fat particles in the blood stream) may become aggregated and form large embolic globules. Fat emboli lodge in the lung obstructing the capillaries and causing pulmonary oedema with hypoxia; the sputum may contain fat. Other emboli may lodge in small coronary vessels, causing hypotension with a rapid feeble pulse; in skin vessels, producing petechiae, especially on the chest; in the brain, causing drowsiness and confusion; or in the kidney, causing fat in the urine. Fat emboli are probably not the sole cause; unbound free fatty acids may be partly responsible.

Probably many cases are mild and transient. When the condition becomes clinically apparent the basic disorder is hypoxia; it must be corrected by energetic oxygen ventilation with monitoring of pO_2.

Fluid balance must be maintained, and other supporting measures have their advocates; e.g. steroids to help reduce pulmonary oedema, or aprotinin (Trasylol) which may prevent the aggregation of chylomicrons.

OTHER GENERAL COMPLICATIONS

'FRACTURE FEVER' — This is a doubtful entity, though it is true that the absorption of a haematoma often causes slight pyrexia. If fever persists for more than 72 hours it is wise to presume the presence of infection.

DELIRIUM TREMENS — This may follow injury in a chronic alcoholic, and lead to alarming but characteristic symptoms. Chlormethiazole is useful.

ACCIDENT NEUROSIS — This condition, which can follow even minor injury, is closely associated with compensation. The patient is not a malingerer, but resolutely denies that he is fit for work or that any treatment is helping him. Prophylaxis is largely a social problem; treatment includes legal settlement of the case.

LOCAL COMPLICATIONS OF LIMB FRACTURES

SKIN COMPLICATIONS

The most important local complication is skin damage. The treatment of open fractures has already been described (page 326).

FRACTURE BLISTERS — These are due to elevation of the superficial layers of skin by oedema, and can sometimes be prevented by firm bandaging. They should be covered by a sterile dry dressing.

PLASTER SORES — Plaster sores occur where skin presses directly on to bone. They should be prevented by padding the bony points and by moulding the wet plaster so that pressure is distributed to the soft tissues around the bony points. While a plaster sore is developing the patient feels localized burning pain. A window must immediately be cut in the plaster, or warning pain quickly abates and skin necrosis proceeds unnoticed.

BED SORES — Bed sores occur in elderly or paralysed patients. The skin over the sacrum and heels is especially vulnerable. Careful nursing and early activity can usually prevent bed sores; once they have developed treatment is difficult, and it may be necessary to excise the necrotic tissue and apply skin grafts.

MUSCLE COMPLICATIONS

TORN MUSCLE FIBRES — Torn muscle fibres are common with any fracture. Unless the muscle is actively exercised the torn fibres may become adherent to untorn fibres, capsule or bone; if adhesions have been allowed to develop, lengthy rehabilitation will be necessary after the fracture has consolidated. The fracture and the torn muscles both need treatment: it is better to serve two sentences concurrently than consecutively.

DISUSE ATROPHY — Like adhesions, disuse atrophy is largely the result of neglect in treatment, and is usually preventable by repeated active muscle exercises.

TENDON COMPLICATIONS

TORN TENDON — A torn tendon is rare in association with a closed fracture, except in transverse fractures of the patella or olecranon process; in these fractures, the loss of continuity of the extensor mechanism of the joint is the essential feature.

AVULSION FRACTURES — Avulsion fractures in which the tendon remains intact but pulls off a small flake of bone, occur at the shoulder (supraspinatus tendon), the fingers (mallet finger), the knee (patellar tendon) and the lesser trochanter (psoas tendon).

LATE RUPTURE — Late rupture of the extensor pollicis longus tendon may occur 6–12 weeks after a fracture of the lower radius, and late rupture of the long head of biceps after a fractured neck of humerus.

TENDINITIS — Tendinitis may affect the tibialis posticus tendon following medial malleolar fractures.   It should be prevented by accurate reduction, if necessary at open operation.

NERVE COMPLICATIONS

NERVE INJURY — Nerve injury (Chapter 10) is not uncommon in association with a fracture.   Usually the lesion is a neurapraxia which quickly recovers.   Axonotmesis is liable to occur when the injury (fracture or dislocation) imposes severe traction on the nerve.   Neurotmesis is rare with closed fractures.

Nerve damage should be diagnosed during the initial examination of the patient.   In closed fractures recovery is usual and should be awaited.   If recovery has not occurred by the expected time, the nerve should be explored as soon as the fracture has consolidated; but preliminary electromyography is a useful safeguard against unnecessary exploration.

COMPRESSION — Nerve compression may damage the lateral popliteal nerve if an elderly or emaciated patient lies with the leg in full external rotation.   Radial palsy may follow the faulty use of crutches.   Both conditions are due to lack of supervision.

LATE ULNAR NEURITIS — This condition results from a valgus elbow following an ununited lateral condyle fracture (*see* page 371).

COMPLICATIONS INVOLVING THE ARTERY TO THE LIMB
GANGRENE

Gangrene occurs if the limb or part of it is completely deprived of arterial blood for several hours.   The arteries may have been divided, thrombosed or in spasm, or constricted by oedema, especially if an encasing plaster prevents the limb from swelling.   If the circulation to a limb is impaired, prompt reduction of a fracture or dislocation is imperative and is sometimes followed by return of pulsation; should this not occur immediate arteriography is worth considering, with a view to possible arterial suture or grafting.

VOLKMANN'S ISCHAEMIA OF THE FOREARM

If arterial obstruction is incomplete or not too long-lasting, Volkmann's ischaemia (as distinct from gangrene) is the danger.   The brachial artery or both the radial and ulnar arteries may be cut, compressed or contused; even with a closed injury, damaged intima may plug the lumen or promote formation of a thrombus which will fill the lumen back to the next collateral branch.   Transmitted pulsation through thrombus proximal to the site of injury, together with an empty vessel distal to it, produces a spurious appearance of spasm.   True spasm is rare and to base management on the possibility is exceedingly dangerous, for effective treatment is thereby delayed.

The effects of ischaemia vary.   Nerve tissue can survive only 2–4 hours, but is theoretically capable of regeneration.   Muscle can survive longer (probably 6–8 hours), but not in a rigid-walled compartment; the danger is that ischaemic muscle swells (because of congestion and metabolic changes) but its expansion is restricted by strong fascial planes; necrosis soon follows.

SYMPTOMS AND SIGNS

Following an injury or its treatment, the patient complains of forearm pain which is severe, and often agonizing.   The signs are as follows.

LOOK — The fingers may look pale, bluish or mottled.

FEEL — The radial pulse is usually absent.   Sensation in the fingers may be diminished. The forearm is tense and tender.

MOVE — Attempts to straighten the fingers are painful and resisted.

X-RAY — Immediate x-ray will determine whether the fracture has displaced.

PAIN — No single sign is to be relied upon for diagnosis, but severe pain, if associated with any one of the signs described, is the signal for urgent action.

TREATMENT

IMMEDIATE MEASURES — (1) The front half of any encircling splints or bandages, which might be causing compression, must at once be removed; the skin of the entire front of the limb should be exposed.   (2) The elbow, if acutely flexed, is straightened a little to ensure that the artery is not unduly kinked.   (3) The fracture is x-rayed and, if the position of the bones suggests that the artery is being compressed or kinked, prompt reduction is necessary.   (4) The limb is kept cool to reduce its metabolic requirements.   (5) The theatre staff are warned to prepare for emergency operation.

OPERATION — One hour after the immediate measures were taken the patient is re-examined.   Unless the signs of ischaemia have abated immediate operation is necessary.

Technique — The skin and fascia are divided over a considerable length, and the artery exposed.   Excision or by-passing of the damaged segment must be performed, after fixation of any unstable fracture.   If swelling is marked the wound is not closed; delayed primary suture is performed after a few days.

AFTER-CARE — Treatment in a hyperbaric oxygen chamber is a valuable method of mini-mizing ischaemia.   If this has not been averted, prolonged physiotherapy (wax baths, exercises and prolonged passive stretching on a 'banjo' splint) may help to minimize contracture.

VOLKMANN'S CONTRACTURE OF THE FOREARM

Volkmann's contracture is the sequel to ischaemia of the forearm muscles.   They become fibrosed and subsequently contract.   Nerves damaged by ischaemia may recover.   Long after an injury associated with severe pain, the patient may present with deformity, stiffness, weakness and possibly numbness of the hand.

SIGNS

LOOK — The forearm is thin and the hand clawed; all the fingers are flexed at the proximal and distal interphalangeal joints.

FEEL — Sensation in the fingers may or may not have recovered.

MOVE — Because the contracture is due to shortening of the flexor muscles the patient can extend his fingers only when he flexes the wrist.   Gripping with the fingers can be accomplished by extending the wrist, but the function of the hand is poor.

X-RAY — This may show evidence of the old injury.

TREATMENT

MUSCLE SLIDE — The origin of the flexor muscles may be moved distally.   Though this reduces the deformity it does not increase the total excursion of the muscle fibres, and there may be no improvement in function.

EXCISION AND TRANSPLANTATION — In suitable cases remarkable improvement in function can be obtained (Seddon).   Necrotic muscles are excised and contracted tendons divided. The wrist dorsiflexors or other available functioning tendons are transplanted to the cut distal ends of the finger flexors.   If necessary, the median nerve is grafted.

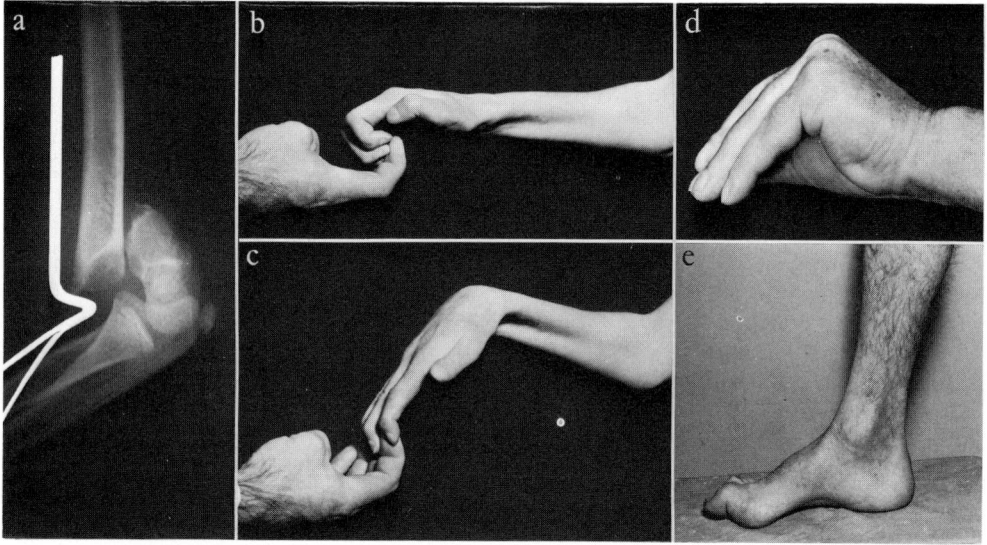

21.21   VOLKMANN'S ISCHAEMIA
(a) Kinking of the main artery is an important cause. (b, c) Volkmann's contracture of the forearm; the fingers can be straightened only when the wrist is palmarflexed (the constant-length phenomenon). (d) Ischaemic contracture of the small muscles of the hand (Bunnell). (e) Ischaemic contracture of the calf muscles with clawing of the toes.

ISCHAEMIA AT OTHER SITES

Ischaemia of the hand may follow forearm injuries, or swelling of the fingers associated with a tight forearm bandage or plaster. The intrinsic hand muscles fibrose and shorten, pulling the fingers into flexion at the metacarpo-phalangeal joints, but the interphalangeal joints remain straight. The thumb is adducted across the palm (Bunnell's 'intrinsic-plus' position).

Ischaemia of the calf muscles may follow injuries or operations involving the popliteal artery or its divisions. It is not as rare as is usually supposed. The symptoms, signs and subsequent contracture are similar to those following ischaemia of the forearm. Occasionally, ischaemia may affect the intrinsic muscles of the foot.

Wherever ischaemia occurs the principles of treatment are those outlined above.

COMPLICATIONS INVOLVING THE ARTERY TO THE BONE
AVASCULAR NECROSIS

Bone dies when deprived of its blood supply. The bones affected are as follows.

FEMORAL HEAD — Avascular necrosis of the femoral head may follow cervical fracture or traumatic dislocation. Segmental necrosis may follow nailing a cervical fracture.

CARPAL BONES — The proximal portion of the carpal scaphoid and the lunate may become avascular following carpal fracture or dislocation (pages 391 and 393).

OTHER SITES — Part of the talus may become avascular after a fracture, or the whole bone after a dislocation. The head of the humerus rarely becomes avascular. Following fractures into joints, small fragments of bone not infrequently become avascular.

Avascular necrosis is not exclusively a complication of fractures and dislocations. Thus, the femoral head may become avascular after forcible reduction of a congenital hip dislocation or a slipped epiphysis, and ' spontaneously ' in Perthes' disease. Other sites of avascular necrosis are described in the section on osteochondritis (page 55).

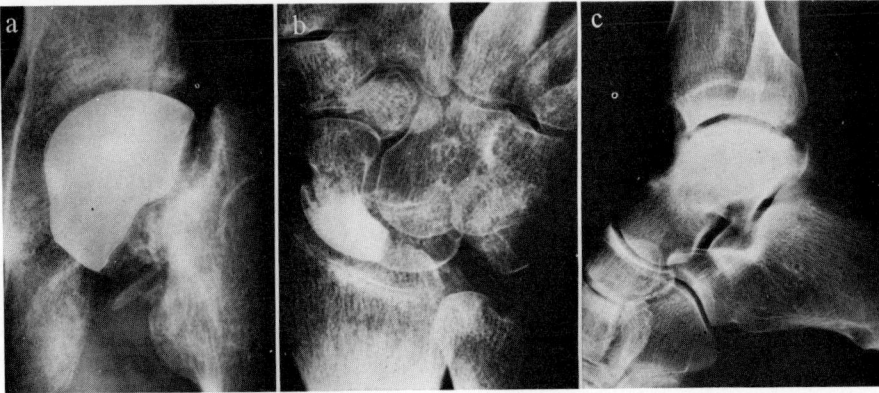

21.22 AVASCULAR NECROSIS
If the fracture cuts off the blood supply to part of the bone the avascular part appears dense on x-ray. 3 common sites are: (a) head of femur, (b) proximal portion of scaphoid, (c) posterior half of talus.

EFFECTS

At first there are no radiological changes, but within a few months the avascular bone may look dense if the area has been immobilized; this is a relative change because the affected bone cannot share in the rarefaction of the surrounding bones which follows immobilization. Still later, absolute increase of density occurs as new bone is laid down on top of dead trabeculae.

UNION — Delay is inevitable in the presence of avascular necrosis, but union follows if the bones can be held together until revascularization has taken place; otherwise non-union is likely.

Osteoarthritis is always liable to follow avascular necrosis, especially if dead bone is allowed to crush with stress.

BONE COMPLICATIONS

DELAYED UNION

The formulae on page 323 are no more than a rough guide to the length of time in which a fracture may be expected to unite and consolidate. They must never be relied upon in deciding when treatment may be discontinued. If the time is unduly prolonged, the term 'delayed union' is used.

CAUSES

INADEQUATE BLOOD SUPPLY — Whenever a fracture occurs through bone which is bare of muscle fibres there is the risk of delayed union. The vulnerable bones include those which are liable to avascular necrosis, and also the lower tibia (especially a double fracture), and the lower ulna.

INFECTION — An open fracture is slow to join, probably because there is little fracture haematoma in which ensheathing callus can form; infection delays union still further.

INCORRECT SPLINTAGE — This includes (a) insufficient splintage; thus, a standard below-knee plaster does not hold a fractured shaft of tibia adequately; and (b) excessive traction, which pulls the bones apart.

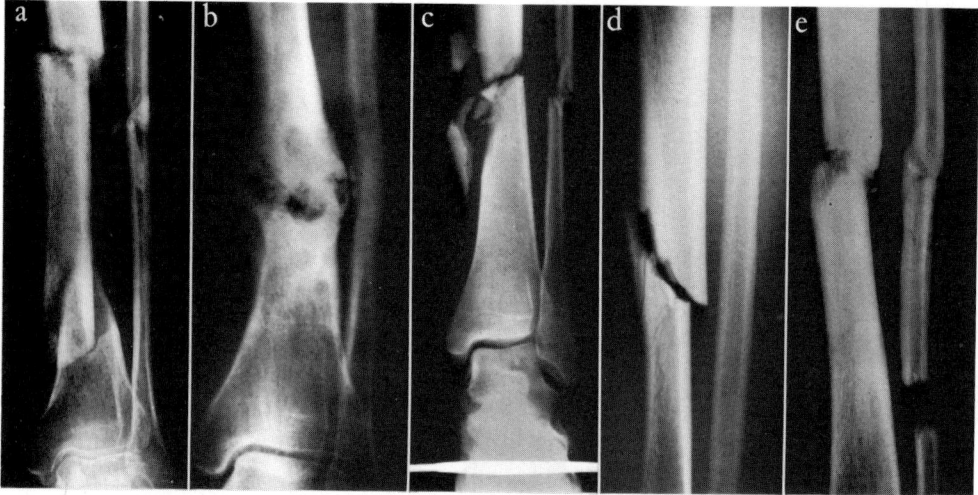

21.23 DELAYED UNION
Causes of delay include (a) a double fracture, (b) infection, (c) excessive traction, and (d) an intact fibula: in (e) both bones were fractured but the fibula joined first and splinted the tibia apart; the delayed union is obvious — an inch of fibula was therefore excised.

INTERNAL FIXATION — Open reduction with internal fixation of a fracture delays union, partly because the fracture haematoma escapes.

INTACT FELLOW BONE — If one bone in the forearm or leg is unbroken, the fractured ends of the other may be held apart, and some delay then follows.

SIGNS

LOOK — There may be no abnormality.

FEEL — The fracture site is tender.

MOVE — The bone may appear to move in one piece; if, however, it is subjected to stress, pain is immediately felt and the bone may angulate; the fracture is not consolidated.

X-RAY — The fracture site is still clearly visible, but the bone ends are not sclerosed.

TREATMENT

CONSERVATIVE — Delayed union is the signal to continue treatment of the fracture, and to continue it efficiently until consolidation is complete. If plaster is being used, it must be sufficiently extensive and must fit accurately. If traction is being used it must not be excessive; it is sometimes better replaced by plaster splintage. Functional bracing is an effective method of promoting bony union.

OPERATIVE — If a fractured tibia is being held apart by a fibula which was not fractured or which has united quickly, it is worthwhile excising 2·5 cm of fibula and reapplying plaster.

NON-UNION

The term 'non-union' implies that bony union cannot occur without operation. Usually the fragments are joined by fibrous tissue.

CAUSES

NON-TREATMENT OF DELAYED UNION — Unless delayed union is recognized, and the fracture adequately treated, non-union is liable to result. Some fractures (for example, those of the carpal scaphoid, lower ulna, and lower tibia) are especially prone to non-union unless splintage is adequate. With these fractures the term 'adequate' means that splintage is sufficiently extensive to prevent movement and uninterruptedly prolonged until consolidation is complete.

TOO LARGE A GAP — If the fracture surfaces are too widely separated union takes a very long time or may never occur. The gap may be due to a gunshot fracture which destroys a large section of bone, to muscle retraction, in which the patient's own muscles pull the fragments apart (as in a fractured patella), or to treatment with excessive traction.

INTERPOSITION — Non-union may develop when any one of the following tissues is interposed between the bone ends: periosteum (for example, a flap of periosteum in association with a fractured medial malleolus); muscle (for example, a fractured femur may spike through the quadriceps muscle, which is consequently interposed between the bone ends); cartilage (for example, a fractured lateral condyle of humerus may be so rotated that its cartilaginous articular surface faces the shaft, and unless the condyle is replaced non-union is inevitable).

21.24 NON-UNION (a) of carpal scaphoid—? from avascular necrosis; (b) of medial malleolus—? from interposition of a flap of periosteum.

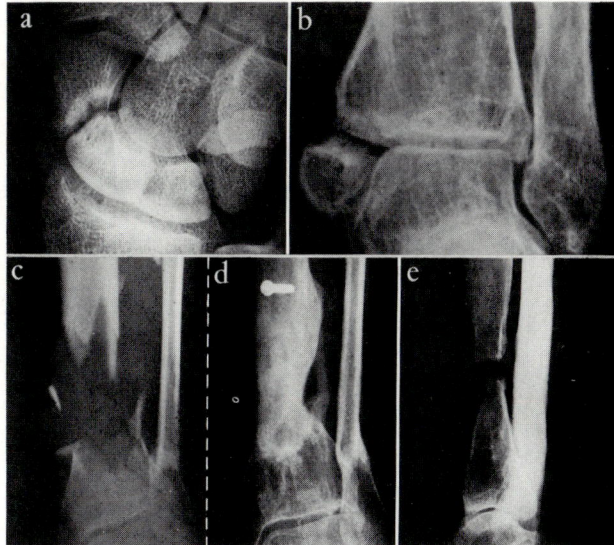

(c) Gap fracture which has been grafted (d) to prevent non-union. (e) Non-union of tibia treated conservatively with a leather gaiter—note the fibular hypertrophy.

SIGNS

LOOK — There may be no abnormality, or there may be deformity.
FEEL — A gap may be palpable. The fracture is not tender.
MOVE — The bone does not move in one piece. Moving the fracture through a few degrees is painless; this painless movement is diagnostic.
X-RAY — The fracture is clearly visible, and often the bone ends are sclerosed.

TREATMENT

Non-union can nearly always be avoided by efficient treatment; established non-union is treated as follows.

CONSERVATIVE — An external splint may permit useful function. It may be all that is necessary or, indeed, all that is possible.

OPERATIVE — Splintage, no matter how extensive and prolonged, can never lead to union once non-union is established (that is, a painless hinge of movement and sclerosis of the bone ends visible on x-ray). To obtain union operation is necessary.

If there is deformity the fibrous tissue and the sclerosed bone at the fracture site are best excised; the fracture is then correctly aligned, bridged by a cortical bone graft (plus cancellous chips), and held by screws or a plate. Suction drainage and plaster splintage are used. Even with infected non-union good results are possible.

If the fragments are in acceptable position it is not essential to disturb the fracture site. Thick onlay grafts may be applied (possibly fixed with screws), or thin slivers of cancellous bone laid across the fracture (Phemister) combined with 'feathering' the host bone; in either case plaster splintage is essential. Alternative methods include rigid fixation with strong plates and screws (Hicks), or screwing and plating combined with compression (Müller).

Electrical stimulation (which promotes osteogenesis) is being tried.

MAL-UNION
CAUSES

PRIMARY — The fracture was never reduced and has united in a deformed position.

SECONDARY — The fracture was reduced but reduction was not held. Redisplacement may occur during the first week, and a check x-ray at one week is advisable.

GROWTH DISTURBANCE — Disturbance of growth does not occur with fracture-separation of an epiphysis: the epiphysis and growth disc are displaced together; the line of fracture is immediately next to the growth disc on its metaphyseal side, and the growth disc is consequently undamaged. An apparently minor injury to the epiphyseal plate, however (especially a vertical fracture through it), may well disturb growth.

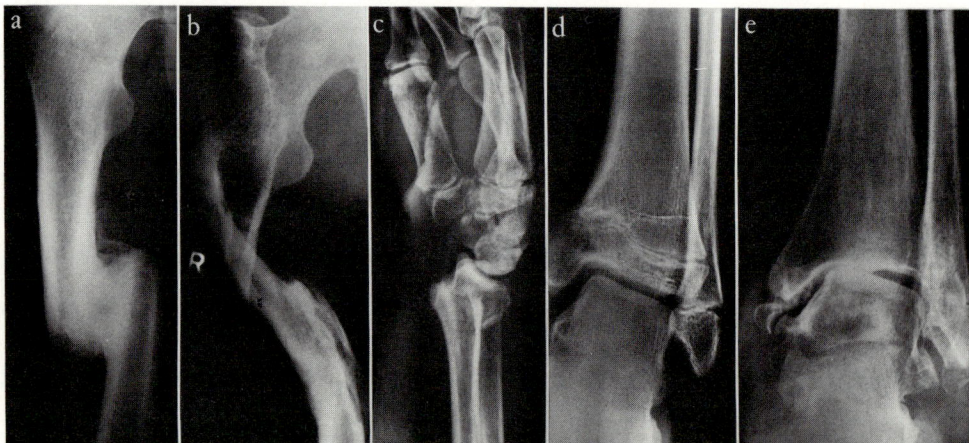

21.25 MAL-UNION
Primary mal-union (a) with overlap, (b) with angulation. (c) Secondary mal-union —this Colles' fracture was reduced satisfactorily, but displaced in plaster. (d) Secondary mal-union following damage to the lower tibial epiphysis. (e) Osteoarthritis, the sequel to mal-union.

SIGNS

The deformity is usually obvious. There may be painful limitation of joint movement (for example, osteoarthritis of the ankle years after a mal-united Pott's fracture). At the elbow valgus deformity may present with delayed ulnar palsy.

TREATMENT

CONSERVATIVE — If shortening is the main feature a raised shoe is usually sufficient. Often no treatment is required, either because a bone may grow straight, or because a neighbouring ball-and-socket joint compensates for the deformity.

OPERATIVE — Osteotomy may be necessary if deformity is unsightly or to prevent the development of osteoarthritis.

JOINT COMPLICATIONS

A fracture or a joint injury may be accompanied by haemarthrosis, which is best aspirated. An open fracture may communicate with a joint (*see* page 326), and a penetrating wound may infect a joint.

As the sequel to injury a joint may be too wobbly (unstable) or too stiff.

INSTABILITY

With a gunshot fracture, there may have been extensive bone loss and consequent flailness. Usually the only treatment possible is an external splint.

A joint may be unstable in the sense that recurrent dislocation occurs following an injury, particularly at the shoulder or ankle. Recurrent dislocation may possibly be preventable by splintage, but can be cured only by operation.

STIFFNESS

Limited movement at a joint, one of the commonest complications of a fracture, has a variety of causes.

INFECTION — Infection of a compound fracture nearly always causes considerable stiffness of long duration.

ADHESIONS — Adhesions of muscle to capsule or bone are likely to follow prolonged splintage or persistent oedema. If stiffness persists, the joint is manipulated under anaesthesia when the fracture has consolidated; at the knee a quadriceps-plasty should be considered.

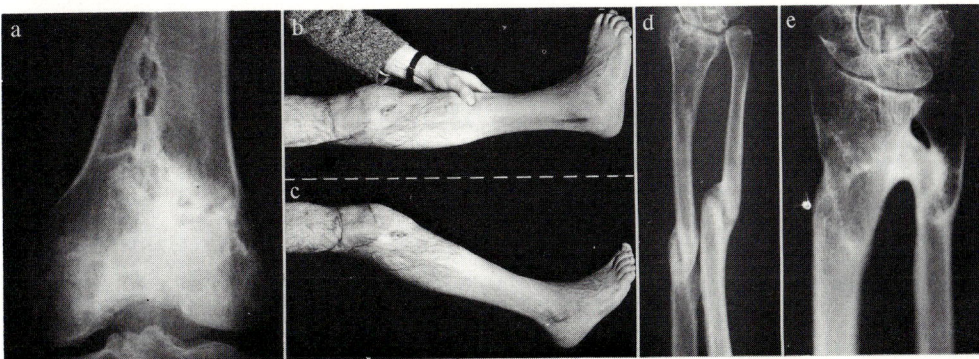

21.26 JOINT STIFFNESS (1)
(a) This heavily compound fracture inevitably caused gross knee stiffness (b, c), which was eventually treated by quadriceps-plasty. (d) Mal-union caused limited rotation of this forearm. (e) Cross-union here abolished rotation.

MAL-UNION — Mal-union may restrict movement; for example, mal-union of the radius and ulna limits forearm rotation; cross-union, which is rare, prevents all rotation.

MYOSITIS OSSIFICANS — This is a post-traumatic condition in which calcium is deposited outside the bone, and joint movement is restricted. Nowadays it is usually called 'traumatic subperiosteal ossification'. It is assumed that movement spreads bone cells further afield within the subperiosteal haematoma. This is unlikely to be the complete explanation, for myositis ossificans rarely follows operations on bone. However, movement, even if not the sole cause of myositis ossificans, probably increases its severity. Passive movement in particular is dangerous and should never be permitted in the treatment of any bone or joint injury.

The commonest site of myositis ossificans is the elbow. A few weeks after injury, movement, instead of increasing, is found to be getting less. The elbow may be painful and almost totally stiff. X-rays show a fluffy mass of calcification in front of the elbow.

At the first hint that movement is decreasing, the elbow should be rested in a plaster gutter. Months later, the fluffy mass of callus appears smaller and more discrete; its removal then is sometimes followed by increased movement.

Myositis ossificans may occur without bony injury, as after a kick on the front of the thigh. A large haematoma of the thigh should if possible be aspirated; ice-packs and ultra-sound may reduce the risk of myositis ossificans in such injuries.

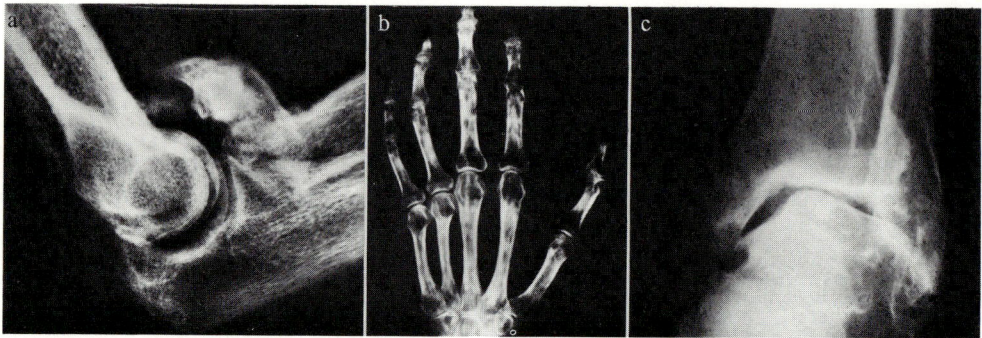

21.27 JOINT STIFFNESS (2)
(a) Myositis ossificans following a fractured head of radius. (b) Sudek's atrophy following a relatively minor injury of the wrist. (c) Osteoarthritis following mal-union.

SUDECK'S ATROPHY — Sudeck's atrophy occasionally affects the foot, but more usually the hand, often after relatively trivial wrist or forearm injuries. Pain and stiffness of fingers come on a few weeks after injury. The fingers are puffy, patchily discoloured, unduly moist, hyperaesthetic and stiff. X-rays show patchy rarefaction of the bones.

With prolonged physiotherapy (heat, elevation and graduated exercises) recovery is slow but steady over many months. Intra-arterial injection of Novocain, or stellate ganglionectomy, has been claimed to accelerate recovery; but a short course of steroids in fairly high dosage (especially if given early) is more likely to be effective.

OSTEOARTHRITIS — Osteoarthritis is liable to follow mal-union when the joint surfaces remain incongruous, or when the direction of stress transmission is abnormal. Avascular necrosis is another potent factor, for the dead bone may crush, causing further incongruity.

UNREDUCED DISLOCATIONS — With every day that passes reduction of a dislocation becomes more difficult and more dangerous. After a few days or weeks (varying with the joint and the patient's age) closed reduction is unwise; open reduction may still be feasible. Still later, neither should be attempted, but function can sometimes be improved by osteotomy, or by a 'sham reduction' (*see* page 378).

PATHOLOGICAL FRACTURES

Pathological fractures are of two kinds: those occurring in apparently normal bone (stress fractures), and those occurring in bone which is clearly abnormal.

STRESS FRACTURES

A stress or fatigue fracture is one occurring in the normal bone of a healthy patient. It is not caused by a specific traumatic incident, but by frequently repeated forces, which are of two main kinds:

(1) *Bending forces*, which breach one cortex; healing begins, but with repeated stress the breach may extend across the bone. This variety affects young adults and is probably due to muscular action, which tends to deform bone; the athlete in training, or the military recruit builds up muscle power quickly but bone strength only slowly and a stress fracture may result.

(2) *Compression forces*, which act on soft cancellous bone; with frequent repetition an impacted fracture may follow.

NOTE — It has been suggested that a stress fracture is the initial lesion in Freiberg's disease (or infraction), in Sever's disease and that repeated distraction is the cause of traction osteochondritis (see page 57).

SITES AFFECTED — Least rare are the following: shaft of humerus (adolescent cricketers); laminae of fifth lumbar vertebra (causing spondylolysis); pubic rami (inferior in children, both in adults); femoral neck (at any age); femoral shaft (chiefly lower third); patella (children and young adults); tibial shaft (proximal third in children, middle third in athletes, distal third in the elderly); distal shaft of fibula (the 'runner's fracture'); calcaneum (adults); metatarsals (especially the second — see page 459).

CLINICAL FEATURES

There may be a history of unusual and repeated activity. This is followed by ache or pain which tends to increase with successive bouts of similar activity, but is relieved by rest. Occasionally the patient presents after the fracture has healed, complaining only of a bony lump (the callus). By definition the patient is healthy; local signs depend upon the progress of the fracture.

LOOK — Swelling or redness may be evident.

FEEL — The overlying skin may be warm. The fracture site is tender. A lump (callus) may be palpable.

MOVE — The neighbouring joint may have painful limitation of movement. Attempting to elicit movement in the bone itself causes pain.

X-RAY — Despite two or even three views, the fracture may not be revealed until callus develops.

DIAGNOSIS

Many disorders including osteomyelitis, scurvy and the battered baby syndrome, can theoretically be confused with stress fractures, but in practice there are only two difficulties:

(1) A small cortical breach or a hair-line fracture may be invisible; the secret is to align the x-ray beam with the suspected fracture.

(2) A compression stress fracture (especially of the upper tibia or femoral neck) shows as a hazy transverse band of sclerosis with peripheral callus. Limbs have been amputated with a mistaken diagnosis of osteosarcoma. The need for caution or biopsy is evident.

TREATMENT

Most stress fractures need no treatment other than an elastic bandage and avoidance of the painful activity. An important exception is femoral neck fractures which (after reduction if necessary) need to be held; in children 2 threaded pins suffice, in adults more formal fixation is needed.

OTHER PATHOLOGICAL FRACTURES

A great variety of disorders may weaken bone and predispose to pathological fracture. Most of the causal conditions are described elsewhere; they can be classified into easily remembered groups as follows:

Defective bone (Congenital)	Disused bone (or faulty use)	Diseased bone	Displaced bone (i.e. Replaced)	Disordered bone (faulty metabolism)
Brittle bones	Post-traumatic disuse	Paget's disease	Solitary cyst	Osteoporosis
Marble bones	Paralysed limbs	Acute osteo-myelitis	Fibrous dysplasia	Osteomalacia
Congenital pseudarthrosis	Rheumatoid arthritis	Syphilitic osteitis	Deposits	Hyperpara-thyroidism

INVESTIGATIONS

GENERAL SYMPTOMS

A history of many previous fractures may suggest a diagnosis of brittle bones.

An operation, no matter how long ago, may have been performed for the removal of a tumour; the present fracture may be the first evidence of metastasis.

Symptoms such as loss of weight, pain, a lump, cough, or haematuria, suggest that the fracture may be through a secondary deposit.

LOCAL SYMPTOMS

Three questions are important. Was the force insufficient to break normal bone? Was the fracture preceded by pain (for example, of a tumour, or Paget's disease)? Was the bone bent before it fractured (as in Paget's disease)?

GENERAL SIGNS

AGE — Under the age of 20 the three common causes are chondroma (in a finger or toe), cyst (in the metaphysis of a long bone) and stress fracture (usually in a metatarsal).

Over the age of 40 the three common causes are Paget's disease (especially of the upper femur); osteoporosis (in the spine or femoral neck); and secondary carcinoma (in the spine, pelvis, humerus or femur).

GENERAL APPEARANCE — The underlying cause may be suggested by cachexia (malignant disease) or by multiple gross deformities (brittle bones, generalized Paget's disease, or von Recklinghausen's disease).

GENERAL EXAMINATION — A thorough general examination is necessary and it is useful to proceed systematically, in the following manner.

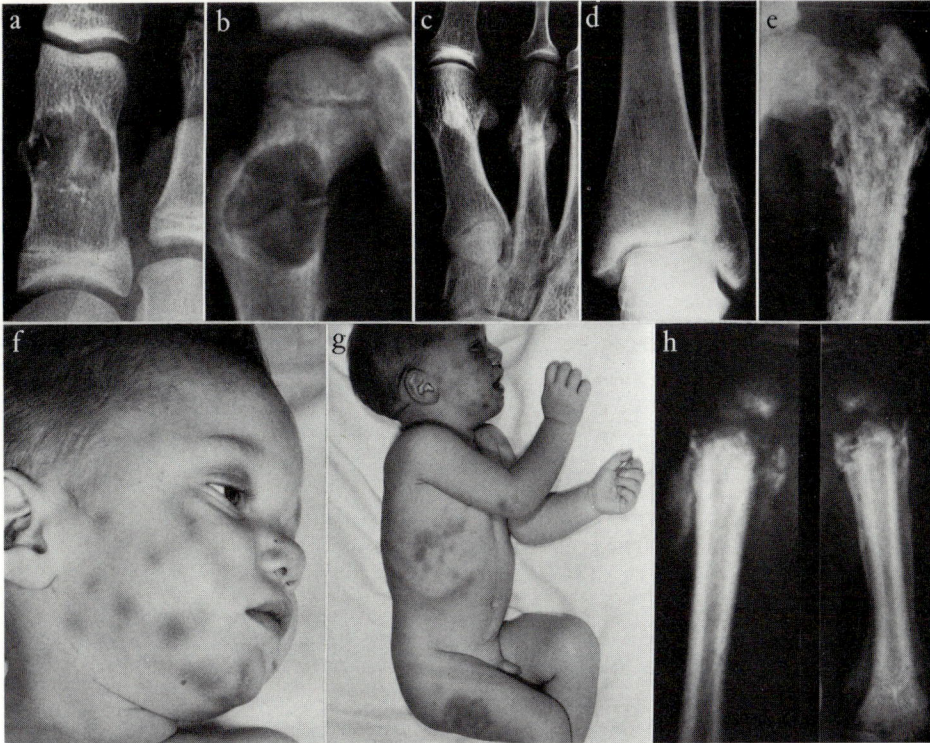

21.28   PATHOLOGICAL FRACTURES (1) IN THE YOUNG
(a) Through a chondroma of the hallux; (b) through a cyst of the femoral neck;
(c) stress fracture of second metatarsal; (d) stress fracture of the fibula — a less
common site; (e) fracture through bone weakened by acute osteomyelitis.
(f, g, h) The battered baby syndrome. The fractures are not pathological but the
family is; the metaphyseal lesions in each humerus (h) are characteristic.

Head — There may be evidence of Paget's disease or rickets.

Neck — Cervical lymph nodes or the thyroid gland may be enlarged.

Chest — Lumps may be palpable in a breast or axilla, and examination of the lung may
suggest a tumour.

Abdomen — The abdominal viscera, kidneys and groins must be palpated.

Pelvis — Examination of the pelvis is incomplete without rectal and vaginal examination.

Central nervous system — There may be evidence of a brain, spinal cord or root tumour,
or of neurosyphilis.

LOCAL SIGNS

SITE — The site of the fracture often suggests the cause.

Spine — Osteoporosis, secondary deposit and myelomatosis.

Femoral neck — Osteoporosis, secondary deposit and irradiation.

Femoral shaft — Paget's disease and secondary deposit.

Near end of a long bone — Solitary cyst, giant-cell tumour, and sarcoma.

Fingers — Chondroma and cyst.

Feet — March (stress) fracture and chondroma.

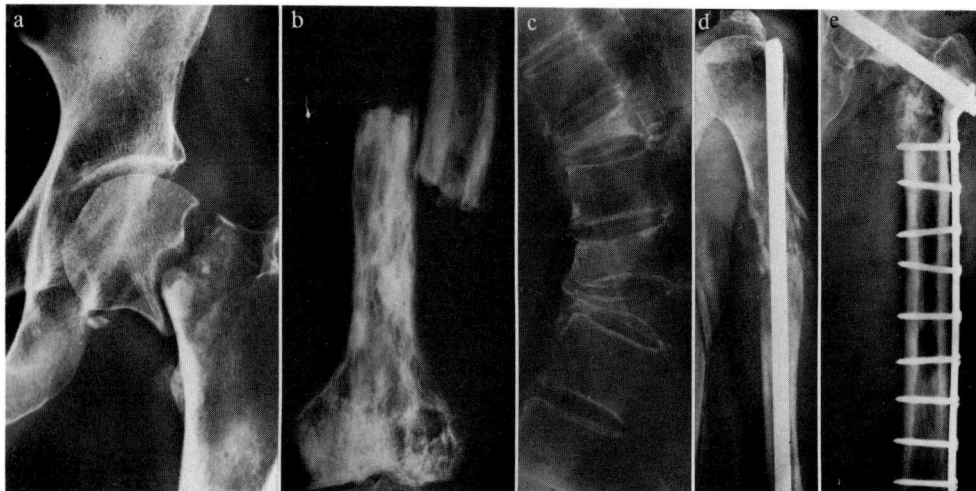

21.29 PATHOLOGICAL FRACTURES (2) IN THE ELDERLY
(a) A fractured femoral neck in a senile patient with osteoporosis is probably the
commonest. Fractures through Paget's disease (b) and through spinal secondaries
(c) are not uncommon. (d) Intramedullary nail for humerus fractured through
secondary deposit. (e) Trochanteric fracture through secondary deposit — the
giant plate was used to anticipate a further fracture through the deposit half way
down the shaft.

X-RAY OF THE BONE AS A WHOLE

Shape — A bent bone suggests brittle bones, Paget's disease, or old rickets.

Density — Generalized decreased density is seen in disuse atrophy, osteomalacia and
osteoporosis.

Architecture — The bone architecture is abnormal in Paget's disease, haemangioma and
fibrous dysplasia.

X-RAY OF THE FRACTURE — The appearance of the bone around the fracture may reveal the
underlying cause.

Periosteum — The periosteum may show callus with a march fracture or sunray spicules
and Codman's triangle with a sarcoma.

Cortex — The cortex may be thinned or eroded by a tumour, or thickened in Paget's
disease.

Medulla — The medulla may contain a rarefied area with well-defined borders (solitary
cyst, giant-cell tumour, chondroma), or a rarefied area with an ill-defined border (malignant tumour), or an area of altered architecture (fibrous dysplasia, Paget's disease).

NOTE ON VERTEBRAE — An ordinary crush fracture is nearly always of the upper border.
With a fracture through malignant disease the anterior border may be eroded; with
osteoporotic fractures the discs are ballooned.

ADDITIONAL INVESTIGATIONS

X-RAY EXAMINATION — X-ray of other bones, the lungs and the urogenital tract may be
necessary to exclude malignant disease.

BLOOD INVESTIGATION — Investigations should always include a full blood count,
a W.R. or Reiter's test and, where necessary, electrophoresis, paper chromatography or
chemical analysis.

URINE EXAMINATION — Urine examination may reveal blood from a tumour, or Bence
Jones protein in myelomatosis.

TREATMENT

The treatment of stress fractures has already been described. With other pathological fractures the underlying disease should if possible be treated.

Nearly all pathological fractures unite, and many at normal speed; most can be treated in the same way as fractures through normal bone.

Fracture through a benign tumour is best treated by curetting or excising the tumour; bone grafting is then often necessary.

Fracture through a sarcoma is often an indication for amputation.

Fractures through secondary deposits may unite with conservative treatment, especially with radiotherapy and control of the hormone environment (by drugs or operation). Internal fixation is, however, often preferred; it enables the patient to enjoy activity during his remaining months of life. With internal fixation for fractures through malignant deposits (or with osteoporosis), the bone may be too weak for the metal to hold securely; one answer is to pack the bone interior with acrylic cement before plating.

Suggestions for further reading

Alms, M. (1961). 'Fracture Mechanics.' *J. Bone Jt Surg.* **43B**, 162

Browse, N. L. (1977). 'What Should I Do About Deep Vein Thrombosis and Pulmonary Embolism?' *Ann. R. Coll. Surg. Eng.* **59**, 138

Charnley, J. (1961). *The Closed Treatment of Common Fractures*, 3rd ed. Edinburgh; Livingstone

Devas, M. (1975). *Stress Fractures.* Edinburgh, London & New York; Churchill Livingstone

J. Bone Jt Surg. (1968). **50A**, 766. Instructional Course Lecture. 'Anatomy, Physiology and Pathology of the Blood Supply of Bone.' (Kelly, P. J.)

Meyer, S. *et al.* (1975). 'The Treatment of Infected Non-Union of Fractures of Long Bones.' *J. Bone Jt Surg.* **57A**, 836

Müller, M. E., Allgower, M., and Willeneger, H. (1965). *The Technique of Internal Fixation of Fractures.* New York; Springer-Verlag

Perkins, G. (1958). *Fractures and Dislocations.* London; Athlone Press

Sarmiento, A. *et al.* (1976). *Instructional Course Lectures.* **25**, 184

Tsuge, K. (1975). 'Treatment of Established Volkmann's Contracture.' *J. Bone Jt Surg.* **57A**, 925.

Watson-Jones, R. (1976). *Fractures and Joint Injuries.* 5th edition. Ed. by Wilson J. N. Edinburgh; Churchill Livingstone

CHAPTER 22

THE MANAGEMENT OF MAJOR ACCIDENTS

THE SCENE OF THE ACCIDENT

MULTIPLE ACCIDENTS

The first duty of a doctor arriving at the scene of a major accident is to introduce calm and order into the prevailing chaos. His actions should be swift yet unhurried, calm yet purposeful. Until the police or other authorities arrive he should assume control and, after rapidly assessing the situation, decide on priorities. If unskilled help is at hand messages are sent to the emergency services (ambulance, police and fire); the nearest accident centre is alerted and, where mobile operating theatres and surgical teams are available, they may need to be summoned.

THE INDIVIDUAL PATIENT

Treatment of the individual patient begins as soon as possible. The doctor who is inexperienced in dealing with accidents will find it useful to follow a routine sequence of actions which may be modified according to circumstances: obtain access; ensure airway; examine; extricate; arrest haemorrhage; combat shock; splint fractures; and transport.

ACCESS — When a patient is trapped or buried, the objects covering him should be moved, rather than pulling him out from beneath them. Priority is given to freeing the head and trunk. If the patient is conscious he will need immediate reassurance.

AIRWAY — If the unconscious patient is breathing stertorously the angle of the jaw is pulled forwards and the head hyperextended; should the difficulty persist a finger is inserted into the mouth to ensure that breathing is not being obstructed by the tongue, false teeth or any other foreign body. If, despite clearing the upper airway the patient still cannot breathe freely, he may have a sucking wound of the chest wall, which should be covered with a dressing strapped firmly in position (*see* page 352).

EXAMINATION — A detailed examination is neither practicable nor essential, but the pulse is felt, the respirations are observed, and the head, chest, abdomen and limbs, if accessible, are quickly palpated.

EXTRICATION — A patient with fractures should not be dragged forcibly from overlying impedimenta. When obstructions have been lifted he can be gently moved. Twisting and flexion must be avoided if there is the possibility of spinal injury.

HAEMORRHAGE — External bleeding can usually be stopped by pressure with a finger, forceps or a firm pad. Tourniquets are rarely necessary; if one must be used a label stating the time of its application is attached to the patient in a prominent position.

SHOCK — Morphine is invaluable and, for a severely injured adult, it is probably best to give both 10 mg ($\frac{1}{6}$ grain) intravenously and 10 mg intramuscularly; again, adequate labelling is essential. Morphine should not be given to patients with abdominal or head injuries. Where facilities are available intravenous fluids may be given (*see* later).

No food or fluids should be given by mouth: if the patient is unconscious these may enter the trachea, and even if he is conscious their presence in the stomach increases the hazards of anaesthesia during the next few hours.

SPLINTAGE — A broken limb should be gently straightened by traction. A fractured arm is easily splinted by bandaging it to the trunk, and a leg by tying it to the other leg if this is intact. Ambulances should carry inflatable splints, and only occasionally are improvised splints needed; an umbrella, walking stick, piece of wood or tubular steel is nearly always available. Open wounds are covered with a clean dressing.

TRANSPORT — To move a severely injured patient on to a stretcher at least two, but preferably three, people are required, so that he is transferred 'in one piece' without serious disturbance; this is particularly important with spinal fractures. The unconscious patient is best transported in the semi-prone position. The airway and pulse should be checked once more before the patient leaves in the ambulance.

Ambulances should be equipped with splints, dressings, airways, oxygen and transfusion apparatus. They should be in two-way radio communication with the accident unit. In difficult terrain helicopter ambulances are almost essential. Ambulance attendants are usually highly trained, but every effort should be made by the staff of the accident unit to keep them continually informed, up to date and interested in their work. Their observations on the patient's state of consciousness and general condition are invaluable.

ACCIDENT CENTRES

Peripheral casualty services (cottage hospitals, health centres and first-aid posts) should deal only with minor injuries. Accident centres are quite different; they must be able to deal with any emergency — medical or surgical. Each centre should therefore be part of a general hospital; but it also needs the support of a central unit with highly specialized services such as neurosurgery, thoracic surgery and dialysis. It is best designed on an open plan system permitting flexibility of use, and needs to be generously supplied with equipment for communications, patient transport and all forms of emergency care. Of particular importance is equipment for resuscitation, airway management, electrolyte investigations and radiology (portable equipment is inadequate, and heavy duty equipment within the centre essential). Staffing also must be generous, but the leader need not be a surgeon. He must be expert in the diagnosis and management of emergencies; he also needs to be a born organizer and a dedicated enthusiast.

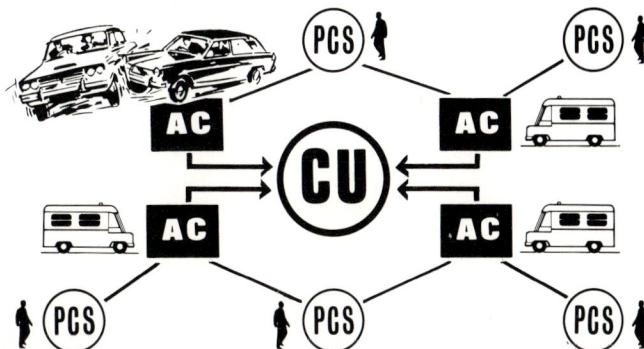

22.1 THE PROBLEM AND THE SOLUTION
PCS — Peripheral casualty services;
AC — Accident centres;
CU — Central unit.

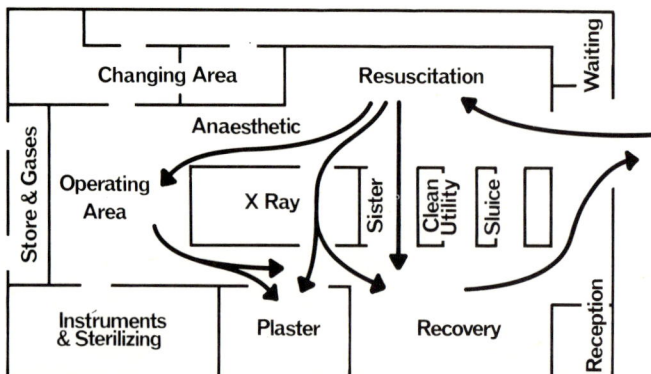

22.2 PLAN OF AN ACCI-DENT CENTRE
Note (1) central position of x-ray department; (2) open planning to permit a variety of flow patterns; (3) operating theatres, though not essential here, must be close by.

THE SEVERELY INJURED PATIENT

The management of the severely injured patient is an urgent and complex task. The greatest problem is to decide on a sequence of procedures and to allot priorities. No rigid rules can apply to every patient and the account which follows aims at providing guidance for those with limited experience. The three essential phases of management, for ease of memory, may be expressed as revive, review, and repair.

REVIVE

The term 'revive' implies rapid appraisal and urgent resuscitation. There are two causes of early death following an accident: (1) circulatory failure from bleeding and shock; (2) respiratory failure from airway obstruction, from paralysis of the respiratory centre (with head injuries), or from insufficient lung ventilation (with major chest injuries). The most urgent necessities are a clear airway, blood transfusion, the closure of a sucking chest wound and the immobilization of a flail segment of the chest wall.

REVIEW

'Review' is a slightly more deliberate procedure. An attempt is made to find out if the patient is a diabetic, or is taking such drugs as steroids or anticoagulants. Then he is stripped, external bleeding arrested and a brief but orderly examination carried out. The head, chest, abdomen, spine and limbs are carefully but rapidly examined in turn. X-ray examination is frequently necessary for injuries of the chest, abdomen and pelvis; with head injuries x-rays are rarely helpful at this early stage, and with limb injuries major fractures are clinically apparent. Throughout the phase of review blood replacement is continuing, and, unless head or abdominal injuries contra-indicate it, morphine is now given.

REPAIR

'Repair' is the term for the emergency operative procedures which resuscitation has made possible. The patient is anaesthetized and transfusion is continued. An orderly sequence is important. (1) Continued bleeding must be stopped; in order of importance are intracranial, intrathoracic and intra-abdominal bleeding. (2) Major chest injuries must be dealt with and this may necessitate tracheostomy. (3) Ruptured abdominal viscera must be repaired. (4) Open wounds are excised and, where possible, closed. (5) Fractures are splinted; where fractures are multiple internal fixation may be necessary, but the temptation to surgical virtuosity should be resisted.

During and after these operations blood replacement is continued as necessary, with the patient's general condition and the central venous pressure as important guides. A fluid balance chart is kept, and electrolyte balance maintained.

SHOCK

NEUROGENIC SHOCK — This occurs with painful injuries, emotional disturbances or both. The blood volume is unchanged but its distribution is faulty, with excess in the non-essential circulation (splanchnic vessels and skeletal muscles) and insufficient in the essential circulation (cerebral and cardiac vessels).

OLIGAEMIC SHOCK — This is the result of bleeding, whether internal or external. The blood volume is reduced, but the harmful effects of this reduction are mitigated, again by re-distribution: the peripheral and splanchnic vessels contract, so that a higher proportion of the reduced volume becomes available for the heart and brain. This compensatory mechanism may fail if the blood loss is great or rapid; the peripheral vessels then become dilated, the cardiac output and blood pressure drop and the circulation fails. This dangerous condition of peripheral vasodilatation is sometimes induced or hastened by heating the patient or giving him alcohol.

The bystander who faints at the sight of an accident is suffering from transient neurogenic shock. The injured man also is suffering from neurogenic shock but, because of blood loss, oligaemic shock may supervene. He becomes ill, apathetic and thirsty, his breathing shallow and rapid: the lips and skin are pale and the extremities feel cold and clammy. As compensation fails the pulse becomes rapid and feeble while the blood pressure drops. Shock must not be diagnosed as purely neurogenic unless careful examination has failed to reveal any serious injury.

TREATMENT

Neurogenic shock is treated by elevating the legs, relieving pain and dispelling fear. If rapid recovery does not occur the patient is suffering from oligaemic shock.

The treatment of oligaemic shock is urgent: the essentials are to arrest bleeding and to replace lost blood. Morphine (preferably given intravenously) is of great value, but must be withheld if there are head injuries or undiagnosed abdominal injuries. Giving oxygen and the early reduction and splintage of fractures are valuable. The intravenous injection of 100 mg of hydrocortisone sodium succinate may relieve a desperate situation, but vasopressor drugs are of doubtful value.

The essential feature of treatment, however, is early and adequate transfusion to restore the volume of circulating blood. Accurate blood grouping takes time, and group 'O' Rh-negative blood may be used in emergency until cross-matched blood is available. Plasma and plasma-substitutes are of much less value; they should be used only as a stopgap and a specimen of blood for cross-matching must be taken first. (With burns, on the contrary, the shock is associated with an initial haemoconcentration, and plasma is the ideal transfusion fluid.)

It is important not only to give blood, but to give enough blood. Even with closed injuries there is far more bleeding into the tissues than is commonly appreciated. Two or three units may be lost with a single major limb fracture and up to 6 units with 3 major fractures; in trunk fractures with visceral damage, as much as half the blood volume may be lost. Rapid transfusion may be important, for which purpose a Martin pump is valuable. In the previously healthy patient 100 ml/min. may be given until the blood pressure reaches 100 mm. With large transfusions the danger of introducing too much sodium citrate must be borne in

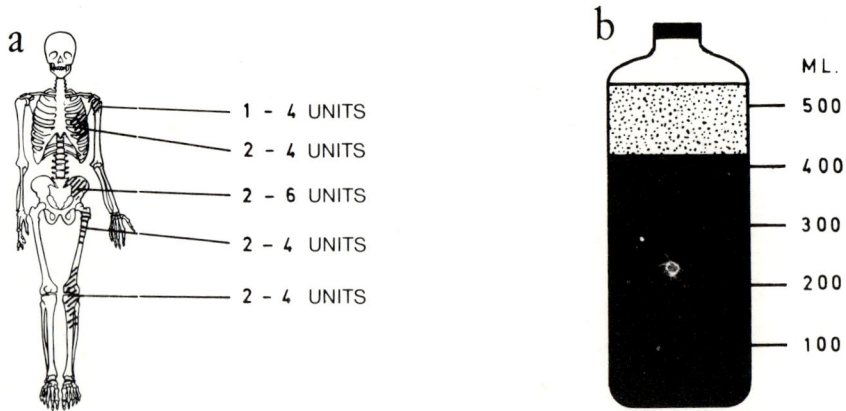

a

1 - 4 UNITS

2 - 4 UNITS

2 - 6 UNITS

2 - 4 UNITS

2 - 4 UNITS

b

ML.

500

400

300

200

100

22.3 SEVERE INJURIES — DANGER POINT (1)
(a) Range of probable blood loss in closed fractures. (b) From a (540ml) container
the patient gets only 400–420 ml of actual blood — the rest is anticoagulant and
space. **Moral** — The severely injured patient may lose more blood than you think,
and get less; do not be afraid of overtransfusion.

mind, and countered by injecting the patient with a solution of calcium gluconate
(1 gm. for each 500 ml. of blood). If shock is not abating despite transfusion,
concealed haemorrhage into the chest or abdomen is probable and must be treated.

HEAD INJURIES

The commonest head injury is concussion. It requires no special treatment beyond
rest, but careful observation is necessary because compression (from intracranial
haemorrhage or oedema) may supervene.

EXAMINATION

(1) The degree of impairment of consciousness is important. A history, usually
obtained from the ambulance attendants, of a lucid interval between unconsciousness
at the scene of the accident and unconsciousness on arrival at the hospital indicates
rising intracranial pressure; so also does increasing depth of unconsciousness.

(2) The head is inspected for external wounds, depressed fracture, and escaping
cerebrospinal fluid.

(3) With generalized increase of intracranial pressure the breathing becomes
stertorous, the pulse slow and bounding, and the pupils dilated. If the pupils
become widely dilated and fixed, or flaccid limb paralysis becomes spastic, a
dangerous level of intracranial pressure has been reached and its treatment is
urgent.

(4) With a depressed fracture, or localized brain damage, the pupils may become
unequal in size or the limbs on the two sides of the body unequal in tone. These
signs also are a signal for urgent action, but it must be remembered that enlargement
of one pupil may be the result of purely local damage to the eye or orbit.

(5) *Special investigations*. Carotid angiography, though valuable, is being sup-
planted by computerized transverse axial tomography (EMI scanning) which is

safe and non-invasive. Lesions such as intra- or extra-cerebral haematomata, contusions and oedema can be diagnosed with precision, thus simplifying management.

EMERGENCY TREATMENT

(1) A clear airway is essential and the administration of oxygen is useful to lessen anoxia, which increases cerebral congestion.

(2) Bleeding from the scalp can be arrested with artery forceps or a stitch. A depressed fracture with localizing signs needs to be elevated.

(3) Restlessness is difficult to control, because sedatives mask the important sign of deepening unconsciousness. A full bladder increases restlessness and should be emptied by catheterization.

(4) Generalized increase of intracranial pressure can sometimes be relieved by intravenous injection of hypertonic solutions, such as triple-strength plasma.

(5) A dangerous rise of intracranial pressure which is not relieved by the above measures may require craniotomy.

(6) The patient with a basal fracture and leaking cerebrospinal fluid is given antibiotics and instructed not to blow his nose.

(7) In all cases careful and regular observation is essential.

RESPIRATORY OBSTRUCTION

The injured and unconscious patient is in danger of suffocation. Respiratory obstruction, probably the commonest single cause of death soon after injury, is preventable. The respiratory passages may be obstructed by the tongue, dentures, blood, mucus or vomit. Breathing becomes laboured and stertorous, and the patient cyanosed.

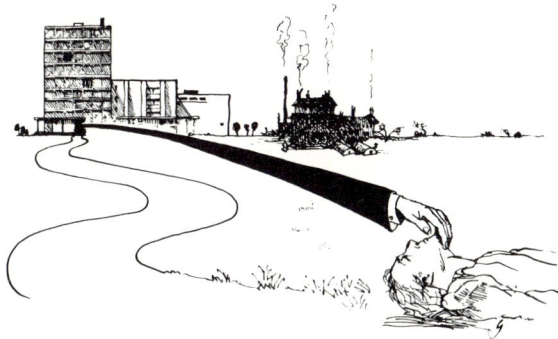

22.4 SEVERE INJURIES —
DANGER POINT (2)
This drawing (reproduced by kind permission of Mr. R. S. Garden and the Editor of *Injury*) emphasizes the vital (literally) importance of a clear airway, and how it can usually be achieved.

TREATMENT

The obstruction must be removed immediately. If pulling the angle of the jaw forwards proves inadequate, a finger in the mouth is used to pull the tongue forwards or to dislodge and remove any other solid obstacle. Fluid is wiped out or aspirated with a sucker. Often these measures prove adequate and the insertion of a simple airway ensures comfortable breathing. If they fail, laryngoscopy or bronchoscopy may be necessary, but when the obstruction cannot be cleared by way of the mouth there should be no hesitation in performing immediate tracheostomy.

CHEST INJURIES

Chest injuries may cause inadequate ventilation through interference with the normal pumping action of the thoracic cage. The effects of the resulting anoxia are made worse by oligaemic shock due to bleeding and by carbon dioxide retention. The most important injuries demanding urgent treatment are (a) lung collapse in closed chest injuries, (b) lung collapse with a valvular wound of the chest wall, and (c) stove-in chest with paradoxical respiration.

EXAMINATION

(1) The skin is inspected for open wounds: the dangerous wounds are often the small ones. The shape of the chest also is noted, a stove-in segment usually being obvious.

(2) Fractured ribs or a stove-in segment can sometimes be palpated.

(3) Movement of the two sides of the chest is observed during breathing. If one side remains still, the lung on that side is probably collapsed; if inspiratory effort is accompanied by indrawing of part of the chest wall, paradoxical respiration is diagnosed.

(4) Percussion reveals pulmonary collapse and mediastinal displacement.

(5) Auscultation confirms lung collapse or paradoxical respiration.

(6) An x-ray film is essential. Even though it may be technically poor and difficult to interpret it may be useful in showing injuries of the skeletal cage, displacement of the trachea and mediastinum, diaphragmatic rupture with abdominal organs in the chest, and it may indicate whether lung collapse is due to air or blood in the pleural cavity.

EMERGENCY TREATMENT

(1) With all major chest injuries, the replacement of blood loss and the administration of oxygen are of paramount importance.

(2) Not all open chest wounds communicate with the thoracic cavity; some involve only cervical or abdominal structures. Those that do communicate must be closed, and if the wound is valvular its closure is urgent. A moist dressing strapped firmly in position is a temporary expedient, but a stitch is much better: the important point is airtight closure. Elective closure is performed later, but, if there is considerable lung damage or bleeding formal thoracotomy will be necessary.

(3) Lung collapse which is causing serious respiratory embarrassment is treated by inserting a needle through the second intercostal space. Often this proves inadequate and must be replaced by a tube which is connected with an underwater seal.

(4) Paradoxical respiration with a stove-in chest may, in a previously fit young patient, cause only moderate respiratory difficulty. The administration of oxygen and possibly strapping a large pack firmly over the mobile segment may be sufficient treatment.

Deteriorating respiratory function due to a stove-in chest with a large unstable segment may be rapidly brought under control in the Accident Department by means of positive pressure ventilation through an endotracheal tube. A chest drain connected to an under-water seal is essential in case there is an associated lung leak. Positive pressure ventilation may be continued for several days until the chest wall becomes stable, but for this a tracheostomy is necessary; alternatively the flail segment can be stabilized by fixing the fractured ribs with intramedullary nails or plates.

(5) The patient who needs no operation may still have reduced lung ventilation which is being accentuated by pain on breathing. Sedation is important but respiratory depressants should not be used; local anaesthetic injections are of great value and they also have a place in post-operative management.

ABDOMINAL INJURIES

The most important abdominal injuries are ruptures of viscera and of blood vessels. There is a real danger that abdominal injuries may be overlooked, either because an unconscious patient can give no history, or because a conscious but shocked patient may not complain even with serious injury.

EXAMINATION

(1) The abdomen is inspected for perforating wounds, for bruising and to observe respiratory movements.

(2) Palpation may reveal localized tenderness, the boggy fullness of extensive bleeding, or board-like rigidity over a ruptured viscus. It must be remembered that considerable bleeding, especially if retroperitoneal, may not be detected on palpation, and rigidity may not develop despite a ruptured viscus if the patient is severely shocked.

(3) Auscultation tends to be forgotten but the complete absence of bowel sounds is an important sign of intra-abdominal damage.

(4) Percussion may disclose the presence of fluid, or of a decreased area of liver dullness due to gas from a ruptured viscus.

(5) Rectal and pelvic examination must not be omitted and, with lower abdominal injuries, the bladder, urethra and urine must be examined.

(6) Intubation of the stomach is often wise; apart from the advantage of aspirating gastric contents prior to anaesthesia, the withdrawing of blood may suggest gastric injury.

EMERGENCY TREATMENT

(1) An open wound needs to be closed. A temporary dressing is sufficient and formal closure must not be performed if the integrity of the abdominal viscera is in doubt, for laparoscopy or laparotomy is then essential.

(2) Continued abdominal bleeding demands emergency transfusion and laparotomy. The patient with oligaemic shock who is not responding to transfusion is probably bleeding into his abdomen and, even if the signs are equivocal, exploration is justified.

(3) A ruptured viscus must be repaired when the patient has been resuscitated.

BURNS

The patient with extensive burns suffers from neurogenic shock because of pain, and from oligaemic shock because (1) fluid exudes copiously from the burnt area, (2) fluid is lost into the tissues, and (3) red cells have been damaged. The amount of fluid loss varies with the area of the burn and can be assessed by a special formula (the rule of 9) or from pyrogram charts. Often the depth of the burn cannot be determined until superficial sloughs separate.

EMERGENCY TREATMENT

(1) Treatment of the shock is urgent. Morphine is given and fluid replacement begun. Every moment of delay in starting the transfusion makes the prognosis

worse. For deep burns, whole blood is given; for superficial burns, plasma is used first, though blood usually becomes necessary later.

(2) With burns of the face or neck, immediate intubation or tracheostomy may be necessary.

(3) With chemical burns, the surface is gently washed. In all other cases the burnt area is not disturbed or treated with topical applications. If the environment is suitable the burn is left exposed, otherwise it is covered with sterile towels.

(4) If transfer to a special burns centre is unavoidably delayed, further measures become necessary. Fluid losses must continually be made good with blood, plasma, or plasma and saline solution as required. Antibiotics are started and sedation is continued. Metabolic requirements are met by oral feeding or, in children, intravenously. At least every 4 hours the patient is examined; the skin colour, pulse, blood pressure and urine output are noted. An indwelling catheter is useful in assessing the all-important fluid balance. In severe cases the blood haemoglobin, electrolytes and urea are examined 4-hourly and used as a guide to further treatment.

Suggestions for further reading

Cole, W. H. and Puestow, C. B. (1972). *Emergency Care*, 7th ed. London; Butterworths

Ellis, M. (1970). *The Casualty Officer's Handbook*, 3rd ed. London; Butterworths

Keen, C. (1974). 'Chest Injuries.' *Ann R. Coll. Surg. Eng.* **54**, 3, 124

Symposium on Blood Volume (1963). *Ann R. Coll. Surg. Eng.* **33**, 3, 137

Symposium on Road Accidents (1966). *Ann R. Coll. Surg. Eng.* **39**, 3, 151

Tindall, G. T. and Fleischer, A. S. (1976). 'Head Injury.' *Hosp. Medicine*, May, 89.

CHAPTER 23

FRACTURES AND DISLOCATIONS IN THE UPPER LIMB

THE SHOULDER

Three principles govern the treatment of injuries around the shoulder.

(1) If reduction is unnecessary or impossible, the fracture is disregarded and treatment concentrated on regaining shoulder movement.

(2) If reduction is necessary and is possible, it may need to be held, and shoulder movements must subsequently be regained by active exercises.

(3) In all shoulder injuries, however treated, the elbow and fingers must be exercised from the start.

FRACTURED CLAVICLE

MECHANISM

A fall on the outstretched hand breaks the clavicle; the outer fragment is pulled down by the weight of the arm and the inner half is held up by the sternomastoid muscle.

SIGNS

LOOK — An obvious lump is present.

FEEL — The lump is tender.

MOVE — The patient is reluctant to move the shoulder.

X-RAY — The fracture is usually in the middle third of the shaft, and is transverse to the length of the bone. The outer fragment lies below the inner; often there is a separate central fragment.

TREATMENT

REDUCE — Accurate reduction is neither possible nor essential. If displacement is considerable, pulling the patient's shoulders firmly backwards (without anaesthetic) may improve the position.

HOLD — A sling worn for 3 weeks is adequate for most cases. The traditional axillary loops, linked posteriorly, can be used for gross instability, extreme pain or maternal over-anxiety.

EXERCISE — The elbow, wrist and fingers must be exercised from the start. Active shoulder movements should also be begun early; the patient feels reassured if the fracture is 'protected' by the physiotherapist's hand.

When the sling is discarded, full shoulder movements are quickly regained.

355

COMPLICATIONS

DAMAGE TO VESSELS OR NERVES — This is very rare.

NON-UNION — Non-union rarely occurs unless a surgeon has been foolish enough to operate on the fracture.

MAL-UNION — Mal-union is invariable and leaves a lump; in a child the lump always disappears in time, and in an adult it usually does. A girl anxious to obtain a good cosmetic result quickly may be willing to undergo more drastic treatment: the fracture is manually reduced under anaesthesia and held reduced by a plaster cuirasse. The patient must remain in bed for 3 weeks.

STIFFNESS — Stiffness of the shoulder is common but temporary; it results from fear of moving a fracture. Unless the fingers are exercised, they also may become stiff and take months to regain movement.

FRACTURE AT EITHER END

Occasionally the clavicle fractures near one or other end. The injury resembles a subluxation or dislocation of the nearby joint and is treated like such an injury (*see* pages 357–358).

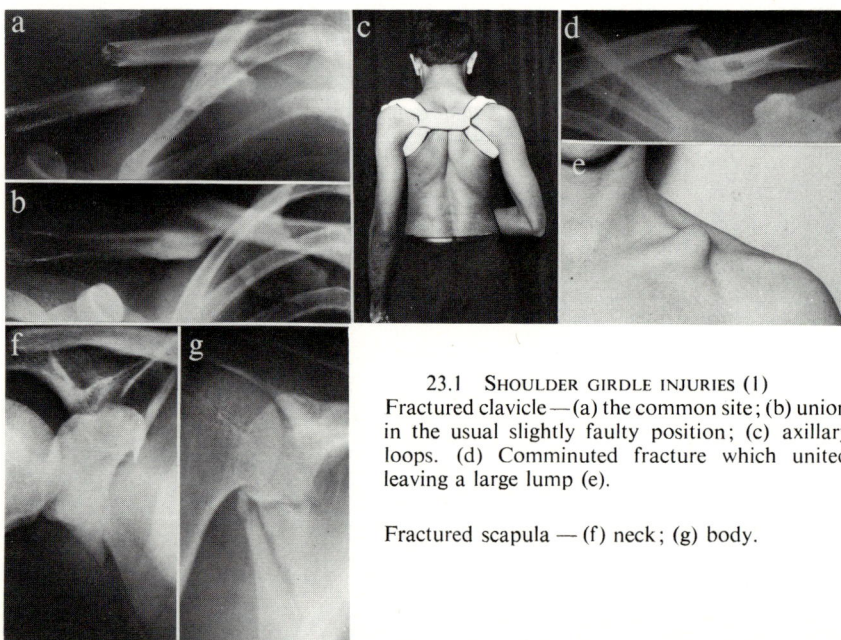

23.1 SHOULDER GIRDLE INJURIES (1)
Fractured clavicle —(a) the common site; (b) union in the usual slightly faulty position; (c) axillary loops. (d) Comminuted fracture which united leaving a large lump (e).

Fractured scapula — (f) neck; (g) body.

FRACTURED SCAPULA

MECHANISM

The body of the scapula is fractured by a crushing force, which usually also fractures ribs. The neck of the scapula may be fractured by a blow or by a fall on the shoulder. The coracoid process may fracture across its base or be avulsed at the tip.

SIGNS

LOOK — Swelling or bruising may be evident.

FEEL — There is localized tenderness.

MOVE — Shoulder movements are painful; breathing also may be painful, and thoracic injury must then be excluded.

X-RAY — The films may show a comminuted fracture of the body of the scapula, or a fractured scapular neck with the outer fragment pulled downwards by the weight of the arm. Occasionally a crack is seen in the acromion or the coracoid process.

TREATMENT

Reduction is impossible and unnecessary. The patient wears a sling for comfort, and from the start practises active exercises to the shoulder, elbow and fingers.

ACROMIO-CLAVICULAR JOINT INJURIES

MECHANISM

A fall on the shoulder tears the acromio-clavicular ligaments, and upward sub-luxation of the clavicle may occur; more severe injury also tears the conoid and trapezoid ligaments, permitting dislocation.

SIGNS

LOOK — An unduly high 'step' is visible, unless swelling obscures it.

FEEL — The step can be felt. Tenderness is localized to the joint.

MOVE — Shoulder movements are limited by pain.

X-RAY — The films show either a subluxation with only slight elevation of the clavicle, or dislocation with considerable elevation.

TREATMENT

REDUCE — Pressure on the outer end of the clavicle effects reduction.

HOLD — Maintaining reduction by closed methods (felt pads over the olecranon and outer clavicle, held approximated with encircling strapping) is rarely effective and may cause skin necrosis. It is better to leave a subluxation untreated (wearing a sling for comfort) and to treat a dislocation by internal fixation using Crawford Adams' pins or a screw.

EXERCISE — The fingers and elbow are exercised from the start, and the shoulder as soon as possible.

COMPLICATIONS

An unreduced subluxation causes no disability.

An unreduced dislocation is common among all-in wrestlers, and clearly need not affect function (the ugly appearance is an advantage in their profession). When it is troublesome the outer 2·5 cm of the clavicle may be excised, or the clavicle anchored down to the coracoid process.

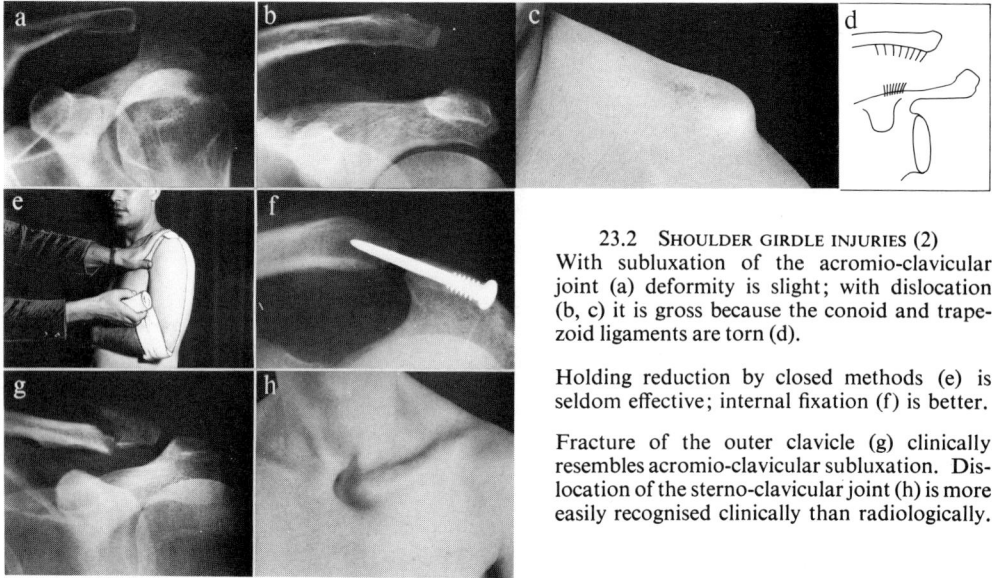

23.2 SHOULDER GIRDLE INJURIES (2)
With subluxation of the acromio-clavicular joint (a) deformity is slight; with dislocation (b, c) it is gross because the conoid and trapezoid ligaments are torn (d).

Holding reduction by closed methods (e) is seldom effective; internal fixation (f) is better.

Fracture of the outer clavicle (g) clinically resembles acromio-clavicular subluxation. Dislocation of the sterno-clavicular joint (h) is more easily recognised clinically than radiologically.

STERNO-CLAVICULAR DISLOCATIONS

MECHANISM

This rare injury is caused by a fall on the shoulder which forces the inner end of the clavicle forwards and upwards.

SIGNS

LOOK — The dislocated inner end of the clavicle forms a prominent lump.
FEEL — Tenderness is localized to the sterno-clavicular joint.
MOVE — Shoulder movements are painful.
X-RAY — The films are difficult to interpret, but enable dislocation to be distinguished from a fractured inner end of clavicle.

TREATMENT

REDUCE — With the patient anaesthetized, the inner end of the clavicle is pushed into position.
HOLD — Strapping, or a firm pad and bandage, is tried. If the pad or strapping holds the reduction, which is unlikely, it is retained for 6 weeks and a sling is worn.
    If the patient is prepared to accept a small lump, a sling worn for a few days is the only treatment necessary. Full function will be regained, though perhaps not for several months.
EXERCISE — Elbow and fingers are exercised from the start, and the shoulder as soon as possible.

COMPLICATIONS

    An unreduced or a recurrent dislocation which is troublesome may be held down, using subclavius as a tenodesis (Burrows, 1951).
    Very rarely the inner clavicle is dislocated backwards by a direct blow. Ribs are broken, shock is profound, and dangerous pressure on the trachea or innominate vein may develop quickly. Reduction is a matter of urgency; the medial end of the clavicle is grasped in bone forceps and pulled forwards.

SHOULDER DISLOCATION: (A) ANTERIOR

MECHANISM

This very common injury is caused by a fall on the hand. The humerus is driven forward, tearing the capsule or avulsing the glenoid labrum. Occasionally the postero-lateral part of the head is crushed. Rarely, the acromion process levers the head downwards and a luxatio erecta position results; nearly always the arm then drops, bringing the head to its usual subcoracoid position. Uncoordinated muscle action, as in an epileptic fit, may also cause dislocation.

SIGNS

LOOK — The patient supports his arm, which is held abducted and appears too long. The contour is angular, because of the unduly prominent acromion process and the flat deltoid muscle.

FEEL — The humeral head is unduly anterior, but is difficult to feel unless the axilla is palpated.

MOVE — Shoulder movements are impossible.

Note — The limb must always be tested for nerve and vessel injury.

X-RAY — Even if the dislocation is obvious, x-rays are taken to see if a fracture co-exists.

TREATMENT

REDUCE — Under anaesthesia with full relaxation reduction is generally easy; an assistant pulls on the arm in abduction while the surgeon thumbs the head into place.

Even without anaesthesia, however, reduction is often possible, and three methods are available. (1) The patient lies prone on a couch with his injured arm hanging vertically for a few minutes; reduction may occur spontaneously, or then be easily achieved. (2) Hippocrates' method: the surgeon places his stockinged foot in the patient's axilla, pulls on the arm, and levers the head of the humerus into position. It is easier if an assistant pulls on the arm while the surgeon thumbs the head back into place. (3) Kocher's method: the surgeon pulls on the flexed elbow, rotates the humerus laterally, then adducts it while rotating it medially.

An x-ray picture is taken to confirm reduction and exclude a fracture.

HOLD — When the patient is fully awake, active abduction is gently tested; if abduction is impossible, there may be a circumflex nerve palsy or supraspinatus tendon avulsion. The complication is noted, but the treatment in any event is a sling for a few days.

EXERCISE — Elbow and finger movements are started at once. Shoulder movements are encouraged, but for three weeks lateral rotation should not be combined with abduction.

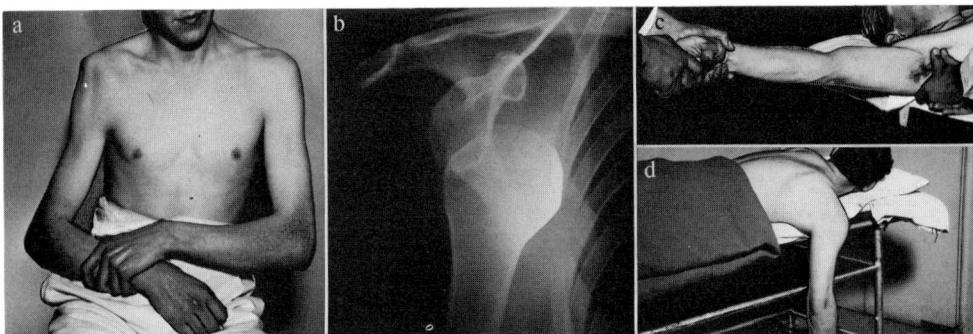

23.3 SHOULDER DISLOCATIONS (1) ANTERIOR
(a, b) Anterior dislocation of the shoulder. (c, d) 2 methods of reduction.

COMPLICATIONS

MUSCLE — A torn supraspinatus tendon should be recognized early, although treatment (surgical re-attachment) is rarely advisable.

NERVE — Injury is common and usually affects the circumflex nerve. It should be recognized before reduction by demonstrating a small patch of anaesthesia over the deltoid muscle insertion, or soon after reduction by the patient's inability to abduct the arm. The lesion is usually a neurapraxia which recovers spontaneously.

BONE — Dislocation may be accompanied by a fracture. (*a*) The greater tuberosity may be sheared off during dislocation. It usually falls into place during reduction, and no special treatment is then required. If it remains displaced, surgical re-attachment is feasible but rarely needed. (*b*) The neck of the humerus may fracture with the initial injury or during unskilled reduction. The combined lesion is known as a fracture-dislocation. The detached head remains dislocated and capsized; it may undergo avascular necrosis. Closed reduction is attempted, using the same method as for an uncomplicated dislocation, and if it succeeds, treatment is similar. If closed reduction fails, open reduction should be attempted only in the young, for it is difficult and dangerous; in the elderly, it is better to leave the dislocation and to try to regain some movement.

JOINT — Following dislocation, the joint may remain unstable (recurrent dislocation) or unduly stiff. These complications are considered separately.

23.4 SHOULDER DISLOCATIONS (2) ANTERIOR — COMPLICATIONS
Associated fractures of (a) great tuberosity; (b) neck of humerus. (c) The ' apprehension test ' for recurrent dislocation; (d) the detached labrum and notch in the humeral head are factors in causing recurrence.

RECURRENT DISLOCATION

If an anterior dislocation tears the shoulder capsule, repair occurs spontaneously and the dislocation does not recur; but if, instead, the glenoid labrum is detached, repair is less likely and recurrence common. Bandaging the arm to the side after reducing the acute dislocation does not seem to influence the outcome. Detachment of the labrum occurs particularly in young patients, and if at injury a bony defect has been gouged out of the postero-lateral aspect of the humeral head, then recurrence is even more likely.

The history is diagnostic. The patient complains that the shoulder dislocates with relatively trivial everyday actions. Often he can reduce the dislocation himself. Any doubt as to diagnosis is quickly resolved by one simple test: if the patient's arm is passively placed behind the coronal plane in a position of abduction and lateral rotation, his immediate resistance and apprehension are pathognomonic.

TREATMENT

Conservative treatment is useless. An operation which uses an anterior approach to the shoulder is almost uniformly successful.

OPERATIONS — A vertical incision along the delto-pectoral groove is the easiest but may leave an unsightly scar; an axillary approach is feasible though more difficult. The deltoid and pectoralis major muscles are separated exposing the coracoid process; this is divided near its base and reflected downwards with its attached muscles. A vertical incision is made through subscapularis and the joint capsule; through this the front of the scapula neck is rawed and the coracoid process screwed to the raw area (Bristow's operation). Movements can safely begin within a few days, but a sling for 5 weeks is wise.

Many other operations are described, the best known being Bankart's (the labrum and capsule are re-attached via drill-holes through the anterior corner of the glenoid), and the Putti-Platt (the capsule and subscapularis are each sutured with 2 cm. of overlap). After either procedure the coracoid process is replaced and the arm bandaged to the side for 5 weeks.

JOINT STIFFNESS AFTER DISLOCATION

There are two reasons why, after dislocation, a shoulder may fail to regain full movement.

IMMOBILIZATION IN SLING POSITION — After a shoulder injury the arm is usually rested in a sling, which necessarily holds the shoulder in medial rotation. Damaged capsule or muscle, if splinted in this position, soon loses the ability to stretch, especially in patients over the age of 40 years. There is consequent loss of lateral rotation, which automatically limits abduction.

Treatment — Early active movements prevent stiffness. Passive exercises are never allowed; they may cause or aggravate traumatic myositis. Active exercises can usually cure stiffness if immobilization has not been prolonged. They are practised vigorously, bearing in mind that full abduction is not possible until lateral rotation has been regained. Manipulation under anaesthesia is advised only if progress has halted and at least 6 months have elapsed since injury. Lateral rotation should be restored before abduction, and the manipulations should be gentle and repeated rather than forceful.

UNREDUCED DISLOCATION — Surprisingly, a dislocation of the shoulder sometimes remains undiagnosed.

Treatment — Closed reduction is worth attempting up to 6 weeks after injury; manipulation later may fracture the bone or tear vessels or nerves.

Operative reduction is indicated after 6 weeks only in the young, because it is difficult, dangerous and followed by prolonged stiffness. An anterior approach is used, and the vessels and nerves carefully identified before the dislocation is reduced. 'Active neglect' summarizes the treatment of unreduced dislocation in the elderly. The dislocation is disregarded and gentle active movements encouraged. Moderately good function is often regained.

SHOULDER DISLOCATION: (B) POSTERIOR

This rare injury is often missed. It is not a complete dislocation but a fracture-subluxation and probably caused by forced internal rotation of the abducted arm. It should be suspected after an epileptic fit or electric shock.

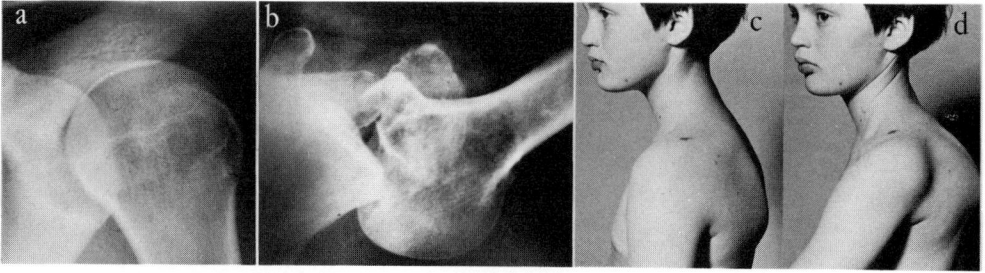

23.5 SHOULDER DISLOCATIONS (3) POSTERIOR
(a) The antero-posterior view may look almost normal, but (b) the lateral view shows obvious subluxation. (c, d) Habitual (voluntary) dislocation: the clue is the unconcerned expression.

SIGNS

LOOK — The arm is held medially rotated. From the front the deformity is obscured by swelling, but from above the anterior aspect of the shoulder appears unduly flat.

FEEL — The posteriorly displaced head of the humerus is difficult to feel, but the coracoid process is unduly prominent.

MOVE — No movement is possible.

X-RAY — In the antero-posterior view the humeral head is abnormal in shape but, because it is in contact with the glenoid fossa, the injury is easily missed. A lateral view is essential; it shows posterior subluxation and a fracture of the humeral head.

TREATMENT

REDUCE — The arm is pulled and rotated outwards while the head of the humerus is pushed forwards.

HOLD — If reduction feels stable a sling is enough; otherwise the shoulder is held widely abducted and laterally rotated in a plaster spica for 3 weeks.

EXERCISE — Shoulder movement is regained by active exercises.

COMPLICATIONS

UNREDUCED DISLOCATION — Unreduced dislocation in the young may be reduced operatively through a posterior incision. In the elderly it is disregarded.

RECURRENT DISLOCATION — Through a posterior approach the capsule is repaired with overlap, and the shoulder held abducted and laterally rotated for 6 weeks.

VOLUNTARY DISLOCATION — This is not the sequel to injury but may be familial and associated with ligament laxity. In other cases (usually adolescent) there is a psychiatric background. The patient can sublux the humeral head backwards painlessly at will. If operation cannot be avoided, a posterior bone block is advisable.

FRACTURED NECK OF HUMERUS

MECHANISM

The patient falls on the outstretched hand. The surgical neck breaks, and the up-thrust may shear off the greater tuberosity. Often the force is sufficient to impact the fragments.

SIGNS

The injury is common in elderly people and not uncommon in adolescents. Between these ages it is rare.

LOOK — The shoulder is swollen and later the arm becomes extensively bruised.

MOVE — Attempted movement is painful unless the fracture is impacted.

X-RAY — In the elderly, a transverse fracture extends across the surgical neck, and often the greater tuberosity also is fractured. The shaft is usually impacted into the head in an abducted position. Occasionally no impaction occurs and the shaft may shift medially.

In adolescents, fracture-separation of the upper humeral epiphysis occurs; the shaft shifts upwards and forwards; the head, with a large triangular piece of the metaphysis attached, remains in position. In young children, fracture through the upper humerus is rare except through a solitary cyst.

TREATMENT

REDUCE — Usually reduction is unnecessary, and with impaction in the elderly it is unwise. But with considerable displacement in the adolescent approaching skeletal maturity, or in the young adult, reduction is worth while, either by manipulation or, very occasionally by open operation (Neer, 1970).

HOLD — Only a sling is necessary, whether or not reduction has been attempted. The weight of the arm tends to correct displacement.

Union occurs in 3 weeks and consolidation in 6 weeks.

EXERCISE — Elbow and finger movements are practised from the start. Pendulum exercises of the shoulder are also begun at once, and the patient is encouraged to abduct the arm actively as soon as possible. In the elderly it is especially important to concentrate on regaining shoulder movements.

COMPLICATIONS

STIFFNESS — Stiffness of the shoulder is common and important, but is minimized by early and persistent exercises. It is important to distinguish stiffness following a fracture from that of a ' frozen ' shoulder (see page 153). Finger stiffness is due to neglect.

MAL-UNION — Mal-union is not uncommon. In the elderly it causes little disability; in the young adolescent the bone grows straight.

FRACTURED GREATER TUBEROSITY

MECHANISM

The greater tuberosity may sustain a 'direct' injury when the patient falls on the abducted arm, and the tuberosity impinges against the acromion process; the fracture is common in association with a dislocated shoulder. Occasionally an 'indirect' or avulsion fracture occurs in a young adult who is trying to save himself from falling, when the action of the supraspinatus muscle is resisted by an obstacle; the tuberosity is then pulled off.

SIGNS

LOOK — The shoulder is a little swollen.

FEEL — The tuberosity is tender.

MOVE — Abduction is impossible or limited.

X-RAY — The tuberosity is usually undisplaced; it is demarcated from the shaft by a fracture line, or is comminuted. Occasionally the tuberosity is avulsed by the supra-

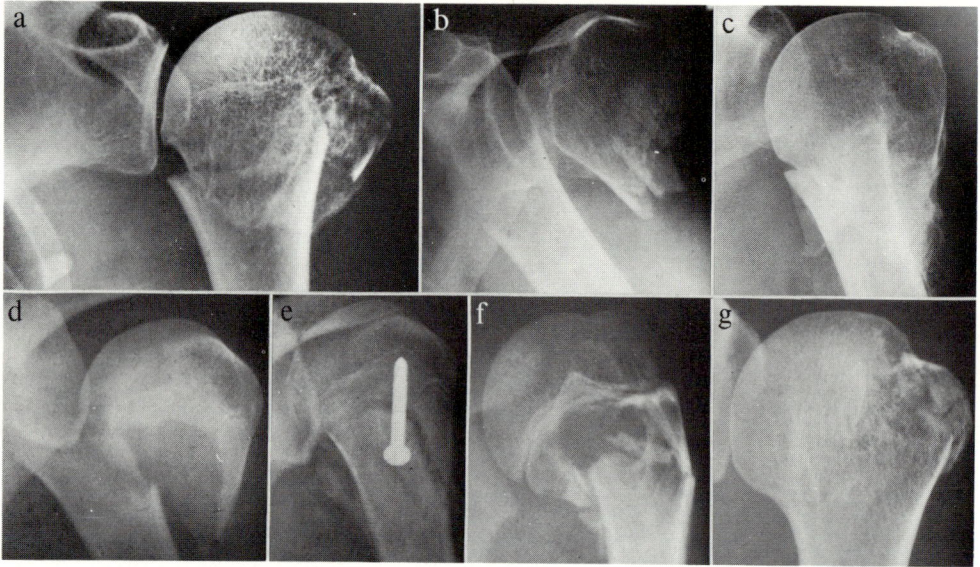

23.6 FRACTURES OF THE UPPER HUMERUS
(a) The common impacted fracture of the neck. (b) A severely displaced fracture which, treated only with a sling, has united (c) in good position.
(d) Fracture-separation of the upper humeral epiphysis with gross displacement which, very unusually, needed (e) open reduction. (f) In a young child fracture is rare except through a cyst. (g) Fractured great tuberosity, usually associated with a dislocation.

spinatus tendon; it is pulled upwards and appears as a thin slice of bone just under the acromion process.

TREATMENT

REDUCE — In the absence of displacement reduction is unnecessary. The rare displaced fracture is difficult to reduce but reduction is important. Watson-Jones advises bringing the humerus into contact with the tuberosity by abducting 90 degrees, laterally rotating 60 degrees, and forwardly flexing 40 degrees.

HOLD — If the reduction described above has been carried out, the arm is maintained in this position by an abduction frame. Union takes 6 weeks, after which the angle of the frame is gradually lowered, and it is discarded at 12 weeks.

The commoner undisplaced fractures do not need to be held; the arm is merely rested in a sling.

EXERCISE — The elbow and fingers are exercised from the start. When a frame has been used, shoulder movements must be regained after the splint has been discarded; but it will be many months before the shoulder moves fully. In all other cases, gentle active shoulder movements should be begun at once, and gradually increased.

SHAFT OF HUMERUS

MECHANISM

A fall on the hand may twist the humerus, causing a spiral fracture. A fall on the elbow with the arm abducted may hinge the bone causing a slightly oblique or transverse fracture. A heavy blow on the arm causes a fracture which is either transverse or grossly comminuted.

SIGNS

LOOK — Deformity, swelling and bruising may be obvious.

FEEL — The arm is tender.

MOVE — The patient is unwilling to move the arm. Finger extension should be tested in order to exclude a musculo-spiral nerve lesion.

X-RAY — The films show the site of the fracture in the shaft, its line (spiral, transverse or comminuted) and any displacement.

TREATMENT OF SPIRAL OR COMMINUTED FRACTURE

REDUCE — Neither anaesthesia nor manipulation is needed for reduction.

HOLD — The distal forearm is supported in a 'wrist sling'. Providing the elbow is unsupported, gravity exerts sufficient traction to effect reduction and to maintain it. The fracture unites in about 3 weeks and is consolidated in 6 weeks, after which the sling is discarded.

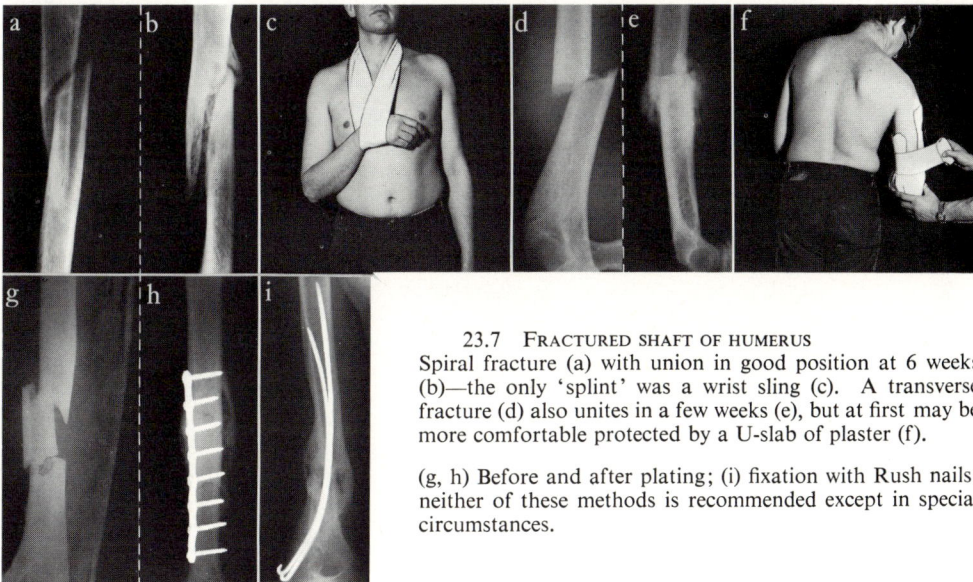

23.7 FRACTURED SHAFT OF HUMERUS
Spiral fracture (a) with union in good position at 6 weeks (b)—the only 'splint' was a wrist sling (c). A transverse fracture (d) also unites in a few weeks (e), but at first may be more comfortable protected by a U-slab of plaster (f).

(g, h) Before and after plating; (i) fixation with Rush nails; neither of these methods is recommended except in special circumstances.

EXERCISE — Wrist and finger exercises are begun at once. To minimize shoulder stiffness the patient is taught to lean forwards at the hips, and, with the arm hanging supported only by its wrist sling, to practise gentle pendulum exercises. When the fracture is 'sticky' active abduction of the shoulder may safely be practised.

TREATMENT OF TRANSVERSE OR SHORT OBLIQUE FRACTURE

REDUCE — Only if the fracture is grossly angulated is manipulative reduction advisable, and it is not essential.

HOLD — To increase the feeling of stability, a U-slab of plaster may be bandaged on; with high fractures the loop of the U is uppermost over the acromion process and with low fractures the loop is round the olecranon process. Alternatively the arm may be bandaged to the trunk. Within a week the slab or trunk bandage is removed, and the forearm is supported in a 'wrist sling'. The patient spends the day sitting bolt upright or standing, and he is propped vertically at night. The fracture unites in about 6 weeks and is consolidated in about 12 weeks, after which the sling is discarded.

Internal Fixation is indicated if closed treatment is impracticable because of associated soft tissue damage or injuries elsewhere. The fracture can be fixed by plating (the radial nerve must be found and protected), or by intramedullary nailing.

EXERCISE — The wrist and fingers are exercised from the start. The patient is taught to contract the elbow flexors and extensors actively. Pendulum exercises of the shoulder are begun within a week, but active abduction of the shoulder is postponed until the fracture is clinically and radiologically consolidated.

COMPLICATIONS

RADIAL NERVE PALSY — Radial nerve palsy is usually temporary. A ' lively ' splint is used to support the wrist and hand while recovery is awaited. If recovery does not occur, nerve repair or tendon transplants may be required (page 124).

DELAYED UNION AND NON-UNION — Delayed union may occur in transverse fractures, especially if excessive traction has been used (for example, a hanging cast) or if the patient has not actively exercised the elbow flexors and extensors. Non-union may follow. The dangerous combination is incomplete union and a stiff joint. If elbow or shoulder movements are forced before consolidation, the humerus refractures, and non-union may occur.

The treatment of established non-union is operative. The bone ends are freshened, bone chips packed around them and an intramedullary nail inserted or a plate screwed on.

JOINT STIFFNESS — Joint stiffness may be minimized by early activity, but transverse fractures (in which shoulder abduction is dangerous) may limit shoulder movement for several months.

THE ELBOW

At the elbow, fractures in children are different from those in adults. Beneath the heading of each individual fracture is indicated whether it occurs in childhood or in adult life.

SUPRACONDYLAR FRACTURE: (A) BACKWARDS
(Children)

MECHANISM

This common injury is caused by a fall on the hand with the elbow bent. The humerus breaks just above the condyles. The distal fragment, with the forearm, is pushed backwards and (because the forearm is usually in full pronation) twisted inwards.

SIGNS

LOOK — The child holds his forearm with the other hand. Until swelling obscures the details, the backward shift just above the elbow is apparent.

FEEL AND MOVE — It is unkind to palpate the fracture or to attempt elbow movement. In every elbow injury, however, it is essential to feel the pulse and to examine the hand for evidence of nerve injury.

X-RAY — The lateral view shows a fracture just above the growth disc. The line of fracture runs obliquely and is lower anteriorly. The fragment and the forearm are shifted backwards and tilted backwards.

An antero-posterior film may be difficult to obtain without hurting the child. If so, it is postponed until the child has been anaesthetized prior to the reduction. It often shows that the distal fragment is shifted and tilted sideways, and is twisted (usually inwards). Occasionally there is only a fine hair-line fracture (easily missed) with no displacement.

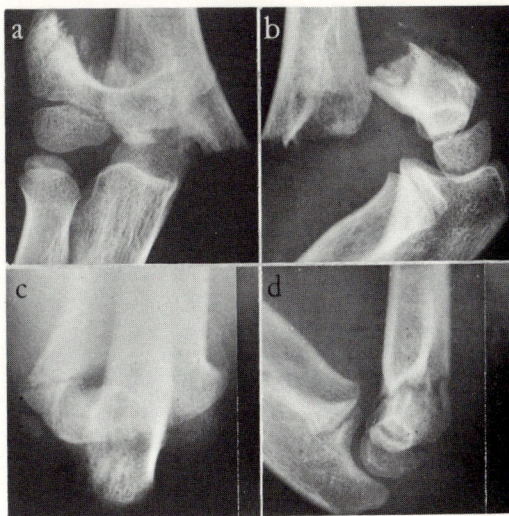

23.8 SUPRACONDYLAR FRACTURES (1)
(a, b) This considerably displaced fracture was reduced (c, d) by the method shown in Fig. 23.9. Note that the antero-posterior view in (c) is taken with the elbow flexed.

TREATMENT

REDUCE — Reduction of the displaced fracture must be carried out methodically with the child relaxed under anaesthesia.   The uninjured arm should first be examined to assess the carrying angle, and to decide how far the arm and forearm together rotate at the shoulder.

(1) With one hand the surgeon then pulls on the injured forearm and maintains traction for 1 minute.   (2) Without releasing traction he grasps the distal fragment with his other hand and corrects sideways shift, tilt and twist.   (3) He then flexes the elbow while pushing the lower humerus forwards with his thumb.   The intact triceps muscle prevents over-reduction.   (4) The radial pulse is then palpated.   If it cannot be felt, the elbow must be extended a few degrees until the pulse returns, then a further 10 degrees for safety. (5) Antero-posterior and lateral films are taken to confirm reduction.   The elbow must not be straightened for the antero-posterior film, which should be taken through the flexed upper forearm.   Slight shift may be accepted, but tilt or twist should be fully corrected.   If necessary, the manipulations are repeated.

Open reduction (held by 2 Kirschner wires) has been advocated but is difficult and hazardous.   If an acceptable position cannot be obtained by manipulation, or if, with the elbow flexed as little as 90 degrees the pulse is obliterated, then Dunlop traction can be used: the child lies supine with the shoulder abducted and the elbow nearly straight; a sling and weights hold the lower humerus; skin traction is applied to the forearm via a metal frame fixed to the bed.

HOLD — A collar and cuff is applied to hold the elbow flexed.   The more the elbow is flexed, the more stable is reduction, and during the next few days, as swelling subsides, the link between the collar and the cuff is tightened, providing the pulse remains palpable.

Occasionally the elbow cannot be sufficiently flexed without obliterating the pulse. A less flexed position, at which the pulse is palpable, must be accepted, and a posterior plaster slab is used in addition to the collar and cuff.   The slab extends two-thirds of the way round the limb, from below the shoulder to above the wrist, and is held on with a crêpe bandage.   A few days later the plaster is removed, the elbow flexed further, and x-rays taken; occasionally remanipulation proves necessary.

Union takes 3 weeks; during this time the hand must not be taken out of the cuff and the limb is kept beneath the shirt.   For the succeeding 3 weeks (until consolidation) the limb is supported outside the clothing.

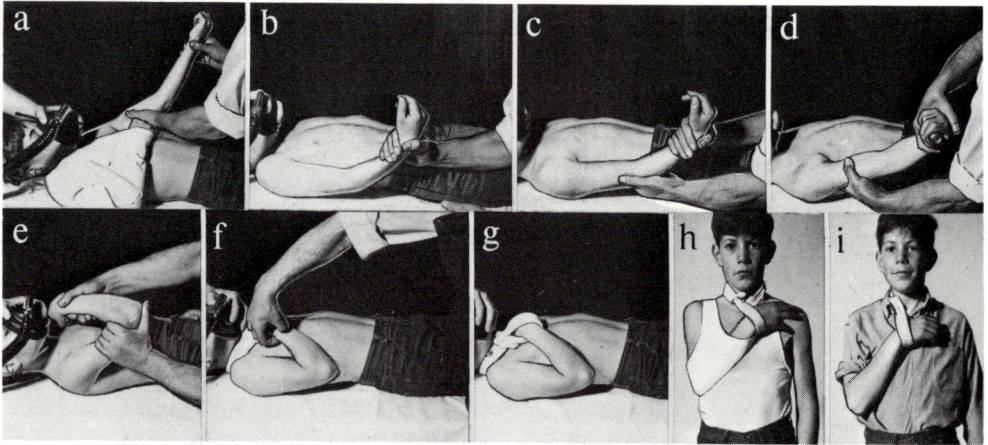

23.9 SUPRACONDYLAR FRACTURES (2) TREATMENT OF DISPLACED FRACTURE
(a) The un-injured arm is examined first; (b) traction on the fractured arm; (c) correcting lateral shift and tilt; (d) correcting rotation; (e) correcting backward shift and tilt; (f) feeling the pulse; (g) the elbow is kept well flexed while x-ray films are taken; (h) for the first 3 weeks the arm is kept under the vest; after this (i) it is outside the vest.

EXERCISE — For the first 3 weeks, only finger and wrist movements are practised.

After 3 weeks the child may take his hand out of the cuff during supervised activities, such as washing, dressing and writing. Elbow flexion is encouraged, but not extension, which returns gradually with use. Passive movements are prohibited at all times; the elbow must never be pulled, pushed or passively stretched by carrying weights.

Note — Occasionally a supracondylar fracture occurs with little or no displacement. Reduction is unnecessary and the child only needs a sling for 3 weeks.

COMPLICATIONS

VOLKMANN'S ISCHAEMIA — This must always be watched for. If there is undue pain, altered colour or diminished sensation of the fingers, or absent pulse, or pain on straightening the fingers, urgent action is necessary (page 333).

JOINT STIFFNESS — Elbow stiffness is common and extension in particular may take months to return. In the first few weeks stiffness may be due to myositis ossificans. Passive or forced movements (and carrying weights is a form of forced movement) are prohibited at all times; if there is a suggestion that movement is diminishing it is wise to rest the elbow in a plaster gutter (page 340).

MAL-UNION — Mal-union is common. With backward or sideways shift, the humerus gradually grows straight. Forward or backward tilt may limit flexion or extension, but consequent disability is slight.

Uncorrected sideways tilt or rotation is more important. It may lead to a varus deformity, which is ugly and sometimes requires osteotomy; or rarely to a valgus deformity, which may cause late ulnar palsy. Epiphyseal damage is often blamed for these deformities, but usually faulty reduction is responsible.

NERVE INJURIES — Nerve injuries are common, but usually recover spontaneously.

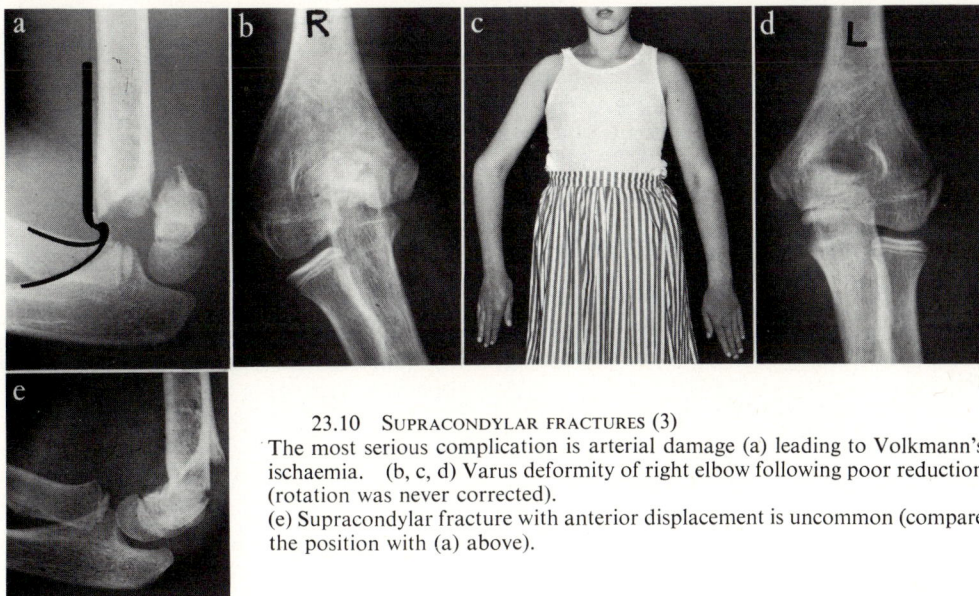

23.10 SUPRACONDYLAR FRACTURES (3)
The most serious complication is arterial damage (a) leading to Volkmann's ischaemia. (b, c, d) Varus deformity of right elbow following poor reduction (rotation was never corrected).
(e) Supracondylar fracture with anterior displacement is uncommon (compare the position with (a) above).

SUPRACONDYLAR FRACTURE: (B) FORWARDS
(Children)

MECHANISM

This rare injury is caused by a fall on the hand with the elbow straight. The humerus breaks just above the growth disc and the fragment is tilted forwards.

SIGNS

LOOK — The elbow is swollen.
FEEL — Tenderness is felt at and above the elbow.
MOVE — The child is asked to move the fingers so that nerve injury can be excluded.
X-RAY — The fracture line is oblique and is lower posteriorly. To assess the forward tilt a line may be drawn down the front of the humeral shaft; normally its projection should bisect the epiphysis.

TREATMENT

REDUCE — The arm is pulled, the elbow fully straightened, and the carrying angle restored.
HOLD — A posterior slab is bandaged on, holding the elbow straight. After 3 weeks the slab is removed.
EXERCISE — The child is allowed to regain elbow flexion gradually.

COMPLICATIONS

If the fracture has not been reduced, extension remains limited but the disability is rarely severe.

T-SHAPED AND Y-SHAPED FRACTURES
(Adults)

MECHANISM

A fall on the point of the elbow drives the olecranon process upwards, splitting the condyles apart.

SIGNS

LOOK — The elbow is grossly swollen.

FEEL — Palpation is painful and unnecessary.

MOVE — The patient is unwilling to move the elbow.

X-RAY — The films show a fracture of the lower humerus extending into the elbow joint. The line of the fracture is a 'T' or a 'Y', or comminution may be seen. Often the condyles are separated, and either may be tilted in any direction.

TREATMENT

ORTHODOX TREATMENT — The forearm is pulled in the straight position and the bones moulded into shape. A posterior plaster slab, bandaged on with the elbow a little straighter than a right angle, is retained for 3 weeks. The shoulder, wrist and fingers are exercised from the start. When the plaster is removed the patient tries to regain elbow flexion.

TREATMENT BY ACTIVITY — The orthodox treatment usually leaves a permanently stiffish elbow, and if flexion is much limited, the disability is considerable. If comminution has occurred, it is probably better to disregard the fracture and to concentrate on the joint. The arm is held above a right angle in a collar and cuff. Active movements are encouraged, and often mould the fragments into reasonable position. The final range is usually better than expected.

OPERATIVE TREATMENT — In the absence of comminution, operation is sometimes worth while. The elbow is approached from the outer side, and the condyles are reduced and held with a screw. Elaborate fixation of comminuted fractures is practised, but considerable stiffness is not uncommon.

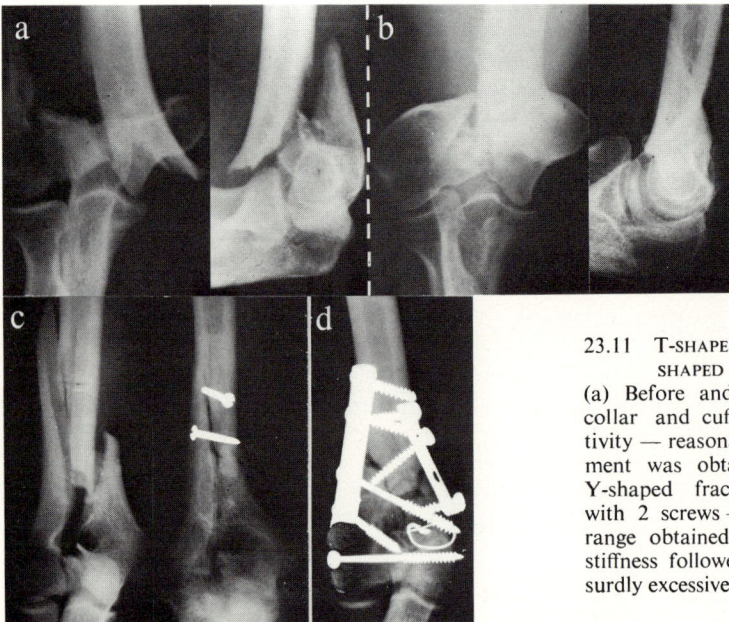

23.11 T-SHAPED AND Y-SHAPED FRACTURES (a) Before and (b) after collar and cuff plus activity — reasonable movement was obtained. (c) Y-shaped fracture fixed with 2 screws — excellent range obtained; (d) total stiffness followed this absurdly excessive fixation.

FRACTURE-SEPARATION OF LATERAL CONDYLAR EPIPHYSIS
(Children)

MECHANISM

The child falls on the hand.   A large fragment, which includes the lateral condyle, breaks off and is pulled upon by the attached wrist extensors.   In severe injuries probably the elbow dislocates postero-laterally; the condyle is 'capsized' by muscle pull and remains capsized while the elbow reduces spontaneously.

SIGNS

LOOK — The elbow is swollen.

FEEL — Tenderness is confined to the outer side.

MOVE — Movements of the elbow and wrist are painful.

X-RAY — Displacement may be slight, or the condyle grossly rotated.   A triangular fragment of metaphysis may be displaced with the condyle.   It is often valuable to compare the films with those of the normal elbow.

TREATMENT

REDUCE — Accurate reduction is important.   Under anaesthesia the forearm is pushed postero-laterally, as if to reproduce the dislocation, then pulled forwards again.   This manoeuvre feels unconvincing but is often successful.

   If closed reduction fails operation is essential.   The fragment is exposed, replaced in position and held with catgut sutures, a small screw or a pin.

HOLD — A posterior plaster slab is applied, extending from below the shoulder to just short of the knuckles, with the elbow just above a right angle and the wrist dorsiflexed

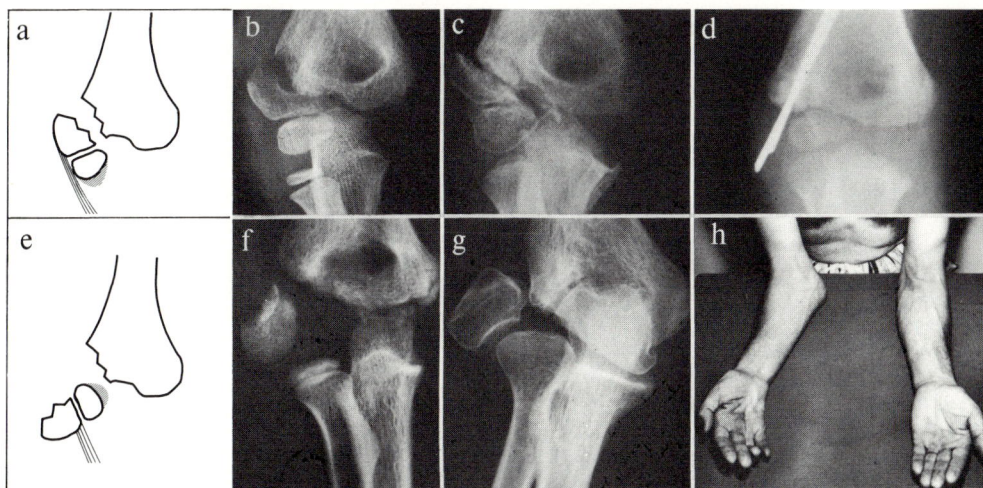

23.12   FRACTURED LATERAL CONDYLE
(a, b) A large fragment of bone and cartilage is avulsed; even with reasonable reduction, union is not inevitable (c), and open reduction with fixation (d) is often wise. (e, f) Sometimes the condyle is capsized: if left unreduced non-union is inevitable (g) and a valgus elbow with delayed ulnar palsy (h) the likely sequel.

(to relax the extensor muscles).   After 3 weeks, the plaster is removed but a collar and cuff is worn for a further 3 weeks.

EXERCISE — The fingers and shoulder are exercised from the start.   Elbow and wrist movements are regained later.

COMPLICATIONS

If the condyle is left capsized non-union is inevitable; with growth the elbow becomes increasingly valgus, and ulnar nerve palsy is then likely to develop, requiring anterior transposition.   Even minor displacements sometimes lead to non-union, and even slight mal-union may lead to ulnar palsy; it is for these reasons that open reduction (and internal fixation) is being increasingly used.

FRACTURED CAPITULUM
(Adults)

MECHANISM

The patient falls on the hand usually with the elbow straight.   The anterior half of the capitulum and the trochlea are broken off and displaced proximally.

SIGNS

LOOK — Fullness is seen in front of the elbow.

FEEL — The elbow is tender.

MOVE — Flexion is grossly limited and painful.

X-RAY — In the lateral view the capitulum is seen in front of the lower humerus, and the radial head no longer points directly towards it.

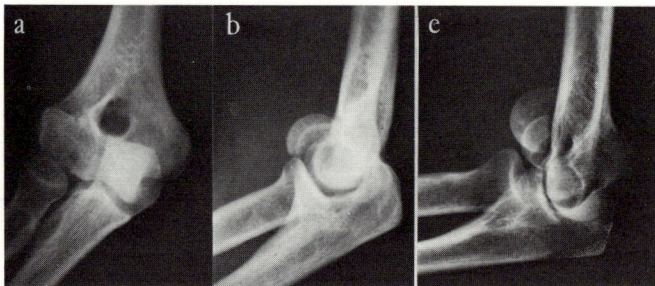

23.13 FRACTURED CAPITULUM (a, b) Antero-posterior and lateral views showing proximal displacement and tilting; in (c) the capitulum has been sheared off vertically.

TREATMENT

REDUCE — While the arm is being pulled straight an attempt is made to thumb the fragment back into position.

If closed reduction fails operation is essential, or flexion will remain permanently limited.   The elbow is approached from the outer side and the capitulum sutured in position with catgut; but if there is difficulty the fragment can be removed.

HOLD — A collar and cuff is sufficient.

EXERCISE — The shoulder, wrist and fingers must be exercised from the start.   Elbow movements are regained when active movement is comfortable.

SEPARATION OF MEDIAL EPICONDYLAR EPIPHYSIS
(Adolescents)

MECHANISM

The medial epicondylar epiphysis begins to ossify at the age of about 9 and fuses to the shaft at about 16; between these ages it may be avulsed by a fall on the hand. The epiphysis is pulled distally by the attached wrist flexors. With more severe injuries the joint dislocates laterally and the epiphysis is pulled into the joint. The elbow may remain dislocated, or may reduce spontaneously and trap the epicondyle.

SIGNS

LOOK — If the joint is dislocated deformity is obvious.

FEEL — The inner side of the joint is tender. The ulnar fingers should be palpated to exclude ulnar nerve damage.

MOVE — Attempted movement is painful.

X-RAY — In the antero-posterior view, the medial epicondylar epiphysis may be seen tilted or shifted downwards; if the joint is dislocated the epiphysis lies distal to the lower humerus. A lateral view may show the epicondyle looking like a loose body in the joint.

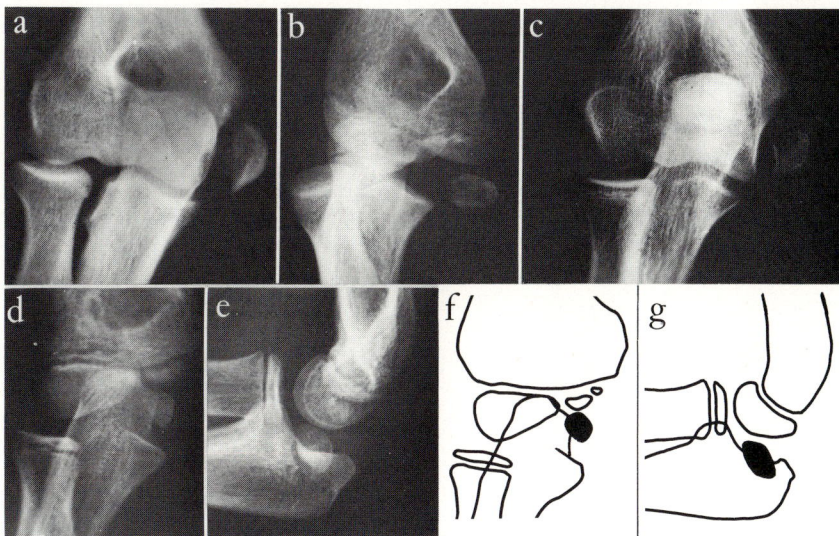

23.14   FRACTURED MEDIAL EPICONDYLE
(a) Avulsion of the medial epicondyle following valgus strain. (b) Avulsion associated with dislocation of the elbow — (c) after reduction.
Sometimes the epicondylar fragment is trapped in the joint (d, e); the serious nature of the injury is then liable to be missed unless the surgeon specifically looks for the trapped fragment, which is emphasized in the tracings (f, g).

TREATMENT

REDUCE — Minor displacement may be disregarded; but an epicondyle trapped in the joint must be freed. Manipulation with the elbow pulled into valgus position is sometimes successful. Another possible manoeuvre is to hold the fingers extended and apply a faradic current to the forearm flexors, which may then pull the fragment out of the joint. If closed methods fail operation is essential. An incision is made on the medial aspect of the elbow and the ulnar nerve, which may be kinked into the joint, is carefully exposed.   The epicondyle is replaced in position or excised and the ulnar nerve transposed to the front of the elbow.

HOLD — A collar and cuff is worn for 3 weeks.

EXERCISE — The shoulder is exercised from the start and elbow range is regained when the collar and cuff has been removed.

COMPLICATIONS

ELBOW STIFFNESS — Stiffness of the elbow is common.   Extension may remain limited for several months, but must not be forced.   Full movement returns eventually, providing the epicondyle has not been left in the joint.

ULNAR NERVE DAMAGE — The ulnar nerve usually recovers unless it is left kinked in the joint.   Occasionally a late palsy develops because of friction against the roughened bony groove.

FRACTURED NECK OF RADIUS
(Children)

MECHANISM

The child falls on the outstretched hand while the elbow is slightly valgus.

SIGNS

LOOK — The elbow is only slightly swollen.

FEEL — There is tenderness over the outer side.

MOVE — Rotation is painful.

X-RAY — The fracture line is transverse.   It is either situated immediately distal to the growth disc, or there is true separation of the epiphysis with a triangular fragment of shaft.   The proximal fragment is tilted distally, forwards and outwards.   Sometimes the upper end of the ulna is also fractured.

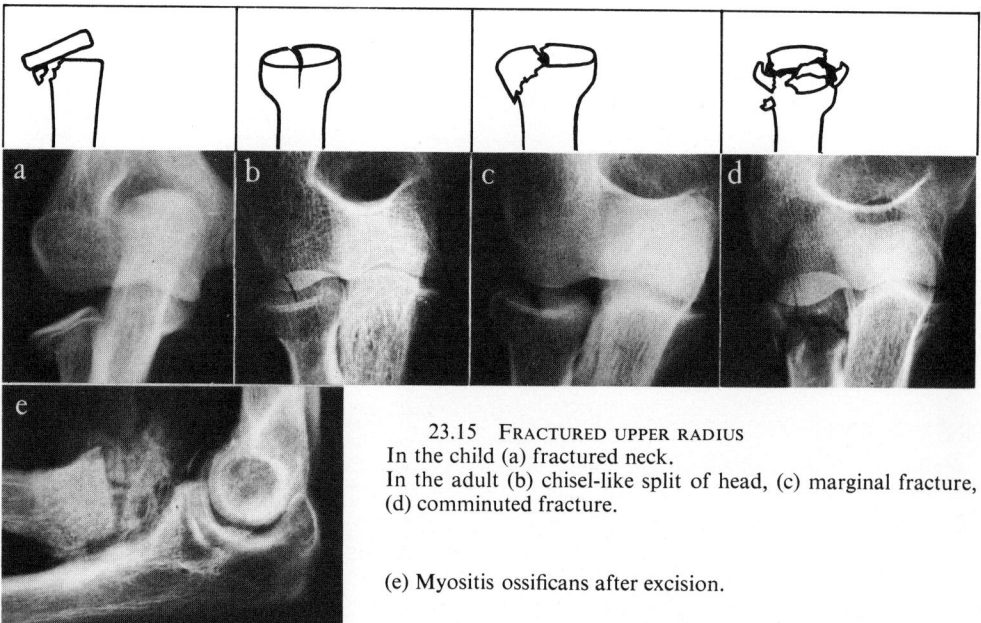

23.15   FRACTURED UPPER RADIUS
In the child (a) fractured neck.
In the adult (b) chisel-like split of head, (c) marginal fracture,
(d) comminuted fracture.

(e) Myositis ossificans after excision.

TREATMENT

REDUCE — Up to about 15 degrees of tilt is acceptable. Beyond that reduction is needed. The arm is pulled into extension and slight varus. With his thumb the surgeon pushes the displaced radial fragment proximally, medially and backwards. If necessary the manoeuvre is repeated in varying positions of pronation and supination.

If this fails, open reduction is performed. The head of the radius must never be excised in children or the ulna will outgrow the radius; the inferior radio-ulnar joint then sub-luxates and rotation becomes limited.

HOLD — A posterior plaster slab extending two-thirds of the way round the limb is ban-daged on. It is usual for the elbow to be held in 90 degrees of flexion, but the angle at which reduction seems stable should be maintained.

The slab is worn for 3 weeks, and a collar and cuff for a further 3 weeks.

EXERCISE — The elbow is allowed to regain movement spontaneously after the collar and cuff has been removed.

FRACTURED HEAD OF RADIUS
(Adults)

MECHANISM

A fall on the outstretched hand forces the elbow into valgus and pushes the radial head against the capitulum. The radial head may be split or broken. In addition, the articular cartilage of the capitulum may be bruised or chipped; this cannot be seen on x-ray but is an important complication.

SIGNS

LOOK — The elbow may look normal.

FEEL — The head of the radius is tender.

MOVE — Rotation of the forearm is painful.

X-RAY — The films may show (a) a vertical split in the radial head; or (b) a single fragment of the lateral portion of the head broken off and usually displaced distally; or (c) the head broken into several fragments.

TREATMENT

When the injury is an undisplaced split the arm is held in a collar and cuff for 3 weeks. Active flexion and extension may be encouraged, but rotation is allowed to return by itself.

A severe fracture should be treated by excision of the entire radial head.

TECHNIQUE — A tourniquet is applied, the elbow is flexed and an incision 5 cm. long is made extending from the lateral epicondyle towards the thumb. The capsule is incised and the radial head removed. The excised portions should be fitted together to ensure that no fragment has been left behind. The capsule and the skin are sutured. After-care is the same as that following closed treatment.

COMPLICATIONS

JOINT STIFFNESS — Joint stiffness is common and may involve both the elbow and the radio-ulnar joints. Occasionally myositis ossificans develops. Stiffness may occur whether the radial head has been excised or not. Probably, however, the prognosis with a comminuted fracture is better after operation.

FRACTURED OLECRANON: (A) COMMINUTED FRACTURE
(Adults)

MECHANISM

A direct blow or fall on the point of the elbow causes a comminuted fracture of the olecranon process with little displacement.

SIGNS

    LOOK — The point of the elbow is bruised or grazed.
    FEEL — There is localized tenderness.
    MOVE — The triceps muscle is intact and the elbow can be extended against resistance.
    X-RAY — The olecranon process may be broken into several fragments, but usually there is little displacement.

TREATMENT

    The injury should be treated as a bruise and the fracture disregarded. A sling is worn for comfort and active movements encouraged.

FRACTURED OLECRANON: (B) TRANSVERSE ('GAP')
(Adults)

MECHANISM

The patient falls onto the hand while the triceps muscle is in action. The olecranon process fractures transversely and its proximal portion is pulled upwards by the triceps muscle.

SIGNS

    LOOK — Swelling behind the elbow may be seen.
    FEEL — The gap in the bone is sometimes palpable.
    MOVE — The patient cannot extend the elbow against resistance.
    X-RAY — The fracture is transverse and the avulsed fragment is pulled proximally.

TREATMENT

    The fracture can usually be reduced by straightening the elbow, but reduction can be held only if the straight position is maintained in plaster for several weeks, and stiffness in the straight position is a disaster. This method is therefore rarely employed. If the fracture is disregarded and the arm rested in a sling, a long fibrous

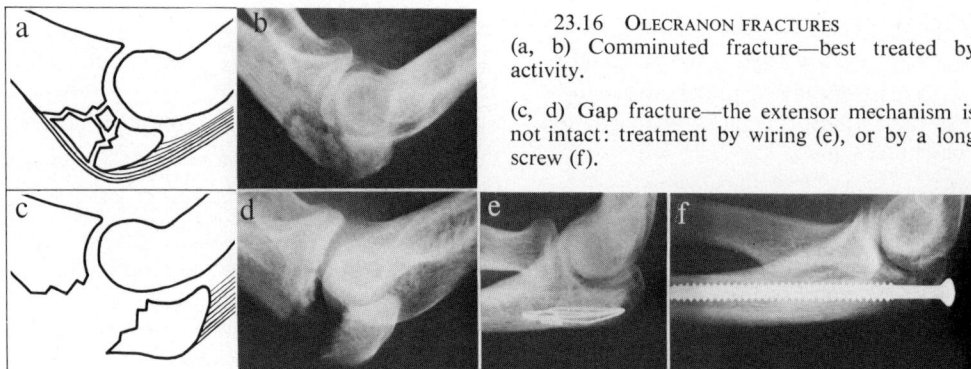

23.16 OLECRANON FRACTURES
(a, b) Comminuted fracture—best treated by activity.

(c, d) Gap fracture—the extensor mechanism is not intact: treatment by wiring (e), or by a long screw (f).

union results; the elbow regains full range but loses power. This method is suitable only for elderly patients unfit for operation.

Operative treatment is the method of choice; its aim is to repair the extensor mechanism. The olecranon process is exposed, carefully reduced, and held by internal fixation (a screw or wire). If the fragment is small it may be excised and the triceps tendon re-attached to the ulna. After operation a sling is worn for 3 weeks.

ELBOW DISLOCATION

(Children or Adults)

MECHANISM

A fall on the hand may dislocate the elbow. The forearm is pushed backwards. Once posterior dislocation has taken place, lateral shift may also occur.

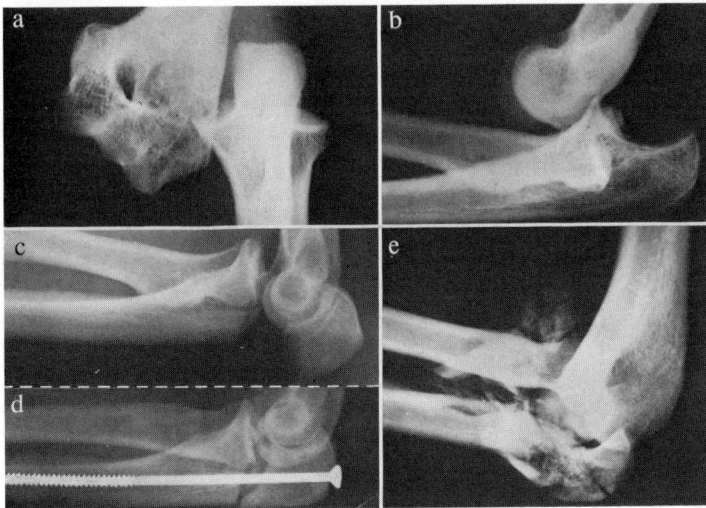

23.17 ELBOW DISLOCATIONS (a, b) The usual uncomplicated dislocation.

(c) Forward dislocation with fractured olecranon; this needs (d) reduction, with stabilization of the olecranon. (e) Side-swipe fracture-dislocation.

SIGNS

LOOK — The patient supports the forearm with his other hand. Deformity and swelling are obvious.

FEEL — The olecranon process can be readily felt out of its normal position. The pulse must be examined and sensation in the fingers tested.

MOVE — No elbow movement is possible.

X-RAY — Even though the dislocation is clinically obvious, x-ray films must be taken to exclude an associated fracture.

TREATMENT

REDUCE — The patient should be fully relaxed under anaesthesia. The surgeon pulls on the forearm while the elbow is slightly flexed. With one hand, sideways displacement is corrected, then the elbow is further flexed while the olecranon process is pushed forward with the thumbs. Unless almost full flexion can be obtained, the olecranon is not in the trochlear groove.

HOLD — The arm is held in a collar and cuff with the elbow flexed above 90 degrees. After 1 week the patient gently exercises his elbow; at 3 weeks he discards the collar and cuff.

EXERCISE — Shoulder and finger exercises are begun at once. Elbow movements are allowed to return spontaneously and are never forced.

COMPLICATIONS

ASSOCIATED FRACTURES — These are common.

Coronoid process — Small flake fractures of the coronoid process are unimportant and require no special treatment.

Medial epicondyle — The association of this fracture with a lateral dislocation of the elbow has already been described (page 373).

Head of radius — This fracture, combined with dislocation, is a serious injury. The dislocation is first reduced; 3 weeks later the head of the radius may need to be excised.

Olecranon process — Rarely, the elbow dislocates forwards, leaving the proximal 2 cm of the olecranon process behind as a separate fragment. Although the combined injury can be treated by reduction and plaster in full extension, it is probably better to ensure stability by fixing the olecranon process internally.

'Side-swipe' fracture-dislocation — This describes the injury sustained when a driver sticks his elbow out of the window and the elbow is struck by another car. The result is forward dislocation with fractures of any or all of the bones. It is best to reduce the dislocation first, then hold it reduced in a split plaster, and treat the fractures when the joint becomes stable.

JOINT STIFFNESS — This may be due to:

Myositis ossificans — To minimize the risk of this complication, passive movements must be prohibited. If movement is diminishing, or if x-rays show calcification, the elbow should be rested in a plaster gutter.

Unreduced dislocation — A dislocation may not have been diagnosed; or only the backward displacement corrected, leaving the olecranon process still displaced sideways. Up to 6 weeks from injury, manipulative reduction is worth attempting. After that a 'sham reduction' can be tried; under anaesthesia the elbow is manipulated to a more flexed position, held in a sling and activity encouraged. Often a useful range of movement is regained, but if the elbow remains stiff and painful, arthroplasty may be considered.

NERVE INJURIES — These are not uncommon. They usually recover.

THE FOREARM

FRACTURED RADIUS AND ULNA

MECHANISM

A twisting force (commonly a fall on the hand) causes a spiral fracture with the bones broken at different levels. A direct blow or an angulating force causes a transverse fracture of both bones at the same level. Additional rotation deformity may be produced by the pull of muscles attached to the radius: they are the biceps and supinator muscles to the upper third, the pronator teres to the middle third, and the pronator quadratus to the lower third.

SIGNS

LOOK — Deformity is usually obvious. The fracture may be compound.

FEEL — The fracture sites are tender. The pulse should be tested.

MOVE — Movement should not be attempted.

X-RAY — Both bones are broken, either transversely and at the same level, or obliquely with the radial fracture usually at a higher level. In children, the fracture is often incomplete (greenstick) and only angulated. In adults, displacement may occur in any direction—shift, overlap, tilt or twist.

CLOSED TREATMENT

REDUCE — A greenstick fracture is easily straightened by firm pressure.

A complete fracture, whether spiral or transverse, is reduced by traction and rotation. The elbow is bent and the surgeon pulls on the hand while an assistant resists the pull by holding the upper arm. While traction is maintained the hand is rotated until the fragments are aligned; the forearm usually needs to be supinated when the radial fracture is high, pronated when it is low, and neutral between the two.

In adults, perfect reduction is essential; in children slight overlap is unimportant, providing no angulation or rotation deformity persists.

HOLD — While traction is maintained, plaster is applied from just below the axilla to just above the knuckles. The elbow is held at 90 degrees, the wrist dorsiflexed and the forearm in that degree of rotation at which reduction was obtained. X-ray films are taken to confirm reduction.

As soon as the plaster has set it is split from top to bottom to expose the skin. The patient is returned to the ward, and his arm elevated. When swelling has subsided, the plaster is completed or renewed.

In adults, a spiral fracture consolidates in about 6 weeks, and a transverse fracture in 12 weeks; in children, these times are considerably shorter. When consolidation may be expected to have occurred, the plaster is removed and the fracture assessed clinically and radiologically. Unless consolidation has occurred a complete plaster must be re-applied.

EXERCISE — Shoulder and finger movements are practised from the start. When the plaster is removed the patient wears a sling and regains elbow and radio-ulnar movements by graduated activity.

Sarmiento (1975) has shown that functional bracing can be used for forearm fractures. The brace permits movements at the elbow and wrist but controls rotation.

OPERATIVE TREATMENT

In open fractures wound toilet is, of course, necessary. The fracture is reduced under direct vision; if reduction is stable the skin is closed and the fracture treated in

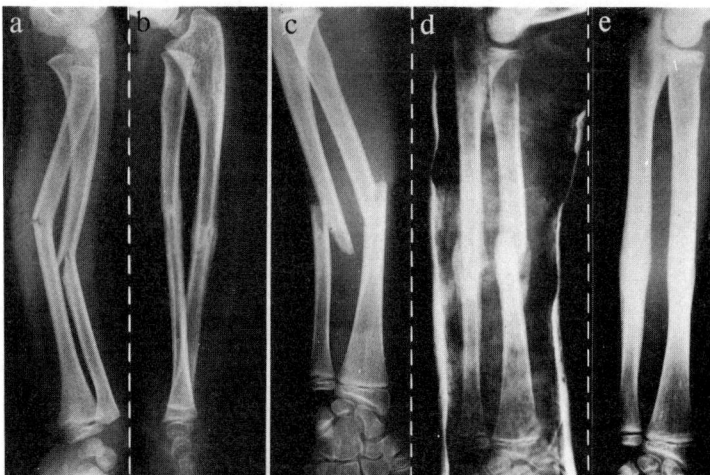

23.18 FRACTURED RADIUS AND ULNA IN CHILDREN
Green-stick fractures (a) only need correction of angulation (b), and plaster.
Complete fractures (c) are harder to reduce: but providing alignment is corrected and held in plaster (d) slight lateral shift remodels with growth (e).

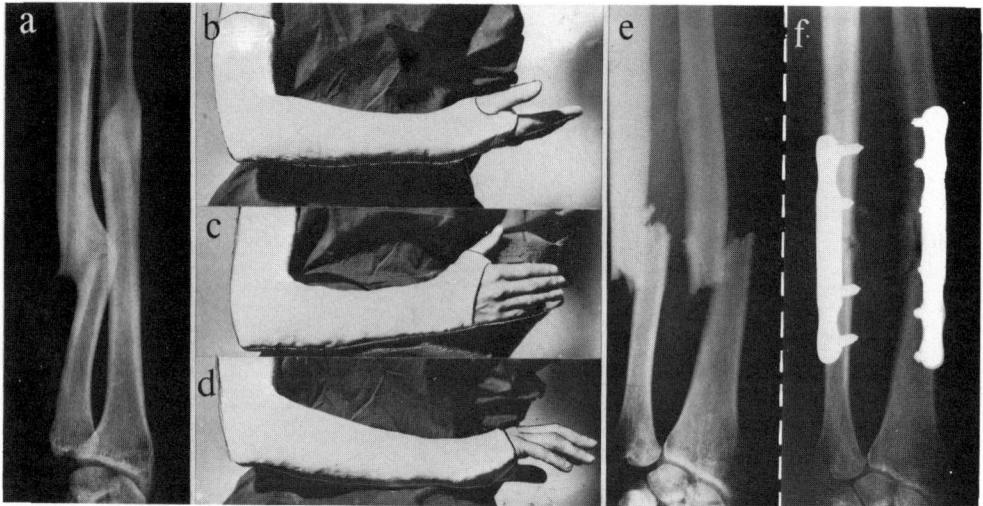

23.19   FRACTURED RADIUS AND ULNA IN ADULTS

Adult fractures also can be treated in plaster, but the danger is mal-union (a).   The radius is the difficult bone: with high fractures the forearm usually needs to be supinated (b); in the middle third usually in mid-rotation (c), and in the lower third pronated (d).   If closed reduction is imperfect, open reduction and plating (e, f) is the answer.

plaster as above; if reduction is unstable, the patient an adult, and the wound not heavily contaminated, then the fractures are plated.

With closed fractures in adults, perfect function cannot be ensured unless perfect reduction has been achieved.   If closed reduction fails or redisplacement occurs in plaster, then operation is advisable; it is probably best performed 2 weeks after injury.

REDUCE — The fractures are exposed by two separate incisions, one for each bone (if one incision only is used, there is danger of cross union).   An assistant pulls on the arm and rotates it, while the surgeon reduces the fracture under direct vision.

HOLD — The fracture in each bone is held by means of a plate and screws.   A plaster slab is bandaged on if the patient cannot be trusted to exercise reasonable care.

Consolidation takes at least as long as if the fractures had not been plated, and the usual practice, once the wounds have healed, is to replace the plaster slab by a complete plaster for at least 8 weeks.

EXERCISE — Plated forearm fractures are eminently suited to the ' delayed splintage ' technique: the day after operation a physiotherapist shows the patient how to exercise all the joints of the injured limb.   This is repeated twice daily until the wounds have healed.   A complete plaster is then applied and, when it is removed, full movement is rapidly regained.

Very occasionally open reduction may be desirable in a child, but plating is never essential.

COMPLICATIONS

ISCHAEMIA — Ischaemia of the hand must be watched for.

NON-UNION — This may occur if the plaster has been removed before consolidation. It is particularly liable to follow plating, especially of comminuted fractures.   Non-union is treated by freshening the bone ends and screwing on a cortical bone graft, or by applying cancellous bone strips around the fracture; plaster splintage is, of course, also necessary.

MAL-UNION — Mal-union is usually due to redisplacement within a loose plaster. The arm looks ugly and rotation is limited. Operative correction and plating may be necessary.

JOINT STIFFNESS — Temporary stiffness of the elbow and radio-ulnar joints may be unavoidable but, unless there is mal-union, full movement will be regained with activity. Shoulder and finger stiffness result from neglect.

FRACTURES OF ONE BONE ONLY

Fracture of the radius alone or of the ulna alone is uncommon and usually caused by a direct blow. It is important for two reasons: (a) an associated dislocation may be undiagnosed; if only one forearm bone is broken and there is displacement, one or other radio-ulnar joint must be dislocated; as a precaution the entire forearm must always be x-rayed; (b) non-union is liable to occur unless it is realized that one bone takes just as long to consolidate as two.

SIGNS

LOOK — Slight swelling is seen, but no obvious deformity.

FEEL — Tenderness is localized to the fracture site.

MOVE — With a fracture of the radius rotation is painful.

X-RAY — The fracture may be anywhere in the radius or ulna. The fracture line is transverse and displacement is slight (or else there must be a fracture-dislocation—see below).

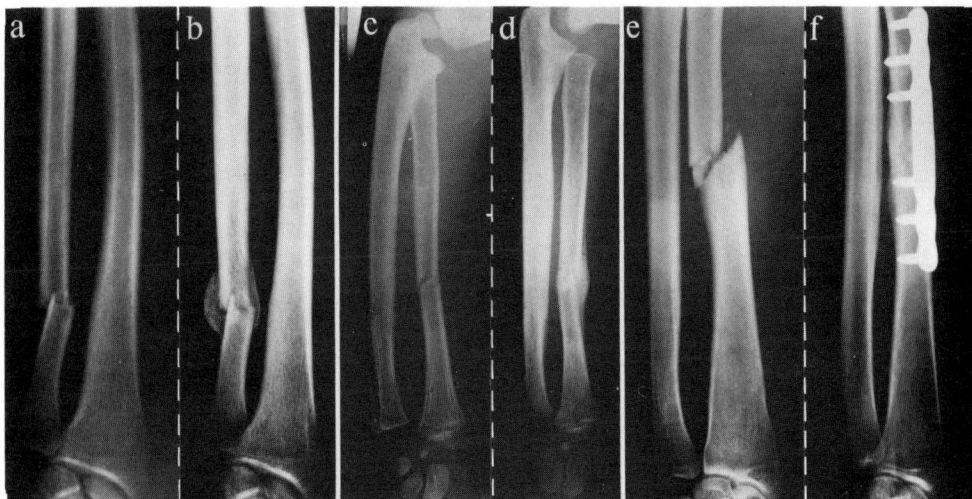

23.20 FRACTURED RADIUS OR ULNA
A fracture of the ulna alone (a) usually joins satisfactorily (b) with treatment in plaster. This fracture of the radius alone in a child (c) also joined (d) in plaster; but in adults a fractured radius (e) is sometimes better treated by plating (f); delayed splintage is then used.

TREATMENT

REDUCE — Displacement is slight and reduction may not be necessary.

HOLD — A complete plaster is applied, to include the elbow and wrist joints, exactly as though both forearm bones were broken. The fracture is transverse; therefore it may be 12 weeks before consolidation is complete.

EXERCISE — Exercises, as for fractures of both bones, are carried out.

Because one bone is intact the ends of the broken bone cannot impinge upon one another; union is liable to be delayed and many surgeons therefore advise internal fixation by a plate and screws. A plated ulna probably needs no plaster, but a plated radius in a manual worker must be protected by a plaster which includes the elbow and wrist.

FRACTURE-DISLOCATION: (A) UPPER (Monteggia)

MECHANISM

Usually the cause is a fall on the hand; if at the moment of impact the body is twisting, its momentum may forcibly pronate the forearm. The radial head dislocates forwards and the upper third of the ulna fractures and bows forwards. Sometimes the causal force is hyperextension.

SIGNS

LOOK — The ulnar deformity is usually obvious but the dislocated head of the radius is masked by swelling.

FEEL — Both the fracture and the dislocation can usually be felt.

MOVE — Attempted movement is painful.

X-RAY — The head of the radius, which normally points directly to the capitulum, is dislocated forwards; and there is a fracture of the upper third of the ulna with forward bowing.

CLOSED TREATMENT

REDUCE — An assistant holds the arm while the surgeon pulls on the forearm, supinates it fully, and tries to thumb the radial head back into place. The manoeuvre rarely succeeds except in children.

HOLD — If reduction is successful plaster is applied, from the axilla to the knuckles, with the elbow at a right-angle and the forearm fully supinated.

Consolidation of the ulnar fracture takes about 12 weeks, and the plaster must be retained until it occurs.

EXERCISE — The shoulder and fingers are exercised from the start. Elbow and radio-ulnar movements take many months to return; they must not be forced.

OPERATIVE TREATMENT

If closed reduction fails, or cannot be held stable, operation is necessary. Moreover, operation with firm internal fixation lessens the period of disability.

The ulna is exposed and reduced under direct vision. It is held reduced by a plate and screws or by an intramedullary nail. With perfect reduction of the ulna, the dislocation of the radial head is reduced automatically; but if the ulna cannot be perfectly reduced, the radial head should be exposed; it may need to be levered back through the orbicular ligament. Then the ulna is plated. After operation, the delayed splintage method is employed, the application of a complete plaster being postponed until movements have been regained.

COMPLICATIONS

MAL-UNION — Mal-union of the ulna causes little disability but, unless the ulna has been perfectly reduced, the radial head remains dislocated and limits elbow flexion. In children no treatment is advised. In adults excision of the head of the radius may be needed.

NON-UNION — Non-union of the ulna should be treated by bone grafting. If the radial head is dislocated it should be excised.

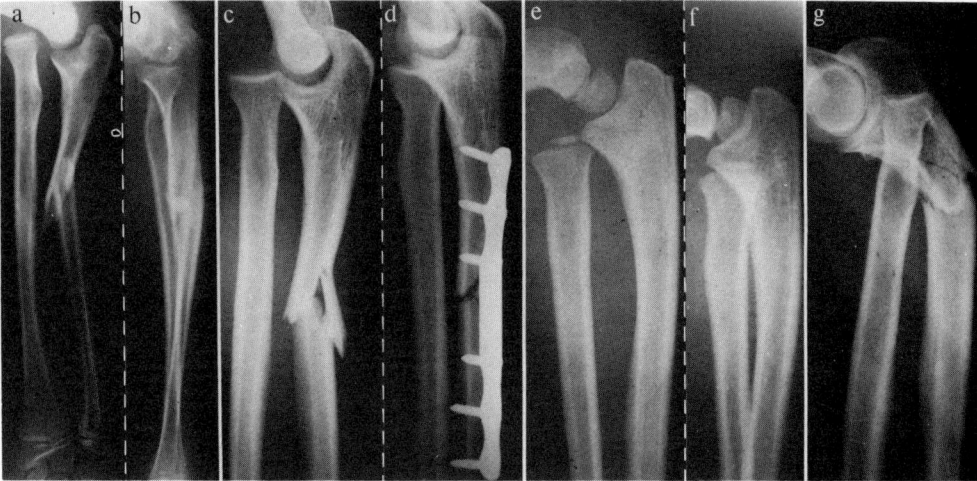

23.21 FRACTURE-DISLOCATION (1) MONTEGGIA
In the child (a) closed reduction and plaster is usually satisfactory (b). In the adult (c) open reduction and plating (d) is often advisable. Forward dislocation of the radial head without an ulnar fracture (e) can also follow pronation injury; (f) shows the dislocation reduced by supination. (g) The rare backward type of Monteggia injury with posterior dislocation of the radial head.

BACKWARD MONTEGGIA

In this variety the head of the radius dislocates backwards and the ulnar fracture bows backwards. Although manipulative reduction is relatively easy, it can only be held in plaster with the elbow extended, and disabling stiffness is likely. Operative treatment with internal fixation of the ulna is therefore better.

DISLOCATION OF THE RADIAL HEAD

This may follow a pronation injury without fracture of the ulna. The dislocation is reduced by supination and direct pressure, and the arm held supine in plaster for 6 weeks.

Dislocation of the radial head may be congenital and if the patient injures his elbow, the unwary surgeon may attempt an impossible reduction. Congenital dislocation may be forward or backward, and is usually bilateral; but in all cases the radial head is dome-shaped, distinguishing it from traumatic dislocation (page 162).

PULLED ELBOW

A child aged 3 or 4 is brought up with a painful elbow which he supports with the other hand. The probable cause is distal subluxation of the radial head which becomes impacted in the orbicular ligament, preventing rotation. Spontaneous recovery occurs if the arm is rested in a sling for a few days; dramatic improvement may follow forcible supination in the course of examination.

FRACTURE-DISLOCATION: (B) LOWER (Galeazzi)

MECHANISM

The usual cause is a fall on the hand; probably a rotation force is superimposed. The radius fractures in its lower third and the inferior radio-ulnar joint dislocates. The injury is an almost exact counterpart of the Monteggia fracture-dislocation.

SIGNS

LOOK — The lower end of the ulna is unduly prominent.

FEEL — It is important to test for an ulnar nerve lesion, which is common.

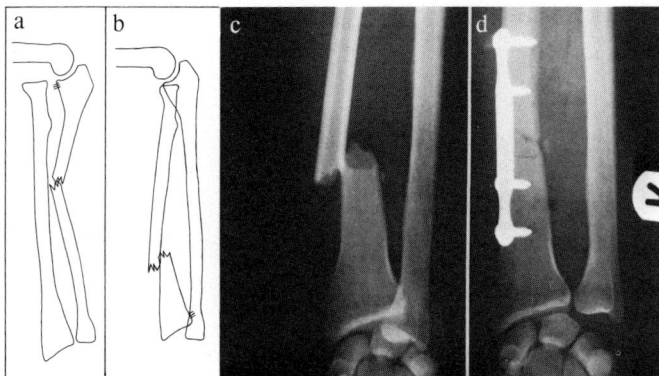

23.22 FRACTURE-DISLOCATION (2) GALEAZZI
The diagrams show the contrast between (a) Monteggia and (b) Galeazzi fracture-dislocations.

(c, d) Galeazzi type before and after reduction and plating.

MOVE — Movement should not be attempted.

X-RAY — A transverse or short oblique fracture is seen in the lower third of the radius, with angulation or overlap. The inferior radio-ulnar joint is dislocated.

TREATMENT

Closed reduction is sometimes successful and can be held by a full above-elbow plaster, which must be maintained for at least 3 months. It is probably better, however, to reduce and plate the radius at open operation. Accurate reduction of the radius ensures replacement of the radio-ulnar dislocation.

THE WRIST

COLLES' FRACTURE

MECHANISM

This injury, the commonest of all fractures, is probably due to a supination force. The patient is usually an elderly woman, often osteoporotic. She falls on the dorsi-flexed hand, breaking the radius transversely just above the wrist. Probably the momentum of the body imposes a supination force and the lower radius, with the hand, is twisted and tilted backwards and radially.

23.23 Colles' Frac-
    ture (1)
(a) Dinner-fork deformity.
(b, c) The fracture is not
into the wrist joint: the
chief displacements are
backwards and radially.

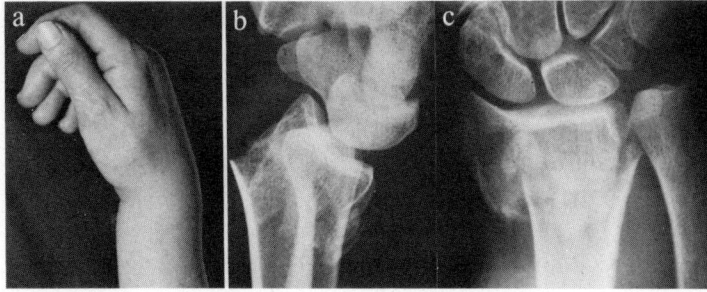

SIGNS

LOOK — The normal slight concavity on the back of the wrist is obliterated, and a depression is seen in front of the lower radius; this 'dinner-fork deformity', however, is seen only with gross displacement.

FEEL — The bony displacement may be palpated, and tenderness elicited.

MOVE — Wrist movements are limited and painful.

X-RAY — There is a transverse fracture of the radius less than one inch from the wrist, and often the ulnar styloid process is broken off. The radial fragment is (a) shifted and tilted backwards, (b) shifted and tilted radially, and (c) impacted.

TREATMENT

REDUCE — Under anaesthesia the fracture is reduced in 3 stages.

(1) *Disimpaction* — Disimpaction may be achieved by pulling on the hand. If this fails, the backward tilt should be temporarily increased and then traction resumed.

(2) *Pronation* — The patient's wrist is palmar-flexed and the forearm strongly pronated.

(3) *Pressure* — To ensure that reduction is complete, the surgeon presses the lower radius firmly forwards and towards the ulna.

HOLD — While the forearm is still held pronated and the wrist slightly palmarflexed and ulnar deviated, a plaster slab is applied. It extends from just below the elbow to the metacarpal necks and two-thirds of the way round the circumference of the wrist. It is held in position by a crêpe bandage. While the plaster slab is setting the surgeon holds the reduction by firm pressure with his thenar eminences. Post-reduction x-rays are taken.

Next day, if the fingers are swollen, cyanosed or painful, there should be no hesitation in splitting the bandage. At 7 days fresh x-rays are taken; re-displacement in the relatively young patient requires re-reduction; in the elderly it is best to abandon splintage and concentrate on activity.

23.24 Colles' Frac-
    ture (2)
Reduction: (a) disimpac-
tion (not always neces-
sary), (b) pronation and
forward shift, (c) ulnar deviation.
Splintage: (d) stockinette,
(e) wet plaster slab, (f)
slab bandaged on and re-
duction held till plaster
set.

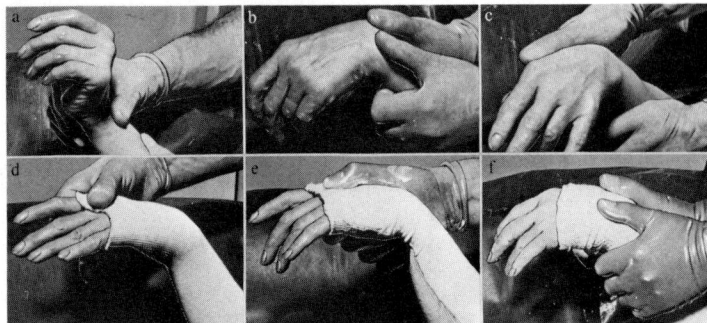

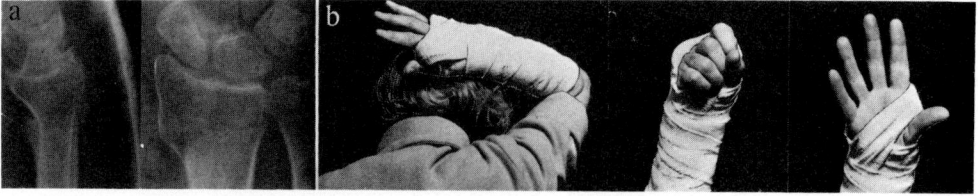

23.25 COLLES' FRACTURE (3)
(a) Post-reduction films are satisfactory (Fig. 23.23 were the pre-reduction films of this patient); (b) before going home she is taught these movements and persuaded to practise them regularly.

The fracture unites in 6 weeks and, even in the absence of radiological proof of union, the slab may safely be discarded and replaced by a temporary crêpe bandage.

EXERCISE — The patient should not be allowed to go home until she can comb her hair and move her fingers fully. Regular active exercises of the shoulder and fingers must be insisted upon — they are more important than treatment of the broken bone.

When the plaster has been removed, return of wrist and radio-ulnar movements is encouraged by the regular practice of such normal activities as washing up.

COMPLICATIONS

MAL-UNION — Mal-union is common, either because reduction was not complete or because displacement within the plaster was overlooked. The appearance is ugly, and weakness and loss of rotation may persist. In most cases treatment is not necessary. Where the disability is severe and the patient relatively young, the lower inch of the ulna may be excised to restore rotation and the radial deformity corrected by osteotomy.

DELAYED UNION AND NON-UNION — Delayed union and non-union of the radius do not occur, but the ulnar styloid process often joins by fibrous tissue only and remains painful and tender for several months.

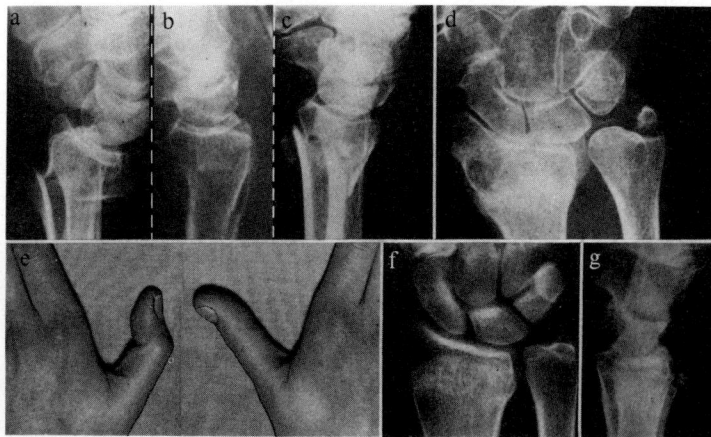

23.26 COLLES' FRACTURE (4)
Mal-union: backward shift (a) was reduced (b), but recurred (c). Slight mal-union of radius with non-union of ulna (d). Delayed rupture of extensor pollicis longus (e) is not a complication of a true Colles' fracture, but of this apparently trivial fracture (f, g).

STIFFNESS — Stiffness of the shoulder, from neglect, is probably the commonest complication.   Stiffness of the wrist may follow persisting with splintage despite poor position in plaster—the patient has the worst of both worlds.   Finger stiffness can nearly always be avoided by active use but, rarely, Sudeck's atrophy (page 340) develops and stiffness then persists for months.

NERVE INJURY — Nerve injury is rare, and even median compression in the carpal tunnel is surprisingly uncommon.

TENDON INJURY — The extensor pollicis longus tendon occasionally ruptures a few weeks after an apparently trivial undisplaced fracture of the lower radius.   The patient should be warned of the possibility and told that operative treatment is available (page 176). Helal believes rupture follows swelling within the tight compartment between bone and ligament; with displaced fractures the ligament ruptures and consequently there is no tension so that tendon rupture does not occur.

OTHER FRACTURES OF LOWER RADIUS

JUVENILE COLLES' FRACTURE

The force which in an older person causes a Colles' fracture may, in a child, cause a fracture-separation of the lower radial epiphysis.   The epiphysis is shifted and tilted backwards and may also be shifted and tilted radially.   As it displaces it carries with it a triangular fragment of the radial metaphysis.   The fracture is reduced and held in the same way as a Colles' fracture.

Fracture-separation of the lower radial epiphysis does not interfere with growth of the bone; but a minor crush of the radial epiphysis without displacement may do so, and premature epiphyseal fusion then occurs.   The ulna outgrows the radius and the ulnar head dislocates.   It may subsequently be necessary to excise the lower inch of the ulna.

FRACTURED RADIAL STYLOID

This injury, formerly called chauffeur's fracture, is caused by forced radial deviation of the wrist and may occur after a fall, or when the starting handle of a lorry 'kicks back'.   The fracture line is transverse, extending laterally from the articular surface of the radius; the fragment, much more than the radial styloid, is often undisplaced.

If there is displacement it is reduced, and the wrist is held in ulnar deviation by a plaster slab round the outer forearm extending from below the elbow to the metacarpal necks.   Imperfect reduction may lead to osteoarthritis; therefore if closed reduction is imperfect the fragment should be screwed back.

COMMINUTED FRACTURES

Instead of the lower radius breaking transversely above the wrist as in a true Colles' fracture, there may be a T-shaped fracture into the joint, or the lower radius may be comminuted.   Accurate reduction can sometimes be achieved by manual traction, and possibly held in an above-elbow plaster for 6 weeks.   If the patient is young and reduction is inaccurate, traction by means of Kirschner wires through the metacarpals and olecranon has been suggested.   Usually the patient is elderly and it is then best to apply a plaster slab (purely for comfort), removing it after a few days for active exercises; the carpal bones mould the radial fragments into reasonable position and quite good function is regained.

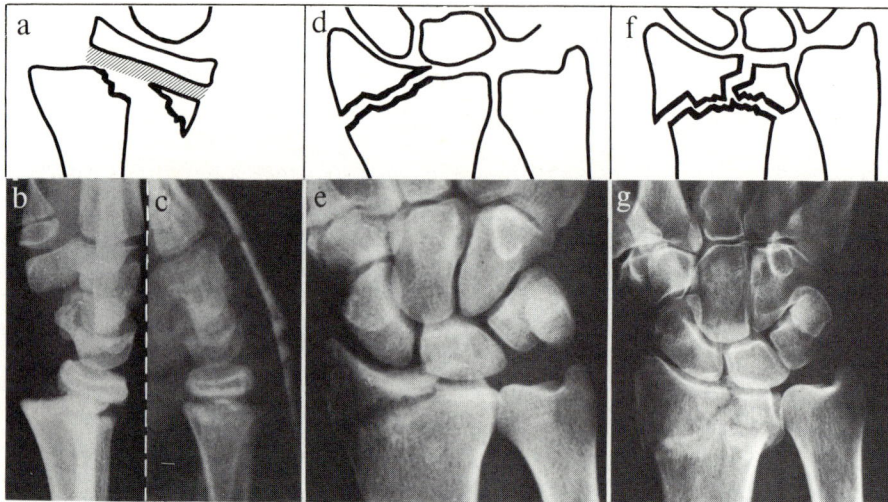

23.27 OTHER FRACTURES OF THE LOWER RADIUS
(a, b) Juvenile Colles' fracture — lateral view. Note that displacement is not through the growth disc but just proximal to it; (c) after reduction. (d, e) Radial styloid. (f, g) Comminuted fracture into the wrist joint.

FRACTURES WITH FORWARD DISPLACEMENT

The terms reversed Colles' and Smith's fracture are used misleadingly. In 1847 Smith described a transverse fracture just above the wrist — a true reversed Colles' fracture. The injury to which his name is usually applied is a fracture-dislocation, and was described in 1839 by Barton.

A true *reversed Colles' fracture* (a transverse fracture of the lower radius with forward shift and tilt) is rare, and occurs mainly in elderly women. It is reduced by disimpaction and held dorsiflexed, preferably in supination and in an above-elbow plaster, for 6 weeks.

23.28 FRACTURES WITH FORWARD DISPLACEMENT
(a, b) True reversed Colles' fracture. (c, d) Fracture dislocation and (e) reduction held with Ellis plate.

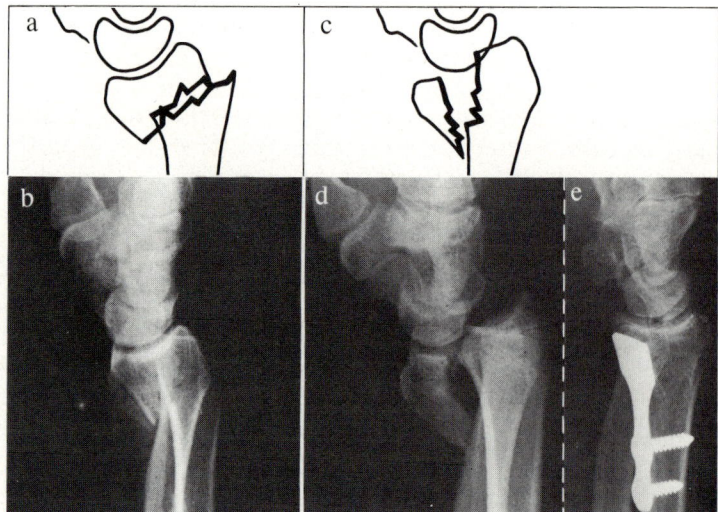

Fracture-dislocation is commoner. The radial fracture is oblique, extending upwards and forwards from the wrist joint; the separated anterior fragment of radius shifts proximally carrying the hand with it. Reduction can usually be achieved by strong traction and supination; if so it may be possible to hold reduction in an above elbow plaster with the forearm supinated. Union takes at least 6 weeks and, if perfect reduction has not been obtained and maintained by closed methods, the fracture can be reduced openly and held by a small anterior plate.

FRACTURED CARPAL SCAPHOID

MECHANISM

A fall on the dorsiflexed hand may fracture the scaphoid. Probably the force is a combination of dorsiflexion and radial deviation. The deviation occurs between the two rows of carpal bones; the scaphoid, lying partly in each row, fractures across its waist. The injury is rare in children and in the elderly.

SIGNS

LOOK — The appearance may be deceptively normal, but the astute observer can usually detect fullness in the anatomical snuff box.

FEEL — There is localized tenderness over the scaphoid.

MOVE — Wrist movements are slightly painful and limited, and the grip is weak.

X-RAY — Antero-posterior, lateral and oblique views are all essential; often a recent fracture shows only in the oblique view. Usually the fracture line is transverse, and through the narrowest part of the bone (waist), but it may be more proximally situated (proximal pole fracture). Sometimes only the tubercle of the scaphoid is fractured. There is rarely much displacement.

DIAGNOSIS

Sprains of the wrist are rare and must not be diagnosed unless repeated x-rays have excluded a fracture. Immediately after injury a fracture of the scaphoid may be

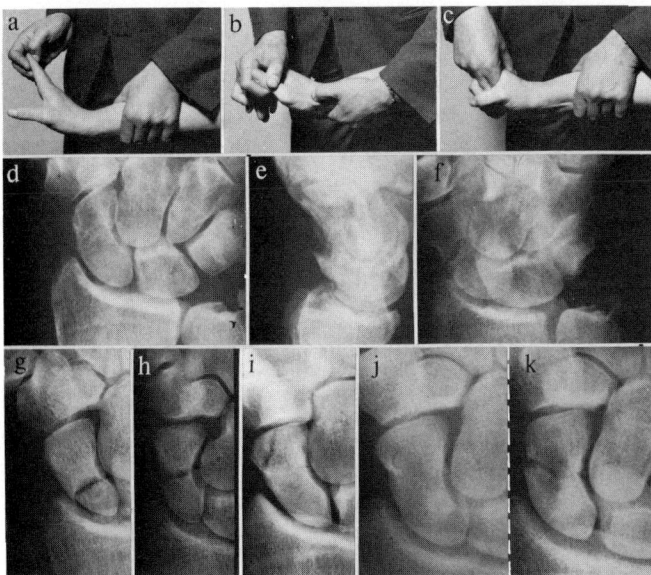

23.29 SCAPHOID FRAC-
TURES (1) DIAGNOSIS
Clinical signs: (a) pain on dorsiflexion (b) localized tenderness (c) pain on gripping.

X-ray signs: the AP view (d) and the lateral (e) often fail to show the fracture; even in an oblique view (f) it may be difficult to see.

Fracture may be through (g) the proximal pole, (h) the waist, or (i) the tubercle. Even when no fracture is seen at first (j) a repeat film at two weeks (k) shows it clearly.

almost invisible; where there is the slightest doubt, further x-rays must be taken 2 to 3 weeks after the injury, when the fracture can be clearly seen.

Wrist sprains may remain uncomfortable for many weeks, but splintage is not helpful. A crêpe bandage for a few days is comforting, but activity should be encouraged. Sometimes a lateral x-ray shows a flake fracture off the back of the triquetrum; this injury also should be regarded as a sprain and treated by active use.

TREATMENT

Fracture of the scaphoid tubercle needs no splintage and should be treated as a wrist sprain (see above). All other scaphoid fractures are treated as follows.

REDUCE — Displacement is not common, but when it is present an attempt should be made to reduce it by manipulation under anaesthesia. Rarely manipulation fails, and if displacement is substantial, open reduction is worth considering; it can usefully be followed by inserting a screw across the fracture (Maudsley, 1972).

HOLD — A complete plaster is applied from the upper forearm to just short of the meta-carpo-phalangeal joints of the fingers, but incorporating the proximal phalanx of the thumb. The wrist is held dorsiflexed and the thumb forwards in the 'glass-holding' position. The plaster must be carefully moulded into the hollow of the hand, and is not split. It is retained (and if necessary repaired or renewed) for 6 weeks.

After 6 weeks the plaster is removed and the wrist examined clinically. A further plaster for 4 weeks is applied only if the wrist is tender and uncomfortable, or with a proximal pole fracture. Otherwise the wrist is left free; often radiological union becomes obvious only after several months. It is possible that too short a time in plaster occasionally leads to non-union; but the risk of painful non-union is smaller than the risk of painful stiffness after prolonged splintage.

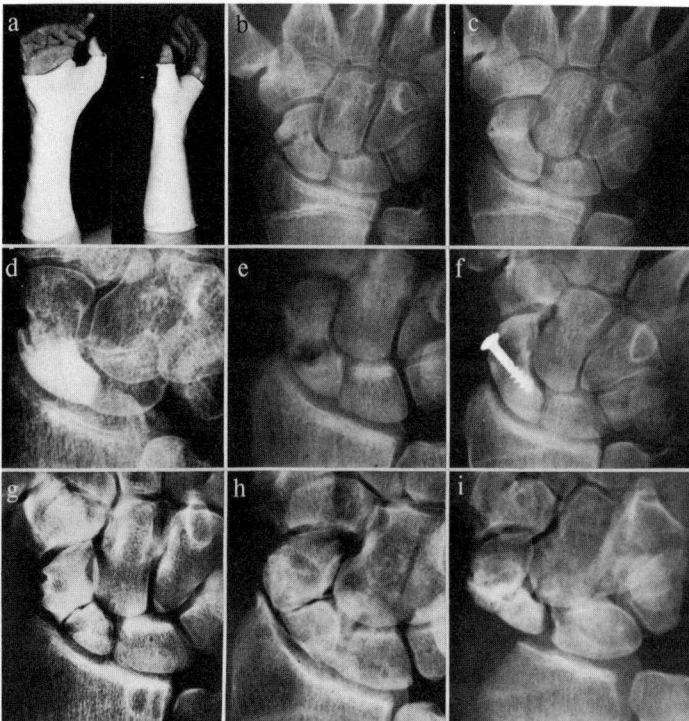

23.30 SCAPHOID FRACTURES (2) TREATMENT AND COMPLICATIONS

(a) Scaphoid plaster—position and extent.

(b, c) Before and after treatment: in this case radiological union was visible at 10 weeks.

(d) Avascular necrosis of proximal half; (e) early non-union, treated successfully by (f) inserting a screw.

(g) Established non-union with sclerosis; (h) non-union with localized osteoarthritic changes; (i) osteoarthritis treated by excising the radial styloid.

EXERCISE — Shoulder movements are practised from the start, and the plaster is so designed that function of the hand is limited as little as possible. Wrist movements are regained when the plaster is removed.

COMPLICATIONS

AVASCULAR NECROSIS — The proximal fragment may die, especially with proximal pole fractures, and then at 2–3 months it appears dense on x-ray. Although revascularization and union are theoretically possible, they take a period of years. The dead fragment and the radial styloid should therefore be excised forthwith.

EARLY NON-UNION — It may be apparent in 3–6 months that the bone ends at the fracture are becoming sclerosed. The fracture may be fixed in compression with a screw, or a bone graft inserted. Plaster is worn for 3 months.

ESTABLISHED NON-UNION — A patient may be seen because of a recent injury, but x-rays show an old, ununited fracture with sclerosed edges. He may recall a previous 'sprain' which was in reality an undiagnosed scaphoid fracture. The wrist soon became painless, fortifying both patient and doctor in their error. Providing avascular necrosis has not occurred, non-union of the scaphoid does not necessarily cause symptoms, but there is an increased likelihood of pain following overuse or further injury.

The patient who presents with a wrist sprain and established non-union is put in plaster for 2–4 weeks; often the wrist becomes painless and strong again. If symptoms persist, or repeated sprains occur, the radial styloid process should be excised.

OSTEOARTHRITIS — Osteoarthritis of the wrist may be a sequel to non-union of the scaphoid, especially when there has been avascular necrosis. The patient may complain of repeated sprains and later of weakness, stiffness and pain. If a wrist strap or polythene splint fails to relieve symptoms, the wrist may need to be arthrodesed.

CARPAL DISLOCATIONS

MECHANISM

A fall on the dorsiflexed hand may displace the hand and most of the carpus backwards, leaving only the lunate in contact with the radius (*perilunar dislocation*); this may be associated with fractures of the radial styloid or any carpal bone. Usually the hand immediately snaps forwards again but, as it does so, the lunate is levered forwards out of position (*lunate dislocation*). A lunate dislocation can possibly occur without preceding perilunar dislocation; during forced dorsiflexion the bone might conceivably be ejected like an orange pip.

If the dorsiflexion injury has also fractured the scaphoid, its proximal half remains alongside the lunate in whatever position that bone lies.

SIGNS

LOOK — The displacement itself is obscured by swelling which makes the wrist look abnormally thick.

FEEL — It is important to test for diminished sensation in the distribution of the median nerve, which is usually compressed.

MOVE — The wrist is immobile. The patient can move his fingers only with difficulty because the tendons, like the median nerve, are compressed in the carpal tunnel.

X-RAY — In the antero-posterior view, the lunate has lost its normal somewhat quadrilateral shape; instead it comes to a point distally. The scaphoid may also have fractured.

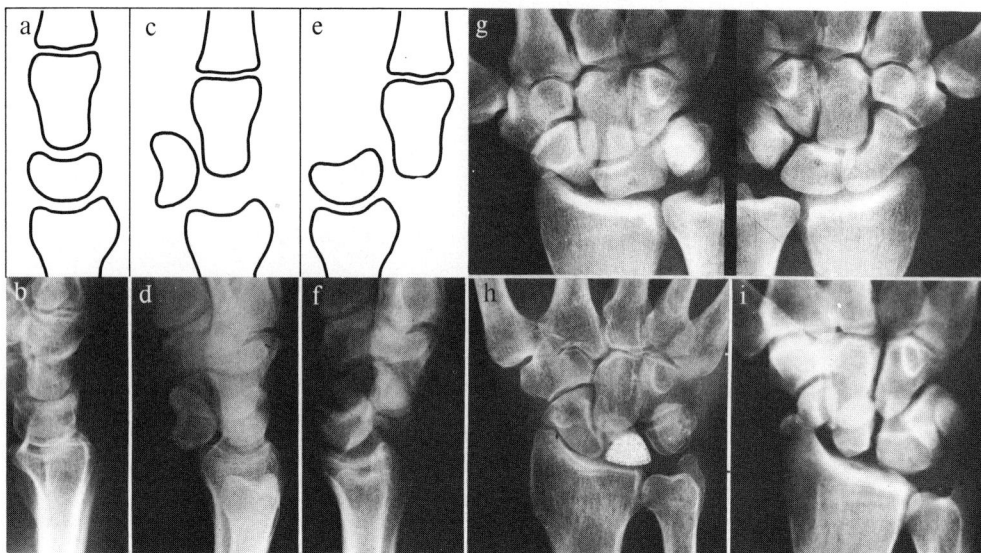

23.31 LUNATE AND PERILUNAR DISLOCATIONS
Lateral view of (a, b) normal wrist; (c, d) lunate dislocation; (e, f) perilunar dislocation. (g) AP of both wrists with dislocated left lunate — note its pointed appearance.
(h) Avascular necrosis following reduction. (i) Associated fracture of scaphoid.

In the lateral view it is easy to distinguish a perilunar from a lunate dislocation. The
dislocated lunate is grossly tilted forwards and is displaced in front of the radius, while
the os magnum and metacarpal bones are in line with the radius. With a perilunar
dislocation the lunate is tilted forwards only slightly, and is not displaced forwards; and
the os magnum and metacarpals lie behind the line of the radius.

TREATMENT

REDUCE — The surgeon pulls strongly on the dorsiflexed hand. While maintaining
traction he slowly palmarflexes the wrist at the same time squeezing the lunate backwards
with his other thumb. These manoeuvres usually effect reduction; they also prevent
conversion of perilunar to lunate dislocation. Reduction is imperative and if closed
reduction fails, the bone is exposed by an anterior approach which has the advantage of
decompressing the carpal tunnel. While an assistant pulls on the hand, the lunate is
levered into place. If at operation the bone is seen to be totally detached, some surgeons
advise its immediate excision, because avascular necrosis is inevitable; but excision leaves
some weakness and silastic replacement is worth considering.

HOLD — Reduction is stable, but a plaster slab holding the wrist neutral is comforting,
and is worn for 3 weeks.

EXERCISE — Finger movements are begun at once.

COMPLICATIONS

NERVE INJURY — Median nerve compression in the carpal tunnel occurs almost invariably, but recovers after reduction.

UNREDUCED DISLOCATION — This presents as a painful stiffish wrist, with median paraesthesia. The lunate should be excised through an anterior incision; it is worth seeing if
a silastic replacement can be fitted into the gap.

FRACTURED SCAPHOID — It is important always to exclude a scaphoid fracture by x-ray after reduction of the dislocation (which will automatically have reduced the fractured scaphoid). Following reduction, an anterior plaster slab is applied which, after one week, is replaced by a full scaphoid plaster; the injury is then treated as a fractured scaphoid.

AVASCULAR NECROSIS — The lunate and the proximal half of the scaphoid may become avascular. Osteoarthritis of the radio-carpal joint is likely to ensue.

THE HAND

MANAGEMENT

In the hand, even more than elsewhere, function is a vital consideration. Fingers stiffen easily and a stiff finger is often worse than no finger. Fractures in the hand almost invariably unite and even if angulation persists, mal-union is less disabling than stiffness.

The guiding principles of treatment are as follows.

SWELLING — Swelling must be controlled by elevating the hand and by early and repeated active exercises.

SPLINTAGE — Splintage must be kept to a minimum. If it is essential it is best to attach the injured finger to its neighbour (by strapping or by a double tubigrip), so that both move as one. Apart from this, only the injured finger should be splinted and then only in the correct position — with the knuckle joint flexed 90 degrees and the finger joints straight (page 185). Sometimes an external splint, to be effective, would need to immobilize other fingers: if so it is preferable to use internal splintage with Kirschner wires. The wires can conveniently be cut short enough to close the skin and subsequently removed under local anaesthesia.

SKIN DAMAGE — Skin damage demands wound toilet followed by suture or skin grafting. Treatment of the skin takes precedence over treatment of the fracture. (Open injuries of the hand are discussed in full on page 183).

FRACTURES

BASE OF THUMB METACARPAL

An unskilled boxer may, while punching, sustain a fracture of the first metacarpal base. Localized swelling and tenderness are found, and x-ray shows a transverse

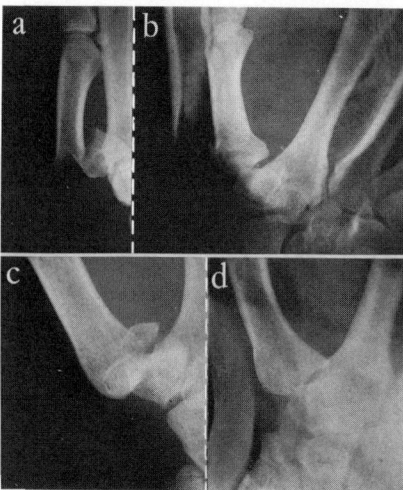

23.32 FRACTURES OF THE FIRST METACARPAL BASE
A transverse fracture (a) can be reduced and held in plaster (b).

A Bennett's fracture-dislocation can often be reduced and held in plaster (c, d): alternative methods are internal fixation (e, f), or treatment by activity (g, h).

fracture a quarter of an inch distal to the carpo-metacarpal joint, with outward bowing and usually impaction.

TREATMENT

To reduce the fracture, the surgeon pulls on the abducted thumb and, by levering the metacarpal outwards against his own thumb, corrects the bowing. A firm crêpe bandage usually suffices to prevent redisplacement, but if the fracture feels unstable a plaster slab is applied, extending from the forearm to just short of the interphalangeal thumb joint; the thumb is in the position of function where the index finger can make pulp-to-pulp contact with it. The slab is removed after 3 weeks and movement usually recovers rapidly.

BENNETT'S FRACTURE-DISLOCATION

This fracture, too, occurs at the base of the first metacarpal bone and is commonly due to punching; but the fracture is oblique, extends into the carpo-metacarpal joint and is unstable. The thumb looks short and the carpo-metacarpal region swollen. X-rays show that a small triangular fragment has remained in contact with the medial half of the trapezium, while the remainder of the thumb has subluxated proximally.

TREATMENT

REDUCTION AND SPLINTAGE — The fracture is easily reduced by pulling on the thumb, abducting it, and extending it. To hold reduction is difficult and 3 methods are available. (1) *Plaster* may be applied with a felt pad over the fracture, and the thumb held abducted and extended. If x-ray shows that perfect reduction is being held the plaster is worn for 3 weeks; otherwise the method is abandoned. (2) *Continuous skin traction* can be employed using a strong wire splint incorporated in plaster. Again 3 weeks' treatment is needed and the method is abandoned if reduction is not successful. (3) *Internal fixation* can be achieved by inserting a small screw, or by driving short lengths of Kirschner wire through the metacarpal base (by-passing the fracture) into the carpus; the protruding ends are incorporated in a small plaster slab. After 3 weeks the slab is removed and the wires pulled out.

FUNCTIONAL TREATMENT — If the fracture is disregarded and active use encouraged, painless function is quickly regained. The fracture unites but in faulty position. It is widely supposed (with little evidence) that osteoarthritis is the inevitable sequel.

METACARPAL SHAFTS

A direct blow may fracture one or several metacarpal shafts transversely, often with associated skin damage. A twisting or punching force may cause a spiral fracture of one or more shafts. There is local pain and swelling, sometimes deformity, and one knuckle may have receded.

TREATMENT

If the fracture is open, wound toilet must be performed and the skin sutured or grafted.

Spiral fractures or transverse fractures with slight displacement require no reduction. Splintage also is unnecessary, but a crêpe bandage worn for a few days may be comforting; this should not be allowed to discourage the patient from active movements of the fingers, which should be practised assiduously.

Transverse fractures with considerable displacement are reduced by traction and pressure. Reduction can be held by a plaster slab extending from the forearm over

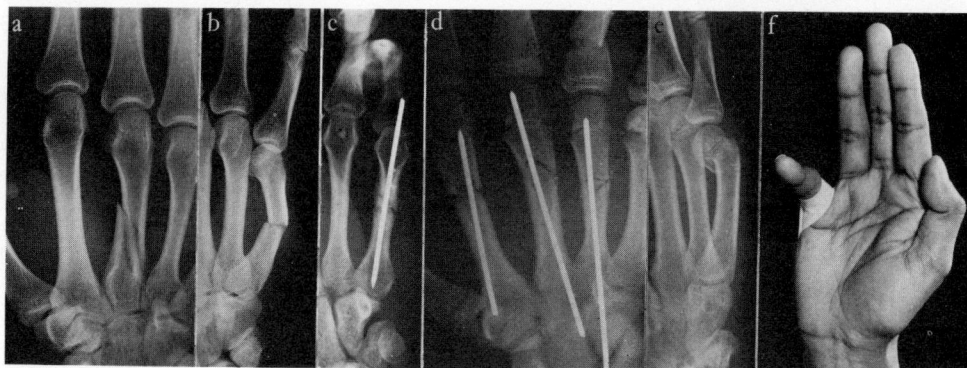

23.33 OTHER METACARPAL FRACTURES
(a) A spiral fracture of a single metacarpal (especially an ' inboard ' one) is adequately held by neighbouring bones and muscles; (b) a displaced fracture (especially an ' outboard ' one) is often best held by a wire (c). With several adjacent metacarpals fractured (d), internal fixation may be the only safe way to avoid stiffness. With a fractured neck of the fifth metacarpal (e), if reduction feels stable, strapping in this position (f) is useful (*see also* page 185).

the fingers (only the damaged ones). The slab is maintained for 3 weeks and the undamaged fingers exercised. A more elegant method is to insert a short length of Kirschner wire across the fracture through a dorsal incision; alternatively the distal fragment, after reduction, may be transfixed to the neighbouring undamaged meta-carpal by a transverse wire. In either case no external splint is necessary and early movements are encouraged.

It sometimes happens that an undetected rotational deformity becomes apparent as movement returns; the patient cannot properly close the fist and osteotomy may be needed.

METACARPAL NECKS

A blow may fracture the metacarpal neck of the fifth finger or occasionally of the index finger. A lump is visible and x-rays show a transverse fracture with backward angulation.

TREATMENT

Slight displacement may be disregarded and the patient is encouraged to use his hand; a small lump may remain, but full function is rapidly regained.

If displacement is considerable it is reduced by direct pressure between the surgeon's finger on the front of the metacarpal head and his thumb on the dorsum of the fracture. The reduction can be held by a plaster slab which extends from the wrist to the proximal finger joint, but no further; if the reduction feels stable, plaster is unnecessary, and strapping may suffice. If, however, the plaster is ineffective, the small distal fragment can (after reduction) be transfixed by a small piece of Kirschner wire anchoring it to the neighbouring metacarpal head.

PHALANGES

Fractures of the proximal or middle phalanx result from direct violence, and may be open. The phalanx fractures transversely, often with forward angulation which may damage the flexor tendon sheath.

The fracture is reduced by pulling on the bent finger and thumbing the phalanx straight. A flexed position must be maintained to hold the reduction, and is most simply achieved by placing a rolled bandage in the palm and holding the flexed finger over it with a crêpe bandage. To prevent rotation deformity, the flexed finger must point towards the scaphoid bone. It is unwise to keep finger joints flexed for long, and after 10 days the bandage should be removed. A removable posterior plaster slab is substituted; it is taken off several times a day and the patient exercises the finger while he protects the fracture with his other hand.

The terminal phalanx may be struck by a hammer, or caught in a door, and the bone shattered. The fracture is disregarded and treatment is focused on controlling swelling and regaining movement.

FRACTURES INTO JOINTS

Any finger joint may be injured by a direct blow (often the overlying skin is damaged), or by an angulation force, or by the straight finger being forcibly stubbed. The affected joint is swollen, tender and too painful to move. X-rays may show that a fragment of bone has been sheared off or avulsed.

It is usually best to disregard the fracture, to strap the finger to its neighbour with a garter, and to concentrate on regaining movement. If a bone fragment is grossly displaced, recovery of function may be hastened by fixing it back in position with a Kirschner wire, or by removing the fragment and repairing the soft tissue defect.

With *mallet finger* (*see also* page 176) the extensor tendon may avulse a fragment from the base of the terminal phalanx; but there are two distinct varieties. With the bed-making type of injury only a tiny flake is avulsed and treatment in an Oatley splint for 6 weeks is satisfactory. With a stubbing injury, such as mis-catching a cricket ball, the avulsed fragment is much larger; unless it reduces accurately with hyperextension, the fragment should be fixed back with a small piece of Kirschner wire, otherwise painful stiffness is likely to develop.

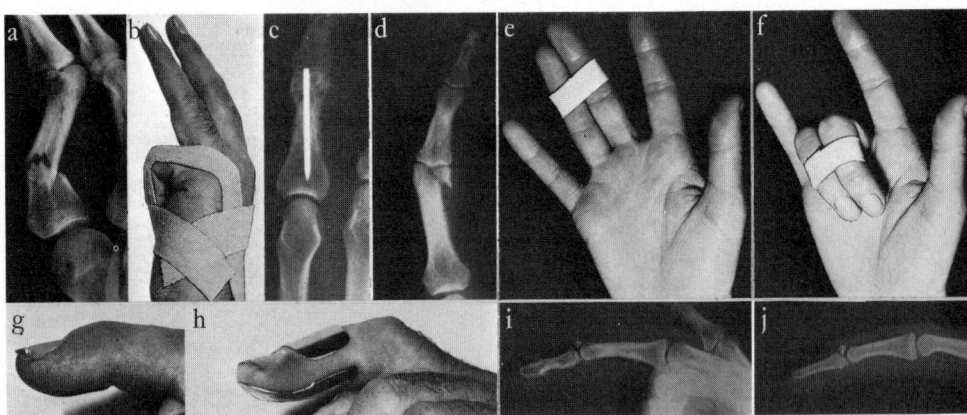

23.34 PHALANGEAL FRACTURES
Fractured proximal phalanx (a), held reduced by strapping in flexion (b), or with a wire (c). A fracture into a joint (d) can either be treated by internal fixation, or by movement with the finger strapped to its neighbour (e, f).
Mallet finger (g) treated by a splint (h); this is adequate when the bony fragment (if any) is small (i), but a large fragment (j) needs fixation.

DISLOCATIONS

CARPO-METACARPAL

The thumb is most frequently affected and clinically the injury then resembles a Bennett's fracture-dislocation; but x-rays show proximal subluxation of the first metacarpal bone without a fracture. The dislocation is easily reduced by traction, but reduction is unstable and can be held only by one of the methods used for a Bennett's fracture-dislocation, namely, plaster, skin traction, a wire splint, or Kirschner wires driven through the metacarpus into the carpus. Splintage is discontinued after 3 weeks.

Dislocations at the other carpo-metacarpal joints occur typically when a motorcyclist holding the handlebars strikes an object; one hand is driven backwards leaving the carpus, thumb and forearm projecting forwards. Closed manipulation is usually successful and a protective slab for 6 weeks restores stability.

METACARPO-PHALANGEAL

Usually the thumb is affected, sometimes the fifth finger, and rarely the other fingers. A hyperextension force may dislocate the phalanx backwards, and the capsule and muscle insertions in front of the joint may be torn. If the metacarpal head has been forced like a button through the hole, closed reduction may be impossible.

Closed reduction is first attempted by pulling on the thumb and levering the phalanx forwards. If this fails, the joint is exposed from behind and, while strong traction is applied, the metacarpal head is levered into place. The joint is then strapped in the flexed position for 1 week.

INTERPHALANGEAL

Backward dislocation at the distal joint is common and is easily reduced by pulling. The joint may be strapped flexed for a few days.

SPRAINS

Sprains of the finger joints are common, and usually due to an angulation force. Sometimes a small bony fragment is avulsed.

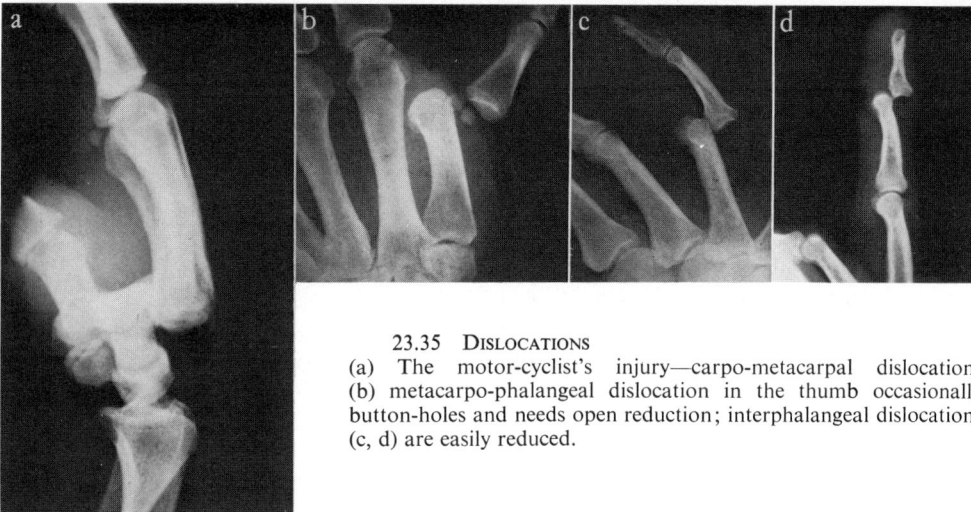

23.35 DISLOCATIONS
(a) The motor-cyclist's injury—carpo-metacarpal dislocation: (b) metacarpo-phalangeal dislocation in the thumb occasionally button-holes and needs open reduction; interphalangeal dislocations (c, d) are easily reduced.

The injured finger should be strapped to its neighbour by means of a garter and active movements encouraged. The patient must be warned that, following a sprain, the joint is likely to remain swollen, slightly painful and stiffish for 6–12 months.

Sprain of the metacarpo-phalangeal joint of the thumb ('gamekeeper's thumb') is more serious. If the ulnar collateral ligament ruptures completely (usually at its proximal attachment), it may not repair even with several weeks in plaster. Injury to this joint merits careful examination; if instability is demonstrable, immediate operative repair is advised. The neglected injury leads to weakness of pinch, which is probably best treated by arthrodesis, although in early cases without articular damage, stability may be preserved by advancing the insertion of adductor pollicis to the base of the phalanx or by re-inforcing the ligament with the tendon of extensor pollicis brevis.

Suggestions for further reading

Barton, N. (1977). 'Fractures of the Phalanges of the Hand.' *The Hand,* **9,** 1, 1

Burrows, H. J. (1951). 'Tenodesis of Subclavius in the Treatment of Recurrent Dislocation of the Sterno-Clavicular Joint.' *J. Bone Jt Surg.* **33B,** 240

Maudsley, R. H. and Chen, S. C. (1972). 'Screw Fixation in the Management of the Fractured Carpal Scaphoid.' *J. Bone Jt Surg.* **54B** 432.

Mikić, Z. (1975). 'Galeazzi Fracture-Dislocations.' *J. Bone Jt Surg.* **57A,** 1071

Neer, C. S. (1970). 'Displaced Proximal Humeral Fractures.' *J. Bone Jt Surg.* **52A,** 1077 and 1090

Rowe, C. R. *et al.* (1973). 'Voluntary Dislocation of the Shoulder.' *J. Bone Jt Surg.* **55A,** 445

Sarmiento, A. *et al.* (1975). 'Forearm Fractures.' *J. Bone Jt Surg.* **57A,** 297

Smith, R. J. (1977). 'Post-Traumatic Instability of the Metacarpophalangeal Joint of the Thumb.' *J. Bone Jt Surg.* **59A,** 14

CHAPTER 24

INJURIES OF THE SPINE AND PELVIS

FRACTURES AND DISLOCATIONS OF THE SPINE*

Spine fractures resemble skull fractures in one respect: the fracture itself is less important than the possibility of associated damage to the nervous system. Because the question of cord damage is dominant, spine fractures are best classified as stable or unstable. In *stable fractures* the cord is rarely damaged and movement of the spine is safe. In *unstable fractures* the cord may have been damaged but, if it has escaped, it may be injured by subsequent movement.

Stability depends, not on the fracture itself, but on the integrity of the ligaments and in particular the posterior ligament complex; this complex consists of the supraspinous ligament, the interspinous ligaments, the capsules of the facet joints and possibly also the ligamentum flavum.

MECHANISM OF INJURY

In order to understand which fractures are stable it is necessary to consider the forces which produce injury. Their study is simplified if we exclude avulsion injuries; these should not be regarded as fractures of the spinal column for essentially they are muscle injuries.

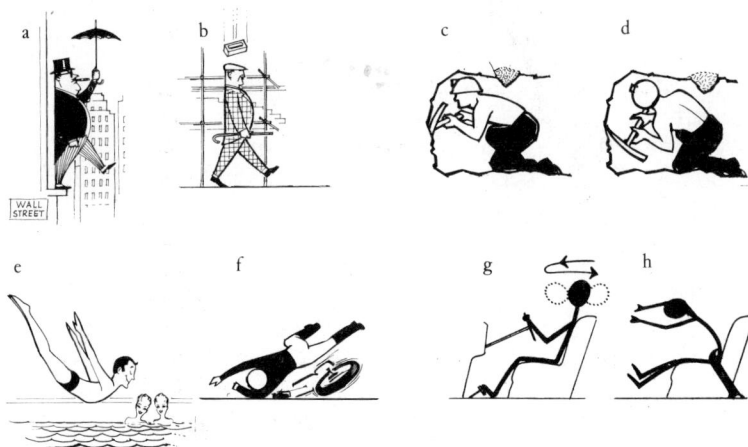

24.1 MECHANISMS OF SPINAL INJURIES
Examples of the forces producing spine fractures: (a) and (b) may cause 'burst' fractures; (c) a fall of roof in this position might cause an anterior wedge fracture; (d) the trunk is twisted and a fracture-dislocation may result; (e) might cause an extension hinging injury to the neck; (f) with rotation a fracture-dislocation is likely to occur; (g) whip-lash injury and (h) a seat-belt fracture — both involve forward shearing forces.

* Based on a postgraduate lecture given by the author at the Royal College of Surgeons of England and reproduced here by kind permission of the Editor of the *Annals*.

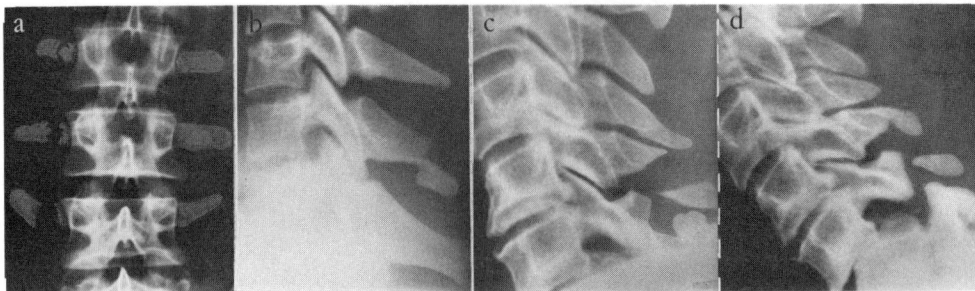

24.2 AVULSION INJURIES
(a) Fractured lumbar transverse processes; (b) clay-shoveller's fracture. (c) This
patient was at first thought to have a simple avulsion, but a subsequent flexion film
(d) showed the serious nature of the injury — a severe fracture-dislocation.

In the lumbar spine resisted muscle effort may avulse transverse processes; in the
cervical spine usually the seventh spinous process is avulsed ('clay-shoveller's
fracture'). Avulsion fractures should alert the doctor to inspect the x-ray films with
even more than usual care so as to exclude other and more important injuries; but in
themselves these 'muscle injuries' require no splintage and are best treated by activity.

The important damaging forces are: (1) compression; (2) hinging; and (3) shearing
(especially rotation).

COMPRESSION FORCES

Compression can be applied only to a straight portion of the spine. The thoracic
spine is always kyphosed and cannot suffer compression, but the cervical and lumbar
spines may sometimes be straight. The lumbar spine may be compressed by a fall
from a height, and the cervical spine when a weight falls on the head. The nucleus
pulposus splits the vertebral end-plate and fractures the vertebra vertically; with
greater force, disc material is forced into the vertebral body, causing a 'burst'
fracture.

HINGING FORCES

A backward hinging force may damage the neural arch but does not tear the
posterior ligaments. In the neck a hyperextension force (caused, for example, by
diving into shallow water) may fracture the arch of the atlas or of the axis. The
injury, though alarming, is stable. Occasionally, instead of the bone breaking, the
anterior common ligament tears; this injury also (unlike a tear of the posterior
ligaments) is stable.

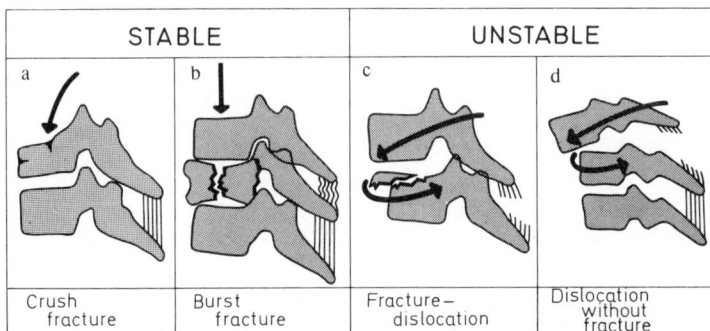

STABLE		UNSTABLE	
a	b	c	d
Crush fracture	Burst fracture	Fracture– dislocation	Dislocation without fracture

24.3 STABILITY
If the posterior ligaments
are intact, the spine is
stable: if they are torn it
is unstable.

Lumbar extension injuries are less common than cervical. Backward hinging can, however, occur and may result in a fractured lamina. It seems possible that the young toddler who falls repeatedly on to his buttocks may sustain just such an injury; this might well be the starting point of a spondylolisthesis which remains unrecognized until a later age.

Forward hinging (flexion) injuries are most common in the lumbar spine following a fall in the bent position or a weight falling on the bent back. The posterior ligaments remain intact, so that the injury is stable, but the front of the vertebral body crumples. Forward hinging less often damages the cervical spine because the chin abuts against the sternum, and rarely involves the thoracic spine which is secured by the ribs.

SHEARING FORCES

Shearing forces tear ligaments and cause instability. Rotation is a particularly important cause of ligamentous damage. Usually the rotation is associated with flexion. In the lumbar spine likely causes are a weight falling asymmetrically on to the back, or a fall from a height with the body twisted.

The posterior ligament complex tears as the spine rotates and shears forward. Bony injury is liable to occur at the same time; a slice of bone may be sheared off the top of one vertebra and the posterior facets may be fractured. In the neck a comparable injury can follow a fall from a motor-cycle or horse.

It may well be that a similarly unstable injury can result, not from rotation, but from the combination of a flexion force with purely forward shearing. A whip-lash injury of the neck, for example, may tear the posterior ligaments and permit forward dislocation; it should be noted that the facets are relatively horizontal in the neck, so that forward dislocation can readily occur without facet fracture. In the lumbar spine a comparable mechanism occurs in the so-called seat-belt fracture; the pelvis is anchored by the lap strap and, following a collision, the body is thrown forwards and jack-knifed forwards. The posterior ligaments are torn but there may be no bony fracture. The spine, however, is angulated and the upper facet may leap-frog over the lower.

CERVICAL SPINE INJURIES

DIAGNOSIS

The most important diagnostic aid is clinical awareness. The force producing a serious head injury (e.g. a road traffic accident or a fall from a height on to the head) may also injure the neck. Consequently it should be a rule that in every patient unconscious from a head injury, a fractured cervical spine should be excluded.

An abnormal position of the neck may be suggestive, but palpation is rarely helpful and movement is dangerous; x-ray examination is mandatory. With the conscious patient the neck can be examined, but the gap where the posterior ligament has been torn is much less easy to detect than in the lumbar spine. Movements should be extremely gentle and, if painful, are best postponed until the neck has been x-rayed. Pain or paraesthesia in the limbs is significant, and the limbs should always be examined for evidence of cord or root damage. X-ray films must be of high quality and should be inspected methodically, beginning at the top and working distally, noting the following points.

(1) Routine AP films may fail to show an odontoid fracture; for this tomograms and an open-mouth view are valuable. The same open-mouth view reveals the rare bursting-fracture of the atlas (if the lateral masses have spread significantly this

implies a torn transverse ligament). The opportunity to inspect the back of the pharynx is too good to miss — a visible prominence suggests a spinal fracture.

(2) Lateral films show the distance between the odontoid peg and the back of the anterior arch of the atlas; this should be no more than 4·5 mm in children or 3 mm in adults and does not vary with flexion. The posterior aspects of all the vertebral bodies (the odontoid can be regarded as a vertebral body) and the bases of the spinous processes should each form a smooth curve; any irregularity suggests injury. A soft tissue shadow in front of the bodies may be a haematoma from a fracture.

(3) To avoid missing a dislocation without fracture lateral films in flexion and extension are taken. Flexion should be guided by the doctor himself and must stop immediately if the patient experiences any arm or leg symptoms.

(4) Forward shift of a vertebral body on the one below is important. Displacement of less than half the vertebral body width suggests unilateral facet dislocation and oblique views are needed to show the involved side; greater displacement suggests bilateral displacement.

(5) C.7 may not be visible on the routine lateral film and injuries are therefore missed. The answer is to count the vertebrae. If necessary the doctor applies traction to the arm; C.7 and the upper border of Th.1 must be displayed.

MANAGEMENT OF FRACTURES OF C.1 AND C.2

NEURAL ARCHES

Hyperextension is the likely cause of neural arch fractures, which are probably stable; but the appearance and situation are sufficiently alarming to justify wearing a polythene collar for 3 months.

A similar force may fracture the pedicles of the axis ('hangman's fracture'). This sinister term is applied to two different injuries, one in which hyperextension is associated with distraction and which is lethal. The other, caused by hyperextension and compression, frequently has no neurological damage; a collar should however be worn for 3 months.

The ring of the atlas may, under load, fracture at its weakest point, where the posterior arch and the lateral masses join (the bursting fracture of Jefferson). Again the survivors often escape neurological damage and need only a collar. But if x-ray shows sideways spreading of the lateral masses, then the transverse ligament has ruptured; this injury is unstable and fusion (C.2 to skull) is needed.

ODONTOID FRACTURES

These result from high velocity accidents or severe falls; the precise mechanism is unknown but rotation or shearing forces may be involved. Diagnosis usually requires open-mouth views and possibly tomograms. The odontoid peg ossifies from a separate epiphysis; fracture-separation can occur, but the normal growth disc should not be mistaken for a fracture. Clinicians find that cord damage is suprisingly uncommon, because only the fortunate patients present to them; those with major cord damage rarely survive.

Blockey and Purser (1956) have shown that, providing the fracture is treated early, is reduced accurately, and is held securely, firm union occurs in about 12 weeks and no late displacement follows. Reduction is best achieved by skull traction. After 3–6 weeks an extensive (Minerva) plaster is applied. Once the lower half has been completed the skull caliper can be removed, and then plaster is extended to the head. The aim is sufficient fixation to hold the neck and head quite still but to leave enough room for jaw movement while eating. Usually six weeks in this irksome plaster is sufficient, followed by a less cumbersome plaster collar.

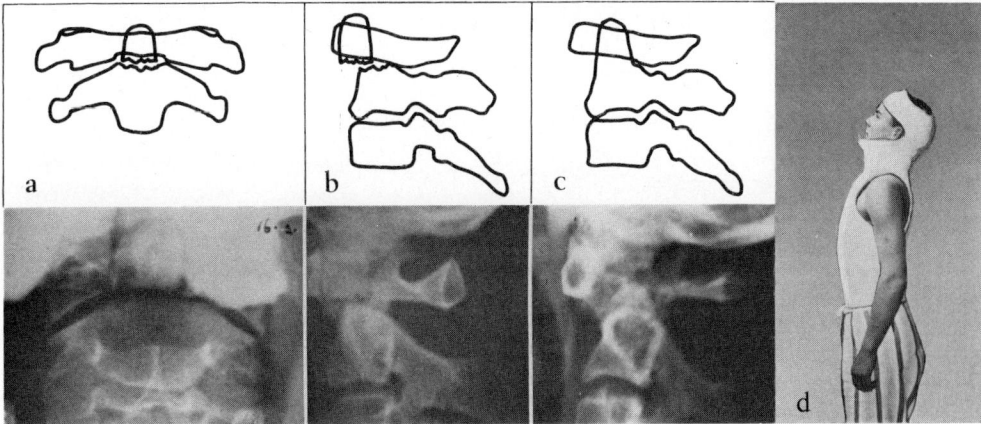

24.4 ODONTOID FRACTURES
(a, b) Fractured base of odontoid peg, permitting forward shift of the atlas and skull. Similar forward shift follows (c) rupture of the transverse ligament. (d) Minerva plaster.

Other authorities believe that non-union is common. Certainly if the fracture is seen late, or has redisplaced, then cord damage may follow and therefore fusion is indicated without delay. Fixing C.1 to C.2 is adequate; through a posterior approach grafts and wires are inserted. Traction is maintained during the operation and is continued afterwards until the wound has healed; the traction is then removed and a collar worn until x-rays show that the grafts are incorporated.

MANAGEMENT OF FRACTURES OF C.3—C.7

ANTERIOR WEDGE FRACTURE

This uncommon injury is stable. A collar may be worn for comfort but can safely be removed to allow washing.

BURST FRACTURES

These also are stable, but they are painful and the bony fragments are close to the cord; it is therefore prudent to restrict movement. A plaster collar is the safest; after 6 weeks it can be replaced by a polythene collar which is worn until inter-body fusion is seen on x-ray.

Some burst fractures ' pancake ' causing cord damage, possibly tetraplegia. These severe injuries need skull traction for 6 weeks, after which a polythene collar is worn until inter-body fusion is seen on x-ray.

NOTE ON TRACTION — All cervical fractures associated with paraplegia should (like unstable fractures even without paraplegia) be treated on traction. Halter traction

24.5 STABLE NECK INJURIES (a) Anterior wedge fracture; (b) burst fracture; (c) extension injury (which is stable in flexion).

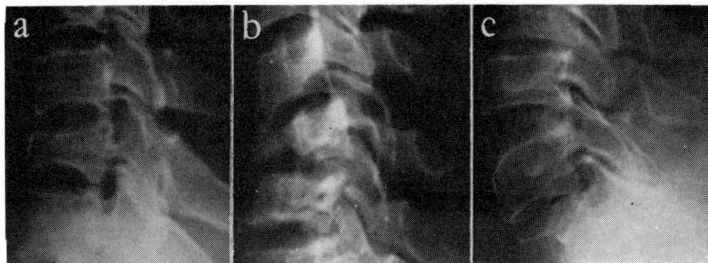

becomes uncomfortable within a few hours and skeletal skull traction is better; techniques include the halo device, Crutchfield's tongs, the cone caliper or Blackburn's caliper. X-ray control is needed; as traction is applied an excessive pull may exacerbate the neurological signs.

HYPEREXTENSION INJURIES

The bone is undamaged, but the anterior common ligament may be torn. The history and facial bruising or lacerations often suggest the mechanism. Neurological damage is variable and probably due to compression between the disc and the ligamentum flavum; oedema and haematomyelia may cause the acute central spinal cord syndrome. X-rays show no fracture, but an extension film shows a gap between the front of two vertebral bodies. These injuries are stable in the neutral position, in which they should be held by a collar for 6 weeks.

Sometimes no gap is seen, even in extension; instead the films show spondylosis. Again there may be cord or root damage. The neck should be held in a collar in the neutral position for 6 weeks.

DISLOCATION WITHOUT FRACTURE

The posterior ligaments are ruptured and the spine is unstable unless the facets are locked. Skull traction is applied; it maintains reduction in those who have reduced spontaneously, and usually achieves reduction in those with locked facets, though occasionally manipulation also is needed. Traction is kept on for 3 weeks. Some surgeons then apply a plaster collar, but ligaments heal poorly and late displacement may occur. Consequently fusion is safer. The spinous processes above and below the ruptured ligament are rawed, bone grafts applied and the processes fixed together with wires. The skull traction is maintained throughout the grafting operation and is continued afterwards until the wound has healed. Then a collar is applied and the traction removed. The collar is retained until the graft is incorporated, as demonstrated by lateral films taken in flexion and extension.

FRACTURE-DISLOCATIONS

These are extremely unstable and often associated with cord damage. They are most satisfactorily reduced by skull traction. The method advocated by Evans (1966) is to anaesthetize the patient, pass an endotracheal tube, and then to x-ray the neck and see if the fracture is reduced. If not, gentle manual traction associated with rotation may achieve reduction; but, whether or not the fracture is reduced, skull traction is then applied.

Many surgeons prefer to apply skull traction as the first manoeuvre. The next step depends upon the precise nature of the injury; with unilateral facet dislocation traction is maintained while the neck is tilted slightly away from the dislocated side,

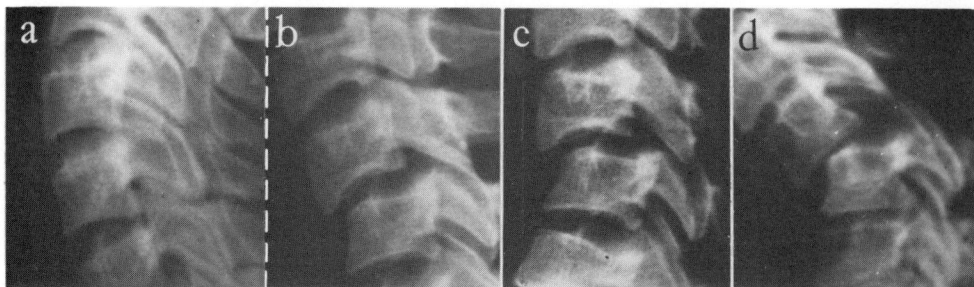

24.6 UNSTABLE NECK INJURIES
In (a) the cervical spine looks normal, but the film in flexion (b) shows forward subluxation — the posterior ligaments are torn. (c) Fracture-dislocation with moderate forward shift; (d) another fracture-dislocation with severe forward shift.

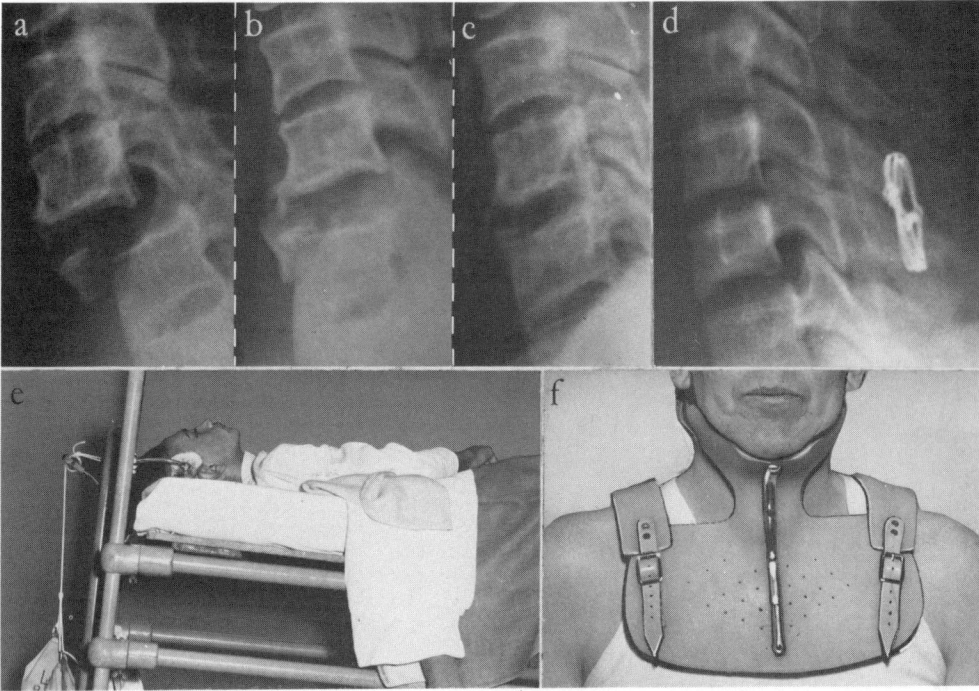

24.7 TREATMENT OF CERVICAL SPINE FRACTURES
(a, b, c) Stages in the reduction of a fracture-dislocation by skull traction; (d) subsequent wiring to ensure stability. (e) The patient was kept on skull traction until the wound was healed. A polythene collar as in (f) was then applied.

then twisted towards it; with fractured facets or bilateral facet dislocation a straight pull may be sufficient to obtain reduction. By adjusting the angle and the amount of traction, and judging the results on lateral films, reduction can usually be achieved within a few hours. Once reduction is satisfactory the neck is held slightly extended with only light traction (10 lb).

Whichever method of reduction is used the patient remains on traction for three weeks and then a lateral x-ray is taken. If this shows that callus is forming (and therefore that spontaneous inter-body fusion will follow) the traction is retained unchanged for a further three weeks, after which it is removed and a collar applied. If the film taken at three weeks shows no callus then inter-body fusion is not likely to occur; the injury is mainly ligamentous and a bone grafting operation is performed as for a pure dislocation. Again the traction is maintained during the operation and afterwards until the wound is healed. Following grafting a polythene collar is sufficient until the graft is incorporated.

24.8 TREATMENT OF CERVICAL SPINE FRACTURES (continued)
(a) Late re-displacement some months after treatment by external splintage alone; (b) stability has been restored by posterior fixation. Sometimes an anterior bone graft, as in (c), is preferred.

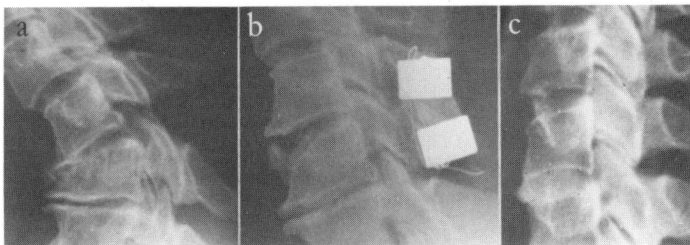

THORACIC SPINE INJURIES

Between T.1 and T.8 the rib cage imparts great stability to the spinal column. Only two varieties of injury occur:

(1) *Anterior wedge fractures* — These of course are stable and can safely be treated by activity. It should be borne in mind, however, that a considerable proportion of anterior wedge fractures in the thoracic spine are pathological in nature, occurring as a result of osteoporosis or malignant deposits.

(2) *A true fracture-dislocation* — Almost invariably paraplegia results and, in any event, the displacement is quite irreducible. Consequently it is the paraplegia which should be treated rather than the fracture itself.

THORACO-LUMBAR INJURIES

Management clearly depends upon precise diagnosis, but in one respect it must precede diagnosis. When the patient is seen at the site of the accident it is essential that he is handled in such a way that, even if he has an unstable fracture, displacement will not be increased. He must be moved on to the stretcher 'in one piece': traction is applied to the head and legs and the spine is kept straight.

DIAGNOSIS

Usually the patient is first seen lying supine on a stretcher or trolley. The opportunity should be taken to examine the chest and abdomen first for associated injuries. It must be remembered that, while abdominal pain and tenderness are suggestive of intra-abdominal damage, they can occur with a purely spinal injury. Next, the lower limbs are examined for evidence of neurological damage.

To examine the back, the patient is carefully turned (at least two and preferably three people are needed) on to one side. First, the skin of the back is inspected for abrasions or bruising; either indicates the probable level of injury. Next, the spinous processes are palpated systematically. With unstable injuries a gap can be felt where the ligament has been torn; this important physical sign is surprisingly easy to elicit. Spinal movements should not be examined; the attempt may imperil the cord.

Finally, x-rays are taken. As they must be of high quality, portable apparatus is quite inadequate. The minimum requirements are antero-posterior and lateral views, but two laterals are better, one centred over the vertebral bodies and the other over the spinous processes: oblique views and tomograms also may be helpful. Interpreting films is not always easy and it is important in both the antero-posterior and lateral views to inspect carefully: (1) The alignment of the vertebrae—is there any angulation or shift at any one point? (2) The shape of the individual vertebral bodies—is there any loss of the normal box-like appearance? (3) The neural arches —is there any evidence of fracture or of dislocation?

MANAGEMENT OF STABLE FRACTURES

ANTERIOR WEDGE FRACTURES

These result from forward hinging and are stable. The best treatment is by activity. For the first few days, while the back is painful and the muscles are in spasm, the patient is turned on to his face several times each day, radiant heat is applied and he is taught to use his spinal muscles. As soon as he is comfortable he is got up and encouraged to use his back fully and actively.

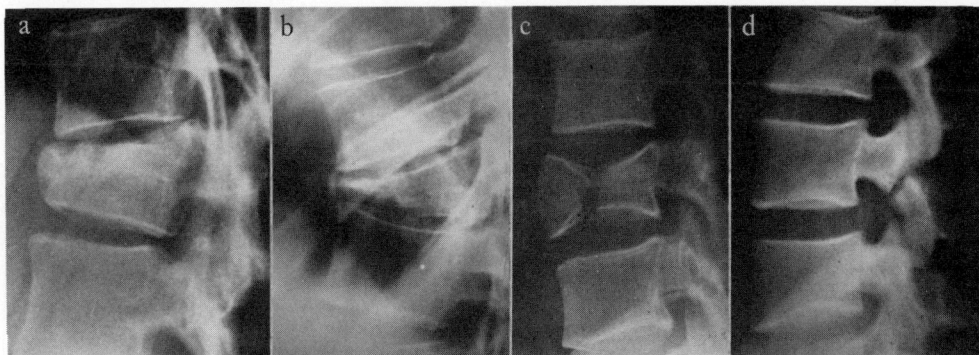

24.9 STABLE THORACO-LUMBAR FRACTURES
(a) Anterior wedge; (b) pathological fracture through a secondary deposit — such fractures are usually stable even though cord involvement is a possibility; (c) burst fracture; (d) fractured lamina.

BURST FRACTURES

Burst fractures also are stable because the posterior ligament complex is undamaged. They are, however, associated with considerable pain and the posterior portion of the vertebral body is perilously close to the dura and nerve roots. Consequently these fractures are usually treated in a plaster jacket despite their stability. The jacket should be applied, not with the spine hyperextended, but in the neutral position. After six weeks it can safely be replaced by a polythene jacket which is taken off for washing and sleeping; and at 12 weeks from the time of injury it can be discarded altogether.

LAMINAR FRACTURES

These probably result from hinging the back into extension and are frequently missed. It has been shown that some patients thought to have sustained disc prolapse have, in fact, sustained laminar fractures which can best be demonstrated on oblique radiographs. If these fractures are untreated, non-union is likely and, at L.4 or L.5, forward displacement may subsequently occur which results in spondylolisthesis. Consequently these injuries too are best treated in a plaster jacket; after six weeks this can be replaced by a polythene jacket which should not be discarded until x-rays demonstrate union.

MANAGEMENT OF UNSTABLE FRACTURES

In these the problem of paraplegia dominates management.

FRACTURES WITH PARAPLEGIA

In the presence of anaesthetic skin, treatment in plaster is not safe, because pressure sores are likely to develop rapidly. Two methods of management are available:

(1) *Conservative* — The patient is turned every two hours on to his side; three nurses are needed so that he is moved in one piece. While on his side his skin is carefully cleaned and the sheets meticulously smoothed. In this way pressure sores can be avoided and, after a few days or weeks, the patient can be moved more easily and without discomfort.

(2) *Operative* — The spine is fixed without delay; plates are attached on each side of the spinous processes and fix two processes above and two below the torn ligament; alternatively 2 small Harrington rods may be used. Fixation facilitates

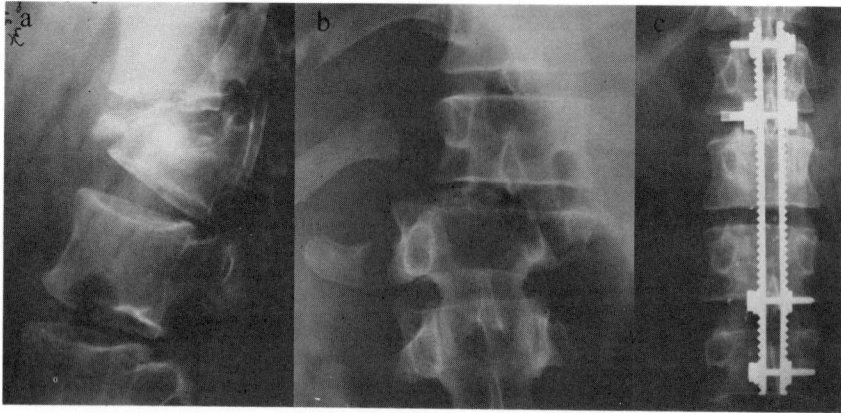

24.10 THORACO-LUMBAR UNSTABLE FRACTURES
(a) Fracture-dislocation with considerable forward shift; (b) AP view of another patient with gross displacement and paraplegia; such fractures are well treated by (c) open reduction and internal fixation.

nursing and turning is made comfortable; moreover, it is conceivable that if divided nerve roots are held in apposition they may regenerate.

The advocates of closed treatment point out that plating often fails; the plates break out of the spinous processes, the fracture re-displaces, the plates press on the skin, and sepsis follows. It may well be that poorly applied plates break out but, in the hands of a skilled spinal surgeon, plating is safe and on the whole is the more satisfactory method.

UNSTABLE FRACTURES WITHOUT PARAPLEGIA

The spine must be held still because movement may damage the cord. Stability can be achieved by plating as already described; but, in the absence of paraplegia, closed treatment in plaster is safe. A reasonable routine is as follows. The patient is placed prone on an operating table and in that position re-x-rayed. Providing reduction has been achieved (and it often has) plaster is applied to the back half of the trunk and legs, as the first step towards making a plaster bed. When this is complete the patient lies in the back half, but for cleaning purposes he is turned over into the front half at least once a week. After six weeks the fracture is less unstable and a plaster jacket is applied with the spine in neutral position. The patient is then allowed up. He wears the jacket for a further 6–12 weeks, the precise time being determined by x-ray; the plaster is not discarded until bony fusion is seen between the fractured vertebra and its neighbour.

Sometimes the prone position fails to achieve reduction. This usually indicates locked facets and it is worth while to hinge the operating table at the level of the fracture. If the facets are still locked the patient is anaesthetized. Gentle manipulation combined with traction may achieve reduction but, if not, there should be no hesitation in exposing the fracture operatively and reducing it under direct vision. Facetectomy is not often necessary and laminectomy hardly ever indicated. Following open reduction, internal fixation is used. Where there is considerable bony (as distinct from ligamentous) damage, plates and bolts are sufficient because spontaneous inter-body fusion will occur before the bolts become loose. But if the injury is mainly ligamentous (as in seat-belt fractures) it is wise to apply bone grafts as well, because spontaneous ligament repair cannot be relied upon to prevent late displacement.

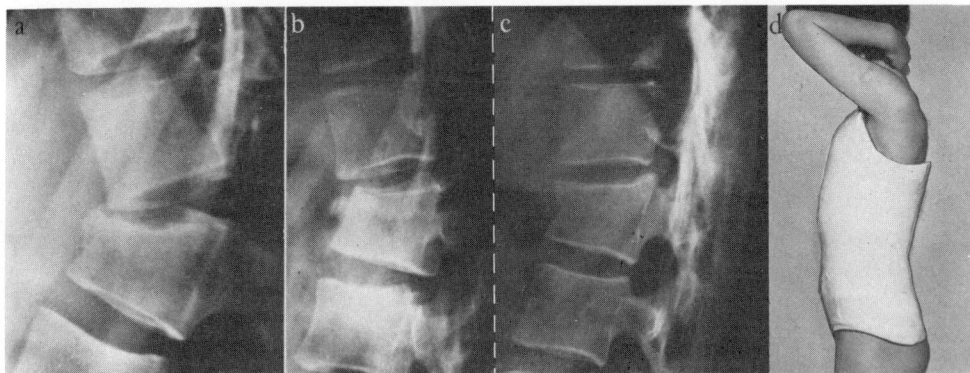

24.11   Unstable thoraco-lumbar fractures without paraplegia
(a) Lap seat-belt injury — locked facets are a possibility; (b) slice fracture-dislocation
at thoraco-lumbar junction treated by (c) open reduction and grafting. Bony damage
was slight, otherwise closed reduction and a plaster bed, followed by a plaster jacket
as in (d) might have been adequate.

FRACTURES WITH PARAPLEGIA

In traumatic paraplegia the displaced structures have damaged the cord, or nerve roots, or both; the damage may be temporary or permanent.   Three varieties of lesion occur.

CORD CONCUSSION — Motor paralysis (flaccid), sensory loss and visceral paralysis occur below the level of the cord lesion.   The disturbance is one of function without a demonstrable anatomical lesion.   Recovery begins within 8 hours and eventually becomes complete.

CORD TRANSECTION — Motor paralysis, sensory loss and visceral paralysis occur below the level of the cord lesion; as with cord concussion the motor paralysis is at first flaccid. This is a temporary condition known as cord shock, but the injury is anatomical and irreparable.

After a time, however, the cord below the level of transection recovers from the shock and acts as an independent structure; that is, it manifests reflex activity.   In a few hours the anal and penile reflexes return, and the plantar responses become extensor.   In a few days or weeks the flaccid paralysis becomes spastic, with increased tone, increased tendon reflexes and clonus; flexor spasms and contractures may develop but sensation never returns.   The presence of anal and penile reflexes in the absence of sensation in the legs is diagnostic of cord transection.

ROOT TRANSECTION — Motor paralysis, sensory loss and visceral paralysis occur in the distribution of the damaged roots.   Root transection, however, differs from cord transection in two ways: (a) regeneration is theoretically possible; and (b) residual motor paralysis remains permanently flaccid.

ANATOMICAL LEVELS

CERVICAL SPINE — With cervical spine injuries, the segmental level of cord transection nearly corresponds to the level of bony damage.   Not more than one or two additional roots are likely to be transected.   High cervical cord transection is fatal because all the respiratory muscles are paralysed.   At the level of the fifth cervical vertebra cord transection isolates the lower cervical cord (with paralysis of the upper limbs), the thoracic cord (with paralysis of the trunk) and the lumbar and sacral cord (with paralysis of the lower limbs and viscera). With injury below the fifth cervical vertebra, the upper limbs are partially spared and characteristic deformities result.

BETWEEN FIRST AND TENTH THORACIC VERTEBRAE — The first lumbar cord segment in the adult is at the level of the tenth thoracic vertebra. Consequently, cord transection at that level spares the thoracic cord but isolates the entire lumbar and sacral cord, with paralysis of the lower limbs and viscera. The lower thoracic roots may also be transected but are of relatively little importance.

BELOW FIRST LUMBAR VERTEBRA — The cord ends at the lower border of the first lumbar vertebra. Fractures below that level can produce only root lesions (of the cauda equina). The lumbar roots, however, stream downwards before emerging at their appropriate intervertebral levels; consequently, all the lumbar and the sacral roots are liable to damage.

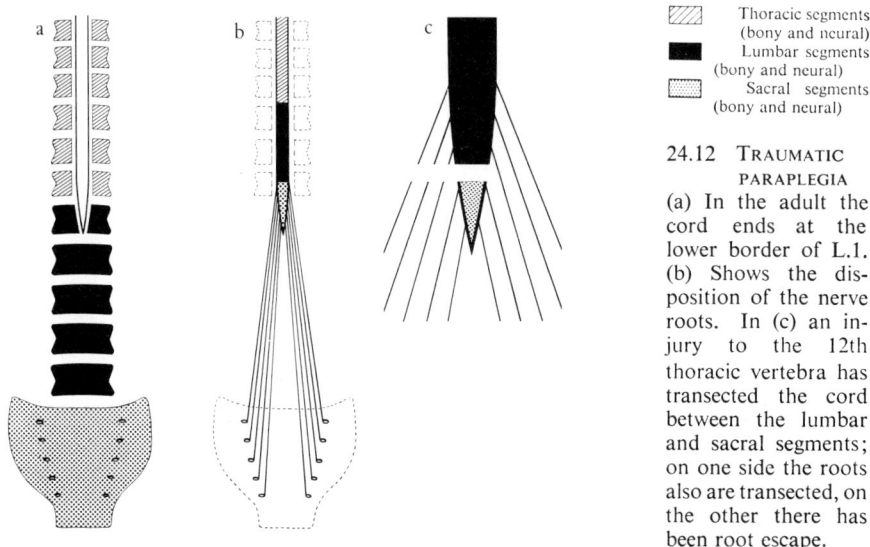

Thoracic segments (bony and neural)
Lumbar segments (bony and neural)
Sacral segments (bony and neural)

24.12 TRAUMATIC PARAPLEGIA
(a) In the adult the cord ends at the lower border of L.1. (b) Shows the disposition of the nerve roots. In (c) an injury to the 12th thoracic vertebra has transected the cord between the lumbar and sacral segments; on one side the roots also are transected, on the other there has been root escape.

BETWEEN TENTH THORACIC AND FIRST LUMBAR VERTEBRAE — A cord lesion may occur at any level in the lumbo-sacral cord. A fracture-dislocation of the twelfth thoracic on the first lumbar vertebra isolates the sacral cord; although the lumbar cord is spared, the lumbar roots may be transected.

The sacral cord innervates (a) sensation in the 'saddle' area, a strip down the back of the thigh and leg, and the outer two-thirds of the sole; (b) motor power to the muscles controlling the ankle and foot; (c) the anal and penile reflexes, plantar responses and ankle jerks; and (d) control of micturition.

The lumbar roots innervate (a) sensation to the entire lower limb other than that portion supplied by the sacral segment; (b) motor power to the muscles controlling the hip and knee; and (c) the cremasteric reflexes and knee jerks.

It is essential when the bony injury is at the thoraco-lumbar junction to distinguish between *cord transection with root escape* and *cord transection with root transection*. A patient with root escape is much better off than one with cord and root transection.

SIGNS

Clinical examination of the back is unnecessary, for neurological disturbance denotes an unstable fracture. The nature and level of the bone lesion are demonstrated by x-ray.

NEUROLOGICAL SIGNS — These are important, for without detailed neurological examination, precise diagnosis and prognosis are impossible. The expected level of neurological damage can usually be deduced from the x-ray. If below this level any sensation is present, the cord may be merely concussed; if sensation is absent but penile and anal reflexes are present, the cord has been transected.

Sometimes the x-ray appearances do not correspond to the neurological level. In the cervical spine this may be due to a variety of syndromes. The commonest is the acute central cord syndrome with disproportionately more weakness in the upper than the lower limbs, and sometimes sparing of bladder function and perineal sensation. With the less common anterior cord syndrome, pain and temperature sense may be lost in the lower limbs, but light touch and position sense retained. The acute posterior cord syndrome is very rare and the Brown-Séquard syndrome, with signs of cord hemisection, more often associated with thoracic injuries. From the 10th thoracic vertebra distally discrepancy between neurological and skeletal levels is usually due to root transection, in which sensation and power are lost from segments higher than the cord lesion.

MANAGEMENT OF TRAUMATIC PARAPLEGIA

Decompression of the cord seems a tempting possibility, but laminectomy alone has proved a failure; its only effect is to make an already unstable spine even more so. Decompression followed by immediate reduction and fusion is, however, worth considering, though only if cord compression can be demonstrated. Riska (1973), for example, has produced some encouraging results especially with partial paraplegia; he uses an antero-lateral approach and operates only if oxygen myelography shows bone compressing the cord. Unless compression can be demonstrated, operation (except perhaps fixation of the fracture to facilitate nursing) plays little part in the treatment of a paraplegic.

No matter whether the paraplegia is complete or partial, temporary or permanent, it is the overall management which is important, and especially the management in the first 24 hours. The patient must be transported with great care to avoid further damage, and preferably taken to a spinal centre. The strategy is outlined below.

SKIN — Within a few hours anaesthetic skin may develop enormous pressure sores, these must be prevented by meticulous nursing. Immediate fixation of the spine (*see* p. 407) enables these essential nursing procedures to be carried out much more easily and without discomfort to the patient. Creases in the sheets and crumbs in the bed are not permitted. Every 2 hours the patient is gently rolled on to his side and his back is carefully washed (without rubbing), dried and powdered. After a few weeks the skin becomes a little more tolerant and the patient can turn himself. If sores have been allowed to develop they may never heal without excision and skin grafting.

BLADDER AND BOWEL — For the first 24 hours the bladder distends only slowly, but, if the distension is allowed to progress, overflow incontinence occurs and infection is probable. In special centres it is usual to manage the patient from the outset by intermittent catheterization under sterile conditions. If early transfer to a paraplegia centre is not possible, continuous drainage through a fine silastic catheter is advised. The catheter drains in a closed manner into a disposable bag, and is changed twice weekly to avoid blockage. When infection supervenes, antibiotics are given.

Bladder training is begun at 1 week if possible. Although retention is complete to begin with, partial recovery may lead to: (a) an automatic bladder which works reflexly, or (b) an expressible bladder which is emptied by manual suprapubic pressure.

A few patients are left with a high residual urine after emptying the bladder. They need special investigations including cystography and cystometry; transurethral resection of the bladder neck or sphincterotomy may be indicated but should not be performed until at least 3 months of bladder training have been completed.

The bowel is more easily trained, with the help of enemas, aperients and abdominal exercises.

MUSCLES AND JOINTS — The paralysed muscles, if not treated, may develop severe flexion contractures. These are usually preventable by moving the joints passively through their full range twice daily. Later, splints become necessary.

With lesions below the cervical cord, the patient should be up within 3 months; standing and walking are valuable in preventing contractures. Calipers are usually necessary to keep the knees straight and the feet plantigrade. The calipers are removed at intervals during the day while the patient lies prone, and while he is having physiotherapy. The upper limbs must be trained until they develop sufficient power to enable the patient to use crutches and a wheelchair.

If flexion contractures have been allowed to develop, tenotomies may be necessary. Painful flexor spasms are rare unless skin or bladder infection occurs. They can sometimes be relieved by tenotomies, neurectomies, rhizotomies or the intrathecal injection of alcohol.

Heterotopic ossification may restrict or abolish movement, especially at the hip. It is doubtful whether ossification can be prevented, but once the new bone is mature it can safely be excised.

MORALE — The morale of a paraplegic patient is liable to reach a low ebb, and the restoration of his self-respect and self-confidence is an important part of treatment. Constant enthusiasm and encouragement by doctors, physiotherapists and nurses is essential. Their scrupulous attention to his comfort and toilet are of primary importance; the unpleasant smells associated with skin or urinary infection must be avoided. The earlier the patient gets up the better, and he must be trained for a new job as quickly as possible.

FRACTURES OF THE PELVIS

Fractures of the pelvis fall into four groups.

ISOLATED PELVIC RING FRACTURES — The ring is broken in only one place, displacement is slight and complications are rare.

PELVIC RING DISRUPTIONS — The ring is broken in two places, displacement may be severe and complications are more likely to occur.

AVULSION FRACTURES — These are relatively unimportant traction injuries.

SACRO-COCCYGEAL INJURIES

ISOLATED PELVIC RING FRACTURES

A direct blow on the side or front of the pelvis may fracture the ilium, the acetabulum, or the pubic rami on one side. The pelvic ring is broken in only one place, displacement is slight and intrapelvic structures are usually undamaged. The patient may feel unsteady on attempting to walk, and often has groin pain.

SIGNS

LOOK — Bruising may be evident.

FEEL — There is tenderness at the site of impact.

MOVE — Usually the patient can lift his leg and as a rule he can stand on it.

X-RAY — The films show one of three injuries: (*a*) a fractured wing of the ilium, often with displacement; (*b*) a fractured acetabular floor, possibly in association with a central dislocation of the hip; or (*c*) a fracture of the front of the pelvis on one side only; in this, the commonest pelvic fracture, one or both pubic rami may be fractured.

It is important to be sure that the sacro-iliac joints are undamaged, for if a fracture in front is combined with sacro-iliac subluxation, pelvic ring disruption has occurred.

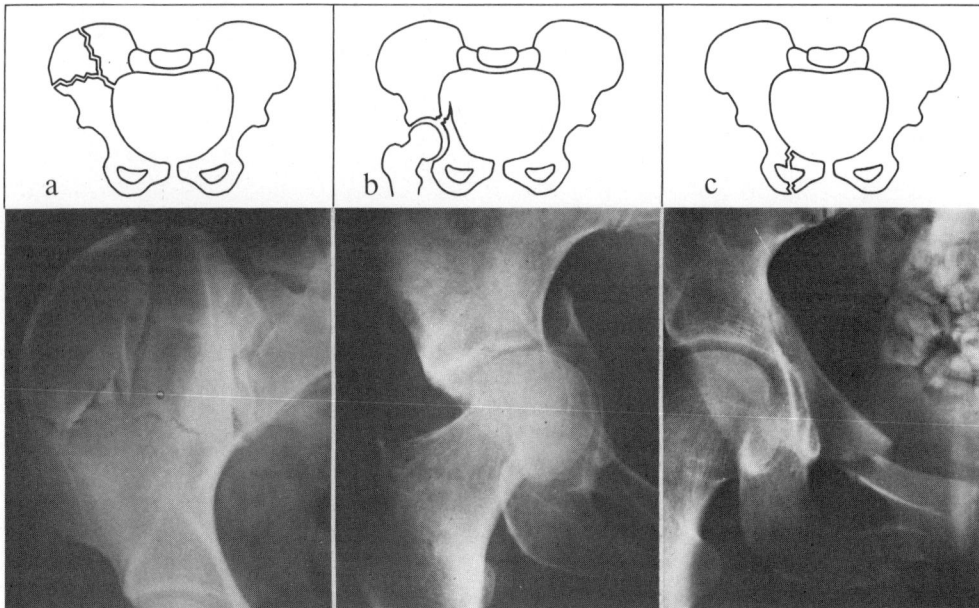

24.13 ISOLATED PELVIC RING FRACTURES
The ring is broken in only one place. (a) Blade of ilium; (b) floor of acetabulum with central dislocation of hip (*see also* page 421); (c) ischio-pubic rami.

TREATMENT

Isolated fractures of the ilium and pubis need not be reduced or held.   The patient stays in bed until he is comfortable, and is then taught to stand and walk.   Acetabular fractures need careful radiography including two 45 degree oblique films; if a large posterior fragment is out of step, reduction and screw fixation may be indicated. Central dislocation of the hip requires skeletal traction (see page 421).

PELVIC RING DISRUPTIONS

The ring is broken in two places; displacement may be considerable.   Perkins has pointed out that there are three distinct varieties of disruption, each caused by a different force.

COMPRESSION — An antero-posterior crushing force fractures both pubic rami on both sides, and the central segment may be pushed backwards, endangering the urethra.

A lateral force may fracture the side wall of the pelvis in two places; medial displacement of the hip is inevitable (page 421).

HINGE — The force is applied to one blade of the ilium and 'opens' the pelvis; for example, when a patient is partially run over. One half of the pelvis is intact; the other half is damaged both in front (the symphysis is forced apart) and at the back (the sacro-iliac joint is hinged open).

VERTICAL FORCE — The patient falls from a height onto one leg. The pubis and ilium on the same side are both fractured; the portion of pelvis lateral to the fractures is pushed upwards.

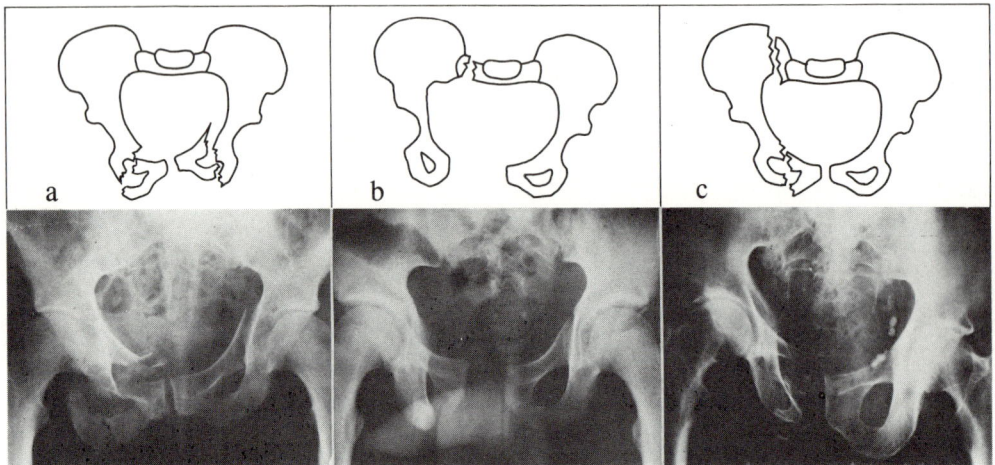

24.14 PELVIC RING DISRUPTIONS
The ring is broken in more than one place. (a) Antero-posterior crush; (b) hinge type of injury; (c) vertical force fracture.

SYMPTOMS AND SIGNS

Pain is considerable and is worse on coughing or moving. The patient is aware of severe pelvic damage; he cannot stand and may be unable to pass urine. Haemorrhage is often considerable and shock may be severe. Urogenital damage may be indicated by the presence of blood at the external meatus. The local signs are as follows.

LOOK — There may be a graze or perineal bruising and swelling.

FEEL — Although tenderness is often too great or too diffuse to be of diagnostic value, marked suprapubic tenderness suggests urogenital damage (mainly in compression fractures). A gap at the symphysis is occasionally felt (in hinge fractures) and one leg may be partly anaesthetic because of sciatic nerve damage (in vertical force fractures).

MOVE — Movements are painful and should not be attempted.

X-RAY — The films show the type of fracture.

Compression — Both pubic rami are fractured on both sides.

Hinge — There is a gap at the symphysis, and sacro-iliac subluxation.

Vertical force — The pubis and the ilium on the same side are fractured; there is upward shift of one side of the pelvis lateral to the fractures.

EMERGENCY TREATMENT

SHOCK — This will need treatment (page 349).

UROGENITAL DAMAGE — Compression fractures are the usual cause of urogenital tract damage; but with all pelvic ring disruptions damage must be excluded. However, all that needs to be provided urgently in a seriously ill patient is adequate urinary drainage, which is accomplished by suprapubic cystostomy. Definitive repair may well be delayed whilst the patient's general condition improves and expert urological advice is sought.

The patient is asked to pass urine; providing he can, and if the urine is clear, all is well. If he cannot, or if there is blood at the external meatus, the temptation to pass a catheter in the less-than-ideal surroundings of the casualty reception room should be resisted for fear of converting a partial to a complete rupture of the urethra. Gentle retrograde urethrography using dilute aqueous contrast-medium will establish the presence and site of a urethral leak. If the urethra is intact, the bladder will be outlined. The uncommon condition of gross upward dislocation of the prostate may be safely demonstrated by intravenous urography, as will ruptures of the bladder.

Intrapelvic rupture of the urethra is treated by suprapubic cystostomy for urinary drainage, a retropubic corrugated or suction drain, and an indwelling fenestrated urethral catheter to provide alignment of the urethra as well as drainage of blood and secretions from its lumen. If the bladder is floating high it is repositioned and held down by a sling-suture passed through the apex of the prostate, through the perineum lateral to the urethra, and anchored to the thighs by elastic bands.

Rupture of the bladder is treated by suprapubic cystostomy with, in addition, suture of the tear if it is intraperitoneal or drainage of the retropubic space if extraperitoneal.

TREATMENT OF THE FRACTURE

COMPRESSION TYPE — Reduction is neither possible nor necessary; consequently splintage is not required. The patient lies free in bed for 3 weeks; active movements of the hip and spine are encouraged. He is then allowed to walk normally; weight-bearing is quite safe because the line of weight transmission does not pass through the fracture area.

HINGE TYPE — Under anaesthesia the patient is rolled on to his unaffected side. The surgeon leans on the upper half of the pelvis and by this means 'closes' the pelvis. Reduction is stable, and a firm binder or lumbo-sacral corset is sufficient protection. If reduction fails (or if urogenital surgery is being done) internal fixation with wire may be used; the wire is inserted through drill holes or through the obturator foramina.

For the first 3 weeks the patient remains in bed, but is encouraged to move his limbs. He is then allowed up, using crutches at first, and within 6 weeks should have regained full activity. The corset is discarded after 3 months.

VERTICAL FORCE TYPE — Under anaesthesia, the leg on the side of the pelvis which has shifted upwards is forcibly pulled down. Skeletal traction is applied and the patient remains on traction for 6 weeks. He is then allowed up with crutches but should not take weight for 3 months from the injury.

COMPLICATIONS

The complications common to all types of ring disruptions are shock, intrapelvic haemorrhage and paralytic ileus.

The complications specific to each type of fracture are urogenital damage in compression fractures, especially in run-over accidents, persistent sacro-iliac pain after hinge fractures (arthrodesis of the sacro-iliac joint may prove necessary), and sciatic nerve injury in vertical force fractures (usually the nerve recovers, but occasionally exploration later proves necessary).

AVULSION FRACTURES

MECHANISM

Violent muscle action in an athletic adolescent may avulse a traction epiphysis (apophysis). The muscles concerned are the sartorius, rectus femoris and the hamstrings.

SIGNS

LOOK — The appearance is normal.

FEEL — The site of avulsion is tender.

MOVE — Resisted action of the affected muscle is painful.

X-RAY — Avulsion may be seen at one of three sites: (*a*) anterior superior iliac spine (sartorius avulsion); (*b*) anterior inferior iliac spine (rectus avulsion, which must be distinguished from an os acetabuli); or (*c*) ischial tuberosity (hamstrings avulsion).

TREATMENT

Reduction is unnecessary. The patient is rested for a few days with the injured muscle in a relaxed position for comfort. Then normal activities are resumed. Ultimately function becomes normal.

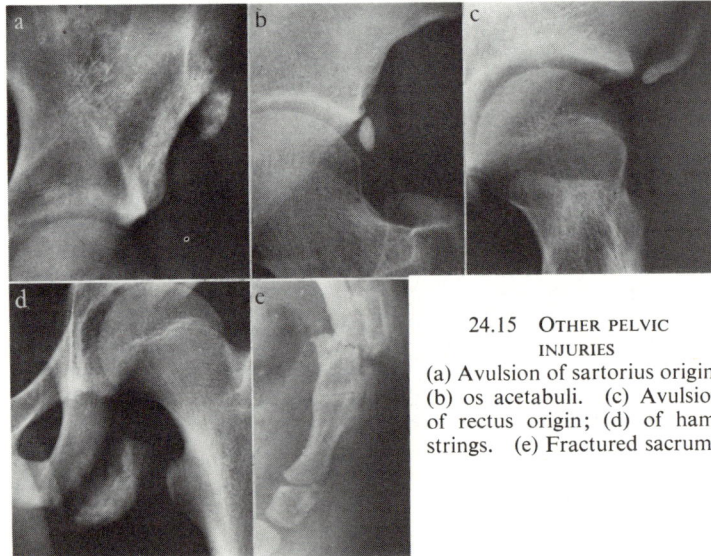

24.15 OTHER PELVIC INJURIES
(a) Avulsion of sartorius origin; (b) os acetabuli. (c) Avulsion of rectus origin; (d) of hamstrings. (e) Fractured sacrum.

INJURIES TO SACRUM AND COCCYX

MECHANISM

A blow from behind, or a fall on to the 'tail' may fracture the sacrum or coccyx, or sprain the joint between them.

SIGNS

LOOK — With a sacral fracture bruising is considerable.

FEEL — Tenderness is elicited when the sacrum or coccyx is palpated from behind or per rectum. Sensation may be lost over the distribution of sacral nerves.

MOVE — Movement is unaffected.

X-RAY — The films may show (*a*) a transverse fracture of the sacrum, in rare cases with the lower fragment pushed forwards; (*b*) a fractured coccyx, sometimes with the lower fragment angulated forwards; or (*c*) a normal appearance if the injury was a sprain of the sacro-coccygeal joint.

TREATMENT

REDUCE — If the fracture is displaced, reduction is worth attempting. The lower fragment may be pushed backwards per rectum.

HOLD — The reduction is stable, which is fortunate.

EXERCISE — The patient is allowed to resume normal activity, but is advised to use a rubber ring or Sorbo cushion when sitting.

COMPLICATIONS

Persistent pain, especially on sitting, is common after coccygeal injuries. If the pain is not relieved by the use of a Sorbo cushion or by the injection of local anaesthetic into the tender area, excision of the coccyx may be considered.

Suggestions for further reading

Anderson, L. D. (1974). 'Fractures of the Odontoid Process of the Axis.' *J. Bone Jt Surg.* **56A,** 1663

Blockey, N. J. and Purser, D. W. (1956). 'Fractures of the Odontoid Process of the Axis.' *J. Bone Jt Surg.* **38B,** 794

Evans, D. K. (1966). In *Clinical Surgery*, Vol. 12 (Fractures and Dislocations), Ed. by R. Furlong. London: Butterworths

Hardy, A. G. and Rossier, A. B. (1975). *Spinal Cord Injuries*. Stuttgart; Georg Thieme

Holdsworth, Sir F. W. (1970). 'Fractures, Dislocations and Fracture–Dislocations of the Spine.' *J. Bone Jt Surg.* **52A,** 1534

Lewis, J. and McKibbin, B. (1974). 'The Treatment of Unstable Fracture-Dislocation of the Thoraco-Lumbar Spine Accompanied by Paraplegia.' *J. Bone Jt Surg.* **56B,** 603

Perkins, G. (1966). 'Fractures of the Pelvis.' *Clinical Surgery*, Vol. 12 (Fractures and Dislocations), Ed. by Rob, C. and Smith, Rodney. London; Butterworths

Riska, E. B. (1973). 'Antero-Lateral Decompression as a Treatment of Paraplegia Following Vertebral Fractures.' *Acta Orth. Scand.* **44,** 89

Turner-Warwick, R. (1973). 'Traumatic Urethral Injuries.' *Br. J. Surg.* **60,** 775

CHAPTER 25

FRACTURES AND DISLOCATIONS IN THE LOWER LIMB

DISLOCATIONS OF THE HIP

POSTERIOR DISLOCATION

Four out of five traumatic hip dislocations are posterior. Usually the bent leg is violently thrust backwards, as when a car hits a tree and the passenger's knee is struck by the dashboard. The impact is liable to fracture the acetabular roof, which displaces with the femoral head; only when the hip is adducted at the moment of impact is dislocation likely to occur without fracture.

SIGNS

LOOK — The leg is short and lies adducted, medially rotated and slightly flexed.

FEEL — The femoral head cannot be felt in its socket, but may be palpable on the dorsum ilii.

MOVE — No movement is possible.

X-RAY — In the antero-posterior film the femoral head is seen out of its socket and above the acetabulum. A segment of acetabular roof may have been broken off and displaced upwards; two oblique films are useful in demonstrating the size of the fragment.

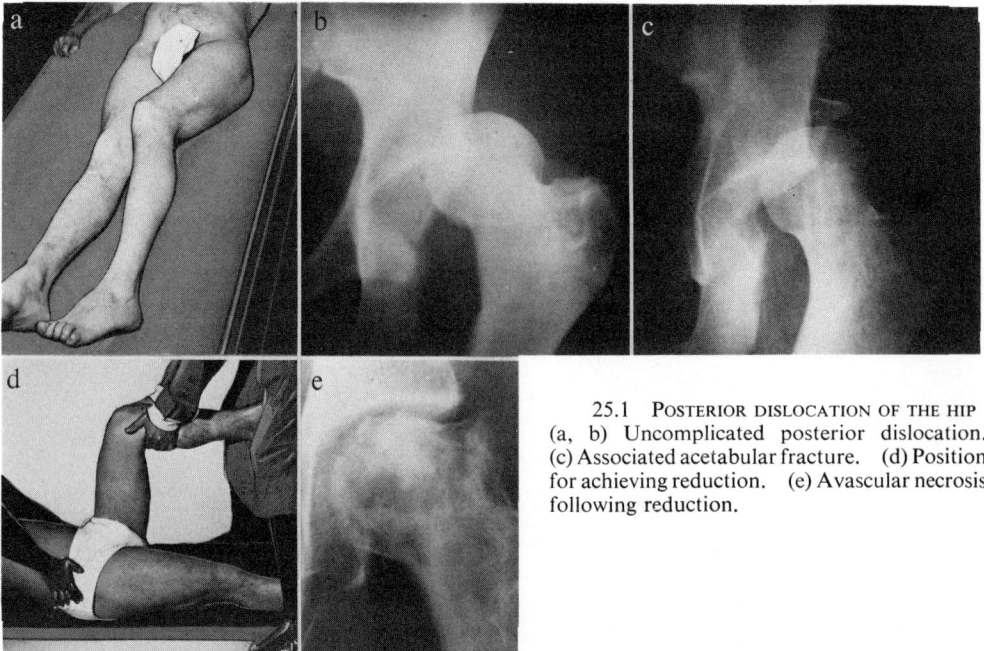

25.1 POSTERIOR DISLOCATION OF THE HIP (a, b) Uncomplicated posterior dislocation. (c) Associated acetabular fracture. (d) Position for achieving reduction. (e) Avascular necrosis following reduction.

TREATMENT

REDUCE — Deep anaesthesia is essential, preferably with a relaxant. Reduction is more easily effected with the patient lying on a mattress on the floor. An assistant steadies the pelvis; the surgeon flexes the patient's hip and knee to 90 degrees and pulls the thigh vertically upwards. Usually this manoeuvre effects reduction, but sometimes it is necessary also to abduct the flexed hip. X-ray examination is essential to confirm reduction and to exclude a fracture.

HOLD — Reduction is stable, but the hip has been severely injured and needs to be rested. The simplest treatment is to apply skeletal traction behind the tibial tubercle and maintain it for 3 weeks. Alternatively, a plaster spica may be applied with the hip in the neutral position.

EXERCISE — If the patient is being treated on traction active exercises are permitted, but passive movements are prohibited for fear of myositis ossificans.

At the end of 3 weeks, plaster or traction is removed and the hip x-rayed. In the absence of an associated fracture, myositis ossificans, or avascular necrosis, weight-bearing is permitted.

COMPLICATIONS

ASSOCIATED FRACTURE

Fractured acetabulum — A triangular fragment of the acetabulum may have been sheared off during dislocation. If the fragment is small and falls into place when the hip is reduced, traction for 6 weeks and avoiding weight-bearing for a further 6 weeks is probably adequate. But if it is large or imperfectly reduced it should be fixed in place by screws.

Fractured femoral shaft — When this occurs at the same time as hip dislocation, the dislocation is commonly missed. It should be a rule that with every femoral shaft fracture the buttock and trochanter are palpated, and the hip clearly seen on x-ray. Even if this precaution has been omitted, a dislocation should be suspected whenever the proximal fragment of a transverse shaft fracture is seen to be adducted (Helal and Skevis, 1967).

Fractured femoral head — The dislocation may have sheared off a segment of the femoral head. As a rule reduction of the dislocation automatically reduces the fracture, but weight-bearing must be deferred for at least 12 weeks. If the head fragment has not been correctly reduced its replacement or excision provides the only hope of regaining reasonable movement at the hip.

JOINT STIFFNESS

Avascular necrosis — The blood supply of the femoral head is seriously reduced in at least 20 per cent of traumatic hip dislocations; if reduction is delayed by more than a few hours, the figure rises to 50 per cent. Avascular necrosis shows on x-ray as an increase in the density of the femoral head; but this change is not seen for at least 6 weeks, and sometimes very much longer.

The avascular head crushes if weight is taken through it; degenerative arthritis soon follows. If avascular necrosis is diagnosed before the head has begun to collapse, and the patient is relatively young, it is conceivable that the avoidance of weight-bearing for a period of up to 2 years might allow the head to revascularize without undue deformation. In most cases, however, the avascular necrosis quickly leads to degenerative arthritis; an attempt can be made to arthrodese the hip, or the head may be excised and replaced by a metal prosthesis.

Myositis ossificans — It is essential after any injury to prohibit passive movements. Even if they are not the sole cause of myositis ossificans they probably increase its severity.

At the first suggestion of calcification around the hip, the joint should be rested in a hip spica. The final range will inevitably be restricted.

Unreduced dislocation — After a few weeks an untreated dislocation cannot be reduced by closed manipulation. Heavy skeletal traction through the femur, or open reduction offers the best hope. If joint stiffness or avascular necrosis supervenes the femoral head or the hip joint can then be replaced.

NERVE LESIONS — The sciatic nerve is sometimes damaged but usually recovers. If, after reducing the dislocation, a sciatic nerve lesion and an unreduced acetabular fracture are diagnosed, the nerve should be explored and the fragment correctly replaced.

ANTERIOR DISLOCATION

Anterior dislocation is rare compared with posterior. The usual cause is a road accident or air crash. Dislocation of one or even both hips may occur when a weight falls onto the back of a miner or building labourer who is working with his legs wide apart, knees straight and back bent forwards.

SIGNS

LOOK — The leg lies laterally rotated, abducted and slightly flexed. It is not short, because the attachment of the rectus femoris prevents the head from displacing upwards. Seen from the side the anterior bulge of the dislocated head is unmistakable. Occasionally the leg is abducted almost to a right angle.

FEEL — The head feels too prominent.

MOVE — Movements are impossible.

X-RAY — In the antero-posterior view the dislocation is usually obvious, but occasionally the head is almost directly in front of its normal position; any doubt is resolved by a lateral film.

TREATMENT AND COMPLICATIONS

The manoeuvres employed are almost identical with those used to reduce a posterior dislocation, except that while the flexed thigh is being pulled upwards, it should be adducted. The subsequent treatment is similar to that employed for posterior dislocation. Avascular necrosis is the only complication.

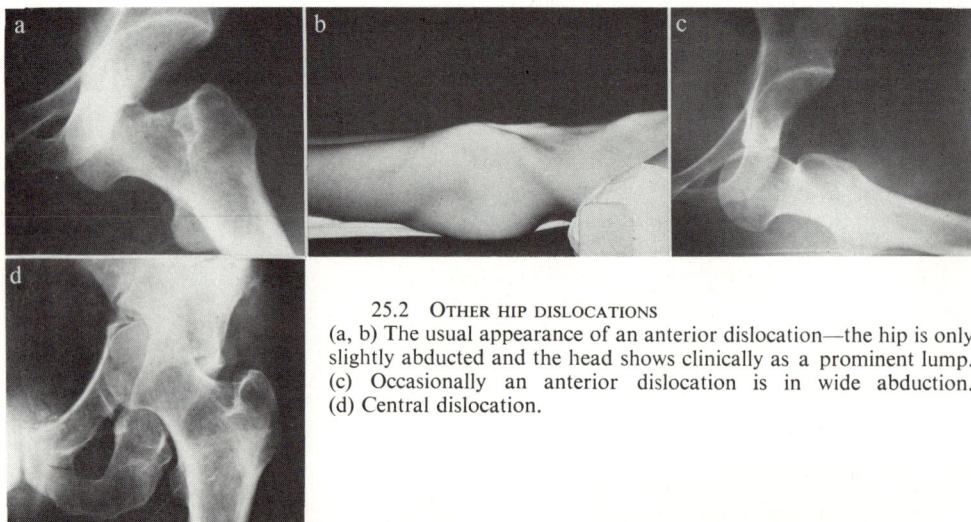

25.2　OTHER HIP DISLOCATIONS
(a, b) The usual appearance of an anterior dislocation—the hip is only slightly abducted and the head shows clinically as a prominent lump.
(c) Occasionally an anterior dislocation is in wide abduction.
(d) Central dislocation.

CENTRAL DISLOCATION

A fall on the side, or a car smash, may fracture the acetabular floor and thrust the femoral head into the pelvis. The force is probably transmitted through the great trochanter.

SIGNS

LOOK — The trochanteric region is grazed or bruised, but the leg lies in normal position.
FEEL — The trochanter and hip region are tender.
MOVE — Little movement is possible.
X-RAY — The femoral head is displaced medially, and the acetabular floor fractured.

TREATMENT

REDUCE — The surgeon pulls strongly on the thigh and then tries to lever the head outwards by adducting the thigh, using his foot as a fulcrum. In the middle aged or elderly patient it is wise to be content with even imperfect reduction. In a young patient, if closed reduction fails, the displacement can theoretically be reduced openly and the fragment fixed with screws; but usually shock or comminution of the fracture precludes useful intervention. Lateral traction with a pin or screw through the greater trochanter rarely succeeds.

HOLD — Whether or not the fracture has been reduced, skeletal traction behind the tibial tubercle is applied and a 15-lb. pull maintained for 3 weeks.

EXERCISE — Active use is encouraged from the start. When traction is removed the patient is allowed up with crutches. Weight-bearing is permitted after 6 weeks. The functional result is better than the x-ray appearance would suggest; but unless displacement was only trivial, all movements except flexion and extension remain considerably limited, and degenerative arthritis ultimately develops.

FRACTURES OF THE FEMORAL NECK

The injury occurs mainly among elderly women (fractures in the young are discussed on page 424). The patient may fall, but often merely catches her foot while walking; the foot twists and the femoral neck is broken by the rotation force. Senile osteoporosis and trabecular fatigue fractures may have weakened the bone, or it may be the site of a secondary deposit. On the rare occasions that an osteoarthritic hip breaks the fracture site is trochanteric, not transcervical.

SIGNS

LOOK — The leg is short and laterally rotated. With trochanteric fractures the line of fracture is lateral to the insertion of the joint capsule and displacement is much greater.
FEEL — The great trochanter is too high and too far posterior.
MOVE — The patient cannot lift her leg.
X-RAY — The fracture may be high (sub-capital), or lower (transcervical or basal). The angle of the fracture line is difficult to determine, but the more vertical it is the less favourable is the prognosis. Displacement is best expressed in terms of Garden's (1961) classification (see Fig. 25.3).

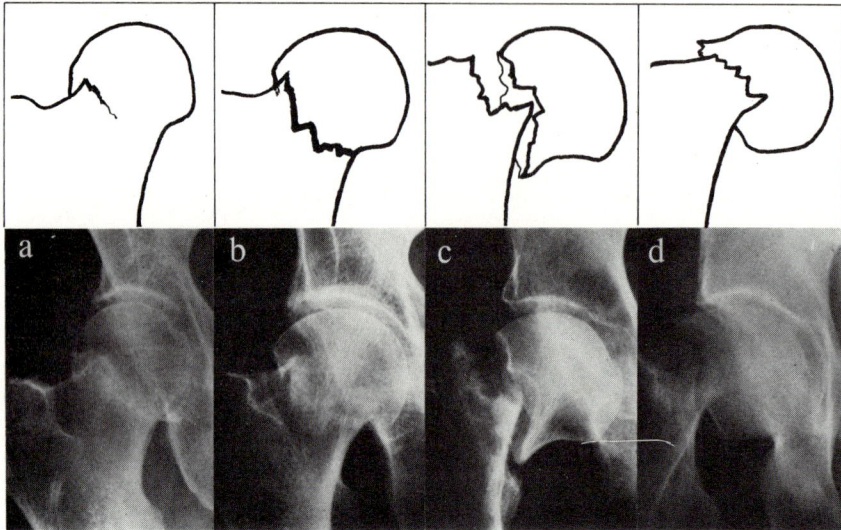

25.3 FRACTURES OF THE FEMORAL NECK (1) CLASSIFICATION
Garden's Classification of Subcapital Fractures. (a) Stage I Incomplete (so-called abducted or impacted); (b) Stage II Complete Without Displacement; (c) Stage III Complete With Partial Displacement — fragments still connected by posterior retinacular attachment; (d) Stage IV Complete With Full Displacement — the distal fragment is in front of the proximal and fully rotated laterally.

TREATMENT

Operative treatment is almost mandatory because old people must be got up and active without delay. Even incomplete fractures (when the patient may be able to walk) are too precarious to be left; they are liable to become complete and to displace. What if operation is considered dangerous? Lying in bed on traction may be even more dangerous, and leaving the fracture untreated too painful. The principles of treatment are simple; accurate reduction, secure internal fixation and early activity; application is more difficult and is controversial.

REDUCE — With the patient on an orthopaedic table, the hip and knee are flexed and the fractured thigh pulled upward, then medially rotated, then extended and abducted; the foot is now tied to a footpiece. X-ray control (preferably with an image intensifier) is used to confirm reduction in AP and lateral views. Accurate reduction is important; to fix an unreduced fracture is to invite failure.

HOLD — The fracture may be held by (1) A trifin nail, the least effective method but adequate for fractures which have never been displaced (Garden I and II). (2) Threaded pins or, better, lag screws — 2 or 3 are required. (3) A sliding device which permits compression or impaction; a stout screw or nail fits inside a sleeve and is attached to a plate screwed to the femoral shaft. (4) Other methods include triangular fixation (Smyth) and angled blade-plate fixation.

In all cases a lateral incision is used to expose the upper femur. Guide wires (which must be radiologically checked in AP and lateral views) are used to ensure correct placement of the fixing device; measuring the protruding portion enables the desired length of implant to be calculated. When a single nail or screw is used it should lie below the middle of the neck and extend into the posterior part of the head.

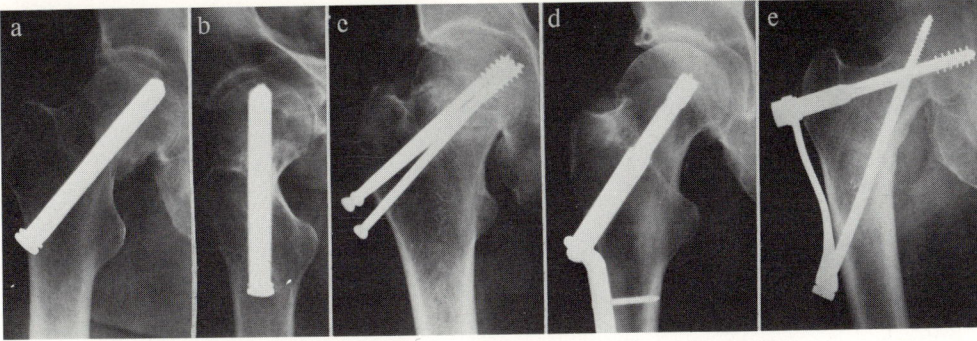

25.4 FRACTURES OF THE FEMORAL NECK (2) EXAMPLES OF TREATMENT
(a, b) Trifin nail; (c) Three screws; (d) Sliding nail-plate; (e) Smyth's triangular
fixation.

EXERCISE — From the first day the patient should sit up in bed or in a chair. She is
taught breathing exercises, encouraged to help herself and to begin walking (with
crutches or a walker) as soon as possible. To delay weight bearing may be theoretically
ideal but is rarely practicable.

PROSTHETIC REPLACEMENT

This carries a high complication and morbidity rate; it should be reserved for subcapital fractures which have proved irreducible and for fractures through secondary
deposits. Performed through an anterior approach the risk of subsequent dislocation is less, and a cemented Thompson prosthesis is probably better than an
uncemented Moore. Total hip replacement is occasionally recommended.

COMPLICATIONS

General complications such as follow any injury or operation in the elderly are
liable to occur, especially calf vein thrombosis, pulmonary embolism, pneumonia,
and bedsores. In some centres anti-coagulants are used routinely. The important
bone complications are avascular necrosis and non-union.

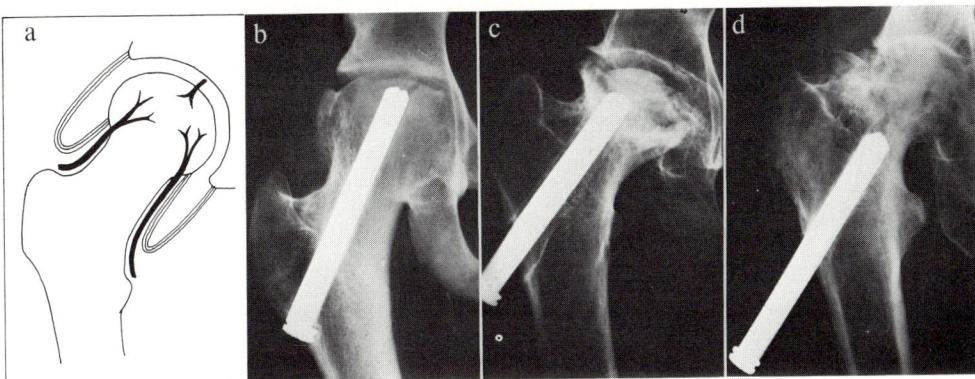

25.5 FRACTURES OF THE FEMORAL NECK (3) AVASCULAR NECROSIS
(a) Apart from the small amount of blood reaching the head through the nutrient
artery and the artery in the ligamentum teres, the main supply is from vessels which
run under the retinacular fibres before entering the bone: in this situation they are
readily damaged. (b) Segmental necrosis. (c) Massive necrosis. (d) The fracture
has united despite avascular necrosis, but the bone has crumbled and the joint is
degenerating.

AVASCULAR NECROSIS — The femoral head is mainly supplied with blood by (a) lateral epiphyseal and inferior metaphyseal branches of the medial femoral circumflex artery; and (b) medial epiphyseal arteries in the ligamentum teres. This second group is small or absent in 20 per cent of adults; if in them the first group is damaged (and this is especially liable to occur with displaced high cervical fractures), then the head becomes avascular. This anatomical explanation fixes the blame firmly on the patient; Garden (1971) maintains that the accurately reduced fracture rarely undergoes the changes ascribed to avascularity.

The increased x-ray density characteristic of dead bone may not become apparent for many weeks, months or even years. The first indication is usually the nail extruding from the head or breaking out of it; the fracture then re-displaces and, if the condition is untreated, non-union occurs. Sometimes the nail is extruded after apparent union of the fracture; a line of separation then develops between living and dead bone, with subsequent re-fracture. The avascular head cannot withstand weight; even when the nail remains in it until the fracture has consolidated, the head will crush and osteoarthritis will result.

NON-UNION — Non-union is likely if the fracture line is unduly vertical; if the operation is unskilfully performed (inaccurate reduction or bad nailing); or if the blood supply to

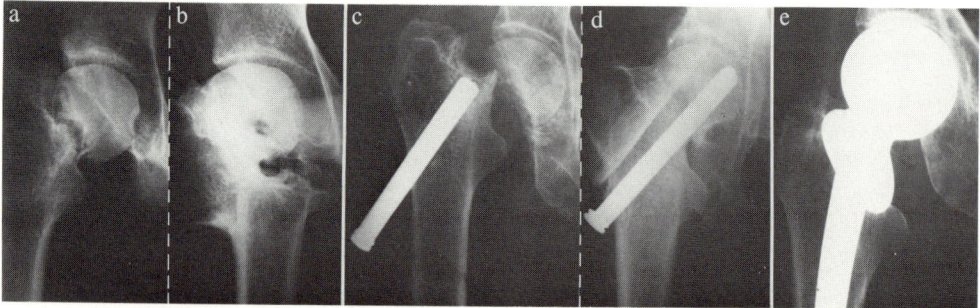

25.6   FRACTURES OF THE FEMORAL NECK (4) NON-UNION
(a, b) In this relatively young patient non-union has been treated successfully by osteotomy.   (c, d) Another patient, treated by nailing and grafting.   (e) In the elderly, replacement by a prosthesis is the usual treatment.

the femoral head is diminished. The method of treatment depends upon the cause of the non-union and the age of the patient.
In the relatively young three procedures are available. (1) If the fracture is unduly vertical but the head is alive, subtrochanteric osteotomy with nail-plate fixation is useful. (2) If the reduction or the nailing was faulty and the head is alive, it is reasonable to remove the nail, reduce the fracture, insert a fresh nail correctly and also to insert a fibular graft across the fracture. (3) If the head is avascular it may be replaced by a metal prosthesis.

In elderly patients only two procedures should be considered. (1) If the pain is not severe, a raised heel and a stout stick or elbow crutch are often sufficient. (2) If the pain is considerable, then, no matter whether the head is avascular or not, it is best removed; if the patient is reasonably fit the head is replaced by a metal prosthesis.

FEMORAL NECK FRACTURES IN THE YOUNG

ORDINARY FRACTURES

In young people the femoral neck breaks only if subjected to considerable force. The child's fracture, if undisplaced, may be treated by closed reduction and plaster, but with displacement, and in young adults, internal fixation is usually preferred. There is a high incidence of avascular necrosis; consequently the patient should not take weight through the leg for 6 months, and then only if the x-ray appearance of the femoral head is normal.

PATHOLOGICAL FRACTURES

In children the neck of the femur may fracture through a cyst. In adolescents the upper femoral epiphysis may slip (page 246), a condition comparable to a fractured neck of femur.

AVULSIONS

In adolescents, the lesser trochanter apophysis may be avulsed by the pull of the psoas muscle; the injury nearly always occurs during hurdling. Less commonly the greater trochanter is avulsed by the abductor muscles. With either injury the patient needs rest in bed for only 2-3 days and may then get up using crutches. As soon as he can balance on the affected leg crutches may be discarded, but he is unlikely to resume athletic activities until the following season.

TROCHANTERIC FRACTURES

The patient is usually old and often unfit. Following a fall she is unable to stand. The leg is shorter and more laterally rotated than with a cervical fracture (because the fracture is extracapsular) and the patient cannot lift her leg. X-ray often shows considerable displacement; the lesser trochanter may be avulsed and the medial cortex just distal to it should be inspected; if it is intact the fracture will, after fixation, be stable to weight bearing.

Early internal fixation is important and several techniques are available, including blade-plate fixation, a sliding nail or screw fixed to a plate, and Ender's condylocephalic nails (inserted through a small incision just above the medial side of the

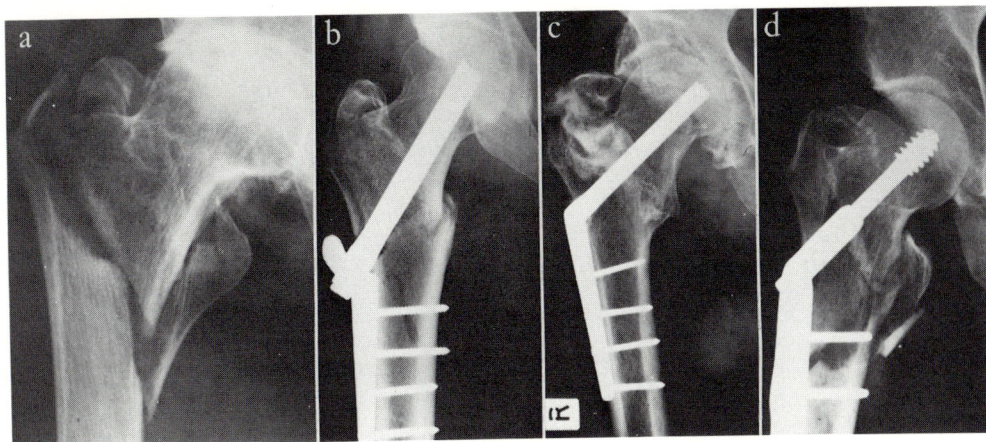

25.7   TROCHANTERIC FRACTURES
(a) The medial femoral cortex just below the lesser trochanter is important for stability; (b) fixation with a McLaughlin pin and plate; (c) with a fixed-angle blade plate; (d) with a sliding screw and plate.

knee). The essential is to get the patient up and walking (with crutches or a walking aid) as soon as possible; hence the need to restore stability by secure fixation. Avascular necrosis is almost unknown; but mal-union is common, resulting in shortening which is best treated by a raised shoe.

NOTE — The potential complications of operation may be unacceptable in younger patients in whom traction is sometimes preferred, despite the economic and social drawbacks.

SUBTROCHANTERIC FRACTURES

MECHANISM
Subtrochanteric fracture may occur at any age if the injury is severe enough; but most occur with relatively trivial injury, in elderly patients with osteoporosis, osteomalacia or a secondary deposit. Blood loss is greater than with femoral neck or trochanteric fractures. The head and neck are abducted by the gluteal muscles, and flexed by the psoas.

SIGNS
LOOK — The leg lies externally rotated, is short, and with a markedly swollen thigh.
FEEL — Palpation is of little value.
MOVE — The patient cannot lift the leg and movement is excruciatingly painful.
X-RAY — The fracture is through or below the lesser trochanter. It may be transverse, oblique, or spiral, and is frequently comminuted. The upper fragment is flexed, and appears deceptively short; the shaft is adducted, and is displaced proximally.

TREATMENT
REDUCE — The fracture is reduced by strong traction in abduction and flexion.

HOLD — Reduction can be held only if the flexed abducted position is maintained. This can be achieved in two ways.

Continuous traction — The lower fragment is in line if the patient is nursed in the sitting position. Traction needs to be maintained for 3 months, so the method is not suited to the elderly.

Internal fixation — This is essential for the elderly, and can be used at any age. If the medial cortex is intact, the fracture can be held with a trifin nail high in the femoral neck and head, attached to a long plate screwed to the shaft above and below the fracture

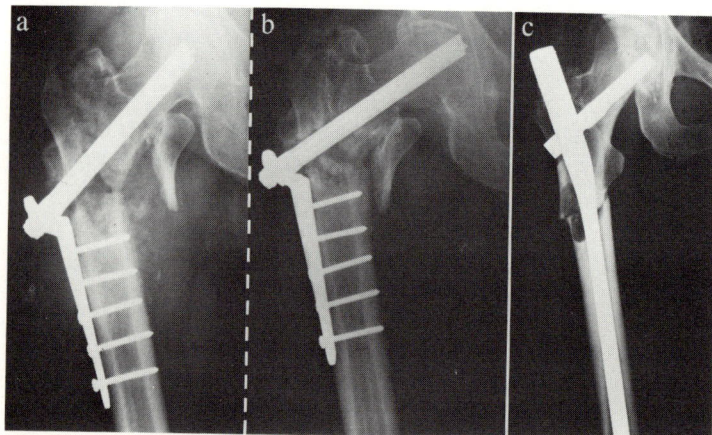

25.8 SUBTROCHANTERIC FRACTURES
Fixation with a pin and plate (a) often fails (b). Zickel nail fixation (c) is better.

line. Low fractures can be fixed with an intramedullary nail. But with neither technique is weight-bearing safe for at least 3 months, and even then coxa vara and shortening are likely to occur. To achieve early weight-bearing (so important for the elderly) without developing coxa vara, the Zickel apparatus or Ender's nails are used. They are mechanically better because they prevent rotation and are secure even without an intact medial cortex.

EXERCISE — During treatment by traction, the muscles are repeatedly exercised; movement is regained when traction is discontinued.

Following internal fixation the patient is allowed up without delay. If Zickel's technique has been used full weight-bearing is safe from the start.

FEMORAL SHAFT FRACTURES

MECHANISM

A spiral fracture is usually caused by a fall in which the foot is anchored while a twisting force is transmitted to the femur. An angulation force or a direct injury may cause a transverse fracture, which is particularly common in motorcycle accidents. A transverse fracture occurring after middle life should be viewed with suspicion; it may be pathological.

SIGNS

Shock is often severe.

LOOK — The leg is usually rotated laterally and may be short and deformed.

FEEL — Palpation is of no value.

MOVE — The patient cannot lift the leg.

X-RAY — The fracture may be situated in any part of the shaft, but the middle third is the most common site. It may be spiral or transverse, or there may be a separate triangular fragment on one side.

Displacement may occur in any direction. Occasionally there are two transverse fractures, so that a segment of the femur is isolated.

EMERGENCY TREATMENT

At the site of the accident shock should be treated and the fracture splinted before the patient is moved. The injured limb may be tied to the other leg or to any convenient splint. For transport a Thomas' splint is ideal: the leg is pulled straight and threaded through the ring of the splint; the shod foot is tied to the cross-piece so as to maintain traction, and the limb and splint firmly bandaged together.

Once in hospital and fit for operation the patient is anaesthetized, the splint removed, (wound toilet is performed if the fracture was open), and definitive treatment instituted.

DEFINITIVE TREATMENT — CHOICE OF METHOD

Unless associated injuries preclude the possibility, open fractures should normally be treated by closed methods. With closed fractures there is a clear choice; as compared with tibial fractures, internal fixation of the femur is safer and closed treatment is more irksome. Nevertheless internal fixation is not without risk and should not be performed unless the necessary expertise and facilities are available. Under these conditions it is often used for transverse fractures of the middle two-fourths of the bone and especially if (a) closed reduction has failed, (b) treatment of the soft tissues is likely to prove difficult because the same tibia also is fractured or because the patient is old and frail, or (*c*) if the fracture is through a secondary deposit.

Closed treatment is safe and reliable; its chief drawback is the length of time spent in bed, and with functional bracing methods this can be considerably reduced. Reduction (usually by manipulation under anaesthesia) is maintained by continuous traction. But — and here controversy begins — is a splint also necessary? In children clearly no splint is needed. In adults a splint usually is employed; either the traditional Thomas' splint with fixed traction, or (since prolonged knee stiffness is the common sequel) with some modification of the splint which allows knee flexion. Perkins, however, has shown that even in adults no splint is needed; skeletal traction with the leg on a pillow is comfortable, exercises ensure knee mobility, and the fractures join at least as quickly as with a splint. Used intelligently (for example traction must not be excessive) this method is very satisfactory; but, since convention dies hard, the techniques of splintage also will be described.

TREATMENT BY FIXED TRACTION

REDUCE — The patient is anaesthetized and manual traction applied by an assistant. The skin is shaved and extension strapping applied. A Thomas' splint of the correct size is threaded over the limb until the ring abuts against the root of the limb. Flannel slings are passed under the limb and secured to the side-bars with safety pins. An attempt is now made to reduce the fracture by manipulation and traction. The traction tapes are pulled tight and tied to the cross-piece of the Thomas' splint. Pads are arranged in front of the flannel slings to maintain the normal forward bow of the femur.

HOLD — The fixed traction is maintained and tightened as necessary. The slings and pads may need adjustment. X-ray films are taken to ensure that reduction is maintained.

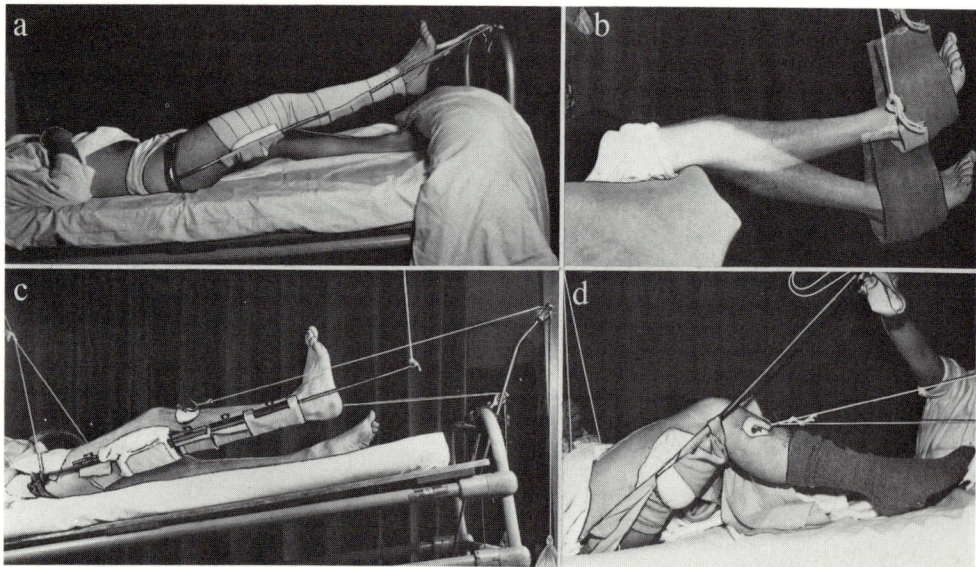

25.9   FRACTURED SHAFT OF FEMUR (1)
(a) Fixed traction on a Thomas' splint: the splint is tied to the foot of the bed which is elevated. This method should be used only rarely because the knee may stiffen; (b) this was the range in such a case when the fracture had united. One way to minimise stiffness is to use skeletal balanced traction (c); the lower slings can be removed to permit knee flexion (d) while traction is still maintained.

To avoid undue pressure by the ring of the splint against the ischial tuberosity, the splint is slung from an overhead beam or tied to the foot of the bed which is raised on blocks.

In adults union may be expected to take 6 weeks for a spiral fracture and 12 weeks for a transverse fracture; consolidation takes twice as long. Once union is fairly well advanced the patient may be allowed up using crutches; but he must take no weight through the leg until consolidation is clinically and radiologically complete.

EXERCISE — The patient is taught to lift himself by a ' monkey pole ' and to exercise all joints not immobilized. He is also taught quadriceps exercises which he must practise assiduously. When the splint is removed knee bending exercises also are started, but it will be many months before a good range of knee flexion is restored.

TREATMENT BY BALANCED TRACTION ON A SPLINT

As with fixed traction, a Thomas' splint with slings and pads is used; this is suspended from an overhead beam. The traction, however, is skeletal, through a Steinmann or Denham pin behind the tibial tubercle. Weights (20 lb. for an adult) are attached, but are not fixed to the cross-piece of the splint; they hang over pulleys at the foot of the bed. Counter-traction is provided by elevating the foot of the bed. The position of the limb is carefully watched and x-ray films taken as necessary. From time to time the pads, slings, or pulleys need adjustment. With transverse fractures it is especially important to avoid overpulling, which inevitably delays union.

As soon as the patient can lift the straight leg from the splint, knee-flexion exercises are begun, for alignment is maintained by the weights. Once union is well advanced the patient may be allowed up non-weight-bearing with crutches. For fractures in the lower half of the femur cast-bracing is suitable; in such a brace the patient can usually be allowed up at 6 weeks from injury.

TREATMENT BY BALANCED TRACTION WITH NO SPLINT

In adults the patient is anaesthetized, the fracture reduced by manipulation, and a Denham pin inserted behind the tibial tubercle. A freely swivelling hook is fixed to each end of the pin and a cord attached to each hook. The 2 cords pass over pulleys at the foot of the bed and a 10 lb. weight is attached to each. The leg is

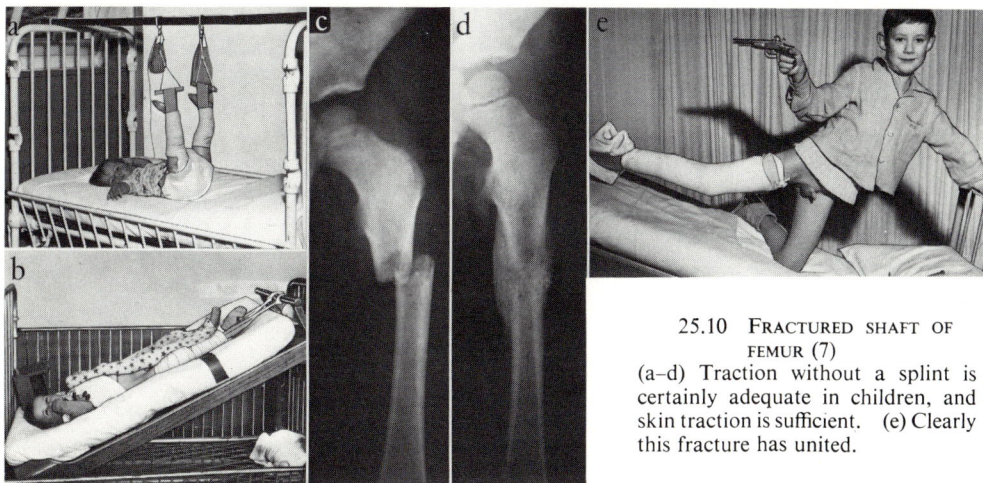

25.10 FRACTURED SHAFT OF FEMUR (7)
(a–d) Traction without a splint is certainly adequate in children, and skin traction is sufficient. (e) Clearly this fracture has united.

cradled on pillows which also prevent backward sag. Exercises are begun without delay; not only quadriceps exercises but also knee-bending which is facilitated by a split mattress (Fig. 25.11).

With fractures in the distal half, the pin can be removed at 6 weeks, but only if functional bracing is then used; this technique is demanding and some shortening may result. If this method is not used, and with more proximal fractures, skeletal traction is retained until union is well advanced. The patient then gets up with crutches, but must not take weight through the leg until the fracture is consolidated.

In children skin traction is usually enough. As soon as the leg feels in one piece, and a little callus is visible on x-ray, a hip spica may be applied and worn until consolidation is complete. Knee movement returns rapidly in children.

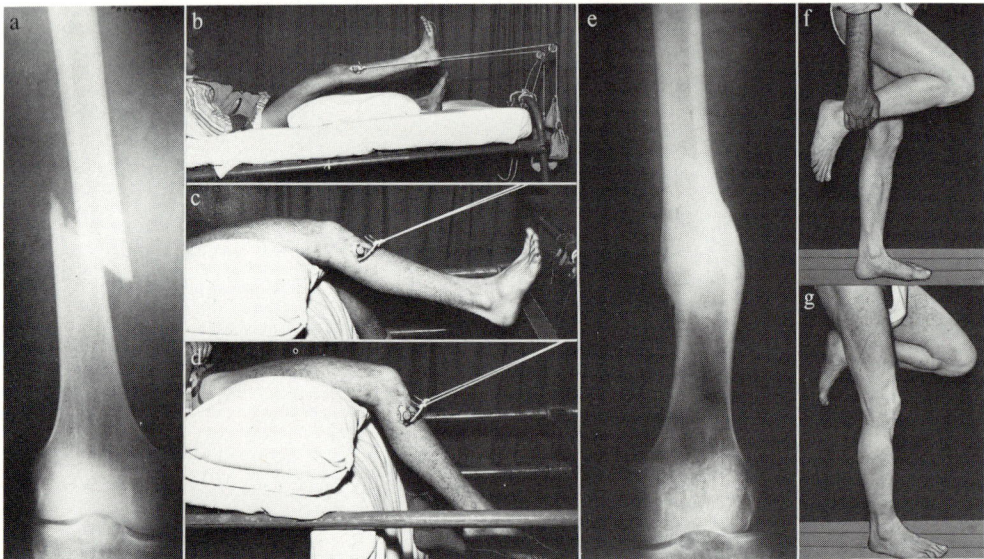

25.11   FRACTURED SHAFT OF FEMUR (3)
Even in the adult traction without a splint can be satisfactory, but skeletal traction is essential. The patient with this rather unstable fracture (a) can lift his leg and exercise his knee (b, c, d). At no time was the leg splinted, but clearly the fracture is consolidated (e), and the knee range (f) is only slightly less than on the uninjured left leg (g).

TREATMENT BY INTERNAL FIXATION

REDUCE — The patient lies on the uninjured side. Through a lateral approach the fracture is exposed and the bone ends cleaned.

HOLD — Much the most efficient method of holding the reduction is by an intramedullary (Küntscher) nail which is introduced as follows.

(1) Long drills are driven upwards and downwards from the fracture to make sure that the medulla is wide enough for the proposed nail (which must fit snugly).

(2) A long guide is pushed up the proximal fragment until, with the hip flexed and adducted, it emerges in the buttock.

(3) A nail of appropriate length (measured on the other leg before operation) is threaded over the guide and hammered down until it emerges at the fracture.

25.12 FRACTURED SHAFT OF
FEMUR (4)

(a) Plating a fractured femur is rarely
satisfactory (though Hicks' very strong
plates may be adequate). Intramedullary
nailing (b) is usually preferred: this young
man also had a fractured tibia in the same
leg.

(c) A delay of 2 weeks before nailing
may explain the exuberant callus in this
case.

(d) Fracture through a secondary
deposit is nearly always treated by nailing.

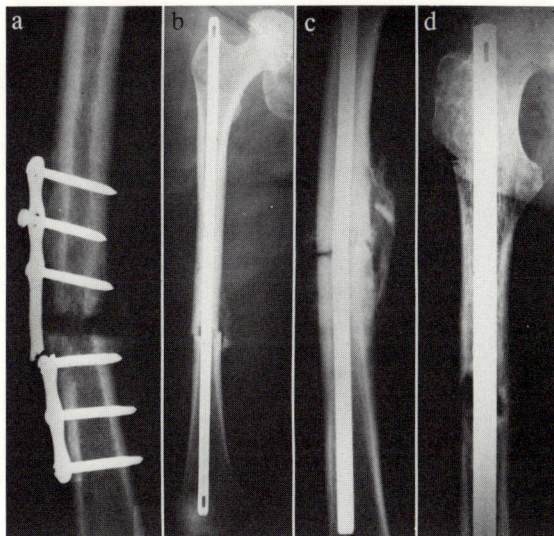

(4) The guide is withdrawn and reinserted down the nail from the upper end; while
the fracture is held reduced the guide is pushed into the distal fragment. The nail is
then hammered home and the guide withdrawn.

NOTE — If the bone is osteoporotic, or the fracture is through a secondary deposit, it is
useful to pack acrylic cement around the nail.

EXERCISE — Immediately after operation, exercises to all the leg joints are begun. Within
a fortnight the patient should have good muscle control of the limb and good movement
of the hip and knee joints. He is then allowed up, weight-bearing if the reduction is
stable and the nail fits snugly; otherwise crutches are used and weight-bearing postponed
until the fixation afforded by the nail is reinforced by callus visible on x-ray.

COMPLICATIONS

SKIN DAMAGE — The fracture may be open and the wound then requires excision. Internal fixation should not be used for an open fracture unless other fractures in the same
limb justify its use.

BONE COMPLICATIONS

Delayed union — Delayed union occurs with open fractures and also if excessive traction
has been used with a transverse fracture. It is essential to ensure that traction is never
excessive and to exercise the longitudinal muscles around the fracture repeatedly.

Non-union — There is a danger that with delayed union splintage may be discarded too
soon. The fracture then angulates and may proceed to non-union. Once non-union
is established, the fracture needs operation: the bone ends are freshened, a Küntscher
nail is inserted and cancellous bone grafts are packed round the fracture.

Mal-union — Mal-union is of little importance unless there is much shortening, and
usually even with shortening the only treatment necessary is a raised shoe.

JOINT STIFFNESS — Stiffness of the knee is the commonest complication of a fractured
femoral shaft. If the muscles have been exercised, knee movement is likely to return
with use even after prolonged splintage. When balanced traction is used, there is no
problem in regaining knee movement. After an infected fracture, considerable knee
stiffness is almost inevitable, and if it is disabling quadriceps-plasty is useful.

THE KNEE

SUPRACONDYLAR FRACTURE

Supracondylar fractures resemble subtrochanteric fractures (page 426) in two respects: (1) While they may occur in adults of any age who sustain a sufficiently severe injury, they often occur through osteoporotic bone in the elderly; (2) continuous traction is suitable for the young, but for the elderly, early mobilization is so important that internal fixation is preferred.

Direct violence is the usual cause. The fracture line is just above the condyles, but may extend between them. When the lower fragment is intact the pull of gastrocnemius may flex it, endangering the popliteal artery.

SIGNS

LOOK — The knee is considerably swollen and deformed.

FEEL — It is important to palpate the anterior and posterior tibial pulses.

MOVE — Movement is too painful to be attempted.

X-RAY — The fracture is just above the femoral condyles and is transverse or comminuted. The fragment may be considerably tilted backwards.

CLOSED TREATMENT

REDUCE — With displacement, reduction is important and with popliteal obstruction it is urgent. A Steinmann or Denham pin is inserted behind the tibial tubercle. Strong traction is applied by an assistant while the surgeon firmly pushes the fragment into place.

HOLD — The patient is returned to bed and 20 lb. traction is maintained with the knee almost straight. The limb is cradled on pillows or on a Thomas' splint.

The fracture takes about 12 weeks to unite and traction must be maintained during that time. The patient is then fitted with a caliper and allowed to take weight. After a further 12 weeks consolidation is usually complete and the caliper may be discarded.

EXERCISE — Quadriceps muscle exercises are encouraged, but knee movements are not permitted until the fracture has united. Then the caliper is removed and active knee movements practised.

OPERATIVE TREATMENT

If closed reduction fails, and the circulation is not restored, urgent open reduction is essential. In elderly patients open reduction with internal fixation, though not essential, reduces the time in bed and the danger of knee stiffness.

Through a lateral incision the fracture is exposed, reduced, and held with intramedullary (Rush) nails or with a specially designed blade plate; with fragile osteoporotic bone it is useful first to pack the interior with acrylic cement. Skin or skeletal traction from below the knee may still be necessary for a few weeks if stability is in doubt but no splint is used and exercises are begun immediately. Unprotected weight-bearing is not permitted until the fracture has consolidated.

COMPLICATIONS

SKIN DAMAGE — Skin damage is common and wound toilet is then necessary.

ARTERIAL DAMAGE — Arterial damage occasionally occurs, and there is danger of gangrene.

KNEE STIFFNESS — Knee stiffness is almost inevitable. A long period of exercises is necessary but full movement is rarely regained.

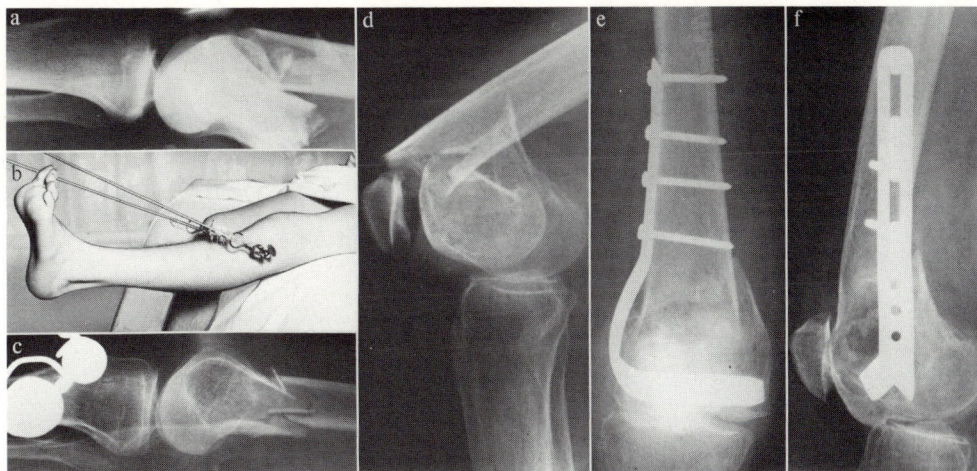

25.13 SUPRACONDYLAR FRACTURES
(a, b, c) Treatment by traction; (d, e, f) treatment by internal fixation. In both cases note the posterior displacement which may endanger the circulation.

NON-UNION — Non-union may be associated with knee stiffness and indeed may be due to forcing knee movement too soon. The fracture is difficult to treat and, unless great care is exercised, the ultimate range of movement at the knee may be less than that at the fracture.

FEMORAL CONDYLE FRACTURES

MECHANISM

A direct injury or a fall from a height may drive the tibia upwards into the inter-condylar fossa. One femoral condyle may be fractured and driven upwards or both condyles split apart.

SIGNS

LOOK — The knee is swollen and may be deformed.

FEEL — There is a tender 'doughy' feel characteristic of haemarthrosis.

MOVE — The knee is too painful to move, but the foot should be examined to exclude nerve damage.

X-RAY — One femoral condyle may be fractured obliquely and shifted upwards, or both condyles may be split apart so that the fracture line is T-shaped or Y-shaped.

TREATMENT

Under anaesthetic the haemarthrosis is aspirated.

REDUCE — A skeletal pin is inserted behind the tibial tubercle. With strong traction and manual compression the fracture can usually be reduced. Only in young people, if closed reduction has failed, is operation advisable; the fracture is then held with intramedullary Rush nails or a transverse bolt.

HOLD — The leg is cradled on pillows and 15 lb. traction maintained for 6 weeks; by this time the fracture has usually united. The patient is then allowed up using crutches, but must not take weight until consolidation is complete, which usually takes 3 months.

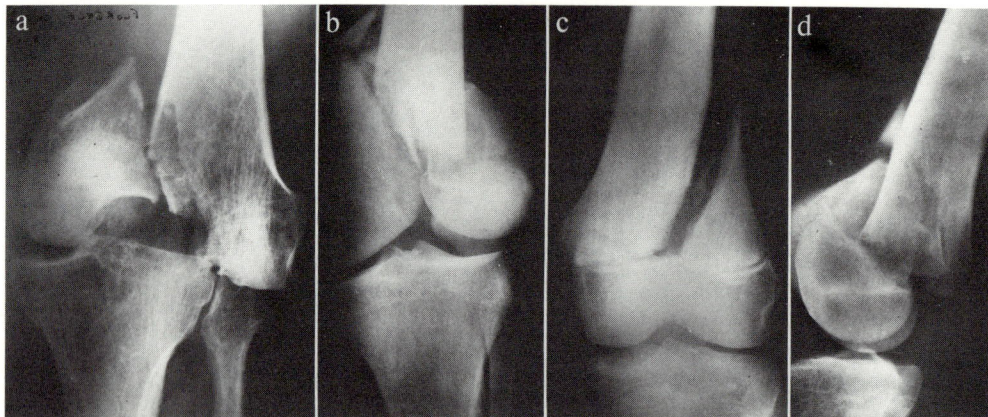

25.14 OTHER FRACTURES OF THE LOWER FEMUR
Manipulative reduction followed by traction is usually the best treatment for con-
dylar fractures (a), inter-condylar fractures (b), and for fracture-separation of the
lower femoral epiphysis (c, d).

EXERCISE — Quadriceps muscle exercises are vigorously practised from the start. Knee
flexion is also encouraged and is facilitated by using a divided mattress; the distal half
of the mattress is removed at intervals and active knee movements practised repeatedly
without removing the traction. Movement often improves a previously imperfect
reduction because the comminuted femoral condyles are 'moulded' by the intact tibia.

FRACTURE-SEPARATION OF LOWER FEMORAL EPIPHYSIS

MECHANISM

In an adolescent the lower femoral epiphysis may be displaced (a) laterally by forced
abduction of the straight knee, as when an opponent falls on a player in a rugger
scrum; or (b) forwards by a hyperextension injury.

SIGNS

LOOK — The knee is swollen and perhaps deformed.
FEEL — The pulses in the foot should be palpated because, with forward displacement of
the epiphysis, the popliteal artery may be obstructed by the lower femur.
MOVE — Movement should not be attempted.
X-RAY — The abduction injury shifts and tilts the epiphysis laterally; the hyperextension
injury shifts and tilts it forwards. In either case, a triangular fragment of the shaft is
displaced with the epiphysis.

TREATMENT

REDUCE — Lateral displacement is corrected by pulling on the straight leg and forcing
the knee into adduction. Forward displacement is corrected by pulling with the knee
bent and thumbing the fragment into position.
HOLD — Plaster is applied from the upper thigh to the malleoli, with the knee straight
if there was lateral displacement, and 60 degrees flexed if there was forward displacement.
The plaster is worn for 6 weeks. The injury may be unstable for much longer than frac-
ture-separations elsewhere; loss of reduction may occur, even in plaster, as late as the
third week.

EXERCISE — Weight-bearing is permitted as soon as the patient can lift his leg. Movement quickly returns when the plaster is removed.

COMPLICATIONS

There is danger of gangrene unless the hyperextension injury is reduced without delay. Interference with growth from damage to the growth disc is uncommon.

TIBIAL CONDYLE FRACTURES

MECHANISM

A fall from a height or a direct blow may fracture one tibial condyle or both. The commonest injury is a fractured lateral condyle, for which the term 'bumper fracture' was coined; but the injury is rarely caused by the impact of a car bumper, it is usually a valgus crush. The patient, nearly always aged 50–60, falls with the knee extended and slightly valgus. The lateral tibial condyle is driven upwards and smashed by the lateral femoral condyle, which remains intact.

SIGNS

LOOK — The knee is swollen and may be valgus.

FEEL — The swollen knee feels 'doughy' because of haemarthrosis.

MOVE — Usually the patient cannot lift the leg or bend it.

X-RAY — Any of the following may be seen: (a) a vertical split of the lateral tibial condyle without displacement; (b) a comminuted crush of the lateral condyle with depression of the fragments; (c) an oblique fracture running downwards and outwards from the tibial plateau; the tibial condyle may be tilted and the upper fibula fractured; or (d) the medial condyle is fractured, and sometimes a transverse line extends across the upper tibia.

TREATMENT BY TRACTION

Treatment by traction is simple and effective and produces uniformly good results. Its sole disadvantage is that the patient must remain in hospital.

REDUCE — If there is much haemarthrosis the joint is aspirated. A Steinmann or Denham pin is inserted through the tibia 5 cm below the fracture. Traction is applied and the condyle manually pushed back into place.

HOLD — The leg is cradled on pillows and 10 lb. traction maintained until the fracture is united, at about 6 weeks. The pin is then removed and the patient is allowed up using crutches. Full weight-bearing should be deferred for a further 6 weeks.

EXERCISE — Quadriceps muscle exercises are vigorously practised from the very beginning. As soon as the patient can lift his leg, knee flexion is permitted while the traction is maintained. There should be fully controlled extension with flexion to 90 degrees within 4 weeks. Movements often improve a previously imperfect reduction.

TREATMENT IN PLASTER

Treatment in plaster also may give good results, though knee movement takes longer to return; it has the advantage that the patient need not remain in hospital for long.

REDUCE — The fracture is reduced by strong traction and lateral compression.

HOLD — Plaster is applied from the upper thigh to the malleoli with the knee straight. It is removed after 6–12 weeks according to the severity of the injury, and weight-bearing is then permitted.

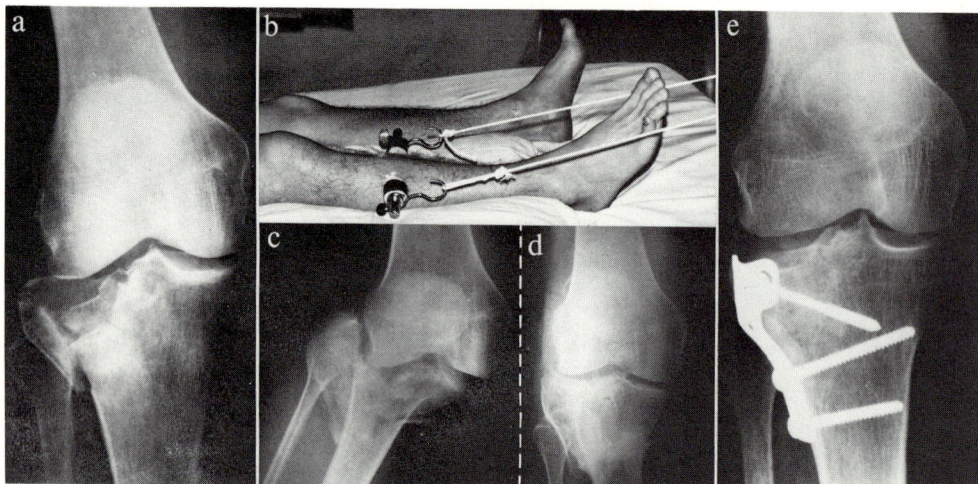

25.15 FRACTURED LATERAL TIBIAL CONDYLE
(a) Typical 'bumper' fracture of the lateral tibial condyle. Skeletal traction applied well below the knee (b) is effective in reducing such a fracture, and in holding it reduced (c, d). Open reduction followed by internal fixation is seldom indicated.

EXERCISE — Quadriceps muscle exercises are practised within the plaster and knee movement is regained when the plaster is removed.

OPERATIVE TREATMENT

If closed reduction fails, and especially if the condyle is much displaced without comminution, open reduction and levering the condyle back into place has been advocated; at operation the condyle may be fixed by a buttress plate and screws. There is no evidence that the results of operative treatment are better than those of treatment by traction.

COMPLICATIONS

Slight valgus deformity may persist but, even so, function is usually very good and late osteoarthritis surprisingly rare. Failure to regain full knee bend is the only important cause of disability, and is avoided by early movements.

FRACTURED TIBIAL SPINE

MECHANISM

A hyperextension injury may tear the anterior cruciate ligament (*see* page 268); sometimes, especially in a child or young adult, the ligament remains intact but the tibial spine is avulsed.

SIGNS

LOOK — The knee is held flexed and is swollen.
FEEL — Because of haemarthrosis the joint feels tense, tender and 'doughy'.
MOVE — Movement is too painful to be attempted.
X-RAY — A lateral film shows the anterior tibial spine elevated from the tibia.

TREATMENT

REDUCE — Under anaesthesia the joint is aspirated; forcing the knee straight reduces the fracture.

Sometimes the true nature of the injury is not immediately realized and after a few weeks it may be impossible to straighten the knee even under anaesthesia. Operative reduction is then essential; the tibial spine is anchored by sutures into a cavity gouged out of the upper tibia.

HOLD — A plaster tube is applied from the upper thigh to the malleoli with the knee straight; it is worn for 6 weeks.

EXERCISE — Weight-bearing is permitted and the quadriceps muscle vigorously exercised. When the plaster is removed, knee flexion is regained by active use.

INJURIES OF UPPER TIBIAL EPIPHYSIS

MECHANISM

In a child, resisted extension of the knee usually strains the insertion of the extensor mechanism into the tibial tubercle (Osgood-Schlatter's disease: *see* page 275). Occasionally a more dramatic avulsion, with displacement, occurs.

SIGNS

LOOK — The knee is swollen.

FEEL — The front of the upper tibia is tender.

MOVE — The knee cannot be actively extended.

X-RAY — The entire upper tibial epiphysis may be tilted forwards. Sometimes, when the ligament is attached to a small apophysis separate from the main epiphysis, this apophysis is avulsed and shifted upwards.

TREATMENT

REDUCE — Under anaesthesia closed manipulative reduction can usually be achieved. If the small separate apophysis remains displaced it is operatively reduced and sutured

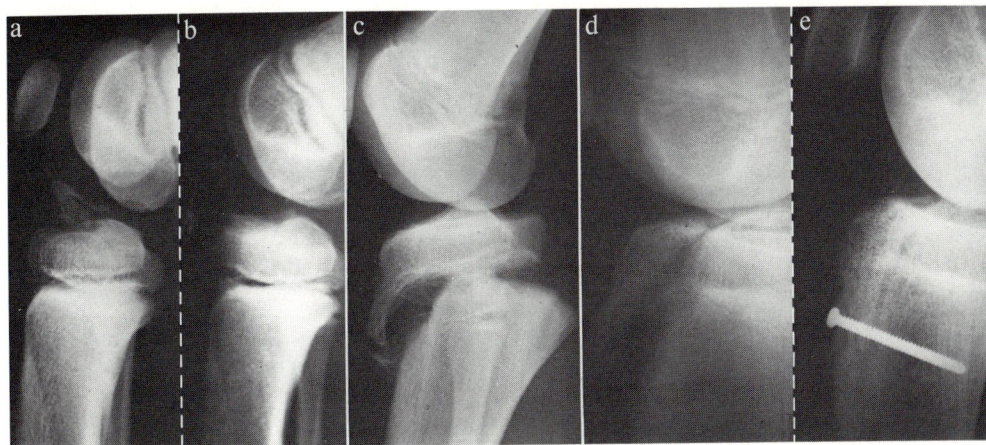

25.16 OTHER FRACTURES OF THE UPPER TIBIA
A fractured tibial spine (a) usually reduces if the knee is straightened fully (b); only when the fracture is missed (which not uncommonly happens) is open reduction sometimes needed. Fracture-separation of the entire upper tibial epiphysis (c) needs urgent reduction because the popliteal artery may be compressed. (d) Avulsion of the patellar ligament insertion (as distinct from Schlatter's disease) is rare: in this case reduction was held with a screw (e).

in position. Occasionally, when the entire tibial epiphysis cannot be accurately reduced by closed manipulation, it is replaced at operation and held by a screw.

HOLD — Following reduction, whether closed or open, a plaster tube is applied from the upper thigh to the malleoli with the knee straight. It is worn for 6 weeks.

EXERCISE — Weight-bearing is permitted at once. Knee flexion quickly returns when the plaster is removed.

FRACTURED PATELLA

DIRECT (STELLATE) FRACTURE

MECHANISM

A fall or a direct blow may smash the patella against the femur. The expansions on each side of the patella usually remain intact.

SIGNS

LOOK — The knee is swollen and held flexed.

FEEL — There is tenderness, and blood in the knee joint.

MOVE — The patient is sometimes able to lift the straight leg.

X-RAY — The films may show (a) one or more fine fracture lines without displacement (the appearance is not to be confused with a bipartite patella in which a smooth line extends obliquely across the superolateral angle of the bone); or (b) multiple fracture lines with irregular displacement.

TREATMENT

ACTIVITY — If there is no displacement, the fracture need not be reduced or held. A tense effusion should be aspirated. A plaster back slab holding the knee straight is worn until quadriceps muscle control is regained. The slab is removed several times a day for active exercises.

OPERATION — If the fragments are displaced the usual treatment is patellectomy, but it is worth attempting wiring, using the technique described for transverse fractures. Patellectomy is then reserved for irretrievable comminution.

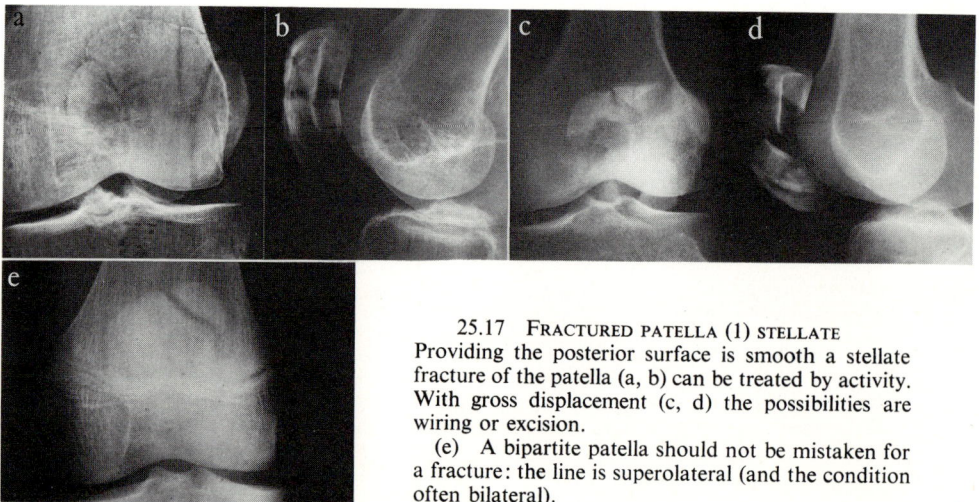

25.17 FRACTURED PATELLA (1) STELLATE
Providing the posterior surface is smooth a stellate fracture of the patella (a, b) can be treated by activity. With gross displacement (c, d) the possibilities are wiring or excision.

(e) A bipartite patella should not be mistaken for a fracture: the line is superolateral (and the condition often bilateral).

INDIRECT (TRANSVERSE) FRACTURE
MECHANISM

Resisted extension of the knee may rupture the extensor mechanism. Typically the patient catches his foot and, to avoid falling, contracts the quadriceps muscle; but the stair or other obstacle prevents straightening of the knee. In middle life this injury usually fractures the patella transversely and tears the lateral extensor expansions.

SIGNS

LOOK — The knee is swollen.

FEEL — At first a gap is palpable, but later it fills with blood.

MOVE — The patient is unable to lift the straight leg.

X-RAY — The patella is fractured transversely; there is a gap between the two halves and the upper fragment is shifted proximally.

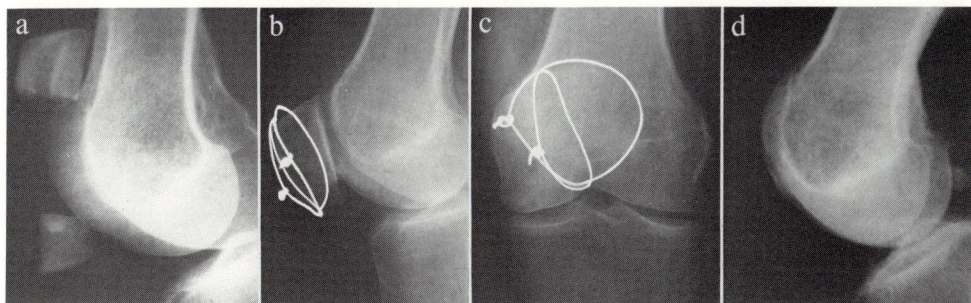

25.18   PATELLAR FRACTURES (2) TRANSVERSE
(a) Gap fracture held together by 2 wires (b, c); it is important that 1 wire is placed anteriorly. This method is preferred to (d) patellectomy.

TREATMENT

Operation is essential. Unless the extensor mechanism is repaired, the last 10 or 20 degrees of active extension will be lost and the knee will be unstable.

TECHNIQUE — Through a transverse incision the fracture is exposed and the lateral expansions are repaired with strong catgut sutures. The patella is reconstituted with 2 wires, one circumferential, the other a tension wire placed anteriorly. Any irregularity of the articular surface may be smoothed away by active use; if patello-femoral signs develop later, the patella can then be excised and the knee recovers more quickly than it does after immediate post-traumatic patellectomy. A plaster back slab is worn until active extension of the knee is regained.

DISLOCATION OF THE KNEE

MECHANISM

The knee can only be dislocated by considerable violence, as in a road accident. The cruciate ligaments and one or both lateral ligaments are torn.

SIGNS

LOOK — There is gross deformity.

FEEL — The circulation in the foot must be examined because the popliteal artery may be obstructed.

MOVE — The patient is asked to move the foot so that possible injury to the lateral popliteal nerve may be detected.

X-RAY — In addition to the dislocation, the films occasionally show a fracture of the tibial spine (cruciate ligament avulsion) or of the tip of the fibula (lateral ligament avulsion).

TREATMENT

REDUCE — Reduction is urgent. Occasionally closed reduction fails because the torn medial ligament lies between the femur and the tibial condyles; open reduction must then be performed and the ligament is sutured back into place.

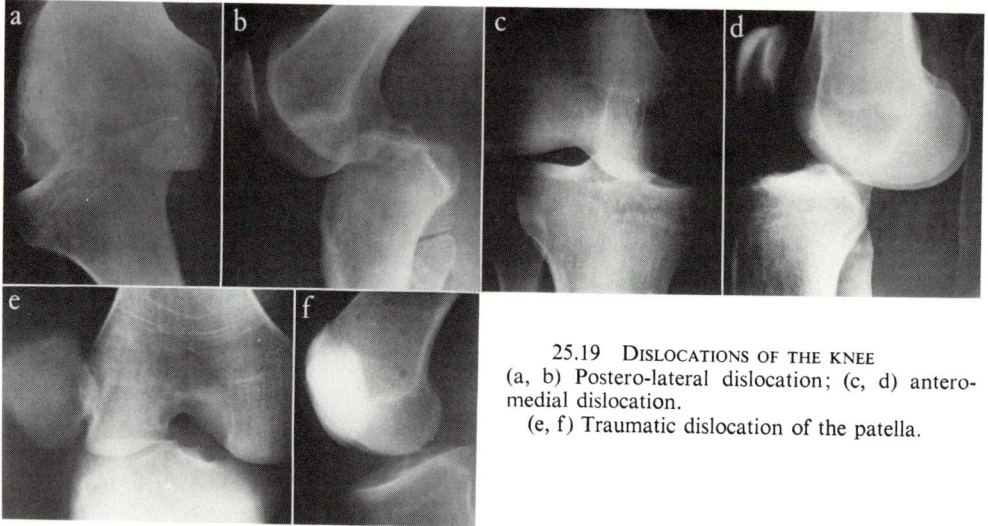

25.19 DISLOCATIONS OF THE KNEE
(a, b) Postero-lateral dislocation; (c, d) antero-medial dislocation.
(e, f) Traumatic dislocation of the patella.

HOLD — Plaster is applied from the upper thigh to the malleoli with the knee slightly flexed. The plaster is split. When swelling has subsided, a new plaster is applied and is worn for 12 weeks from the injury.

EXERCISE — Quadriceps muscle exercises are practised from the start. Weight-bearing in the plaster is permitted as soon as the patient can lift his leg. Knee movements are regained when the plaster is removed.

COMPLICATIONS

ARTERIAL DAMAGE — Popliteal artery damage is common, and early repair is important.
NERVE INJURY — Nerve injury, especially to the lateral popliteal nerve, may occur but usually recovers.
JOINT INSTABILITY — Joint instability (increased antero-posterior glide or lateral wobble) usually remains but, providing the quadriceps muscle is sufficiently powerful, the disability is not severe.

DISLOCATION OF THE PATELLA

MECHANISM

While the knee is flexed and the quadriceps muscle relaxed, the patella may be forced laterally by direct violence. It may perch temporarily on the ridge of the lateral femoral condyle and then either slip back into position or be displaced to the outer side, where it lies with its anterior surface facing laterally.

SIGNS

LOOK — There is obvious deformity. The displaced patella may not be easily noticed but the uncovered medial femoral condyle is unduly prominent.

FEEL — The patella can be felt on the outer side of the knee.

MOVE — Neither active nor passive movement is possible.

X-RAY — The patella is seen to be laterally displaced and rotated.

TREATMENT

REDUCE — The patella is easily pushed back into place, and anaesthesia is not always necessary.

HOLD — With the knee straight, a plaster back slab is applied. It is worn for 3 weeks.

EXERCISE — Quadriceps muscle exercises are begun at once and practised assiduously. As soon as the patient can elevate his leg, walking is allowed. When the back slab has been removed, flexion is easily regained.

COMPLICATIONS

The dislocation may recur, either because the quadriceps muscle has not been redeveloped, or because the torn medial capsule has not healed securely.

THE LEG

FRACTURED TIBIA AND FIBULA

MECHANISM

A twisting force applied to the foot may cause a spiral fracture of both bones. The tibia may puncture the skin.

A direct injury crushes the skin and fractures both bones at the same level. An angulation force also breaks both bones at the same level, usually the mid-shaft, and the tibia often pierces the skin. Motorcycle accidents are the commonest cause.

SIGNS

LOOK — The skin may be undamaged or obviously divided; sometimes it is intact but has been crushed, and there is danger that it may slough within a few days. The foot is usually rolled outwards and deformity is obvious.

FEEL — The pulses are palpated to assess the circulation, and the toes felt for sensation.

MOVE — Movement at the fracture should not be attempted, but the patient is asked to move his toes.

X-RAY — A spiral fracture is usually in the lower third of the tibial shaft; the fibular fracture also is spiral and usually at a higher level; often there is lateral shift, overlap and outward twist below the fracture.

With a transverse fracture both bones are broken at the same level and there may be shift, tilt or twist in any direction; sometimes there is a separate triangular 'butterfly' fragment.

CLOSED TREATMENT

With closed fractures the treatment of choice is closed reduction and plaster; if satisfactory reduction is unobtainable, then open reduction followed by internal fixation becomes a reasonable option. With open fractures, operation (other than wound toilet) is best avoided.

A preliminary period of 14 days traction is useful and, if internal fixation is contemplated, highly desirable. The advantages are: (1) reduction may become sufficiently good to dispense with the need for operation. (2) latent skin damage may become manifest, revealing the hazard of operation; (3) exercises while on traction abolish oedema, restore joint movement and minimize subsequent stiffness; and (4) union occurs more rapidly (Smith, 1974). The technique (termed 'provisional treatment' by Perkins) is to apply a 10 lb pull via a Steinmann pin through the calcaneum; the leg is cradled on a pillow and the foot of the bed elevated.

Provisional treatment is of course not essential. Many surgeons apply plaster without delay. The technique for such fresh fractures is described below. It is slightly more difficult than that following provisional traction, but the principles and after-care are similar in both cases.

REDUCE — Reduction is effected by traction and manipulation, preferably with a skeletal pin through the calcaneum or the lower tibia. The bone ends are first accurately apposed, then the alignment corrected; care must be taken to avoid torsional deformity. Skeletal traction is not essential; manual traction on the foot may be effective in achieving reduction, especially if the knee is bent over the end of the table.

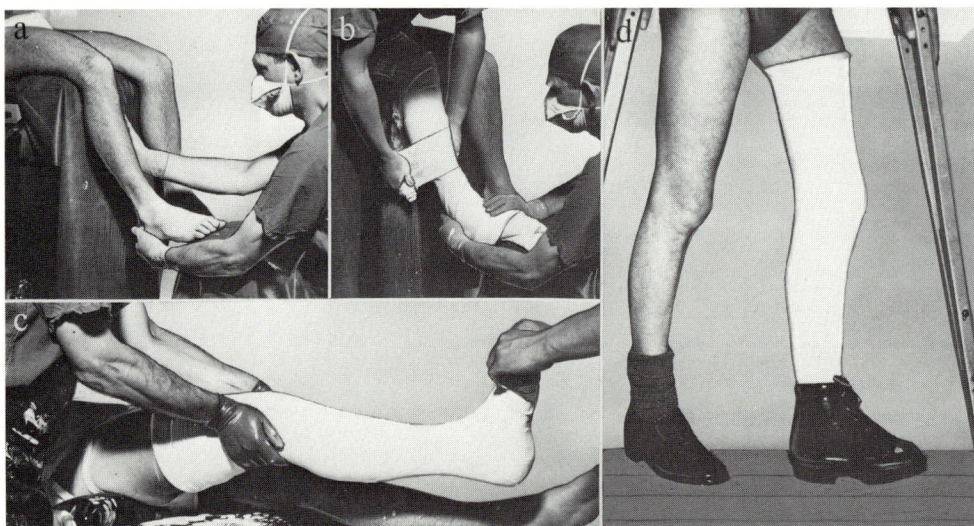

25.20 FRACTURED TIBIA AND FIBULA (1) CLOSED TREATMENT
Reduction is facilitated by bending the leg over the end of the table, with the normal leg alongside for comparison (a). The surgeon holds the position while an assistant applies plaster from the knee downwards (b). When the plaster has set the leg is lifted and the above-knee plaster completed (c); note that the foot is plantigrade, the knee slightly bent, and the plaster moulded round the patella. A rockered boot is fitted for walking (d).

HOLD — (1) An assistant maintains traction while the surgeon applies plaster extending from the upper thigh to the toes with the knee slightly flexed and the foot plantigrade. With fresh fractures the front of the plaster is split.

X ray films are taken and, if necessary, the plaster is wedged. The pin is removed and the patient returned to bed with the leg elevated. When swelling has subsided the plaster is completed.

(2) Spiral fractures take at least 12 weeks to consolidate, transverse or comminuted fractures a few weeks longer, and open fractures may take 24 weeks. Weight-bearing should be graduated, the amount being guided by comfort, not the calendar. The full above-knee plaster is retained until the fracture is clinically and radiologically consolidated, unless functional bracing techniques are used.

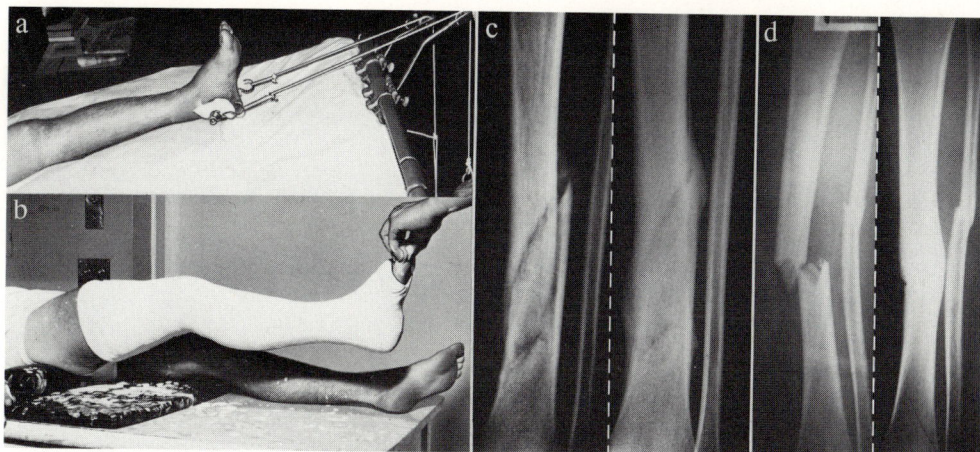

25.21 FRACTURED TIBIA AND FIBULA (2) CLOSED TREATMENT (Continued)
Skeletal traction is useful to reduce overlap, and also as provisional treatment when skin viability is doubtful (a). 10 to 14 days later plaster is applied (b) using the technique shown in the previous illustration, except that the skeletal pin is retained until the plaster has set. (c, d) Examples of spiral and tranverse fractures treated in this way.

EXERCISE — Right from the start, the patient is taught to exercise the muscles of the foot, ankle and knee. When he gets up, an overboot with a rockered sole is fitted, and he is taught to walk correctly; even if weight is not being taken, he must go through the proper motions of walking. When the plaster is removed, a crêpe bandage is applied and the patient is told that he may either elevate and exercise the limb, or walk correctly on it, but he must not let it dangle idly.

FUNCTIONAL BRACING — Sarmiento's technique (1967) is gaining popularity. The full length above knee plaster is worn for only a few days, then changed to a functional plaster cast which liberates the knee and takes some pressure on the patellar tendon; weight-bearing in this is permitted after 48 hours. At 3 to 4 weeks the ankle also is liberated; a splint of plaster or orthoplast holds the leg and is fixed to a special footpiece by links of malleable polypropylene. The surgeon using this method must master an exacting technique and be prepared to accept some shortening.

OPERATIVE TREATMENT

Apart from wound toilet for an open fracture, operative treatment is never essential. But when the surgeon can rely on the aseptic technique of his team, internal fixation has advantages. It is useful when, with closed methods, union is likely to be delayed, i.e. when the fracture is unstable or comminuted, when there is a double tibial fracture, and in the elderly.

After provisional treatment by traction for 14 days the tibia is exposed, the fracture ends meticulously cleaned, and then accurately fitted together. Screws alone may suffice for a spiral fracture; but for most cases it is better to use a long and strong plate (preferably a dynamic compression plate) fixed to the bone by screws which penetrate the opposite cortex.

'Delayed splintage' is now used. The leg is not yet splinted, unless fixation was insecure, when a removable plaster back splint is used. Several times daily the physiotherapist encourages knee, ankle and foot movements. When the wound has

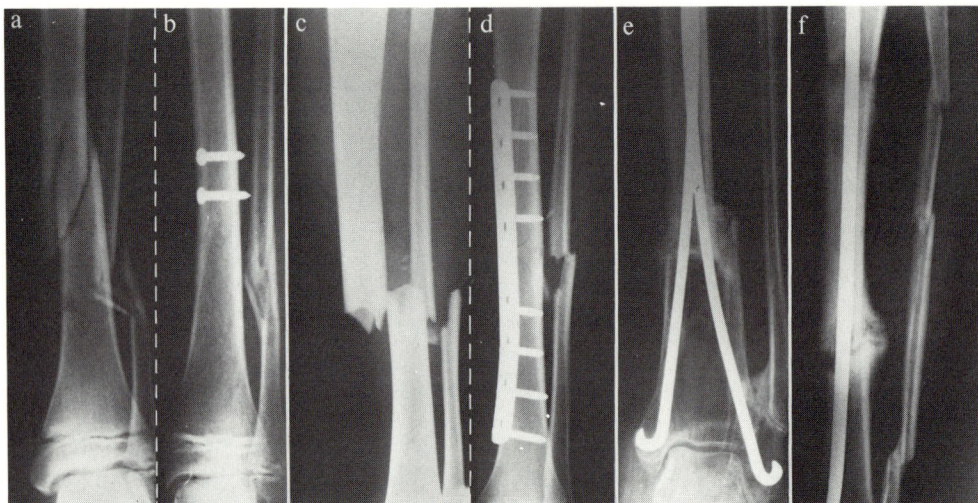

25.22   Fractured tibia and fibula (3) open treatment
(a, b) Spiral fracture stabilized with two screws, facilitating early weight-bearing in plaster. (c, d) Transverse fracture fixed with a plate and screws: movement at the ankle was regained before applying plaster and allowing the patient up. (e) Rush nails were used in this patient because the state of the skin precluded a direct approach (f) An intramedullary nail was used to stabilize this double fracture.

healed an above-knee plaster is applied and worn until the fracture has consolidated. Full weight may be taken. Movements, having once been regained, should return rapidly when the plaster is removed. With mid-shaft fractures, if the fixation is good enough to prevent rotation and overlap, a plaster gaiter may be used instead of the full plaster; this prevents angulation and the patient walks normally.

COMPLICATIONS

SKIN DAMAGE — Skin damage is common. It is important, after wound toilet, to close the skin over the tibia, but tension must be avoided.   If the wound becomes infected union is considerably delayed, and splintage must not be discarded too early.

ARTERIAL DAMAGE — Arterial damage is sometimes severe.   When considerable skin loss is combined with arterial damage, external fixation may be useful (page 322). Volkmann's ischaemia also occurs but, because it is less common in the leg than in the forearm, it is less likely to be diagnosed; and minor degrees of ischaemia probably account for the clawing of the toes which sometimes develops.

MAL-UNION — Mal-union is common and slight shortening is usually of little consequence. Rotation and angulation deformity, apart from being ugly, are disabling, because the knee and ankle no longer move in the same plane. Severe deformity can be corrected by osteotomy.   Backward angulation (caused by allowing the fracture to sag while the plaster is being applied) is common and, if accompanied by a stiff equinus ankle, is dangerous, for when the patient tries to force the foot up in walking the tibia is liable to re-fracture.   This may occur insidiously and lead to non-union.

DELAYED UNION — Union is slow when the fracture is open (especially with infection), if the initial displacement was considerable, if the tibia is fractured in two places, or if the fracture is comminuted.   Union may be hastened by weight-bearing (especially with functional bracing) but if delay seems unduly prolonged, or if the fibular fracture has

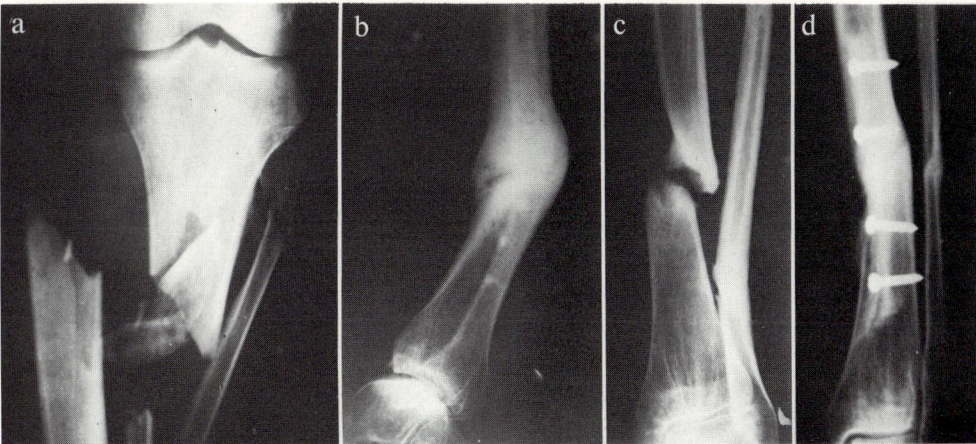

25.23 FRACTURED TIBIA AND FIBULA (4) COMPLICATIONS
(a) With this type of fracture skin damage is inevitable and arterial damage not
unlikely. (b) Mal-union: if the fracture is even slightly angulated in plaster, deformity is liable to increase when weight-bearing begins. (c) Non-union, and (d) a
similar case treated with a sliding bone graft.

joined and is splinting the tibia apart, then an inch of fibula may be excised and a sliding
bone graft screwed across the tibial fracture.

NON-UNION — Non-union is usually the result of faulty treatment.   Either delayed union
has not been recognized and splintage discontinued too soon, or the patient with a recently
united fracture has walked with a stiff equinus ankle.

Once non-union is established the patient must either wear a permanent splint or the
fracture must be operated upon.   Compression plating, with its great rigidity, may be
adequate, but often grafting is preferred.   The bone ends are freshened, fixed with a
cortical bone graft and packed with cancellous bone chips.   An inch of fibula is excised
and the fracture is then treated in plaster.

JOINT STIFFNESS — Joint stiffness is often due to neglect in treatment of the soft tissues;
but with the prolonged splintage necessary, and especially in the presence of sepsis, some
stiffness may be unavoidable.   Limitation of movement at the ankle and foot may persist
for 6–12 months after removal of the plaster, in spite of active exercises.

FRACTURE OF ONE BONE ONLY

FIBULA

Most spiral fibular fractures are associated with injuries of the ankle or knee;
especially with a high fracture the ankle also should be examined.

An isolated fracture of the fibula (usually transverse) may be due to stress or to a
direct blow.   There is local tenderness, but the patient is able to stand and to move
the knee and ankle.   A crêpe bandage is comforting but no other treatment is
necessary.

TIBIA

In children a twisting injury may cause a spiral fracture of the tibia without fracture
of the fibula; this is rare in adults.   At any age a direct injury, such as a kick, may
cause a transverse or slightly oblique fracture of the tibia alone at the site of impact.

Local bruising and swelling are usually evident, but knee and ankle movements are possible. The child with a spiral fracture may be able to stand on the leg, and as the fracture may be almost invisible in an antero-posterior film, unless two views are taken the injury can be missed; a few days later an angry mother brings the child with a lump which proves to be callus. Transverse and slightly oblique fractures are easily seen on x-ray but displacement is slight.

TREATMENT

With displacement reduction should be attempted. An above-knee plaster is applied as with a fracture of both bones; first a split plaster then, when swelling has subsided, a complete one. A fracture of the tibia alone takes just as long to unite

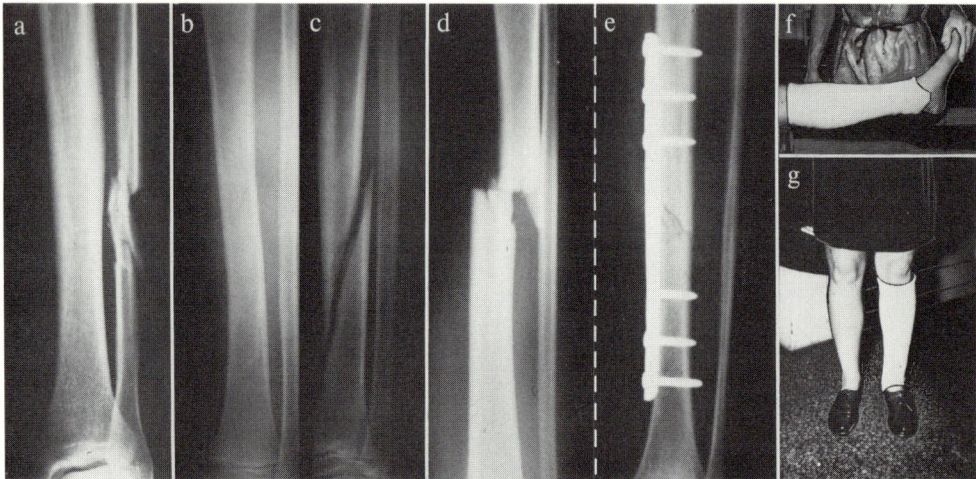

25.24 FRACTURE OF ONE BONE ONLY
(a) Fracture of the fibula alone. (b, c) In this child's leg the spiral fracture of the tibia shows only in one view. (d) Transverse fracture of the tibia alone in the adult: it has been plated (e) and is now so stable that a plaster gaiter (f, g) is the only protection needed.

as if the fibula also was broken; so at least 12 weeks is needed for consolidation and sometimes 24. The child with a spiral fracture, however, can be safely released after 6 weeks; and with a mid-shaft transverse fracture the surgeon may (if he is a skilled plasterer and reduction is perfect) replace the above-knee plaster by a short plaster gaiter.

COMPLICATIONS

An open fracture will, of course, need wound excision; with infection union will be slow. When closed, isolated tibial fractures, especially in the lower third, may be slow to join, and the temptation is to discard splintage too soon. Even slight displacement may delay union so that open reduction with internal fixation is often preferred. In managing delay, union can usually be hastened by excising an inch of the fibula, which allows the tibial fragments to impact.

THE ANKLE

LIGAMENT INJURIES

MECHANISM

The patient falls or stumbles and the foot inverts under him. As a rule, there is only a partial tear of the lateral ligament and the injury is an ankle sprain. Sometimes, however, the ligament is completely torn, and the joint subluxates; the talus momentarily tilts into inversion, then snaps back into position.

SIGNS

LOOK — The ankle is swollen.

FEEL — Tenderness is usually maximal on the lateral aspect of the joint.

MOVE — Inversion is painful, but only with a complete tear of the ligament is the movement excessive. Pain may prevent excessive movement from being demonstrated and, if the injury is severe, inversion must be tested again under local or general anaesthesia.

X-RAY — The x-ray appearance of the resting ankle is normal whether the joint has been sprained or subluxed, for a subluxation reduces itself. X-ray films are taken with both ankles inverted (if necessary using local or general anaesthesia); these, known as 'strain films', show whether the talus tilts unduly on the affected side.

TREATMENT

PARTIAL TEAR — An ankle sprain should be treated by activity. A crêpe bandage is applied and active exercises are begun immediately and persevered with until full movement is regained. The patient is not allowed to dangle the leg and the bandage is worn until swelling has disappeared. Weight may be taken as soon as the patient will walk, but he must be taught to walk correctly with the normal heel-toe gait.

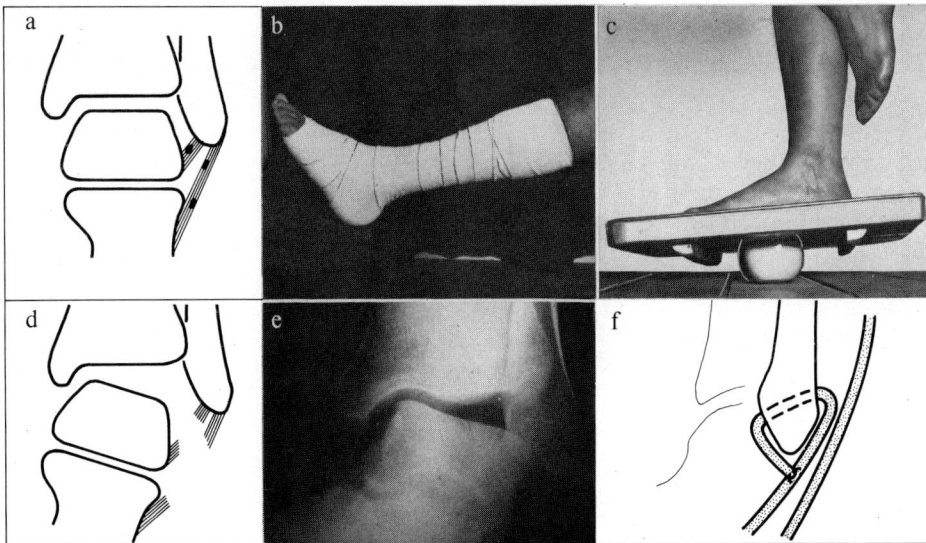

25.25 ANKLE SPRAINS

The commonest is a partial tear of the lateral ligament (a). In treatment a crêpe bandage (b) is more efficient than adhesive strapping. The balancing board (c) is a useful method of strengthening the muscles.

A complete tear of the lateral ligament (d) causes recurrent giving way: a strain film reveals talar tilt (e): Harding's operation (f) is simple and effective.

COMPLETE TEAR — A subluxation must be treated in plaster.   No reduction is necessary. Plaster is applied from just below the knee to the toes, with the foot plantigrade.   If there is swelling, the plaster is split and replaced when the swelling has subsided.   Plaster is worn until the ligament may be expected to have repaired, which takes about 10 weeks. The patient is encouraged to walk normally with the aid of an overboot with a rockered sole.   When plaster is removed, a crêpe bandage is worn and movements are regained by active use.

COMPLICATIONS

ADHESIONS — Following an ankle sprain, adhesions are liable to form unless the foot is actively and correctly used.   The patient complains that the ankle 'gives way' and lets him down.   Following such an incident, there is tenderness on the outer side and pain on inversion, but no excessive inversion.   If active exercises fail to restore full painless movement, the joint should be manipulated under anaesthesia and full range maintained by activity.

RECURRENT SUBLUXATION — If a complete tear of the lateral ligament was undiagnosed, and consequently unsplinted, the ligament fails to repair and subluxation becomes recurrent.   The history is similar to that of adhesions following a sprain; the patient, after an injury, complains that the ankle gives way at intervals.   The talus, however, can be inverted further than that of the normal ankle.   If the diagnosis is in doubt, the patient should be anaesthetized and both ankles x-rayed in full inversion.   If the talus tilts, the injury is a subluxation; if not, the adhesions should be broken down forthwith by manipulation.

Treatment of recurrent subluxation — Raising the outer side of the heel and extending its lower surface laterally ('floated-out heel'), may relieve symptoms; but operation is more reliable.

Technique — A simple and effective procedure is Harding's operation, in which the peroneus brevis tendon is detached from the muscle, threaded through a hole drilled in the fibula and then sewn back to itself, to the peroneus longus, and to the ligamentous structures at the tip of the fibula.   Plaster must afterwards be worn for 8 weeks.

RECURRENT DISLOCATION OF PERONEAL TENDONS — Adhesions and recurrent subluxation are two causes of giving way of the ankle.   A third but uncommon cause is recurrent dislocation of the peroneal tendons.   The condition is unmistakable, for the patient can demonstrate that the peroneal tendons dislocate forwards over the fibula in certain positions.   At operation the superficial cortex of the lower 5 cm of the fibula should be hinged backwards and stitched over the peroneal tendons to hold them in their correct position.

FRACTURES AROUND THE ANKLE

MECHANISM

Usually the foot is anchored to the ground while the momentum of the body continues forwards; the patient may stumble over an unexpected obstacle or stair, or into a small depression in the ground, or he may have fallen from a height.   The momentum of the body may impose any one of a variety of forces upon the ankle, the most important being external rotation, abduction and adduction.   To these may be added an upward thrust if the patient has fallen from a height.

SIGNS

LOOK — The ankle is swollen, and deformity may be obvious.

FEEL — The site of tenderness is important; the ligament on one or other side of the joint may be torn.

MOVE — Attempted ankle movements are painful and limited.

X-RAY — From a study of the fracture pattern the precise type of fracture-dislocation can be deduced, and treatment depends upon correct identification of the injury.

Talus — The most important single feature of an ankle injury is how accurately the talus fits the mortise. If the mortise is widened or the talus shifted or tilted, subluxation is present. Usually there is an accompanying mortise fracture and the injury is called a fracture-subluxation. Injuries are classified according to the direction of the damaging force and its consequences.

25.26 ANKLE FRACTURES (1)
THE TALUS
The position of the talus is all-important. (a) Fracture without subluxation — 1. the surfaces of the tibia and talus are precisely parallel, 2. the distance of the talus from the medial malleolus is normal.
(b) Subluxation — the talus is tilted and unduly separated from the medial malleolus; there is also diastasis (displacement was permitted by a high fracture of the fibula).

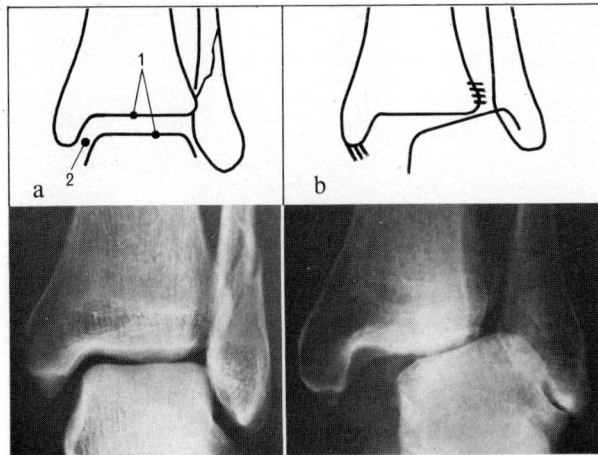

The mortise — (*a*) An external rotation force causes a spiral fracture of the fibula. With continuing force, the medial malleolus may be avulsed and fractured transversely. Further rotation may lead to avulsion of a posterior fragment of the tibia, to which the tibiofibular ligament is attached.

(*b*) An abduction force fractures the fibula transversely 5 cm above the joint and may avulse the medial malleolus.

Diastasis may occur in (*a*) or (*b*). The tibio-fibular ligament tears with or without avulsion of its tibial attachment; the ligament tear allows the tibia and fibula to separate and the talus to be driven up between them.

(*c*) An adduction force causes a near-vertical fracture of the medial malleolus extending upwards from the medial angle of the mortise; the tip of the fibula may also be avulsed.

(*d*) An upward thrust may split the tibia vertically and this vertical fracture often joins a transverse fracture 2–3 inches above the joint. Sometimes a vertical force shears off the anterior or posterior corner of the lower tibia.

In adolescents, similar injuries occur and may cause fracture-separation of the lower tibial epiphysis.

TREATMENT

Union in perfect position is mandatory at the ankle. Unless closed reduction is perfect and the fracture will unquestionably remain undisplaced (both uncommon), open methods are needed.

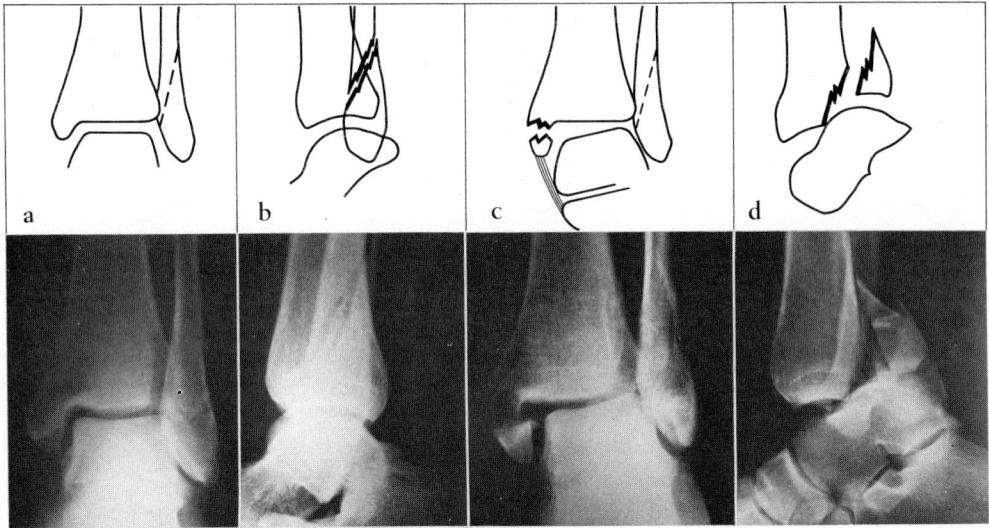

25.27 ANKLE FRACTURES (2) EXTERNAL ROTATION
(a, b) with an undisplaced external rotation fracture the talus fits the mortice accurately; the fibular fracture may show only in the lateral film. (c) With more severe injury the talus tilts laterally, and the medial malleolus may be avulsed; (d) if the posterior margin of the tibia is fractured the talus may be displaced upwards.

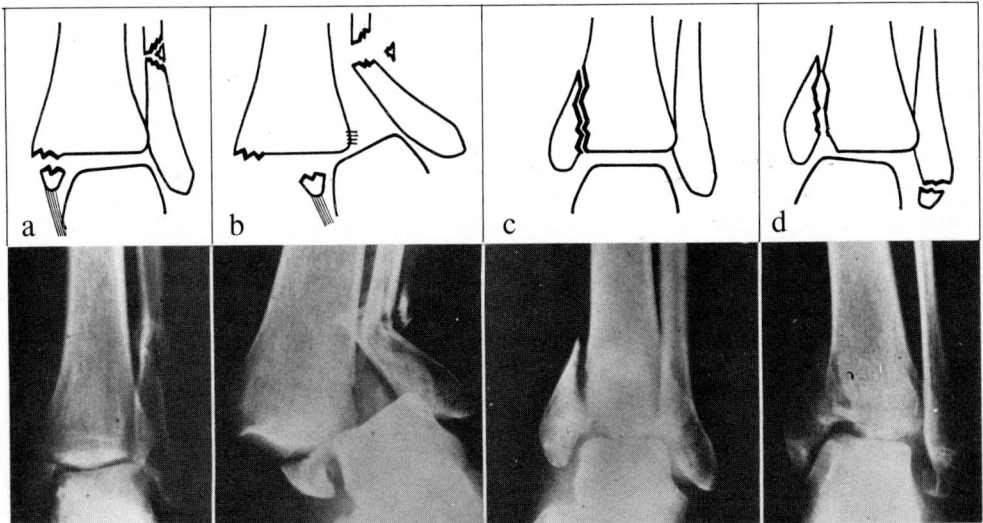

25.28 ANKLE FRACTURES (3) ABDUCTION AND ADDUCTION
(a) Abduction fracture with moderate displacement, (b) with severe displacement and diastasis — note that the fibular fracture is well above the joint. (c) Adduction fracture with slight displacement, (d) with moderate displacement — note that the tibial fracture line is almost vertical.

CLOSED METHODS

Fractures with no trace of displacement clearly require no reduction and are sometimes treated without plaster, the patient being allowed to walk with the ankle in a crêpe bandage. The method is safe only when it is certain that there has not been spontaneous reduction of a displacement. Fractures with displacement are treated as follows:

REDUCE — First manual traction is applied, then a force is applied the reverse of that which caused the injury. Unless the causal force has been correctly deduced and reversed by manipulation, accurate replacement of the talus is unlikely.

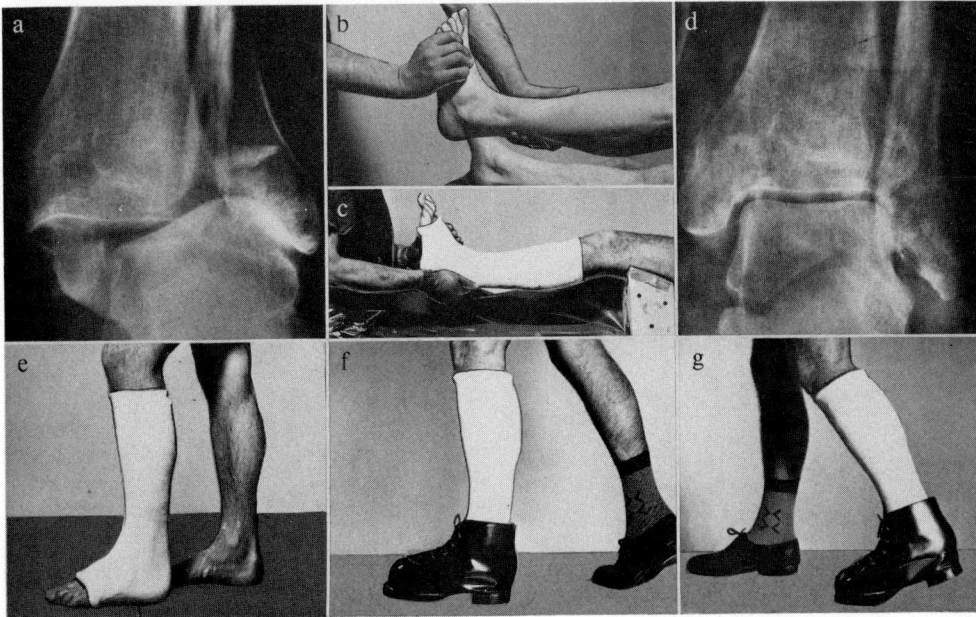

25.29 ANKLE FRACTURES (4) CLOSED TREATMENT
An external rotation fracture (a) is reduced by traction followed by internal rotation (b); a below-knee plaster is applied, moulded and held till it has set (c). The check x-ray is usually satisfactory (d). The plaster must be plantigrade (e): a rockered boot permits an almost normal gait (f, g).

HOLD — A padded plaster is applied from just below the knee to the toes, with the foot plantigrade; that is, with the foot at an angle of 90 degrees to the leg and neither in varus nor valgus position. (There is a tendency to apply the plaster with the foot inverted, and this must be resisted.) The plaster may need to be split and if so it must be completed or replaced when swelling has subsided. An x-ray film to confirm reduction must be taken after the plaster has been applied and another after it has been changed. With an external rotation fracture, 6 weeks in plaster is sufficient; all other fractures should be kept in plaster for 12 weeks.

EXERCISE — An overboot is fitted and the patient is taught to walk correctly as soon as possible. Ankle and foot movements are regained by active exercises when the plaster is removed. As with any lower limb fracture, the leg must not be allowed to dangle idly. It must be exercised or elevated. After removal of the plaster a temporary crêpe bandage is necessary.

OPERATIVE TREATMENT

Operative treatment may be advisable (*a*) to ensure perfect reduction; (*b*) to maintain reduction; or (*c*) to facilitate early movement. When operation is undertaken, internal fixation with a screw is employed, even if the object of the operation was only to obtain perfect reduction. Internal fixation by itself is insufficient to permit unprotected walking. After operation, movements should be regained and then a below-knee plaster worn until the fracture has consolidated.

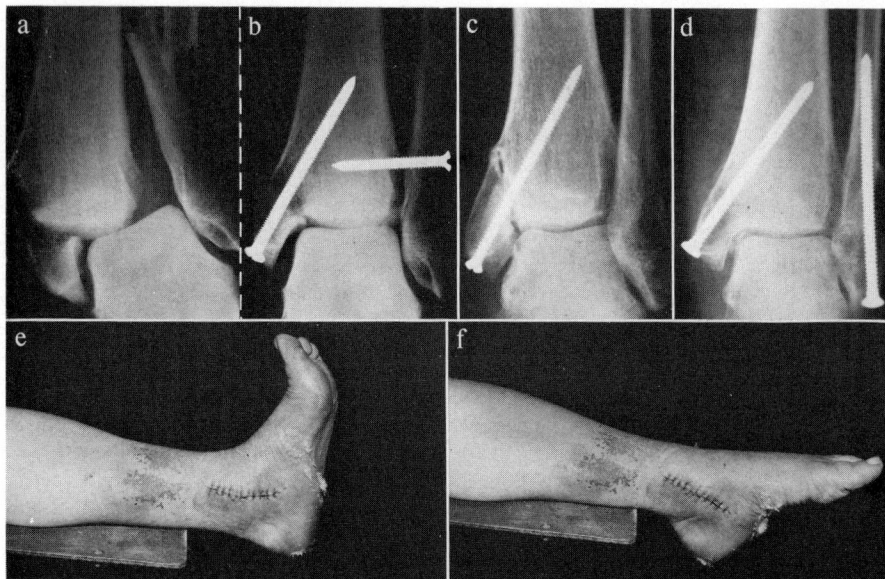

25.30 ANKLE FRACTURES (5) OPEN TREATMENT
(a) Abduction fracture with diastasis; (b) after fixation with 2 screws. (c) Adduction fracture fixed with a single screw. (d) If both malleoli are fixed additional stability is provided and, until the patient gets up, no splint is needed; (e, f) show this patient exercising his ankle a few days after operation, and before the walking plaster was applied.

TO REDUCE — If, after closed reduction, the talus does not fit the mortise accurately, one or other malleolus (usually the medial) is exposed. Sometimes a flap of periosteum is found interposed between the medial malleolus and the tibia, or the peroneal tendons between the lateral malleolus and the shaft of the fibula. The fracture is accurately reduced and held by internal fixation.

TO HOLD REDUCTION — Fractures with diastasis are very unstable. They are most efficiently held if a screw is inserted through the medial malleolus into the tibia and, when necessary, a second screw inserted transversely from the fibula to the tibia; because it is subjected to a shearing strain the transverse screw should be removed after 3 months. In some cases the second screw is better inserted from the lateral malleolus straight up the medulla of the fibula; the fibula is held out to length, and stability enhanced.

TO TREAT SOFT TISSUES — In elderly people it may be unwise to immobilize the foot for a long period in plaster. The fracture may be fixed internally; movement is regained while the patient is in bed, and a walking plaster is then applied until the fracture is consolidated.

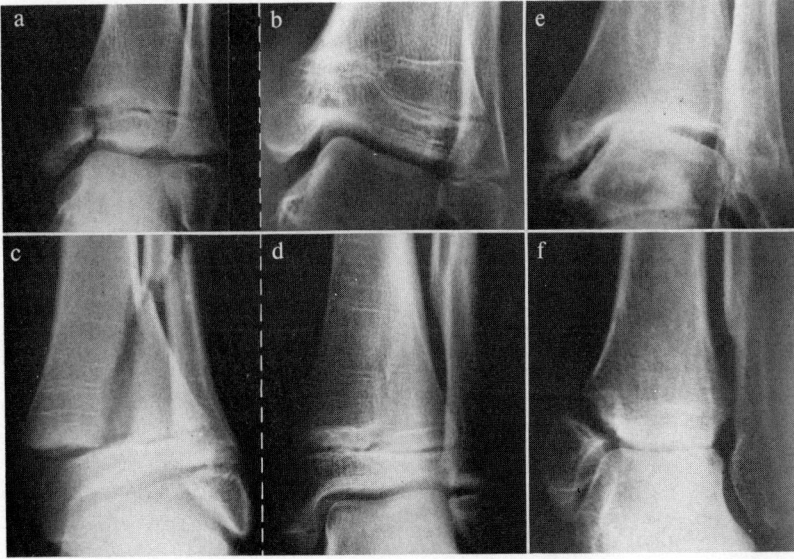

25.31 ANKLE FRACTURES (6) COMPLICATIONS
(a) Fracture through the epiphysis has disturbed growth, and (b) 3 years later the ankle is no longer horizontal. This contrasts with the 2 x-rays below in which fracture-separation of the entire tibial epiphysis (c), has, after reduction, grown normally (d). (e) Mal-union following failure of reduction in the adult. (f) Non-union of the medial malleolus.

COMPLICATIONS

MAL-UNION — Incomplete reduction is common and, unless the talus fits the mortise accurately, degenerative changes may occur. Sometimes degeneration can be halted or prevented by a corrective osteotomy. If osteoarthritis has already developed arthrodesis may prove necessary.

Secondary mal-union from epiphyseal arrest in an adolescent is rare.

NON-UNION — Non-union of the medial malleolus occasionally occurs if a flap of periosteum is interposed between it and the tibia. It should be prevented by operative reduction and screw fixation.

JOINT STIFFNESS — Joint stiffness and swelling of the ankle are usually the result of neglect in treatment of the soft tissues. The patient must walk correctly in plaster and, when the plaster is removed, he must, until circulatory control is regained, wear a crêpe bandage and elevate the leg whenever he is not using it actively. Occasionally, several months after the fracture, manipulation under anaesthesia may be needed to restore full movement.

THE TARSUS AND FOOT
INJURIES OF THE TALUS

MECHANISM

Talar injuries are rare and due to considerable violence, usually a car accident or falling from a height. The injuries include fractures (of the head, neck, body or lateral process of the talus) dislocations (mid-tarsal, subtalar or total dislocation of the talus) and fracture-dislocations (talar fractures combined with dislocation). Mid-tarsal injuries are often missed; they have been classified according to the deforming force: longitudinal compression, plantar and crush varieties are described, as well as medial or lateral displacements, sometimes of a ' swivel ' type (Main and Jowett 1975).

SIGNS

LOOK — The foot is obviously deformed and swollen. The skin may have been split or may rapidly necrose.

FEEL — The dorsalis pedis artery should be palpated.

MOVE — The foot is held immobile.

X-RAY — AP, lateral and oblique views are needed. The talus is first identified (not always easy); then inspected to see if it is fractured (and if so how the fragments are displaced); next its relationship to the tibia, calcaneum and other tarsal bones is studied (to identify dislocation); finally the mid-tarsal joint is carefully inspected — the bones must fit precisely, and comparison with the normal foot is useful.

TREATMENT

UNDISPLACED FRACTURES — When displacement is no more than trivial reduction is not needed. A split plaster is applied and, when the swelling has subsided, is replaced by a complete plaster in the plantigrade position. With fractures of the head weight-bearing is allowed, with body or neck fractures it is avoided. At 6–8 weeks the plaster is removed and function regained by normal use.

DISPLACED FRACTURES AND FRACTURE–DISLOCATIONS — Reduction is urgent (because the stretched skin soon necroses), but may be difficult. Closed manipulation is tried first, and forced plantarflexion is often the key manoeuvre. If this proves ineffective a Steinmann pin through the calcaneum can be used to exert powerful traction while a second Steinmann pin transfixes the displaced bone and is used to reduce it. Should this also fail there must be no hesitation in performing open reduction.

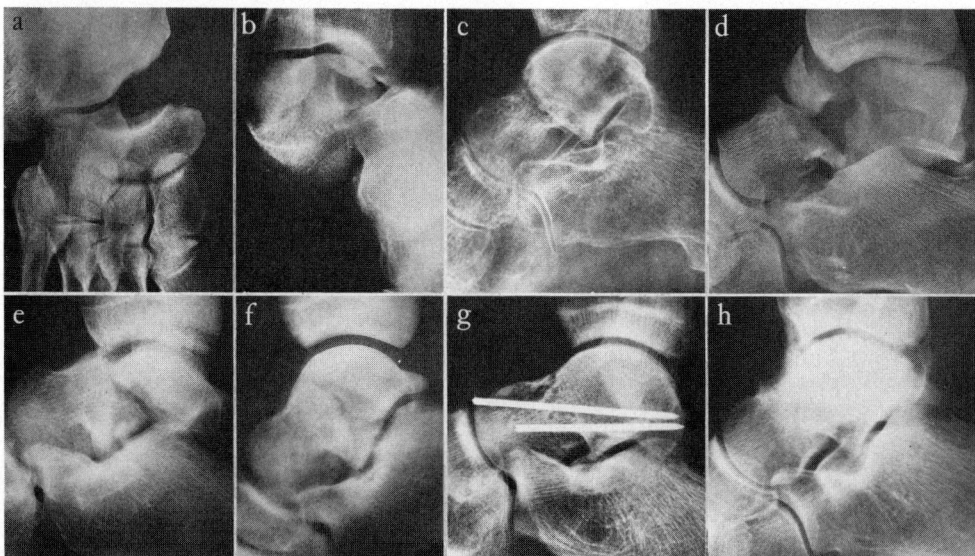

25.32 TALAR FRACTURES AND DISLOCATIONS
(a, b) 2 views of subtalar dislocation. (c) Talar fracture without displacement, and (d) with considerable displacement. (e, f) Talar fracture before and after reduction by forced plantar-flexion. (g) Another method of treatment, by open reduction and internal fixation. (h) Avascular necrosis of the posterior half of the talus following fracture.

It is often expedient to stabilize a reduced fracture with one or two pieces of Kirschner wire, but plaster also is needed. Most of these injuries are stable only with the foot plantarflexed; this unpleasant position is maintained in a split plaster for 2–3 weeks. Then, without anaesthesia, the plaster is removed, and the patient is persuaded to dorsiflex his foot gently; a complete below-knee plaster is then applied with the foot plantigrade and this is worn for a further 6 weeks. When the plaster is removed, the patient is encouraged to exercise the leg and foot, but he should avoid weight-bearing until x-rays show that the talus has not undergone avascular necrosis.

NOTE — An innocuous-seeming flake beneath the lateral malleolus may, on a 20 degree oblique view, prove to be a substantial fragment — the lateral process of the talus. It must be recognized and either fixed back or removed; otherwise considerable loss of function is inevitable.

COMPLICATIONS

SKIN DAMAGE — Skin damage is common either because the skin has been split or because it is tightly stretched and necroses. Even when a totally detached talus is lying in the wound the bone should not be excised but replaced.

AVASCULAR NECROSIS — Avascular necrosis of part or all of the talus may occur. The bone becomes dense on x-ray, but it should be remembered that in the lateral view the overlying malleoli normally cause a dense appearance. An avascular talus crushes with weight-bearing: degenerative changes are then inevitable and the ankle may need to be arthrodesed.

FRACTURES OF THE CALCANEUM

MECHANISM

The patient usually falls from a height, often from a ladder, on to one or both heels. The calcaneum is driven up against the talus and split or crushed. The same accident may also have damaged the spine, which must always be examined in calcaneal injuries.

SIGNS

LOOK — The heel is broad and a D-shaped bruise appears in the sole.

FEEL — The heel is thick and tender and the normal concavity below the lateral malleolus is lacking.

MOVE — The subtalar joint cannot be moved but ankle movement is possible.

X-RAY — Unless every patient with a painful heel after a fall is x-rayed, fractures of the calcaneum will be missed. Lateral and axial films are required. (An axial film is one taken with the x-rays passing obliquely through the sagittal plane of the bone.)

Calcaneal fractures are classified as chip, split, or crush fractures.

Chip fractures — These comprise (*a*) vertical fracture of the medial tuberosity; (*b*) horizontal fracture of the postero-superior corner, sometimes with upward tilt; and (*c*) fracture of the antero-superior corner obliquely into the calcaneo-cuboid joint. All these are rare.

Split fractures — The calcaneum is split into two segments by a vertical fracture which extends from the medial aspect near the back of the bone to the lateral aspect in front. The larger lateral segment is usually shifted laterally and the smaller medial segment displaced upwards. The fracture usually extends into the subtalar joint but the joint may not be severely damaged.

Crush fractures — The fracture line or lines resemble those of split fractures but the portion of the calcaneum which articulates with the talus is driven downwards into the body of the bone. The subtalar joint is grossly damaged.

TREATMENT OF CHIP FRACTURES

If there is no displacement, neither reduction nor splintage is necessary. A crêpe bandage is applied and the patient encouraged to walk.

If there is displacement it is reduced by manipulation under anaesthesia. A below-knee plaster is applied with the foot plantigrade (except when a horizontal fracture can be held reduced only with the foot plantarflexed). An overboot is fitted and the patient is taught to walk. After 6 weeks the plaster is removed, a crêpe bandage is applied and full active use encouraged. If a large fragment of the back of the bone has been avulsed by the tendo achillis, it should be screwed or wired back into position.

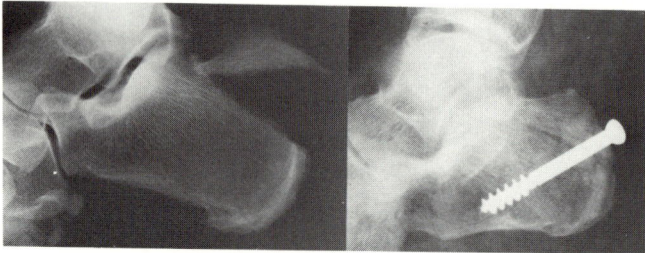

25.33 CALCANEAL FRACTURES (1) Chip fracture of postero-superior corner fixed by screw.

TREATMENT OF SPLIT AND CRUSH FRACTURES

Three methods are available: (1) closed reduction and plaster; (2) open reduction and bone grafting; (3) functional treatment.

CLOSED REDUCTION AND PLASTER — Lateral spreading of the calcaneum is reduced (if possible) by compressing the bone between the thenar eminences; the clamp used formerly is considered unwise. Upward displacement of the back of the heel also is difficult to correct by manipulation; a spike thrust into the bone from behind and used as a lever may help and can be incorporated in the plaster. Following reduction a split plaster is applied and replaced by a complete one when swelling has subsided. It is removed at 6 weeks and exercises are begun, but weight-bearing is not resumed for a further 6 weeks.

OPEN REDUCTION AND GRAFTING — The fracture is exposed from the lateral side and, from within the bone, all articular surfaces carefully re-positioned and the bone restored to as near its original shape as possible. The position can be held by transfixing Kirschner wires, but it is probably better to build up the interior of the bone with cancellous grafts or a bone block. Plaster is used for 6 to 12 weeks.

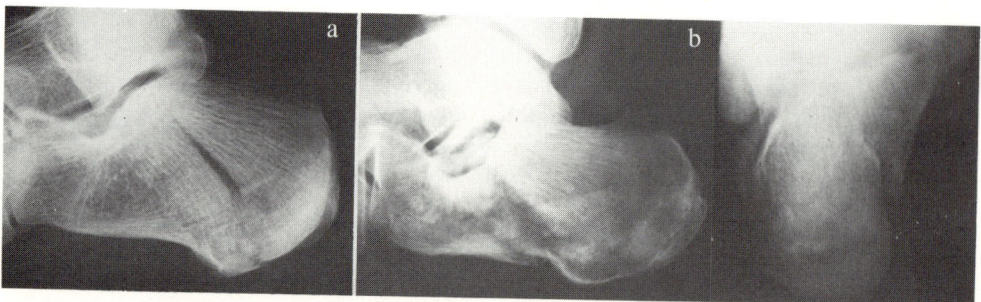

25.34 CALCANEAL FRACTURES (2)
(a) Split fracture with little displacement and no joint involvement, (b) lateral and axial views of severe split fracture with considerable joint involvement.

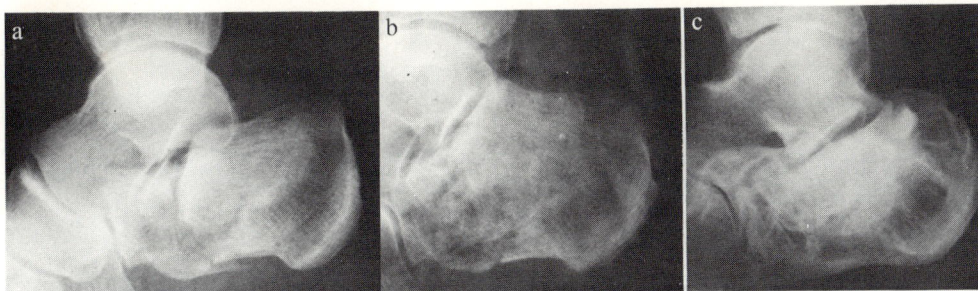

25.35   CALCANEAL FRACTURES (3)
(a) Severe crushed fracture treated by (b) open reduction and bone grafting (by courtesy of Mr.G. R. Fisk who performed the operation); the subtalar joint has been accurately restored and function was good. (c) Another severe crush which was treated by early activity and also regained reasonably good function.

FUNCTIONAL TREATMENT — Under general anaesthesia closed reduction can be attempted, as already described.   More often this stage is omitted, but in either case the patient is put to bed with the leg elevated and swelling kept to a minimum by elastic bandaging or, better, by a pneumatic compressing stocking.   A physiotherapist coaxes the patient to exercise the ankle and foot joints regularly, repeatedly and assiduously.   Within 3 or 4 days he is encouraged to put his foot to the ground and take a little weight.   He begins walking, using crutches at first, but graduating to full weight-bearing as comfort permits.   What he must not do is walk with a stiff foot, or allow the foot to swell; exercise is punctuated by elevation.

CHOICE OF METHOD
   This depends on the prognosis and complications.   The prognosis is not good; few patients can walk or work comfortably in less than 3 months, many take much longer and some have to change jobs permanently.   Stiffness, especially of the subtalar joint, is the bugbear; worse still, the restricted movement may be painful. Consequently the choice of method depends on the prospects of regaining a useful range of comfortable movement.
   Closed reduction is never perfect, so plaster merely perpetuates mal-position and encourages stiffness.   Open reduction can be accurate, it is radiologically rewarding, and it ensures a heel whose shape fits a normal shoe; but to maintain reduction plaster is needed and full movement is rarely regained.   Functional treatment, by insisting on early and repeated activity, moulds the fragments in such a way that a modestly useful range of movement is usually regained; for most patients and most surgeons it is probably the method of choice.
   Persistent pain following split or crush fractures may occur, often just below the lateral malleolus. If local anaesthetic injection or manipulation fails to provide relief, a small piece of the medial side of the lower fibula may be excised.   Pain when walking on rough ground is usually due to restriction of subtalar movement and may justify arthrodesis.   Immediate arthrodesis of all severe calcaneal fractures has been advocated, or even total excision of the calcaneum; such pessimism seems unwarranted.

OTHER TARSAL INJURIES

A crushing force may fracture the scaphoid or cuboid bone or both, and may also cause mid-tarsal dislocation.

Dislocation or displacement is reduced under anaesthesia, and the foot held in plaster for 6 weeks. The patient walks with an overboot. In the absence of displacement, neither reduction nor plaster is required.

INJURIES OF THE METATARSAL BONES

ROTATION INJURY

If the forefoot is violently twisted, abducted or plantarflexed, tarsometatarsal dislocation may occur. The first metatarsal is either dislocated or fractured near its base; the other metatarsal bones are fractured more distally. The injury is serious and may endanger the circulation of the foot.

Reduction is urgent and is maintained by a padded split plaster. The leg is kept elevated until it is certain that the circulation is satisfactory. After 3 weeks plaster is discarded, active exercises are started, and weight-bearing is resumed at 6 weeks.

CRUSH INJURY

Any or all of the metatarsal bones may be fractured by crush injuries. Usually the metatarsal necks fracture and often the overlying skin is damaged. The orthodox treatment is to reduce the fractures by manipulation and to hold them in plaster for a few weeks.

The functional method is as follows. Unless displacement is gross, which is rare, it may be ignored. The leg is elevated and active movements started immediately. As soon as swelling has subsided, and the patient is comfortable, he is encouraged to walk normally. Mal-union rarely results in disability when mobility has been regained.

TRACTION INJURY

Forced inversion of the foot may cause avulsion of the base of the fifth metatarsal. Displacement is slight and the fracture should be disregarded. If early activity is encouraged, and the patient walks as normally as possible in an ordinary shoe, full painless function is rapidly regained.

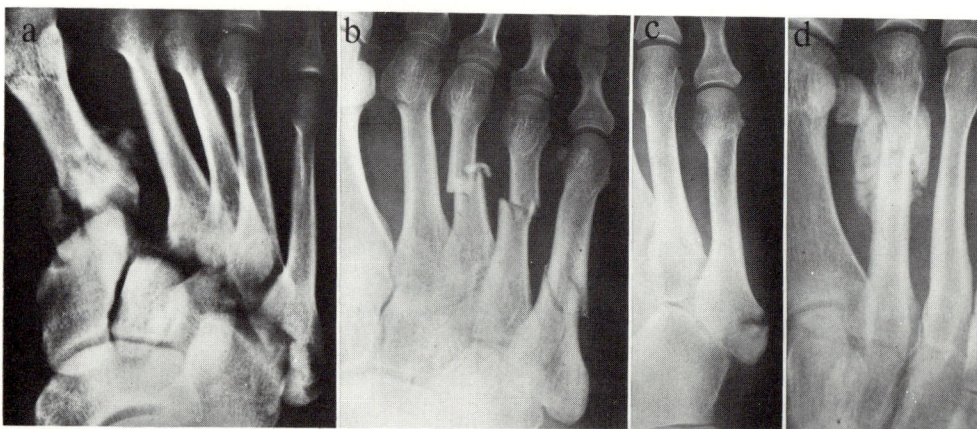

25.36 METATARSAL INJURIES
(a) Tarso-metatarsal dislocation is a serious injury which may endanger the circulation of the foot. (b) Transverse fractures of several metatarsal shafts. (c) Avulsion fracture of the base of the fifth metatarsal. (d) Florid callus in a stress fracture.

STRESS INJURY (MARCH FRACTURE)

In a young adult (often a recruit or a nurse) the foot may become painful after overuse. A tender lump is palpable just distal to the mid-shaft of a metatarsal bone. Usually the second metatarsal is affected, especially if it is much longer than an 'atavistic' first metatarsal. The x-ray appearance may at first be normal, although a hair-line crack is sometimes visible; later a large mass of callus is seen.

No displacement occurs and neither reduction nor splintage is necessary. The forefoot may be supported with Elastoplast and normal walking is encouraged.

FRACTURED TOES

A heavy object falling on the toes may fracture phalanges. If the skin is broken it must be covered with a sterile dressing. The fracture is disregarded and the patient encouraged to walk in a suitably mutilated boot.

Suggestions for further reading

Apley, A. G. (1956). 'Fractures of the Lateral Tibial Condyle treated by Skeletal Traction and Early Mobilisation.' *J. Bone Jt Surg.* **38B,** 699

Barnes, R. *et al.* (1976). 'Subcapital Fractures of the Femur.' *J. Bone Jt Surg.* **58B,** 2

Burwell, H. N. (1971). 'Plate Fixation of Tibial Shaft Fractures.' *J. Bone Jt Surg.* **53B,** 258

Collado, F. *et al.* (1973). 'Condylo-Cephalic Nail Fixation for Trochanteric Fractures of the Femur.' *J. Bone Jt Surg.* **55B,** 774

Colton, C. L. (1976). 'Injuries of the Ankle' in Watson-Jones' *Fractures and Joint Injuries.* (Ed. by Wilson, J. N.) Edinburgh; Churchill Livingstone

Connolly, J. F. and King, P. (1973). 'Closed Reduction and Early Cast-Brace Ambulation in the Treatment of Femoral Fractures.' *J. Bone Jt Surg.* **55A,** 1559 and 1581

Garden, R. S. (1961). 'Low-Angle Fixation in Fractures of the Femoral Neck.' *J. Bone Jt Surg.* **43B,** 647

— (1971). 'Malreduction and Avascular Necrosis in Subcapital Fractures of the Femur.' *J. Bone Jt Surg.* **53B,** 183

Helal, B. and Skevis, X. (1967). 'Unrecognized Dislocation of the Hip in Fractures of the Femoral Shaft.' *J. Bone Jt Surg,* **49B,** 293

Lam, S. F. (1971). 'Fractures of the Neck of the Femur in Children.' *J. Bone Jt Surg.* **53A,** 1165

Main, B. J. and Jowett, R. L. (1975). 'Injuries of the Midtarsal Joint.' *J. Bone Jt Surg.* **57B,** 89

Nicoll, E. A. (1964). 'Fractures of the Tibial Shaft.' *J. Bone Jt Surg.* **46B,** 373

Sarmiento, A. (1967). 'A Functional Below-the-Knee Cast for Tibial Fractures.' *J. Bone Jt Surg.* **49A,** 855

Smith, J. E. M. (1974). 'Results of Early and Delayed Internal Fixation for Tibial Shaft Fractures.' *J. Bone Jt Surg.* **56B,** 469

Soeur, R. and Remy, R. (1975). 'Fractures of the Calcaneus with Displacement of the Thalamic Portion.' *J. Bone Jt Surg.* **57B,** 413

INDEX

Pes planus, 295–298
Peyronie's disease, 178
Phantom limb, 145
Phemister grafts, 138
    (Fig. 11.9), 338
Phenylbutazone, 22, 30, 214
Physiotherapy in rheumatoid
    arthritis, 30
Pirogoff's amputation, 144
Plantar fasciitis, 295
Plasmacytoma, 96
Plaster sores, 331
Plaster technique, 318
    disadvantages of, 319
    plating combined with, 321
    stiffness following, 319
Plastics in bone surgery, 140
Platt's operation at knee, 131,
    132
Platyspondyly, 64
Policeman's heel, 295
Poliomyelitis, 112–114, 234
    affecting hand, 178
    elbow joint affected by, 164
    foot deformity in, 290
    scoliosis in, 206
Polydactyly, 72
Polymyalgia rheumatica, 28
Polyostotic fibrous dysplasia,
    71
Popliteal aneurysm, 281
Popliteal artery injury, in
    knee dislocation, 439, 440
Popliteal cyst, 281
Popliteal nerve lesions, 126
Posterior interosseous nerve
    lesions, 167
Postural flat foot, 297
    kyphosis, 211
    scoliosis, 205
Pott's fracture-dislocation,
    137
Pott's paraplegia, 204
Prednisolone, 30
Prednisone, 30
Pressure sores, 331, 411
Profundus tendon, division of,
    176
Progressive diaphyseal dysplasia
    69
Prolapsed cervical disc,
    191–193
Prolapsed lumbar disc,
    261–221
Proprionic acid, 29
Prostatic secondaries, 13, 98
Prostheses,
    amputation, following, 145
    fractured femoral neck, for,
    423
    elbow replacement for, 131
    finger joint replacement for,
    131
    hip replacement for, 133

Prostheses—contd.
    knee replacement, for, 135
    shoulder replacement for,
    131
Protrusio acetabuli, 252
Pseudarthrosis, clavicle, 74
    tibia, 74
Pseudocoxalgia (See Perthes'
    disease) 243–246
Pseudo-gout, 23, 46, 80
Pubis, fractures of, 412, 413
Pulmonary embolism, 328–330
Pulled elbow, 383
Pulp infection, 180
Putti-Platt operation, 361
Pyle's disease, 68
Pyrford arthrodesis, 130
    (Fig. 11.2), 255 (Fig. 18.31)

Q

Quadriceps, contracture of,
    280
Quadriceps-plasty, 339
    (Fig. 21.26), 431
de Quervain's disease, 172

R

Radial club hand, 169
Radial nerve,
    compression of, 165
    lesions, 124
    palsy, after fractured humerus,
    366
Radial styloid, fracture of,
    387
    excision of, 391
Radial tunnel syndrome, 165
Radiology, 10
    bone, 10
    joints, 13
Radiotherapy in ankylosing
    spondylitis, 215
    in malignant tumours, 92,
    93, 95, 98
Radius,
    absent, 73
    cleido-cranial dysostosis, in,
    67
    congenital subluxation of
    head, 162
    dislocations of head, 162,
    383
    fractured head, 375, 378
    fracture of neck, 374
    fracture of, 378, 381, 387
Rarefaction, 11
Razor back, 208
von Recklinghausen's disease,
    101, 206

Rectus femoris, rupture of, 276
Reduction of fractures,
    315–317
    (see also individual fractures)
Reiter's disease diagnosis, 28
Renal (uraemic) osteodys-
    trophy, 79, 261
Renal rickets, 79
Renal transplant, 46
Replacement of joints,
    131–136
Resistant rickets, 80
Respiratory obstruction, 351
Resuscitation, 348
Reticulocytoma, 94
Reticulum-cell sarcoma, 95
Rhabdomyoma, 101
Rhabdomyosarcoma, 102
Rheumatic fever, 18, 21
Rheumatoid arthritis, 4, 23,
    25–33
    amyloid disease in, 36
    ankle, of, 293
    cartilage in, 45
    cause of, 25
    cervical spine in, 26
    deformities in, 27
    differential diagnosis of,
    28, 42
    elbow joint, of, 163, 167
    joints of hand, of, 177
    osteoporosis in, 82
    pathology of, 25
    radiology of, 28
    signs and symptoms of, 25, 26
    treatment of, 29–33
    general, 20
    local, 30
    surgical, 31
Rheumatoid factor, 25, 26
Ribs, fractured, 352
Rickets, 5, 9, 78–79, 82
    bent bones in, 10, 16
    clinical features of, 79
    coxa vara in, 251
    knee deformities in, 263
    renal osteodystrophy, in,
    79
Rickety rosary, 79
Rigidity in cerebral palsy, 110
Ring sign, 82
Ring's prosthesis, 133
Risser's sign, 205
Robert Jones transplant, 121,
    124
Rocker bottom foot, 298
    (Fig. 20.10)
Rockered sole, 305
von Rosen's lines, 233
von Rosen's splint, 235
    (Fig. 18.7)
von Rosen's x-ray, 234
Rose-Waaler test, 26